Adjunctive Analgesic Strategies for the Bedside Clinician and Beyond

Justin P. Reinert • Donald L. Branam
Michael A. Veronin • Thomas J. Papadimos
Editors

Adjunctive Analgesic Strategies for the Bedside Clinician and Beyond

An Interdisciplinary Approach to Pain Management

Springer

Editors
Justin P. Reinert Pharm.D., MBA, BCCCP
Department of Pharmacy Practice
The University of Toledo College of Pharmacy and Pharmaceutical Sciences
Toledo, OH, USA

Michael A. Veronin Ph.D.
Department of Pharmaceutical Sciences and Health Outcomes
The University of Texas at Tyler
Tyler, TX, USA

Donald L. Branam Pharm.D., FASHP, FTPA
Department of Pharmacy Practice
South College School of Pharmacy
Knoxville, TN, USA

Thomas J. Papadimos M.D., MPH, FCCM, FAIM
Departments of Surgery and Anesthesiology
The University of Toledo College of Medicine and Life Sciences
Toledo, OH, USA

ISBN 978-3-032-21674-8 ISBN 978-3-032-21675-5 (eBook)
https://doi.org/10.1007/978-3-032-21675-5

This Springer imprint is published by the registered company Springer Nature Switzerland AG
The registered company address is: Gewerbestrasse 11, 6330 Cham, Switzerland

For my wife Valerie, my best friend, staunchest supporter,
and fiercest advocate. Nothing that I have accomplished in my life
would have happened were it not for you.
Donald L. Branam

Preface

The human condition is one closely associated with pain. From the earliest historical records, those with the knowledge and ability to relieve suffering of their fellow humans sought to do so. Though we are now millennia from the Sumerian deployment of the opium-containing "joy plant" (*Papaver somniferum*) and several hundred years past the Incan utilization of cocaine (*Erythroxylum coca*) as a topical anesthetic prior to trepanning procedures, we continue to pursue strategies and medications to alleviate the suffering and discomfort of mankind.

The landscape of healthcare has changed significantly since the time of our forebearers in medicine, and the intention of this book is to address pain management through an interdisciplinary lens and through a scope of medication safety. While many parts of the world continue to combat opioid epidemics, clinical perspectives and research have indicated a clear role for adjunctive, non-opioid analgesics in the management of pain. This book will explore these adjunctive analgesic medications in detail, in addition to addressing humanistic considerations and discussing methods for providing total human care for pain outside of pharmaceutical agents.

With the sincere desire of benefiting patients and educating healthcare professionals, I hope this textbook will inform clinical practice and inspire holistic care for people with pain.

Toledo, OH, USA Justin P. Reinert

Acknowledgments Justin P. Reinert wishes to acknowledge and give thanks to the following:

- To my wife, Dr. Samantha Reinert, in recognition of her support, patience, and unwavering encouragement
- To my children, EG, JP, and LJ, for their contagious laughter during times of stress
- To my parents, for inspiration and keeping me grounded
- To my mentors, past and present, for their guidance and critical appraisal
- To my co-editors, for their dedication and hard work in bringing this book to fruition
- To each contributing author for their expertise, perspective, and contribution
- To the publication team at Springer for their vision and assistance for the entirety of this project

Justin P. Reinert

Contents

Contributors

Aliya Abdulla, Pharm.D., BCCCP Houston Methodist Hospital, Houston, TX, USA

Jennifer S. Abeles, DO Department of Medicine, Jacobs School of Medicine and Biomedical Sciences, Buffalo, NY, USA

Canan Akman, M.D. Canakkale Onsekiz Mart University, Department of Emergency Medicine, Canakkale, Turkey

Faith M. Armstrong, M.D. University of Maryland Baltimore Washington Medical Center, Glen Burnie, MD, USA

Abagail Barazi, Pharm.D., BCCCP Bon Secours Mercy Health St. Vincent Medical Center, Toledo, OH, USA

Chelsea K. DiPasquale, Pharm.D., BCPS, BCCP Kaleida Health, Buffalo General Medical Center, Catholic Health, Kenmore Mercy Hospital, Elmwood, NY, USA

Caitlin S. Brown, Pharm.D., MPH, BCCCP, FCCM Department of Pharmacy, Mayo Clinic, Rochester, MN, USADepartment of Emergency Medicine, Mayo Clinic, Rochester, MN, USA

Maya R. Chilbert, Pharm.D., BCCP Department of Pharmacy Practice, University at Buffalo School of Pharmacy and Pharmaceutical Sciences, Wolters Kluwer Health, Buffalo, NY, USA

Mariann D. Churchwell, Pharm.D., BCPS, FCCP Department of Pharmacy Practice, The University of Toledo College of Pharmacy and Pharmaceutical Sciences, Toledo, OH, USA

Nicole E. Cieri-Hutcherson, Pharm.D.,BCPS,MSCP,FCCP,FASHP Department of Pharmacy Practice, University at Buffalo School of Pharmacy and Pharmaceutical Sciences, Buffalo, NY, USA

Marilee Clemons, Pharm.D., BCACP Pharmacy Services, UToledo Health, Toledo, OH, USA

Elizabeth A. Cook, Pharm.D., BCACP, CDCES Robert J. Dole Veterans Affairs Medical Center, Wichita, KS, USA

Alberto Corriero, M.D., Ph.D. Department of Interdisciplinary Medicine, ICU Section, University of Bari Aldo Moro, Bari, Italy

Ryan C. Creek, DMSc, MPAS, PA-C Bayer Medical Affairs, Whippany, NJ, USA

Austin De La Cruz, Pharm.D. University of Houston College of Pharmacy, Houston, TX, USA

Kellyn Engstrom, Pharm.D., MPH, BCEMP Department of Pharmacy, Mayo Clinic, Rochester, MN, USADepartment of Emergency Medicine, Mayo Clinic, Rochester, MN, USA

Grace Erdman, Pharm.D., BCCCP Sinai Hospital of Baltimore, Baltimore, MD, USA

Giacomo Farì, M.D., Ph.D. Department of Experimental Medicine, University of Salento, Lecce, Italy

Norman E. Fenn III, Pharm.D.,BCPS,BCPPS,FASHP,FPPA Manchester University College of Pharmacy & Health Sciences, Manchester, UK
Parkview Women's and Children's Hospital, Fort Wayne, IN, USA

Fiona Emrys Fonseca, MBBChBAO, MS Division of Endocrinology, Transgender and Intersex Specialty Care Clinic, Mayo Clinic, Rochester, MN, USA
Department of Psychiatry and Psychology, Mayo Clinic, Rochester, MN, USA

Christopher Gharibo, M.D. Department of Pain Management, NYU Langone Health, New York, NY, USA

Derek Gyori, Pharm.D., BCOP VA Ann Arbor Healthcare System, Ann Arbor, MI, USA
General Internal Medicine & Pharmacy Practice, University of Toledo College of Pharmacy and Pharmaceutical Sciences, Toledo, OH, USA

Mojdeh S. Heavner, Pharm.D., BCCCP, FCCM, FCCP Department of Practice, Science, and Health Outcomes Research, University of Maryland School of Pharmacy, Baltimore, MD, USA

Peter Iskander, M.D. Nesbitt School of Pharmacy, Department of Gastroenterology, The Wright Center, Scranton, PA, USA

Alena Javurkova, Ph.D. Department of Clinical Psychology, University Hospital Kralovske Vinohrady and 3rd Faculty of Medicine, Prague, Czech Republic

Cole Jerousek, Pharm.D. Cleveland Clinic Akron General, Akron, OH, USA

Ozgur Karcioglu, M.D. University of Health Sciences, Department of Emergency Medicine, Istanbul Education and Research Hospital, Istanbul, Turkey

Danielle M. Kieck, Pharm.D. Nesbitt School of Pharmacy, Wilkes University, Wilkes-Barre, PA, USA

Rachel T. Lazim, Pharm.D., BCCCP, BCNSP South College School of Pharmacy, Knoxville, TN, USA

Matteo Luigi Giuseppe Leoni, M.D. Department of Medical and Surgical Sciences and Translational Medicine, Sapienza University of Rome, Rome, Italy

Susan J. Lewis, Pharm.D., BCPS Department of Pharmacy Practice, University of Findlay College of Pharmacy, Findlay, OH, USA

Troy Lynn Lewis, Pharm.D., BC-ADM Nesbitt School of Pharmacy, Wilkes University, Wilkes-Barre, PA, USA

Juan V. Luciano, Ph.D. Department of Clinical & Health Psychology, Autonomous University of Barcelona (UAB), Bellaterra, Spain
Centre for Biomedical Research in Epidemiology and Public Health (CIBERESP), Madrid, Spain
Research & Innovation Unit, Parc Sanitari Sant Joan de Déu (PSSJD), Sant Boi De Llobregat, Spain, Madrid, Spain

Loulwa Maktabi, Pharm.D., BCPS Department of Pharmacy Practice, The University of Toledo College of Pharmacy and Pharmaceutical Sciences, Toledo, OH, USA

Coral Matus, M.D., FAAFP Department of Family Medicine, The University of Toledo College of Medicine and Life Sciences, Toledo, OH, USA

Andrea L. Miller, DPT Harmony Physical Therapy, Fleetwood, PA, USA

Sophie Mullins, BSc., MbChb., MRCP St. Peter's Hospice, Bristol, UK

Julie A. Murphy, Pharm.D., FASHP, FCCP, BCPS Department of Pharmacy Practice, The University of Toledo College of Pharmacy and Pharmaceutical Sciences, Toledo, OH, USA

Jaime Navarrete, Ph.D. Centre for Biomedical Research in Epidemiology and Public Health (CIBERESP), Madrid, Spain
Research & Innovation Unit, Parc Sanitari Sant Joan de Déu (PSSJD), Sant Boi De Llobregat, Spain, Madrid, Spain

Randy Neblett, MA, LPC PRIDE Research Foundation, Dallas, TX, USA

Edwin E. Nyambi, DMSc, MPAS, PA-C Central Coast Physician Assistant Program, A.T. Still University—College of Healthy Communities, Santa Maria, CA, USA

Olajumoke Olateju, MSc University of Houston College of Pharmacy, Houston, TX, USA

Thomas J. Papadimos, M.D., MPH, FCCM, FAIM Departments of Surgery and Anesthesiology, University of Toledo College of Medicine and Life Sciences, Toledo, OH, USA

Scott M. Pappada, Ph.D. Department of Anesthesiology, University of Toledo College of Medicine and Life Sciences, Toledo, OH, USA

Filomena Puntillo, M.D., Ph.D. Department of Interdisciplinary Medicine, ICU Section, University of Bari Aldo Moro, Bari, Italy

Jaroslava Raudenska, Ph.D. Department of Nursing, 2nd Faculty of Medicine, Charles University, Prague, Czech Republic

Justin P. Reinert, Pharm.D., MBA, BCCCP Department of Pharmacy Practice, The University of Toledo College of Pharmacy and Pharmaceutical Sciences, Toledo, OH, USA

Sarah Aldrich Renner, Pharm.D., BCACP General Internal Medicine & Pharmacy Practice, University of Toledo College of Pharmacy and Pharmaceutical Sciences, Toledo, OH, USA

Dipali Rinker, Ph.D., MA University of Houston College of Pharmacy, Houston, TX, USA

Estíbaliz Royuela-Colomer, Ph.D. Department of Clinical & Health Psychology, Autonomous University of Barcelona (UAB), Bellaterra, Spain
Centre for Biomedical Research in Epidemiology and Public Health (CIBERESP), Madrid, Spain

Juan P. Sanabria-Mazo, Ph.D. Unit for the Study and Treatment of Pain-ALGOS, Department of Psychology, Universitat Rovira i Virgili, Tarragona, Spain
Institut d'Investigació Sanitària Pere Virgili, Universitat Rovira i Virgili, Tarragona, Spain

Kyle A. Schofield, Ph.D. Division of Endocrinology, Transgender and Intersex Specialty Care Clinic, Mayo Clinic, Rochester, MN, USA
Department of Psychiatry and Psychology, Mayo Clinic, Rochester, MN, USA

Stephanie Seyse, Pharm.D., BCPS, FASHP, CACP Kaleida Health, Buffalo General Medical Center, Buffalo, NY, USA

Denver Shipman, Pharm.D., BCPP Robert J. Dole VA Medical Center, Wichita, KS, USA

Mina Shrestha, Ph.D. University of Houston College of Pharmacy, Houston, TX, USA

Laura Sjoquist, Pharm.D. Department of Pharmacy Practice, University of Findlay College of Pharmacy, Findlay, OH, USA

Austin Smith, Pharm.D., BCPP Robert J. Dole VA Medical Center, Wichita, KS, USA

Dakota Smith, Pharm.D. Fisch College of Pharmacy, The University of Texas at Tyler, Tyler, TX, USA

Nathan Smith, Pharm.D., BCPS Division of Pain Medicine and Department of Pharmacy, Mayo Clinic, Rochester, MN, USA

Kharmene Sunga, M.D. Department of Emergency Medicine, Mayo Clinic, Rochester, MN, USA

Brian Tasma, M.D. General Internal Medicine, University of Toledo College of Medicine and Life Sciences, Toledo, OH, USA

Department of Internal Medicine, College of Medicine and Life Sciences, The University of Toledo, Toledo, OH, USA

Miriam Thake, BMBCh., MRCP Department of Medicine, University of Ottawa, Ottawa, ON, Canada
Ottawa Hospital Research Institute, Ottawa, ON, Canada

Emma Thorman, BSc., MBBS., MRCP North Bristol NHS Trust, Bristol, UK

Douglas Thornton, Pharm.D., Ph.D., BCPS University of Houston College of Pharmacy, Houston, TX, USA

Giustino Varrassi, M.D., Ph.D. Fondazione Paolo Procacci, Rome, Italy

Takova D. Wallace-Gay, Pharm.D., BCACP, TTS School of Medicine, Fisch College of Pharmacy, The University of Texas at Tyler, Tyler, TX, USA

Matthew A. Wanat, Pharm.D., BCPS, BCCCP, FCCM Department of Pharmacy Practice and Translational Research, The University of Houston College of Pharmacy, Houston, TX, USA
Houston Methodist Hospital, Houston, TX, USA

Elisabeth M. Wang, Pharm.D., BCCP The University of Houston College of Pharmacy, Houston, TX, USA

Faith S. Wellings, Pharm.D., BCPS Nesbitt School of Pharmacy, Wilkes University, Wilkes-Barre, PA, USA

J. Cole Wilder, Pharm.D., M.Ed., BCPS, BCCCP, The University of Houston College of Pharmacy, Houston, TX, USA

Wenxin Zhuo, Pharm.D., MS, BCPS Department of Pharmacy, UToledo Health, Toledo, OH, USA

Marie C. Ziesat, M.D., FACS University of Maryland Baltimore Washington Medical Center, Glen Burnie, MD, USA

Part I

Introduction to Pain Management and Multimodal Analgesia

Definitions and Classifications of Pain

1

Edwin E. Nyambi and Ryan C. Creek

Introduction

The medical understanding of pain has evolved beyond nociception alone to a complex physical and emotional response influenced by a multitude of factors. The biopsychosocial model of pain recognizes this interplay. Many patients still do not receive adequate or appropriate recognition, diagnosis, and treatment for their pain. However, the inherently subjective experience of pain can also make assessment difficult. This makes it even more crucial to incorporate a thorough approach to pain assessment to ensure that patients' pain is not dismissed and that they receive the most effective treatments. Failure to do so can lead to mismanagement, which may also allow an acute pain complaint to become a debilitating chronic one.

A comprehensive pain assessment includes accurately classifying a patient's pain by severity, duration, and type, and there are a variety of tools available to help accomplish this. It is also vital that the provider recognizes the clues that patients share with them and that the proper terminology is used when describing the type of pain that they are experiencing. For example, differentiating between nociceptive and neuropathic pain elements can help zero in on potential pain generators and directly impact medical decision-making.

Keywords and Definitions

- Biomedical model of pain: The activity of nociceptive neurons in response to a noxious stimulus
- Biopsychosocial model of pain: A new pain model that recognizes the interplay of biological, cognitive, behavioral, and social factors unique to each patient's pain experience
- Pain: An unpleasant sensory and emotional experience associated with, or resembling that associated with, actual or potential tissue damage
- Pain assessment tools: Validated tools to assess the severity, quality, location, or other aspect of the pain, including but not limited to rating scales, questionnaires, and drawings
- Acute pain: Pain less than 1 month in duration
- Subacute pain: Pain between 1 and 3 months in duration
- Chronic pain: Pain for at least 3 months in duration
- Nociceptive pain: Pain from the activation of nociceptors due to actual or perceived insult to tissues
- Somatic pain: A type of nociceptive pain occurring in peripheral tissues
- Visceral pain: A type of nociceptive pain occurring in internal organs
- Nociplastic pain: Nociceptive pain without evidence of an injury or lesion
- Neuropathic pain: Pain caused by injury or lesion of the central or peripheral nervous system, aka neuropathy
- Neuralgia: A type of neuropathic pain without evidence of a cause
- Neuritis: A type of neuropathic pain for which inflammation is suspected
- Paresthesia: An abnormal sensation that is not painful
- Dysesthesia: An abnormal sensation that is painful
- Radicular pain: A type of neuropathic pain due to an identifiable insult to one or more spinal nerves, aka radiculopathy
- Dermatome: An area of skin that receives innervation from a specific spinal nerve root
- Myotome: A muscle group that receives innervation from a specific spinal nerve root
- Hyperesthesia: Increased sensitivity to stimuli
- Hyperalgesia: Pain that exceeds what is expected from a noxious stimulus
- Allodynia: Pain experienced from a stimulus that is not expected to be painful
- Hypoesthesia: Decreased sensitivity to stimuli

E. E. Nyambi (✉)
Central Coast Physician Assistant Program, A.T. Still University - College of Healthy Communities, Santa Maria, CA, USA
e-mail: edwinnyambi@atsu.edu

R. C. Creek
Bayer Medical Affairs, Whippany, NJ, USA
e-mail: ryan.creek@bayer.com

J. P. Reinert et al. (eds.), *Adjunctive Analgesic Strategies for the Bedside Clinician and Beyond*,
https://doi.org/10.1007/978-3-032-21675-5_1

- Psychogenic pain: A debated concept that a patient's pain complaint comes entirely from their mind, aka psychosomatic or nonorganic
- Malingering: Feigning a condition or its severity, often for personal gain or avoidance of a consequence

Understanding and Defining Pain

Pain is intricately more complex than the simple activity of nociceptive neurons in response to a noxious stimulus, which is an overly simplified biomedical view. It is important to learn why pain experts now advocate for a different definition and why it matters. Throughout history, many attempts have been made to define, understand, and classify the subjective human experience of pain. These attempts often involved considerable bias from philosophical, political, cultural, religious, or racial viewpoints, rather than a purely evidence-based approach [1, 2]. As a result, significant disparities developed in the understanding and treatment of pain, many of which persist to this day [2, 3]. For example, it has been shown that Black and Hispanic patients "consistently receive less adequate treatment for acute and chronic pain than non-Hispanic Whites, even after controlling for age, gender, and pain intensity [3] (Fig. 1.1)."

> The savage does not feel pain as we do: nor as we examine the descending scale of life do animals seem to have the acuteness of pain-sense at which we have arrived [2].—a prejudiced statement from influential American neurologist, Dr. Silas W. Mitchell, MD, in 1892

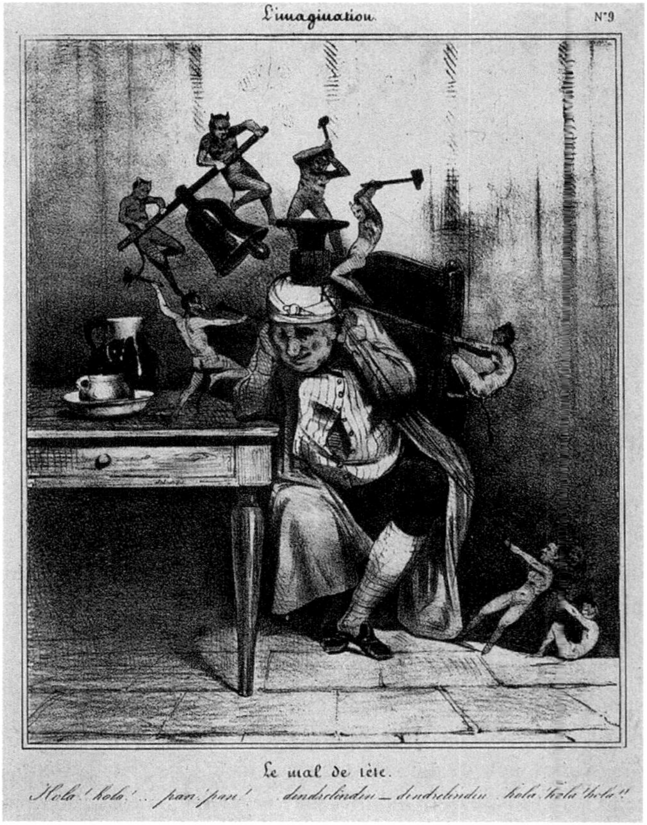

Fig. 1.1 Devils besiege a man's head; symbolizing headache. (Lithograph by C. Ramelet after H. Daumier, c. 1833. Wellcome Collection. Source: Wellcome Collection (PUBLIC DOMAIN) The belief that pain is a punishment, or God's will, has been demonstrated through the ages

Complicating this further, cultural norms and personal expectations have been shown to directly influence the individual experience of pain [4]. The existence of a "mind–body" connection to pain severity is also supported in the medical literature [5–7]. Even the word "pain" can refer to unpleasant but purely emotional sensations without physical stimuli, such as anxiety or grief. Indeed, many patients experience both physical and emotional pain together to varying degrees [7]. As a result of all of this, "pain" remains a highly nuanced word and topic. This renders the purely physiological and biomedical understanding and definition of pain incomplete (Fig. 1.2).

In an attempt to adequately acknowledge and address this complexity, the biopsychosocial model of pain was first proposed in 1977 by internist and psychiatrist Dr. George L. Engel, MD. He argued that the biomedical model alone did not explain why two individuals with the same condition or injury could experience pain and pain-related disability so differently [8]. This new model recognized the interplay of biological, cognitive, behavioral, and social factors unique to each patient's pain experience—acute or chronic. Examples of biological factors may include condition severity, comorbidities, and genetics. Examples of psychological factors may include mood, mental illness, and coping skills. Social factors may include socioeconomic status, ethnic identity, gender norms, biases, and discrimination (Fig. 1.3).

This model is not without challenges, and its limitations and potential for misuse have also been explored [9, 10]. However, it continues to dominate the current scientific community's conversations of pain, is widely cited in the literature, and is utilized by many clinicians—particularly those engaged in the treatment of chronic pain [11].

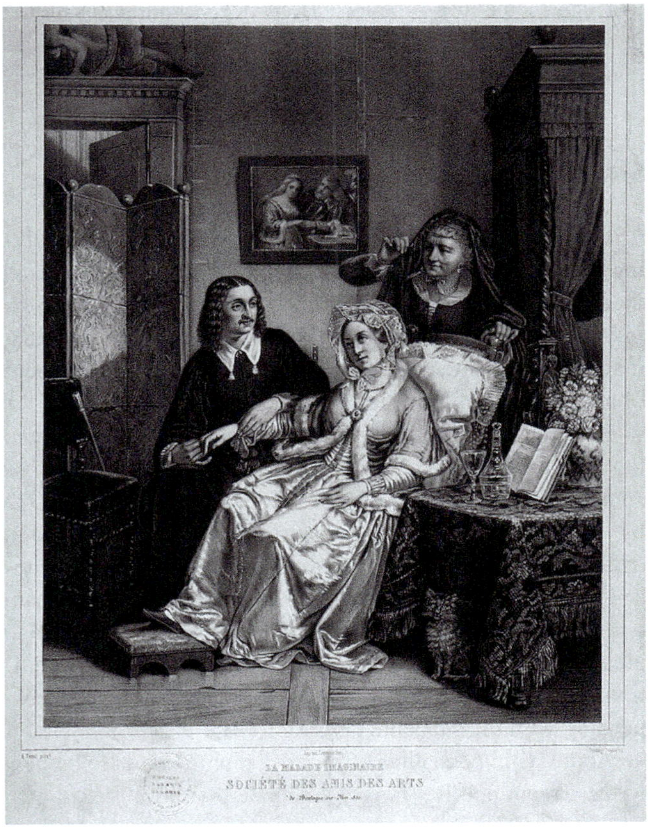

Fig. 1.2 A young physician feeling the pulse of a young woman in pain. (Lithograph by S. Teissier, 1850, after P.L.A.A. Terral. Source: Wellcome Collection (PUBLIC DOMAIN) In this lithograph from 1850 of a physician attending to a woman, the painting of lovers on the wall suggests that her pain is actually grief

A New Definition of Pain

In 2020, a committee of pain experts associated with the International Association for the Study of Pain (IASP) stated the following [12]:

- "Pain is a personal experience that is influenced by many factors."
- "Pain cannot be explained solely by the activity of sensory neurons."
- "Life experience informs an individual's concept of pain."
- "An individual's report of pain should be respected."
- "Pain can be adaptive, but can also adversely affect social and psychological well-being."
- Verbalizing is only one of many ways to express pain. A person's inability to communicate does not negate the possibility of pain.

The following definition of pain was then provided as a common-language definition that reflects this understanding:

> Pain is an unpleasant sensory and emotional experience associated with, or resembling that associated with, actual or potential tissue damage [12].

This definition is both simple and practical. It captures the personal experience and recognizes the interplay of the physical and emotional components of pain. It unequivocally states that actual tissue damage does not need to be present. "Real pain" is that which the patient perceives, independent of an identifiable physical cause. This is also supportive of

Fig. 1.3 Biopsychosocial model of pain

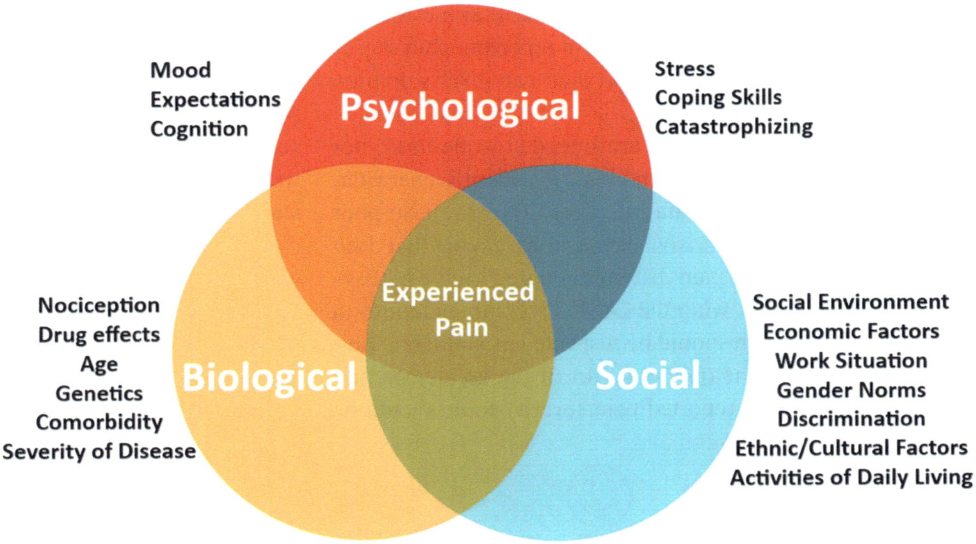

the adoption of a holistic and interdisciplinary clinical approach to pain diagnosis and management, which should encourage the use of multimodal treatment.

Classifying Pain by Severity

Among the most commonly used clinical pain assessment methods are the use of self-reported tools. For pain severity, these may include a visual analog scale, a graphic rating scale, a numerical rating scale, or a verbal rating scale [13]. The Wong–Baker FACES® Pain Rating Scale is another tool often posted near the patient's bedside [14]. Questionnaires have also been developed, such as the Oswestry Disability Index for Low Back Pain [15]. The latter often delves into questions about the effects of pain on quality of life and activities of daily living. For pain location, a pain drawing where the respondent marks the regions of their pain on a human figure is often used (Fig. 1.4).

Such tools have been in use for decades and are widely considered indispensable for the management of pain. While useful, it is important to recognize their drawbacks and limitations. All of these tools are attempts to generate objectivity to guide decision-making around an inherently subjective complaint, as opposed to measuring the heart rate or blood pressure. Indeed, experts have stated that pain scores alone are not an accurate reflection of pain and have critiqued their use [16, 17]. Others have called them a social transaction tied to the inappropriate movement to make pain a fifth vital sign, a practice some believe is partially responsible for the opioid epidemic [18, 19]. They have also been used inappropriately as auditing tools to critique physicians' management of their patients' pain [17] and as direct evidence against them in malpractice suits [20]. Some patients also express difficulty and hesitancy in reporting pain scores for fear that it will negatively affect their caregiver's opinion and treatment of them.

This is not how such tools are intended to be used, nor should they lead to judgments about a patient's character, willpower, toughness, or pain tolerance. They are also poor at drawing patient comparisons because we expect that each patient will experience pain differently based on the biopsychosocial model. Following the IASP's recommendations, a patient's report of pain should be respected as valid, but their verbalization of pain is only one part of the greater picture [12]. When used, self-reported pain severity tools should be just one factor in a broader shared decision-making model incorporating many other factors to best determine how to alleviate an individual's pain.

Classifying Pain by Duration

Chronicity of pain is a straightforward way to begin classifying it, which also has direct implications for the patient and their treatment options. It can also help distinguish post-injury and surgical pain that may be expected from pain that may hint at an unresolved issue or the potential development of a long-standing maladaptive process.

Pain may be categorized as acute, subacute, or chronic, but definitions and time points for these vary greatly across sources [21]. A clinical practice guideline released in 2022 by the Centers for Disease Control and Prevention (CDC) defined acute pain as pain with a duration <1 month, subacute pain with a duration of 1–3 months, and chronic pain with a duration >3 months [22]. Other sources may also incorporate a degree of activity restriction in these definitions or simply determine pain to be acute or chronic, dispensing with the subacute definition [21].

Acute pain, persisting for up to 1 month, tends to be new to the patient and is strongly associated with injury, trauma, or surgery [23]. This is also the type of pain that most clinicians will treat in an inpatient setting. There is a renewed focus on acute pain control, particularly in opioid-sparing analgesic techniques, as effective early pain control is associated with enhanced patient recovery and a reduced transition to chronic pain [23].

Chronic pain, persisting for longer than 3 months, may be the result of a prior injury, an underlying medical condition, or some unknown cause. It is also a very common comorbidity among patients. In 2019, it was found that one in five adults in the United States had a chronic pain complaint, with one in 14 stating that it had limited their life and work activities [24]. Patients with chronic pain may already be well-versed in pain control methods and taking various medications for management prior to their hospital stay. They may also be engaged in various forms of self-treatment and self-medication. This can affect their response to established pain control protocols if they are also being managed for a separate, new, acute pain complaint. In an ideal scenario, chronic pain patients should already be under the care of a

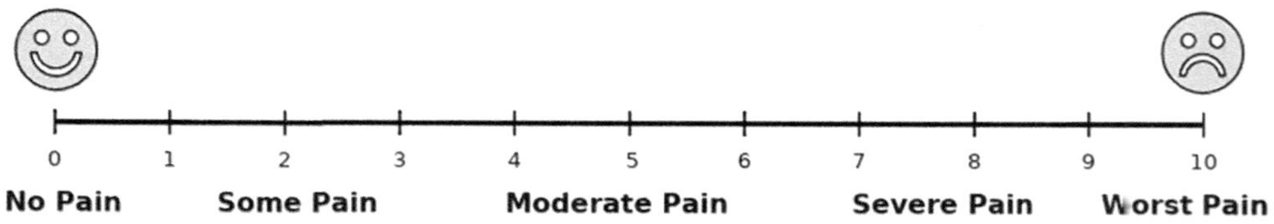

Fig. 1.4 An example of a numerical pain rating scale incorporating descriptors and faces

chronic pain specialist, which may allow an opportunity for consultation and discharge planning.

Subacute pain lies between acute and chronic pain, persisting for greater than 1 month but less than 3 months. Some experts disagree with this and consider it to be a subset of acute pain, begining at 6-weeks, but occuring for less than 3-months (>3 months become chronic) [25]. At any rate, when acute pain moves to this stage, it raises the likelihood that the pain will develop into a chronic one [21]. This warrants enhanced multidisciplinary involvement to avoid the deleterious consequences of chronic pain.

Classifying Pain by Type

The classification of pain by type is less straightforward and often requires thorough history taking and physical examination skills. Patients may also present with multiple types of pain at once. Yet it is essential to be thorough for several reasons. The character of the pain or the descriptors that patients use provide clues that help determine the type of pain that they have. This is important because different types of pain also respond differently to various treatment modalities. A proper diagnosis will narrow down potential causes for the pain, which guides decision-making. Misdiagnosis of their pain type can lead to increased associated healthcare costs and ineffective or delayed treatment [26]. This can also lead to worsening of the pain and cause an otherwise acute condition to be more likely to develop into a debilitating chronic one [26, 27]. Finally, "pain and suffering" are common factors heavily considered in medical malpractice cases. Failure to recognize and treat pain can inevitably lead to patient dissatisfaction and harm.

An introduction to these pain types is provided here, while the physiological processes will be discussed in greater detail in the next chapter.

Nociceptive Pain

Nociceptive pain is the "classic" type of pain that most people are familiar with. This is defined as "pain that arises from actual or threatened damage to non-neural tissue and is due to the activation of nociceptors." [28] There are at least three known subtypes of nociceptive pain: somatic, visceral, and nociplastic (Fig 1.5).

Somatic pain, derived from the Latin word "soma," is a type of nociceptive pain experienced anywhere on the body, excluding the internal organs. It is often due to integumentary or musculoskeletal injury. Due to the high distribution and sensitivity of nociceptors in these tissues, this pain is generally well-localized and more likely to be described as

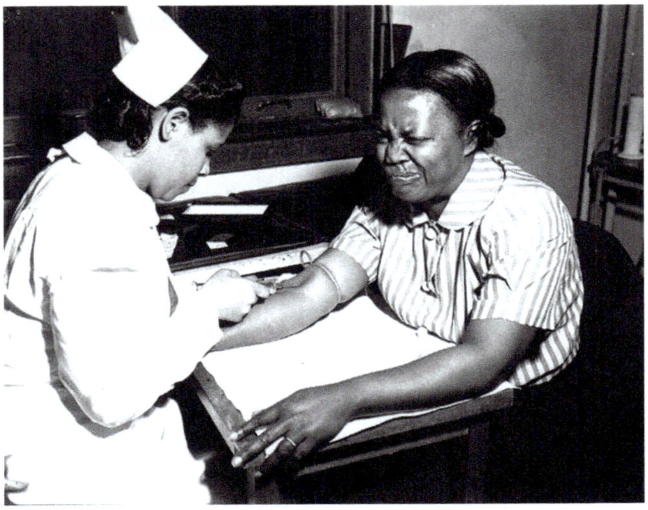

Fig. 1.5 Ouch! Flint Goodrich Shot, New Orleans, 1941. (Source: Works Progress Administration Photograph PUBLIC DOMAIN) A woman makes a pained face during venipuncture due to somatic nociceptive pain

sharp. Depending on the nature and location of the stimulus, patients may also describe it as dull and achy, such as in a joint. The intensity of this pain and the reflexive reactions it causes "underscores the importance of avoiding damaging situations for survival and maintaining homeostasis." [29]

Visceral pain, as the name suggests, is pain that arises from nociceptors associated with internal organs, including the chest, abdomen, and pelvis. In contrast to somatic pain, this pain tends to be more diffuse and poorly localized and often radiates to other body areas. Patients will also describe this in widely variable terms. It can range in severity from simple discomfort due to indigestion to acute debilitation from pyelolithiasis. Visceral pain is also one of the most common medical complaints. For example, abdominal pain is responsible for up to 10% of ER visits [30]. And in many of those cases, no specific cause is found.

Despite its prevalence, visceral pain is less understood than somatic pain. This is largely due to its diverse nature, multitude of potential causes, the presence of confounding variables, and difficulty in establishing an animal model for study [31]. Patients, especially those with chronic visceral pain, can perplex even the most experienced clinicians.

Nociplastic pain is a little-known type of nociceptive pain, which involves the activation of nociceptors but for which there is no clear evidence of tissue damage or lesion [28]. "Nociplastic" is sometimes used in association with "psychogenic pain," although this is going out of favor. Examples of nociplastic pain include myofascial pain syndrome and fibromyalgia. Fibromyalgia is characterized in part by increased pain sensitivity, and there is a growing body of evidence that is beginning to elucidate its pathophysiology far beyond associated psychological factors [32].

Neuropathic Pain

Neuropathic pain, often called neuropathy, is defined as "pain caused by a lesion or disease of the somatosensory nervous system [28]." This may have either a central or a peripheral nervous system origin. It is commonly described as a shooting, burning, electric, or a "pins and needles" sensation. Causative lesions are diagnosed with imaging, electrophysiology, or other tests. Examples include a herniated lumbar disc or a surgery resulting in irritation or injury to a nerve. Disease processes that can also cause this pain include such conditions as stroke, multiple sclerosis (MS), and diabetes. Neuropathy can be further classified depending on the number of nerves affected. Mononeuropathy occurs when only one nerve is involved. Mononeuropathy multiplex occurs when several specific nerves are involved. Polyneuropathy, the type often seen in diabetes and MS, is typically more diffuse and bilateral.

Neuralgia and Neuritis

Neuralgia and neuritis are related but different terms that must not be confused. Neuralgia is used to describe nerve pain, but in contrast to neuropathy, it does not require specific evidence of a nerve lesion or disease process. Primary trigeminal neuralgia is one example, which is diagnosed by its clinical presentation alone [33]. The term neuritis is a subtype of neuropathy, reserved for use only when an inflammatory process is likely. Acute nerve pain from an active varicella zoster infection and the optic neuritis seen in MS are common examples [34, 35]. When the zoster infection has resolved but the nerve pain continues, it is then called postherpetic neuralgia [36].

Paresthesia and Dysesthesia

Neuropathic conditions are often associated with abnormal sensations that may or not be painful, such as paresthesia and dysesthesia. The descriptions and recommendations for use of these terms have been updated by the IASP. It has been agreed that paresthesia describes an abnormal sensation that is not painful, while dysesthesia describes an abnormal sensation that is painful [28]. Furthermore, the concept that paresthesia is spontaneous, while dysesthesia is evoked, is no longer in favor [28]. A body part "falling asleep" due to pressure on the blood supply to a nerve is an example of a transient paresthesia. In contrast, a persistent paresthesia is likely to be caused by a disease process or lesion. This could have a multitude of potential causes, including vitamin deficiency, metabolic disturbances, autoimmune conditions, and focal nerve entrapment, to name a few [37]. Paresthesia may be described as tingling, pins and needles, burning, or numbness. If these sensations are unpleasant, they can then be called dysesthesia. Thus, patients with these abnormal sensations often present with both paresthesia and dysesthesia at different times.

Radicular Pain

Radicular pain, also known as radiculopathy, is a type of neuropathic pain caused by nerve compression, irritation, or injury that is experienced along the route of one or more spinal nerves exiting the spinal cord. In these cases, the symptoms occur in a characteristic pattern and distribution that match the known areas of spinal nerve innervation. The dermatomes involve cutaneous sensation, while the myotomes involve muscular contraction. Nerve entrapment due to vertebral degeneration or disc displacement, as in lumbosacral radiculopathy (sciatica), is a common cause. Radicular symptoms may also include varying degrees of paresthesia and disrupted motor function and reflexes (Fig. 1.6).

Hyper- and Hypoesthesias

Some patients demonstrate hyperesthesia, which simply means increased sensitivity. This sensitivity may be in response to tactile, thermal, or mechanical stimuli and is associated with both nociceptive and neuropathic conditions. It is thought to be largely due to central and/or peripheral sensitization processes that alter sensation and perception [38], which will be covered further in the next chapter. Two types of hyperesthesia are hyperalgesia and allodynia. These terms are often confused and used incorrectly. Hyperalgesia is pain that is exaggerated or prolonged beyond what is expected, generated from a stimulus that is expected to cause some pain [38]. More simply described, it is pain that is out of proportion to the stimulus. Hyperalgesia may also spread beyond the site of the stimulus. This has been tested in the research setting through the application of pressure, cold or warm stimuli, or pinpricks [39].

Allodynia differs from hyperalgesia in that it is pain that is generated from a stimulus that is not expected to be painful [38]. For example, patients with allodynia may experience pain simply from something touching their skin or while combing their hair. Those with trigeminal neuralgia often experience allodynia while brushing their teeth or eating [40]. The pain caused by touching the skin of a severely sunburned area is an example of a transient allodynia that many people have experienced (Fig. 1.7).

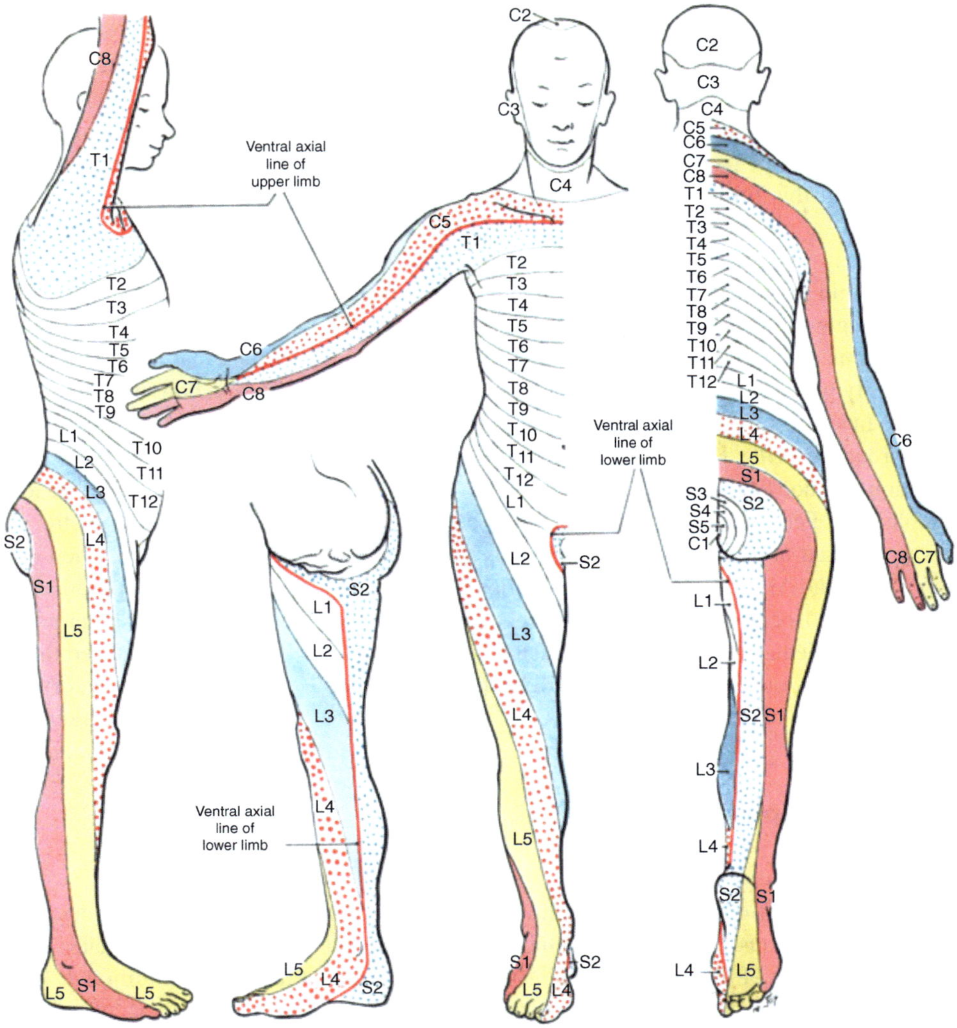

Fig. 1.6 Dermatome map. (Grant, John C.B. An atlas of anatomy by regions, 1962 PUBLIC DOMAIN) Dermatome map of the human body, showing sensory distribution innervated by the afferent nerve fibers of specific spinal nerves

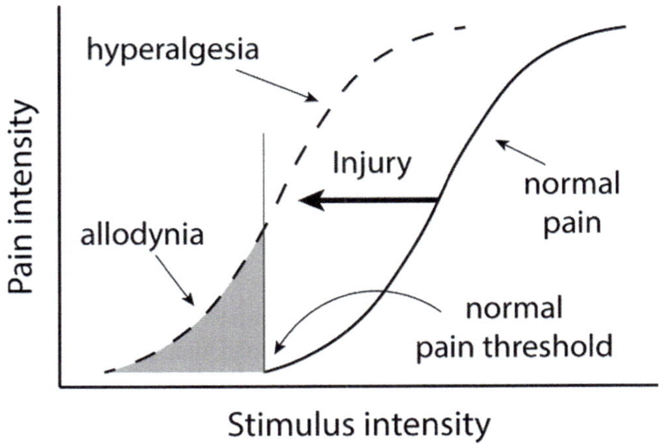

Fig. 1.7 Illustration of hyperalgesia and allodynia. (Richard Lennertz, 2020. CC BY-SA 2.0 license)

Hypoesthesic and hypoalgesic conditions are also prevalent, in which patients have diminished sensation and pain. This is generally due to nerve damage resulting in impaired signaling. Again, diabetic polyneuropathy is a common example. A hallmark finding in many of these patients is reduced sensation during pinprick testing as part of the neurological foot exam. There are also reports in the literature of diabetic patients experiencing severe burns without pain as a result of self-applied heat treatments in an attempt to manage paresthesia/dysesthesia [41].

Psychogenic Pain

The concept of psychogenic pain, also known as psychosomatic, supratentorial, somatization, or nonorganic pain, has generated clinical debate and controversy for many years

[42–44]. Since the IASP's definition of pain recognizes the inherent emotional component, even without actual tissue injury, some have argued that psychogenic pain does not actually exist since all pain is pain [43]. Others believe it is still important to distinguish pain that is more psychological from other types of pain in order to guide treatment [45]. Complicating this further is the patient's perception of the term, as it can come across as dismissive and stigmatizing. Patients may interpret psychogenic pain to mean "since there's nothing wrong with your body, there must be something wrong with *you* [43]."

Factitious disorders and malingering are known to occur, particularly where litigation and the opportunity for personal gain are involved [46]. Nevertheless, such judgments should be approached with a high degree of caution, as clinical detection methods to identify malingering in pain are not reliable [44]. Perhaps the best understanding of this term, if it is to be used at all, is that the mind–body connection in pain is real, and ALL pain includes an emotional component. The biopsychosocial model acknowledges that pain is frequently complicated by a multitude of factors, including psychological ones, the degree of which will be different in each individual's own experience of pain.

Real-World Applicability

There are numerous cases in the media and in the medical literature that highlight the need for clinicians to take their patients' pain seriously and conduct a thorough workup and accurate diagnosis of their patients' pain. We also know that poorly controlled postoperative pain is associated with several negative consequences based on an examination of outcomes [27]. Publicized cases where a patient's pain was dismissed although they had a life-threatening condition have also received considerable attention (and litigation). When we factor in the increased caution surrounding opioid use, there is understandably a renewed interest in better pain education and management techniques across many clinical settings [47]. An unintended consequence, however, is that, sometimes, even well-meaning clinicians, who do take the time to recognize different aspects of their patient's pain, such as neuropathic symptoms, make errors. For these reasons, it is essential to approach pain judiciously and consult a specialist whenever appropriate.

One example of a pain condition that has historically been underdiagnosed and mistreated is complex regional pain syndrome (CRPS). In recent years, more clinicians have become educated about this condition and the diagnostic criteria, and as a result, they have been more vigilant about diagnosing it. But this has also created new problems. In a peer-reviewed article published in 2022, the authors made a plea for clinicians to be more thoughtful about their pain workups for suspected CRPS patients [26]. One case involved a patient who had sustained a traumatic forearm injury. They presented with both spontaneous and evoked pain, cold skin with a bluish tint, and muscle atrophy, all localized to an area of the hand innervated by the ulnar nerve. Those familiar with the criteria may diagnose this as CRPS type II. However, CRPS is a diagnosis of exclusion, and one key requirement is that no other diagnosis better explains the findings. The correct diagnosis in this case was neuropathic pain due to post-traumatic neuralgia of the ulnar nerve, for which anticonvulsant medication and nerve repair were warranted [26]. Surgery would not be advised in CRPS, which is known to lead to exacerbation. In another case published in 2019, a patient was misdiagnosed with CRPS due to hyperalgesia, motor disturbance, and mild edema in the legs years after an motor vehicle accident (MVA), when in fact she was dealing with the consequences of a spinothalamic tract injury [48]. Misdiagnosis occurs in many other pain-related conditions. For example, it has been suggested that as much as half of all US cases of chronic inflammatory demyelinating polyneuropathy (CIDP) are misdiagnosed, with many patients receiving unnecessary, costly, and harmful treatments [49].

Summary

This chapter provides an overview of how pain is defined, understood, and classified in modern medicine. The shift from the traditional biomedical model—which focused solely on nociceptive input—to the more nuanced biopsychosocial model that considers biological, psychological, and social factors is an important development. This perspective acknowledges that pain is a complex and subjective experience that may not always correlate with identifiable tissue damage. The IASP's updated definition reinforces that pain is both a sensory and emotional experience, warranting that each individual's report of pain should be respected.

The classification of pain based on duration (acute, subacute, or chronic) and type (nociceptive, neuropathic, nociplastic, or psychogenic) is helpful in practice. There are also various assessment tools used to evaluate pain, each with its own limitations. Misdiagnosis and inadequate management of pain can lead to significant harm, including chronic disability and unnecessary treatments. The clinical examples and historical context provided underscore the value of a holistic, patient-centered approach. Incorporating careful, empathetic, and evidence-informed pain evaluation and treatment strategies into practice should be a goal for all healthcare providers.

References

1. Duncan G. The meanings of 'Pain' in historical, social, and political context. The Monist. 2017;100(4):514–31. https://www.jstor.org/stable/26370814.
2. Bourke J. Pain sensitivity: an unnatural history from 1800 to 1965. J Med Humanit. 2014;35(3):301–19. https://doi.org/10.1007/s10912-014-9283-7. PMID: 24682629; PMCID: PMC4133135.
3. Mossey JM. Defining racial and ethnic disparities in pain management. Clin Orthop Relat Res. 2011;469(7):1859–70. https://doi.org/10.1007/s11999-011-1770-9. PMID: 21249483; PMCID: PMC3111792.
4. Henschke N, Lorenz E, Pokora R, et al. Understanding cultural influences on back pain and back pain research. Best Pract Res Clin Rheumatol. 2016;30(6):1037–49. https://doi.org/10.1016/j.berh.2017.08.004. Epub 2017 Sep 30. PMID: 29103548.
5. Birch S, Stilling M, Mechlenburg I, Reinholdt MB, Hansen TB. Association between pain catastrophizing, physical function and pain at first visit in the outpatient knee clinic. Knee. 2019;26(6):1286–91. https://doi.org/10.1016/j.knee.2019.08.012. Epub 2019 Oct 15. PMID: 31628075.
6. Gorczyca R, Filip R, Walczak E. Psychological aspects of pain. Ann Agric Environ Med. 2013;20(1):23–7. PMID: 25000837.
7. Lumley MA, Cohen JL, Borszcz GS, Cano A, Radcliffe AM, Porter LS, Schubiner H, Keefe FJ. Pain and emotion: a biopsychosocial review of recent research. J Clin Psychol. 2011;67(9):942–68. https://doi.org/10.1002/jclp.20816. Epub 2011 Jun 6. PMID: 21647882; PMCID: PMC3152687.
8. Engel GL. The need for a new medical model: a challenge for biomedicine. Science. 1977;196(4286):129–36. https://doi.org/10.1126/science.847460. PMID: 847460.
9. Mescouto K, Olson RE, Hodges PW, Setchell J. A critical review of the biopsychosocial model of low back pain care: time for a new approach? Disabil Rehabil. 2022;44(13):3270–84. https://doi.org/10.1080/09638288.2020.1851783. Epub 2020 Dec 7. PMID: 33284644.
10. Mas RR, López-Jiménez T, Pujol-Ribera E, et al. Effectiveness of a multidisciplinary BIOPSYCHOSOCIAL intervention for non-specific SUBACUTE low back pain in a working population: a cluster randomized clinical trial. BMC Health Serv Res. 2019;19(1):962. https://doi.org/10.1186/s12913-019-4810-x. PMID: 31831074; PMCID: PMC6909445.
11. Schwan J, Sclafani J, Tawfik VL. Chronic pain management in the elderly. Anesthesiol Clin. 2019;37(3):547–60. https://doi.org/10.1016/j.anclin.2019.04.012. Epub 2019 Jun 18. PMID: 31337484; PMCID: PMC6658091.
12. Raja SN, Carr DB, Cohen M, et al. The revised International Association for the Study of Pain definition of pain: concepts, challenges, and compromises. Pain. 2020;161(9):1976–82. https://doi.org/10.1097/j.pain.0000000000001939. PMID: 32694387; PMCID: PMC7680716.
13. Haefeli M, Elfering A. Pain assessment. Eur Spine J. 2006;15(Suppl 1):S17–24. https://doi.org/10.1007/s00586-005-1044-x. Epub 2005 Dec 1. PMID: 16320034; PMCID: PMC3454549.
14. Wong-Baker FACES Foundation. Published July 23, 2018. https://wongbakerfaces.org/.
15. Mao G, Aldahak N, Kusyk D, Yeager M, Cook D, Cameron J, Cheng B, Oh M. A consideration for the utility of the post-operative Oswestry Disability Index for measuring outcomes after sacroiliac joint fusion. Orthop Rev (Pavia). 2018;10(2):7549. https://doi.org/10.4081/or.2018.7549. PMID: 30057723; PMCID: PMC6042050.
16. Green SM, Krauss BS. The numeric scoring of pain: this practice rates a zero out of ten. Ann Emerg Med. 2016;67:573–4.
17. Sampson FC, Goodacre SW, O'Cathain A. The reality of pain scoring in the emergency department: findings from a multiple case study design. Ann Emerg Med. 2019;74(4):538–48. https://doi.org/10.1016/j.annemergmed.2019.02.018. Epub 2019 Apr 5. PMID: 30955987.
18. Schiavenato M, Craig KD. Pain assessment as a social transaction: beyond the "Gold Standard". Clin J Pain. 2010;26(8):667–76. https://doi.org/10.1097/AJP.0b013e3181e72507.
19. Levy N, Sturgess J, Mills P. "Pain as the fifth vital sign" and dependence on the "numerical pain scale" is being abandoned in the US: Why? Br J Anaesth. 2018;120(3):435–8. https://doi.org/10.1016/j.bja.2017.11.098. Epub 2018 Jan 19. PMID: 29452798.
20. Rich BA. Physicians' legal duty to relieve suffering. West J Med. 2001;175(3):151–2. https://doi.org/10.1136/ewjm.175.3.151. PMID: 11527832; PMCID: PMC1071521.
21. Banerjee S, Argáez C. Multidisciplinary treatment programs for patients with acute or subacute pain: a review of clinical effectiveness, cost-effectiveness, and guidelines [Internet]. Ottawa (ON): Canadian Agency for Drugs and Technologies in Health; 2019. Available from: https://www.ncbi.nlm.nih.gov/books/NBK546002/.
22. Dowell D, Ragan KR, Jones CM, Baldwin GT, Chou R. CDC clinical practice guideline for prescribing opioids for pain — United States, 2022. MMWR Recomm Rep. 2022;71(3):1–95. https://doi.org/10.15585/mmwr.rr7103a1.
23. Tighe P, Buckenmaier CC, Boezaart AP, et al. Acute pain medicine in the United States: a status report. Pain Med. 2015;16(9):1806–26. https://doi.org/10.1111/pme.12760.
24. Zelaya CE, Dahlhamer JM, Lucas JW, Connor EM. Chronic pain and high-impact chronic pain among U.S. Adults, 2019. NCHS Data Brief. 2020;390:1–8. PMID: 33151145.
25. King W. Acute pain, subacute pain, and chronic pain. In: Gebhart GF, Schmidt RF, editors. Encyclopedia of pain. Berlin: Springer; 2013. https://doi.org/10.1007/978-3-642-28753-4_75.
26. Terkelsen AJ, Birklein F. Complex regional pain syndrome or limb pain: a Plea for a critical approach. J Pain Res. 2022;15:1915–23. https://doi.org/10.2147/JPR.S351099. PMID: 35837543; PMCID: PMC9275500.
27. Gan TJ. Poorly controlled postoperative pain: prevalence, consequences, and prevention. J Pain Res. 2017;10:2287–98. https://doi.org/10.2147/JPR.S144066. PMID: 29026331; PMCID: PMC5626380.
28. International Association for the Study of Pain. Terminology | International Association for the Study of Pain. International Association for the Study of Pain (IASP). Published 2011. https://www.iasp-pain.org/resources/terminology/
29. Dubin AE, Patapoutian A. Nociceptors: the sensors of the pain pathway. J Clin Invest. 2010;120(11):3760–72. https://doi.org/10.1172/JCI42843. Epub 2010 Nov 1. PMID: 21041958; PMCID: PMC2964977.
30. Cervellin G, Mora R, Ticinesi A, Meschi T, Comelli I, Catena F, Lippi G. Epidemiology and outcomes of acute abdominal pain in a large urban Emergency Department: retrospective analysis of 5,340 cases. Ann Transl Med. 2016;4(19):362. https://doi.org/10.21037/atm.2016.09.10. PMID: 27826565; PMCID: PMC5075866.
31. Sengupta JN. Visceral pain: the neurophysiological mechanism. In: Handb Exp Pharmacol, vol. 194; 2009. p. 31–74. https://doi.org/10.1007/978-3-540-79090-7_2. PMID: 19655104; PMCID: PMC3156094.
32. Gyorfi M, Rupp A, Abd-Elsayed A. Fibromyalgia pathophysiology. Biomedicines. 2022;10(12):3070. https://doi.org/10.3390/biomedicines10123070. PMID: 36551826; PMCID: PMC9776089.
33. Araya EI, Claudino RF, Piovesan EJ, Chichorro JG. Trigeminal neuralgia: basic and clinical aspects. Curr Neuropharmacol. 2020;18(2):109–19. https://doi.org/10.2174

/1570159X17666191010094350. PMID: 31608834; PMCID: PMC7324879.
34. Albrecht M, Levin M. Treatment of herpes zoster. 2023. Accessed 19 Jan 2024. https://www.uptodate.com/contents/treatment-of-herpes-zoster.
35. Osborne B, Balser L. Optic neuritis: prognosis and treatment. UpToDate; 2023. Accessed 19 Jan 19 2024. https://www.uptodate.com/contents/optic-neuritis-prognosis-and-treatment.
36. Mallick-Searle T, Snodgrass B, Brant JM. Postherpetic neuralgia: epidemiology, pathophysiology, and pain management pharmacology. J Multidiscip Healthc. 2016;9:447–54. https://doi.org/10.2147/JMDH.S106340. PMID: 27703368; PMCID: PMC5036669.
37. Mehta P, Potter CA, Feinberg JH, Simon JH, Maravilla KR. Paresthesias and dysesthesias. In: Filippi M, Simon JH, editors. Imaging acute neurologic disease: a symptom-based approach. Cambridge: Cambridge University Press; 2014. p. 332–46. https://doi.org/10.1017/CBO9781139565653.022.
38. Latremoliere A, Woolf CJ. Central sensitization: a generator of pain hypersensitivity by central neural plasticity. J Pain. 2009;10(9):895–926. https://doi.org/10.1016/j.jpain.2009.06.012. PMID: 19712899; PMCID: PMC2750819.
39. van den Broeke EN, Lambert J, Huang G, Mouraux A. Central sensitization of mechanical nociceptive pathways is associated with a long-lasting increase of pinprick-evoked brain potentials. Front Hum Neurosci. 2016;10:531. https://doi.org/10.3389/fnhum.2016.00531.
40. Renton T, Wilson NH. Understanding and managing dental and orofacial pain in general practice. Br J Gen Pract. 2016;66(646):236–7. https://doi.org/10.3399/bjgp16X684901. PMID: 27127274; PMCID: PMC4838424.
41. Chang WY, Liu HH, Huang DW, et al. Severe burn injury from the common Asian practice of heat application in patients with diabetic neuropathy. Int Wound J. 2022;19(4):845–52. https://doi.org/10.1111/iwj.13682. Epub 2021 Aug 27. PMID: 34448552; PMCID: PMC9013579.
42. Engel GL. Psychogenic pain. Med Clin North Am. 1958;42(6):1481–96. https://doi.org/10.1016/s0025-7125(16)34200-6. PMID: 13599760.
43. Covington EC. Psychogenic pain—what it means, why it does not exist, and how to diagnose it. Pain Med. 2000;1(4):287–94. https://doi.org/10.1046/j.1526-4637.2000.00049.x.
44. Tuck NL, Johnson MH, Bean DJ. You'd better believe it: the conceptual and practical challenges of assessing malingering in patients with chronic pain. J Pain. 2019;20(2):133–45. https://doi.org/10.1016/j.jpain.2018.07.002. Epub 2018 Jul 20. PMID: 30036608.
45. Isagulyan ED, Makashova ES, Myasnikova LK, Sergeenko EV, Aslakhanova KS, Tomskiy AA, Voloshin AG, Kashcheev AA. Psychogenic (nociplastic) pain: current state of diagnosis, treatment options, and potentials of neurosurgical management. Prog Brain Res. 2022;272(1):105–23. https://doi.org/10.1016/bs.pbr.2022.03.008. Epub 2022 May 18. PMID: 35667797
46. Bass C, Wade DT. Malingering and factitious disorder. Pract Neurol. 2019;19(2):96–105. https://doi.org/10.1136/practneurol-2018-001950. Epub 2018 Nov 13. PMID: 30425128.
47. Nallani R, Fox CC, Sykes KJ, Surprise JK, Fox CE, Reschke AD, Simpson MH, Polivka BJ, Villwock JA. Pain management and education for ambulatory surgery: a qualitative study of perioperative nurses. J Surg Res. 2021;260:419–27. https://doi.org/10.1016/j.jss.2020.11.001. Epub 2020 Nov 28. PMID: 33256986; PMCID: PMC10165861.
48. Jang SH, Kwon YH, Lee SJ. Central pain due to injury of the spinothalamic tract misdiagnosed as complex regional pain syndrome: a case report. Diagnostics (Basel). 2019;9(4):145. https://doi.org/10.3390/diagnostics9040145. PMID: 31597370; PMCID: PMC6963659.
49. Allen JA. The misdiagnosis of CIDP: a review. Neurol Ther. 2020;9(1):43–54. https://doi.org/10.1007/s40120-020-00184-6. Epub 2020 Mar 26. PMID: 32219701; PMCID: PMC7229131.

Pathophysiology of Pain

2

Edwin E. Nyambi and Ryan C. Creek

Introduction

Most of our understanding of pain signaling comes from studies on simple nociceptive pain, but we are learning more about other types of pain with new research. Pain signaling occurs in the stages of transduction, transmission, modulation, and perception. Transduction refers to the process by which a stimulus can trigger an action potential at nociceptor terminals. These first-order nociceptor cell bodies are housed in the dorsal root ganglion for the body or the trigeminal ganglion for the face. There are two main subtypes of nociceptors that transmit either fast or slow pain. The anterolateral system is critical to the transmission of pain signals and is composed of ascending and descending tracts. Here, first-order nociceptors synapse with second-order neurons in the spinal cord. The spinothalamic and spinoreticular tracts make up the ascending tracts, which relay to third-order neurons in the brain. The spinomesencephalic tract is the descending tract most involved in pain modulation.

Pain modulation is an intricate process orchestrated by many different mechanisms and molecules. Modulation can be excitatory or inhibitory and greatly affects the severity of perceived pain. The gate control theory (GCT) may explain how pain signals compete with other sensory signals, only to be transmitted when one outweighs the other. The descending tracts utilize endogenous opioids, autonomic neurotransmitters, a variety of non-opioid peptides, and cannabinoids (CBs). The clinical use of analgesics exploits pain modulation mechanisms for the benefit of the patient. Pain perception is the cerebral process of putting all of the signals into their greater whole as the subjective experience of pain, and it can also serve as a pain modulation mechanism.

Central and peripheral sensitization are examples of pathological, maladaptive responses to pain and are implicated in many chronic pain conditions. They represent an imbalance of various pain modulation systems, as well as reorganized, hypersensitive nociceptor activity that negatively affects the patient's well-being.

Understanding the physiological processes of pain can provide us with greater empathy and understanding toward our patients and inform the research and clinical application of therapeutics.

Keywords and Definitions

- Primary nociceptor: A specialized primary neuron that has terminals situated in the target tissue, the first to respond to a noxious stimulus.
- Afferent nerve fibers: Sensory nerve fibers that direct signals toward the central nervous system (CNS), as opposed to efferent motor fibers that direct them away.
- Transduction: The process by which a noxious stimulus is sensed at the nociceptor terminals and initiates an action potential.
- Transmission: The process by which pain signals propagate and relay from the peripheral to the central nervous system.
- Modulation: The process by which pain signaling can be altered and either increased (excitatory) or decreased (inhibitory).
- Perception: The high-order cerebral mechanism by which pain signals are interpreted as part of a greater whole and given significance.
- Ascending tracts: Pain transmission pathways that travel "up" to the brain.
- Descending tracts: Pain transmission pathways that travel "down" from the brain.

E. E. Nyambi (✉)
Central Coast Physician Assistant Program, A.T. Still University - College of Healthy Communities, Santa Maria, CA, USA
e-mail: edwinnyambi@atsu.edu

R. C. Creek
Bayer Medical Affairs, Whippany, NJ, USA
e-mail: ryan.creek@bayer.com

J. P. Reinert et al. (eds.), *Adjunctive Analgesic Strategies for the Bedside Clinician and Beyond*,
https://doi.org/10.1007/978-3-032-21675-5_2

- Dorsal root ganglion: A cluster of neurons situated near the dorsal root of a spinal nerve, where nociceptor neuron bodies reside.
- Pseudo-unipolar: A type of neuron with a common stalk connected to the axon, which allows for bidirectional transmission.
- A-beta (Aβ) fibers: Large-diameter, myelinated sensory neuron fibers that transmit touch and other sensations.
- A-delta (Aδ) fibers: Small-diameter, myelinated nociceptive fibers that transmit "fast" pain.
- C fibers: Unmyelinated nociceptive fibers that transmit "slow" pain.
- Anterolateral system: Composed of the ascending (spinothalamic and spinoreticular) and descending (spinomesencephalic) tracts.
- First-order neuron: The first neuron to detect and transmit a signal in the periphery, which then synapses to a second-order neuron at the spinal cord.
- Second-order neuron: A neuron in the spinal cord that synapses with a peripheral first-order neuron and transmits signals to a third-order neuron in the brain.
- Third-order neuron: A neuron in the brain that synapses with a second-order neuron from the spinal cord, sending signals directly for processing.
- Gate control theory (GCT): A theory of pain modulation involving afferent signals that describes how we perceive competing sensory and pain information, which share a common pathway.
- Endogenous opioids: Endorphins and enkephalins that are secreted to inhibit pain signaling.
- Autonomic modulation: Serotonergic, noradrenergic, and dopaminergic neurotransmitters that alter pain signaling.
- Non-opioid peptides: Amino acids and other proteins that alter pain signaling, such as glutamate or Gamma-aminobutyric acid (GABA).
- Endocannabinoids: Lipid compounds that interact with the endocannabinoid system (ECS) to modulate pain.
- Central sensitization: A pathological and maladaptive process by which pain signals are transformed into a condition of chronic hypersensitivity in the CNS, with potential whole-body effects.
- Peripheral sensitization: A pathological and maladaptive process by which pain transduction in peripheral tissues is greatly enhanced, isolated to a specific body region.

Background

As previously discussed, pain is a complex process that can cause emotional distress and affect quality of life. The experience, duration, and level of emotional and cellular response are different for every individual [1]. Without appropriate interventions, pain can lead to despair, loss of employment, addiction to pain medications/illicit recreational substances, and disruption of social interactions. These are some of the reasons why it is important for clinicians who treat pain to have an in-depth understanding of the anatomy and physiology of pain pathways.

Much of what we know about the pathophysiology of pain is based on animal models or cutaneous nociception elicited in humans, which has inherent limitations. Compared to nociception, the mechanisms of the different types of pain remain comparatively less clear. However, researchers continue to elucidate pain in new ways, and we are better able to understand the physiological changes that occur as a result. For example, advances in neuroimaging techniques, such as functional magnetic resonance imaging (fMRI), are bridging "the gap between brain activity and the subjective experience of pain [2]."

In terms of physiology, nociception shares much in common with the other body senses. As with touch or taste, for example, it relies on specialized receptors. These pain receptors are associated with nerve endings that are distributed all throughout the body at varying densities [3]. This means that some body regions and tissues are more "sensitive" to pain or generate different perceptions of pain than others. The sensitive nerve ending receptor in the tissue and the nerve cell body it is attached to together comprise what is called a primary nociceptor. Pain stimuli enter the spinal cord via these afferent nerve fibers through the dorsal root and are carried to the central nervous system (CNS) for interpretation at the parietal lobe of the cerebral cortex. Damage to the parietal lobe, as in a stroke, can cause permanent numbness or other altered sensations. It is also interesting to note that in the CNS, the pathways for both pain and depression are also connected and share neurotransmitters [1, 4]. This may help explain why these conditions often overlap and offer clinical insight into the treatment of chronic pain, particularly.

Nociceptive Pain Signaling

A helpful way to better understand nociceptive pain physiology is to first divide it into its stages of signaling and processing: transduction, transmission, modulation, and perception. Transduction occurs at the nociceptor and is how a stimulus is transformed into a signal that can be transmitted [5]. Transmission is what happens to that signal as it is relayed along afferent/ascending pathways to the brain. Modulation refers to processes that alter the sensation, whether excitatory or inhibitory, often using a descending tract. Finally, perception "involves the integration of many sensory messages into a coherent and meaningful whole [5]." It is the subjective awareness of the sensation, which includes cerebral processing and many factors such as attention, expectation, and elements of the biopsychosocial model.

Transduction

Nociceptors are specialized to respond to either mechanical, thermal, or chemical stimuli that reach the threshold to generate an action potential [5, 6]. Numerous stimuli have been found to activate nociceptors, including a wide variety of exogenous and endogenous chemicals (i.e., prostaglandins) and inflammation inducing chemicals such as cytokines [7]. Transduction begins when transient receptor potential (TRP) channels at the terminals allow the escape of intracellular calcium. This depolarizes the cell axon and initiates an action potential that propagates through voltage-gated sodium channels [7, 8].

There are cutaneous, visceral, bronchopulmonary, and musculoskeletal variations of nociceptors, each responsible for pain in those regions [9]. For example, a sharp pain from a cut is sensed by cutaneous nociceptors. The dull, squeezing, and poorly localized abdominal pain from an ulcer comes from visceral nociceptors. With one exception, all nociceptor cell bodies are housed in the dorsal root ganglion, which is a cluster of neurons in the dorsal root of a spinal nerve. The exception is the face, in which the cell bodies lie in the trigeminal ganglion [6]. They are pseudo-unipolar, including a peripheral branch of the axon with sensory terminals in the target tissue and a central axonal branch that leads to the spinal cord [6]. Thus, they have a bidirectional nature to their signaling and response, which directly impacts pain modulation and treatment [6].

There are two pain subtypes of nociceptors, A-delta (Aδ) and C, which differ both in the diameter of their axons and their conduction velocity [7]. Aδ fibers are myelinated and thicker and are responsible for rapid signal transmission, resulting in a sharp pain sensation. Dull pain that transmits slowly comes from the activation of C fibers. This explains why pain is often first felt at a high intensity, followed by a lingering ache (second pain).

Table 2.1 shows the properties of sensory fibers [10]. Aδ fibers are myelinated and transmit rapid/pricking pain (i.e., touching a hot surface or being stung by a bee), while C fibers are unmyelinated and transmit slow/dull pain.

Transmission/Conduction

The transmission of the signal from the nociceptors through the spinal cord to the brain is an example of an ascending neural pathway, which uses the anterolateral system. The anterolateral system itself is composed of three separate tracts: the spinothalamic, spinoreticular, and spinomesencephalic tracts [11]. The spinothalamic tract is the most involved in transmitting pain information to the cerebral cortex, which is essential for awareness of the stimulus. Both fast pain (Aδ fibers) and slow pain (C fibers) use this tract. As fast pain is thought to have evolved later, the portion of the tract these fibers utilize is called the neospinothalamic tract, while slow pain utilizes the paleospinothalamic tract. When the first-order nociceptor neuron enters the spinal cord via the dorsal root ganglion, it encounters a synapse of another neuron. This second-order neuron decussates or crosses to the other side of the spinal cord and then travels up the spinal cord via the spinothalamic tract. It then synapses with another third-order neuron at the ventral posterolateral nucleus of the thalamus, which then travels to the cortex of the brain [11].

The spinoreticular tract is less understood, but it is also responsible for a degree of pain signal transmission. It runs adjacent to the spinothalamic tract and differs further in that it projects fibers not just to the cerebral cortex but also to the reticular formation of the brain stem. It is considered more primitive and appears to be especially involved in automatic reactions to pain [12].

Visceral and somatic pain pathways can be said to share a ride through the spinal cord to the cortex. As a result, pain from visceral organs can be misinterpreted as coming from the skin. A clinical example of this is when myocardial pain from infarction is referred in a segmental distribution to the T1-T5 dermatome in the left shoulder or arm [10].

Table 2.1 Afferent nerve fibers

Fiber type	Detects pain?	Myelination	Diameter (μm)	Conduction velocity (m/s)	Distribution	Key functions
Aδ	Yes	Thin	~1–6	~5–40	Skin, cornea, joints, some organs	"First pain". Fast, sharp, well-localized
C	Yes	None	~0.4–1.2	~0.4–2	Widespread in most tissues	"Second pain. Slow, dull, diffuse
Aβ	No	Heavy	~6–12	~35–90	Dense in skin, especially mechanoreceptors	Touch,vibration, pressure, proprioception

Steeds [10]

Modulation

Pain modulation is a fascinating area of research on the frontiers of neurobiology, and an entire textbook could be written on this topic alone. While pain signals are being sent to the CNS, they are persistently accompanied by endogenous modulating processes, often in the opposite direction, via the descending tracts. This is highly relevant to clinical practice, as defects in these processes are directly implicated in many pain syndromes [13]. It is also a contributing biological factor to the individual differences in pain perception. Furthermore, the medical use of exogenous analgesic modalities directly exploits these processes for the patient's benefit [13].

Gate Control Theory

The gate control theory (GCT) of pain modulation, first published by Melzack and Wall in 1965, was a groundbreaking development in the field of pain research [14]. Some elements of the theory have now been disproven, causing some to propose a revised "leaky gate theory [15]," but as a whole, it continues to be strongly influential to our understanding of pain modulation. We know that large, myelinated afferent sensory fibers (Aβ) are responsible for touch, pressure, and vibration but not pain, which is transmitted via the smaller afferent Aδ and C fibers [6]. All of these neurons synapse at the dorsal horn of the spinal cord with second-order neurons [1]. The dorsal horn is also a site of interneuron and inhibitory fibril interplay [14]. This begs the question: Which peripheral sensory signals are allowed through to the ascending tracts?

The GCT explains that painful and non-painful stimuli compete with one another in the substantia gelatinosa (gray matter of the spinal cord). According to this theory, the Aβ fibers activate the interneurons to "gate" the firing of the second-order neurons associated with afferent pain fibers. If other sensory signals exceed that of nociceptive signals, they are the ones that pass through to the brain. On the other hand, pain is perceived if painful stimuli are intense enough to outweigh the other sensations. This explains why we may instinctively rub or massage a painful area, as the sensation of rubbing competes with the painful stimulus and decreases our perception of it. A similar technique is observed to diminish the itch of a mosquito bite by trading it for pain by pinching it or marking an X in the skin with the edge of the fingernails. Topical capsaicin and the use of transcutaneous electrical nerve stimulation (TENS) units are other examples of the gate control theory in practice.

Descending Tracts

When a pain signal reaches the CNS, the first thing that is likely to occur is a protective motor response. However, there are several additional mechanisms that utilize the descending tracts to modulate pain. The spinomesencephalic tract is the third tract of the anterolateral system, which relays pain signals to an area of gray matter in the midbrain called the periaqueductal gray (PAG). There, it is processed and sent to the rostroventral medulla (RVM) and then the spinal cord (see Fig. 2.1). Several chemicals are involved in this process, each with different effects on pain modulation. These include such things as endogenous opioids, autonomic neurotransmitters (i.e., noradrenalin and serotonin (5-HT)), amino acids and other non-opioid peptides (i.e., GABA), and cannabinoids [10, 13, 16] (see Fig. 2.2 and Tables 2.2 and 2.3).

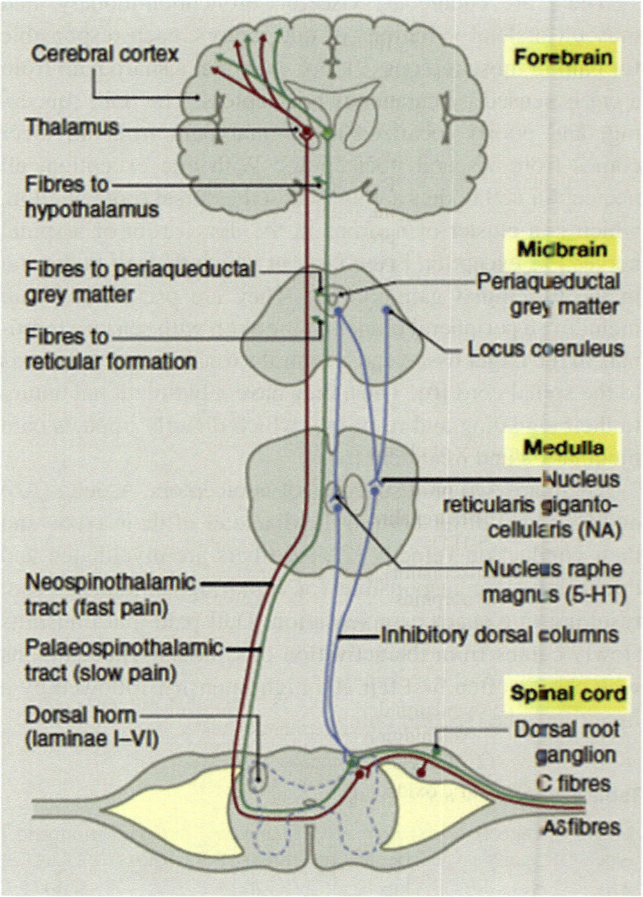

Fig. 2.1 Spinal and supraspinal pathways of pain. Ascending nociceptive fast (red) and slow (green) pathways, NA noradrenaline, 5-HT 5-hydroxytryptamine. (Steeds [10])

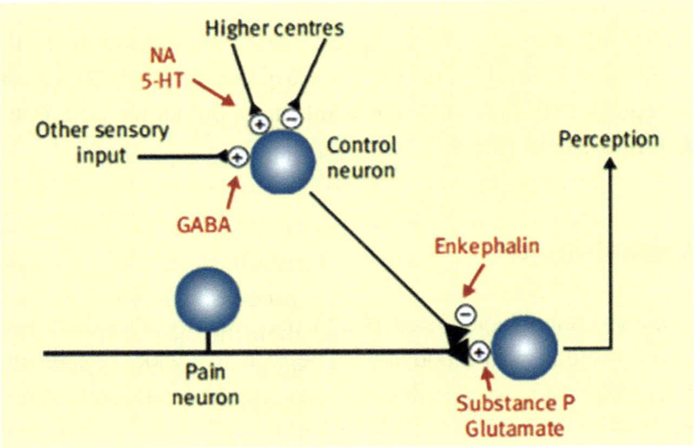

Fig. 2.2 Excitatory and inhibitory interactions at the spinal cord level. NA noradrenaline, 5-HT 5-hydroxytryptamine, GABA g-aminobutyric acid. (Steeds [10])

Endo/Exogenous Opioids

Opioids are the classic example of pain modulation effects in practice. We often think of these only as inhibitory analgesics, but the truth is more complicated. These molecules affect both the central and peripheral nervous systems. Endogenous endorphins and enkephalins, as well as exogenous opioids/opiates, bind to opioid receptors to reduce nerve excitability. The mu-opioid receptors located at synapses are particularly responsive, and binding triggers an inhibitory response that reduces neurotransmitter release presynaptically and hyperpolarizes the neuron postsynaptically [17]. These are demonstrably effective for analgesia in acute pain, but a paradoxical response can occur with high-dose or prolonged use. Opioids have been shown to induce conditions of hyperalgesia in patients [18, 19], which further demonstrates the fact that modulation can be both excitatory or inhibitory.

Table 2.2 The anterolateral system

Tract	Target	Function	Fiber Input
Spinothalamic—Lateral division	Ventral posterolateral thalamus → somatosensory cortex	Sensory-discriminative: precise localization, intensity, quality of pain & temperature	Mostly Aδ
Spinothalamic—Medial division	Medial & intralaminar thalamus → limbic & association cortices	Diffuse, poorly localized pain; affective and motivational aspects	Mostly C
Spinoreticular	Reticular formation (pons, medulla) → intralaminar thalamus → diffuse cortical projections	Arousal, autonomic, and emotional components of pain; contributes to suffering and attention	Aδ and C
Spinomesencephalic	Periaqueductal gray matter in midbrain	Pain modulation (descending inhibitory systems), orienting reflexes (eye/head toward stimulus), defensive behaviors	Aδ and C

Steeds [10]

Table 2.3 Summary of chemicals involved in pain transmission

Class	Chemical	Comments
Amines	Noradrenaline, serotonin (5-HT)	Modulate pain by facilitating or inhibiting nociceptive signaling in the spinal cord and brain stem
Endogenous opioids	Enkephalins, endorphins, dynorphins	Inhibit pain transmission by binding opioid receptors, enhancing descending inhibition, and reducing neurotransmitter release from nociceptors
Non-opioid peptides/ amino acids	Glutamate, GABA, Galanin, Substance P, cholecystokinin, etc.	Primarily excite nociceptive neurons, amplifying and transmitting pain signals. Some are inhibitory
Endogenous cannabinoids	Anandaminde, 2-Arachidonoylglycerol (2-AG), etc.	Suppress pain by activating CB1/CB2 receptors, reducing excitatory neurotransmitter release, and modulating descending pain control
Other	Nitric oxide	Acts as a diffusible messenger that can enhance or modulate nociceptive transmission and contribute to central sensitization

Steeds [10]

Autonomic Modulation

Autonomic modulation occurs via serotonergic, dopaminergic, and noradrenergic processes [13]. Here, pain has considerable overlap with psychiatric conditions such as depression and anxiety. This also offers insight into pain conditions such as fibromyalgia and irritable bowel syndrome, where autonomic dysregulation is suspected [20]. Indeed, the off-label use of selective serotonin norepinephrine reuptake inhibitors (i.e., milnacipran and duloxetine) and tricyclic antidepressants (i.e., amitriptyline) is widely accepted and supported by evidence for the treatment of certain types of chronic pain [21, 22].

In serotonergic modulation, various forms of 5-hydroxytryptophan (the precursor to serotonin) have been shown to have both excitatory and inhibitory effects on pain in several studies [23–25]. Dysregulation of serotonergic pain modulation is therefore likely highly contributory in chronic pain conditions. In contrast, dopaminergic modulation is less understood and likely indirect [13]. However, there is frequent comorbidity of pain in patients with dopamine disorders [26], and a placebo-controlled randomized controlled trial (RCT) investigating the use of a dopamine agonist found that it altered pain sensitivity [27]. Dopamine is also implicated in behavioral responses such as fear and anxiety, as well as reward and addiction, all factors that play a role in the pain response. Finally, noradrenergic modulation of pain has been studied extensively. Norepinephrine release in the descending pathways inhibits nociception, while its presence in peripheral tissues may be pronociceptive in the setting of injury [28].

Non-opioid Peptides

Some of the peptides that are known to affect pain include GABA, glutamate, galanin, substance P, and cholecystokinin [13, 29]. The role of GABA as an inhibitory neurotransmitter is well-established, and it is crucial in descending pain pathways to inhibit pain [13, 30]. Some GABA receptor agonists, such as alcohol [31] and gabapentin, can have potent analgesic effects, while the analgesic effects of others, such as benzodiazepines, are debatable.

In contrast to GABA, glutamate is an abundant excitatory neurotransmitter that acts on ligand-gated ion channels to enhance neurotransmission [32]. It is known to be involved in chronic pain syndromes associated with central sensitization and is the subject of much pain-related research [32]. Additional peptides, galanin and substance P, have been found in the dorsal root ganglion (DRG) and dorsal horn and are associated with both acute and chronic pain modulation [29, 33]. Substance P appears to influence glutamate, and exogenous galanin administration has antinociceptive effects [29, 33]. Finally, cholecystokinin, a hormone produced by the gastrointestinal (GI) tract, has been shown for years to impair the endogenous opioid system and is also linked to states of chronic nerve injury and inflammation [34]. Continued research into the role of these peptides and their receptors may provide significant therapeutics for pain control in the near future.

Cannabinoids

The endocannabinoid system (ECS), only recently elucidated, also plays a role in pain modulation. The ECS is a widely expressed neuromodulatory system distributed in both the central and peripheral tissues [35]. It is directly involved in "CNS development, synaptic plasticity, and the response to endogenous and environmental insults [35]." Cannabinoid receptors (CB1 and CB2) are G-protein-coupled receptors that have been located in such regions as GABA and glutamate synaptic terminals and cholecystokinin-positive interneurons [35], peptides that are also involved in pain modulation, as previously described. CB1 receptors are primarily found in the CNS, while CB2 receptors are more common in the periphery. They are acted upon by endogenous cannabinoid lipids, such as anandamide and 2-arachidonyl glycerol, as well as the exogenous cannabinoid Tetrahydrocannabinol (THC). Several high-quality studies have demonstrated ECS-mediated antinociceptive effects [36]. Other cannabinoids found in the cannabis plant, such as Cannabidiol (CBD), are modulators rather than antagonists of CB receptors. They have also been shown to affect ion channels completely independent of CB receptors. Cannabinol (CBN), for example, was recently shown to inhibit sodium channel activity and thus the excitability of DRG neurons [37]. It is therefore understandable that such compounds are being used and researched for the treatment of pain and other conditions.

Perception

The perception of pain is highly subjective and is where the collection of many sensory messages is interpreted as a whole, influenced by various patient factors [5]. This is the highest and most complex stage of processing of the pain experience. Attention, cognitive appraisal, emotional reactions, and behavioral responses all directly influence pain [13]. An anxious and fearful response may create a feedback loop, which has an excitatory autonomic effect, thus increasing the perception of pain. Likewise, a calmer response may reduce autonomic activity and have an inhibitory effect on pain modulation. Studies have shown that increased pain scores are positively correlated with increased attention to a painful stimulus, as well as pain catastrophizing appraisals and statements [38, 39]. Thus, pain perception is also a pain-modulating mechanism and one for which we have a degree of control and can be trained to improve. For these reasons, there is an emerging specialty of pain psychologists [40].

Sensitization Syndromes

With a foundational understanding of pain, pain signaling, and pain modulation mechanisms, the pathology of various pain syndromes can be better appreciated. One of the most significant maladaptive responses by the body to pain is central sensitization, a driving factor in many types of chronic pain. This is described as "a phenomenon of synaptic plasticity and increased neuronal responsiveness in central pain pathways after painful insults [41]." It was first described in 1989 when rats exposed to painful stimuli were observed to develop hyperexcitable neurons in the dorsal horn of the spinal cord [42]. It is marked by hyperalgesia, allodynia, global hypersensitivity, fatigue, and other symptoms [41]. Central sensitization involves structural, functional, and chemical changes and is thought to occur via a few mechanisms. It may include the co-opting of larger Aβ mechanoreceptor neurons, normally responsible for sensations such as touch, so that these now also relay nociception [43]. Changes in the gray matter of the CNS involved in pain processing have also been observed, as have increased levels of excitatory neurotransmitters such as glutamate and decreased levels of inhibitory neurotransmitters such as GABA [44]. Additional observations include enhanced sodium channel activity along axons and the presence of cytokines and neuroinflammation [41, 43, 44]. These changes lead to a persistent state of hyperexcitable pain pathways. Previously innocuous or mild stimuli can be amplified, or in many cases, pain can arise from no stimuli whatsoever (nociplastic pain).

Central sensitization may be best thought of as a spectrum that varies in severity [44]. It can occur as a result of a prior injury or disease process. It can also occur without an inciting event, with fibromyalgia being an example. This condition features many of the symptoms of central sensitization, frequently co-occurs with psychiatric conditions, and could have a genetic predisposition component as well [44]. Although some previous findings suggested a peripheral nerve issue such as "small fiber neuropathy," the current body of evidence suggests a central mechanism [44].

Peripheral sensitization is often confused with central sensitization, as it also presents with hyperalgesia, but its mechanisms are different. Peripheral sensitization represents an increased responsiveness of nociceptors at the terminals and is restricted to the site of injury [43]. However, a patient can present with both central and peripheral sensitization. Persistent peripheral pains have also been shown to contribute to the development of central sensitization, as has been suspected in many cases of complex regional pain syndrome (CRPS), chronic pelvic pain, low back pain, and other conditions [45].

Neuropathic pain is regularly associated with sensitization, sharing many of the same anatomical and physiological changes. Neuropathic pain is caused by a lesion or disease of the nervous system, and patients often complain of ongoing, intermittent, or spontaneous numbness, burning, shooting, or pins-and-needles sensations [46]. Hyperalgesia, allodynia, paresthesias, and dysesthesias are all findings seen in neuropathic pain conditions [10, 46]. These conditions may include trigeminal neuralgia, polyneuropathy, postherpetic neuralgia, radiculopathy, or central and peripheral nerve injury (which can also cause sensitization) [46]. Sensitization after an injury or surgery is a common cause, as evidenced in cases of damage to the ilioinguinal, sciatic, or intercostal nerves [47]. When this occurs, observations of the damaged area show compensatory changes to adjacent receptors, axonal growth and sprouting, remyelination, and remodeling of synapses, all of which are adaptive and beneficial [47]. However, other changes are not, including "abnormal stimulus thresholds and sensitivity, ectopic impulse generation, conduction slowing or block, reduced inhibition, inappropriate connectivity, abortive growth, neuronal loss, and glial scarring [47]."

References

1. Gore DG. The anatomy of pain. Anesth Intensive Care Med. 2022;23(7):355–9. https://doi.org/10.1016/j.mpaic.2022.04.002.
2. Morton DL, Sandhu JS, Jones AK. Brain imaging of pain: state of the art. J Pain Res. 2016;9:613–24. https://doi.org/10.2147/JPR.S60433. PMID: 27660488; PMCID: PMC5019436.
3. Mancini F, Bauleo A, Cole J, Lui F, Porro CA, Haggard P, Iannetti GD. Whole-body mapping of spatial acuity for pain and touch. Ann Neurol. 2014;75(6):917–24. https://doi.org/10.1002/ana.24179. Epub 2014 Jun 6. PMID: 24816757; PMCID: PMC4143958.
4. Bair MJ, Robinson RL, Katon W, Kroenke K. Depression and pain comorbidity: a literature review. Arch Intern Med. 2003;163(20):2433–45. https://doi.org/10.1001/archinte.163.20.2433. PMID: 14609780.
5. Institute of Medicine (US) Committee on Pain D, Osterweis M, Kleinman A, Mechanic D. The anatomy and physiology of pain. National Academies Press (US); 1987.
6. Basbaum AI, Bautista DM, Scherrer G, Julius D. Cellular and molecular mechanisms of pain. Cell. 2009;139(2):267–84. https://doi.org/10.1016/j.cell.2009.09.028. PMID: 19837031; PMCID: PMC2852643.
7. Kendroud S, Fitzgerald LA, Murray IV, et al. Physiology, nociceptive pathways. [Updated 2022 Sept 26]. In: StatPearls [Internet]. Treasure Island (FL): StatPearls Publishing; 2024. Available from: https://www.ncbi.nlm.nih.gov/books/NBK470255/.
8. Samanta A, Hughes TET, Moiseenkova-Bell VY. Transient receptor potential (TRP) channels. Subcell Biochem. 2018;87:141–65. https://doi.org/10.1007/978-981-10-7757-9_6. PMID: 29464560; PMCID: PMC6038138.
9. Nikolenko VN, Shelomentseva EM, Tsvetkova MM, et al. Nociceptors: their role in body's defenses, tissue specific variations and anatomical update. J Pain Res. 2022;15:867–77. https://doi.org/10.2147/JPR.S348324.
10. Steeds CE. The anatomy and physiology of pain. Surgery (Oxford). 2016;34(2):55–9. https://doi.org/10.1016/j.mpsur.2015.11.005.
11. Nwonu CNS. Neuronal cell mechanisms of pain. West Afr J Med. 2022;39(10):1075–983. PMID: 36260866.
12. Kang JH, Im S. Functional anatomy of the spinal tracts based on evolutionary perspectives. Korean J Neurotrauma. 2023;19(3):275–87. https://doi.org/10.13004/kjnt.2023.19.e43. PMID: 37840623; PMCID: PMC10567534.

13. Kirkpatrick DR, McEntire DM, Hambsch ZJ, Kerfeld MJ, Smith TA, Reisbig MD, Youngblood CF, Agrawal DK. Therapeutic basis of clinical pain modulation. Clin Transl Sci. 2015;8(6):848–56. https://doi.org/10.1111/cts.12282. Epub 2015 May 11. PMID: 25962969; PMCID: PMC4641846.
14. Melzack R, Wall PD. Pain mechanisms: a new theory. Science. 1965;150(3699):971–9. https://doi.org/10.1126/science.150.3699.971. PMID: 5320816.
15. Pereira PJS, Lerner EA. Gate control theory springs a leak. Neuron. 2017;93(4):723–4. https://doi.org/10.1016/j.neuron.2017.02.016. PMID: 28231458; PMCID: PMC5474310.
16. Palazzo E, Luongo L, Novellis V, Rossi F, Maione S. The role of cannabinoid receptors in the descending modulation of pain. Pharmaceuticals (Basel). 2010;3(8):2661–73. https://doi.org/10.3390/ph3082661. PMID: 27713370; PMCID: PMC4033943.
17. Reeves KC, Shah N, Muñoz B, Atwood BK. Opioid receptor-mediated regulation of neurotransmission in the brain. Front Mol Neurosci. 2022;15:919773. https://doi.org/10.3389/fnmol.2022.919773. PMID: 35782382; PMCID: PMC9242007.
18. Watanabe C. Mechanism of spinal pain transmission and its regulation (Japanese). Yakugaku Zasshi. 2014;134(12):1301–7. https://doi.org/10.1248/yakushi.14-00203. PMID: 25452239.
19. Lee M, Silverman SM, Hansen H, Patel VB, Manchikanti L. A comprehensive review of opioid-induced hyperalgesia. Pain Physician. 2011;14(2):145–61. PMID: 21412369.
20. Chalaye P, Goffaux P, Bourgault P, Lafrenaye S, Devroede G, Watier A, Marchand S. Comparing pain modulation and autonomic responses in fibromyalgia and irritable bowel syndrome patients. Clin J Pain. 2012;28(6):519–26. https://doi.org/10.1097/AJP.0b013e31823ae69e. PMID: 22673485.
21. Obata H. Analgesic mechanisms of antidepressants for neuropathic pain. Int J Mol Sci. 2017;18(11):2483. https://doi.org/10.3390/ijms18112483. PMID: 29160850; PMCID: PMC5713449.
22. Dharmshaktu P, Tayal V, Kalra BS. Efficacy of antidepressants as analgesics: a review. J Clin Pharmacol. 2013;52(1):6–17.
23. Ossipov M, Morimura K, Porreca F. Descending pain modulation and chronification of pain. Curr Opin Support Palliat Care. 2014;8(2):143–51.
24. Treister R, Pud D, Ebstein RP, Laiba E, Raz Y, Gershon E, Haddad M, Eisenberg E. Association between polymorphisms in serotonin and dopamine-related genes and endogenous pain modulation. J Pain. 2011;12(8):875–83.
25. Kim YS, Chu Y, Han L, Li M, Li Z, LaVinka PC, Sun S, Tang Z, Park K, Caterina MJ, Ren K, Dubner R, Wei F, Dong X. Central terminal sensitization of TRPV1 by descending serotonergic facilitation modulates chronic pain. Neuron. 2014;81(4):873–87. https://doi.org/10.1016/j.neuron.2013.12.011. Epub 2014 Jan 23. PMID: 24462040; PMCID: PMC3943838.
26. Grashorn W, Schunke O, Buhmann C, Forkmann K, Diedrich S, Wesemann K, Bingel U. Influence of dopaminergic medication on conditioned pain modulation in Parkinson's disease patients. PLoS One. 2015;10(8):e0135287. https://doi.org/10.1371/journal.pone.0135287. PMID: 26270817; PMCID: PMC4536013.
27. Treister R, Pud D, Eisenberg E. The dopamine agonist apomorphine enhances conditioned pain modulation in healthy humans. Neurosci Lett. 2013;548:115–9. https://doi.org/10.1016/j.neulet.2013.05.041. Epub 2013 May 30. PMID: 23727387.
28. Pertovaara A. Noradrenergic pain modulation. Prog Neurobiol. 2006;80(2):53–83. https://doi.org/10.1016/j.pneurobio.2006.08.001.
29. Zieglgänsberger W. Substance P and pain chronicity. Cell Tissue Res. 2019;375(1):227–41. https://doi.org/10.1007/s00441-018-2922-y. Epub 2018 Oct 3. PMID: 30284083; PMCID: PMC6335504.
30. Reichl S, Augustin M, Zahn PK, Pogatzki-Zahn EM. Peripheral and spinal GABAergic regulation of incisional pain in rats. Pain. 2012;153(1):129–41. https://doi.org/10.1016/j.pain.2011.09.028. Epub 2011 Nov 3. PMID: 22054599.
31. Davies M. The role of GABAA receptors in mediating the effects of alcohol in the central nervous system. J Psychiatry Neurosci. 2003;28(4):263–74. PMID: 12921221; PMCID: PMC165791.
32. Pereira V, Goudet C. Emerging trends in pain modulation by metabotropic glutamate receptors. Front Mol Neurosci. 2019;11:464. https://doi.org/10.3389/fnmol.2018.00464. PMID: 30662395; PMCID: PMC6328474.
33. Fonseca-Rodrigues D, Almeida A, Pinto-Ribeiro F. A new gal in town: a systematic review of the role of galanin and its receptors in experimental pain. Cells. 2022;11(5):839. https://doi.org/10.3390/cells11050839. PMID: 35269462; PMCID: PMC8909084.
34. Wiesenfeld-Hallin Z, Xu XJ, Hökfelt T. The role of spinal cholecystokinin in chronic pain states. Pharmacol Toxicol. 2002;91(6):398–403. https://doi.org/10.1034/j.1600-0773.2002.910619.x. PMID: 12688385.
35. Lu HC, Mackie K. An introduction to the endogenous cannabinoid system. Biol Psychiatry. 2016;79(7):516–25. https://doi.org/10.1016/j.biopsych.2015.07.028. Epub 2015 Oct 30. PMID: 26698193; PMCID: PMC4789136.
36. Anthony AT, Rahmat S, Sangle P, Sandhu O, Khan S. Cannabinoid receptors and their relationship with chronic pain: a narrative review. Cureus. 2020;12(9):e10436. https://doi.org/10.7759/cureus.10436. PMID: 33072446; PMCID: PMC7557112.
37. Ghovanloo MR, Effraim PR, Tyagi S, et al. Functionally-selective inhibition of threshold sodium currents and excitability in dorsal root ganglion neurons by cannabinol. Commun Biol. 2024;7:120. https://doi.org/10.1038/s42003-024-05781-x.
38. Quevedo AS, Coghill RC. Attentional modulation of spatial integration of pain: evidence for dynamic spatial tuning. J Neurosci. 2007;27(43):11635–40.
39. Severeijns R, Vlaeyen JWS, van den Hout MA, Weber WEJ. Pain catastrophizing predicts pain intensity, disability, and psychological distress independent of the level of physical impairment. Clin J Pain. 2001;17(2):165.
40. Wandner LD, Prasad R, Ramezani A, Malcore SA, Kerns RD. Core competencies for the emerging specialty of pain psychology. Am Psychol. 2019;74(4):432–44. https://doi.org/10.1037/amp0000330. Epub 2018 Aug 2. PMID: 30070541.
41. Ji RR, Nackley A, Huh Y, Terrando N, Maixner W. Neuroinflammation and central sensitization in chronic and widespread pain. Anesthesiology. 2018;129(2):343–66. https://doi.org/10.1097/ALN.0000000000002130. PMID: 29462012; PMCID: PMC6051899.
42. Woolf CJ, King AE. Subthreshold components of the cutaneous mechanoreceptive fields of dorsal horn neurons in the rat lumbar spinal cord. J Neurophysiol. 1989;62(4):907–16. https://doi.org/10.1152/jn.1989.62.4.907.
43. Latremoliere A, Woolf CJ. Central sensitization: a generator of pain hypersensitivity by central neural plasticity. J Pain. 2009;10(9):895–926. https://doi.org/10.1016/j.jpain.2009.06.012. PMID: 19712899; PMCID: PMC2750819.
44. Harte SE, Harris RE, Clauw DJ. The neurobiology of central sensitization. J Appl Behav Res. 2018;23:e12137. https://doi.org/10.1111/jabr.12137.
45. De Schoenmacker I, Mollo A, Scheuren PS, Sirucek L, Brunner F, Schweinhardt P, Curt A, Rosner J, Hubli M. Central sensitization in CRPS patients with widespread pain: a cross-sectional study. Pain Med. 2023;24(8):974–84. https://doi.org/10.1093/pm/pnad040.
46. Finnerup NB, Kuner R, Jensen TS. Neuropathic pain: from mechanisms to treatment. Physiol Rev. 2021;101(1):259–301. https://doi.org/10.1152/physrev.00045.2019.
47. Costigan M, Scholz J, Woolf CJ. Neuropathic pain: a maladaptive response of the nervous system to damage. Annu Rev Neurosci. 2009;32:1–32. https://doi.org/10.1146/annurev.neuro.051508.135531. PMID: 19400724; PMCID: PMC2768555.

Evaluation of Pain Scales and Definitions of Outcome Measures from Primary Literature

3

Ozgur Karcioglu

Abbreviations

CRIES	Crying, requires oxygen, increased vital signs, expression, and sleeplessness
ED	Emergency department
FLACC	Face, Legs, Activity, Cry and Consolability
NRS	Numeric Rating Scale
VAS	Visual Analog Scale
VRS/VDS	Verbal Rating/Descriptor Scale
PROM	Patient-reported outcome measures

Introduction

Most studies demonstrated that pain—more specifically, acute pain—is the most common chief complaint reported by most patients in the acute and primary care settings [1]. The definition of pain by the International Association for the Study of Pain (IASP) as "an unpleasant sensory and emotional experience associated with actual or potential tissue injury, or defined in terms of such damage" is accepted worldwide [2]. Subjectivity and multidimensional characteristics of pain make its evaluation and measurement extremely difficult.

Scientific bodies from the Veterans Health Administration (VHA), The Joint Commission (TJC), and others have been involved in an intense debate on rigid regulations for recording pain in the clinical evaluation of patients in the past decades [3]. The VHA created an extensive tool kit to implement pain assessment and management in all its patients [4]. In 1995, the American Pain Society urged that healthcare providers treat pain as the "fifth vital sign" (P5VS) [5]. Implementation of this standard in clinical practice comprised the addition of pain as the "fifth" vital sign to be noted in the context of initial evaluation, the use of pain intensity recording, and a statement on pain management in all medical settings. Perception of pain should be documented during the initial assessment of each patient. Pain estimations are obtained to record both the severity of pain and the effect of pain management. Pain is mostly viewed as a subjective experience that cannot be objectively measured.

The latest guidelines recommend that pain must be assessed and intervened within around 15–25 min of initial evaluation in the emergency department (ED) [6, 7]. Provided that regular pain reassessments are performed, reassessment should be planned in line with the recorded severity of the experience [8, 9]. On the other hand, pain treatment should be targeted to a goal of reducing the pain score (e.g., by 50%, below 4/10, or referred to as mild/moderate or severe) rather than prescribing a specific analgesic dose [8].

Characteristics of Pain Patterns

(a) *Somatic pain* arises from the skin, connective, and musculoskeletal systems and tends to be a sharp, localized pain.
(b) *Visceral pain* emerges from the internal organs and structures of the thorax, abdomen, and pelvis. This kind of pain is mostly dull and diffuse, while the gut endothelial tissue can trigger somatic-type pain (i.e., acute and localized) [10].
(c) *Neuropathic pain*, on the other hand, is accompanied by an injury to the neural tissue [11]. Neuropathic pain mostly follows chronic pain, whereas it can also appear acutely [12]. Acute neuropathic pain may appear with nerve transection (e.g., amputation or tissue loss peripherally), while a cerebrovascular accident may also cause injury to the central neurons [13]. *Nociplastic pain* is defined as multifocal, diffuse, and/or more intense than

O. Karcioglu (✉)
University of Health Sciences, Department of Emergency Medicine, Istanbul Education and Research Hospital, Istanbul, Turkey
e-mail: Ozgur.Karcioglu@saglik.gov.tr

J. P. Reinert et al. (eds.), *Adjunctive Analgesic Strategies for the Bedside Clinician and Beyond*,
https://doi.org/10.1007/978-3-032-21675-5_3

Table 3.1 Categories of pain

Nociceptive pain	Pain arising from actual or threatened damage to nonneural tissue. Its main source is the nociceptor activation. It is often divided into somatic and visceral pain
Neuropathic pain	Pain stems from an injury or disease of the somatosensory nervous system
Nociplastic pain	Pain caused by altered nociception despite no clear evidence of tissue injury that activates peripheral nociceptors or evidence for lesion of the somatosensory system triggering the pain

expected by the severity of the clinical findings (Table 3.1) [14]. Fatigue, sleep, and mood problems can accompany the perception of pain in most patients. Fibromyalgia and tension-type headaches can be comorbid conditions in those with nociplastic pain. It should be kept in mind that multiple pathophysiological processes triggering pain may coexist in the same patient, described as "*mixed pain*" [15]. Of note, patients may experience and complain of different types of pain concurrently; thus, healthcare workers should be cognizant of the distinguishing features of various pain syndromes.

Documentation of Pain and Obtaining a Patient History

The physician must rely on the patient's reports to obtain critical data on the localization, quality, and severity of the pain, especially when he or she cannot get access to objective measurements (Table 3.2). Patients' self-reports are viewed as the most accurate data of the presence and severity of pain, which is also valid for all ages, irrespective of problems of communication or cognition [17]. On the other hand, validated pain scales are important aids to provide the best possible assessment of a given patient. Providers often question the reported severity and rely on their own estimates, but the value of the patients' description of the location and nature of the discomfort has been proven on a theoretical basis and in daily practice [9, 18].

Measuring pain using specific scoring systems has been accepted as the most accurate and reliable tool used to assess patients' pain and response to the treatment given [19]. Scoring systems developed to gauge the intensity of patients' experience can be divided into two groups: unidimensional (describing only one perspective, such as the magnitude of pain intensity as perceived by the patient) and multidimensional (addressing sensation, including intensity, location, and affective and sensory qualities) measures [20]. Of note, unidimensional scales measure intensity; thus, they are not used to provide pain assessment comprehensively, which should encompass both the unidimensional measurement of pain intensity and the multidimensional evaluation of the pain perception.

Table 3.2 Essential elements of history in the evaluation of pain

Pain location	Primary location of pain, using description and pain diagram Pain radiation from the primary location
Triggering events attributed to pain onset	Injuries and/or surgical procedures
Focused medical history	Previous or concurrent painful conditions, syndromes, and treatment outcomes
Characterization of pain in relation to descriptors of sensation	Descriptors: Sharp, burning, throbbing, etc. MPQ: Sensory and affective descriptors Characteristics of NP using specific NP questionnaires, e.g., NPQ, DN4, LANSS, PainDETECT, and ID pain
Severity of pain in different situations	Does it hurt at rest or on movement Pain duration: pain over time: Current, past week, highest intensity Characteristics of pain: Continuous or intermittent
Associated symptoms	Complaints such as nausea, interruptions to sleep Inability to undertake normal activities
Factors affecting the management process	Beliefs in regard to the causes of pain Understanding, knowledge, expectations, and preferences for pain management Expectations of the outcome of treatment The reduction in pain required for patient satisfaction The patient's typical coping strategies for stress and pain (in relation to the patient's anxiety, depression, or psychiatric conditions) Family/carer expectations and beliefs about pain, stress, and management course
Treatment	Current and previous medications, including dose, frequency, efficacy, and side effects Other treatment for pain Which healthcare professionals have been consulted in relation to pain

Adapted from Schug et al. [16]
MPQ McGill Pain Questionnaire, *NP* neuropathic pain, *DN4* Douleur Neuropathique en 4 Questions, *NPQ* Neuropathic Pain Questionnaire, *LANSS* Leeds Assessment of Neuropathic Symptoms and Signs

There are at least three major foundations for prioritizing pain assessment:

(a) Quality of medical care.
(b) Patient satisfaction.
(c) Compliance with regulatory requirements for assessing and documenting pain levels [21].

The Unidimensional Pain Scales Commonly Used Worldwide

They include (Fig. 3.1a–d):

- Visual Analog Scale (VAS)
- Numeric Rating Scale (NRS)
- Verbal Rating/Descriptor Scale (VRS/VDS)
- Thermometer Pain Scale (TPS)

(a) *The Visual Analog Scale (VAS)* is the most commonly employed scale to estimate the intensity of pain and measure the treatment response [22]. The physician or nurse asks the patients to mark a point on a line drawn between two ends to show how intense they perceive the experience (Fig. 3.1a). The VAS is a continuous scale comprising a *horizontal* or *vertical* line, usually 100 mm long, anchored by two verbal descriptors (i.e., "no pain" and "worst imaginable pain") [23, 24]. Patients are asked to rate their pain intensity perceived "currently" or "in the past 24 hours."

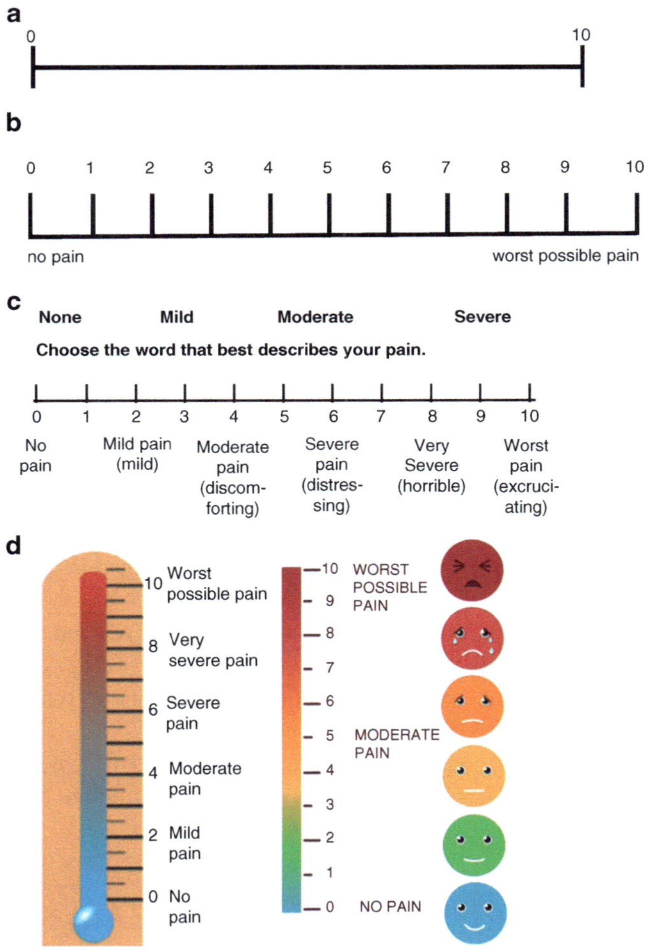

Fig. 3.1 (**a**) Visual Analog Scale (VAS). The patient is asked to mark his/her pain on the line. (**b**) The Numerical Rating Scale (NRS). The patient needs to rate his/her pain as a number from 0 to 10, without using a pen or paper. (**c**) Verbal Rating Scale (VRS) or Verbal Descriptor Scale (VDS) and Verbal Numerical Rating Scale (VNRS) (**d**) Example of Thermometer Pain Scale

The VAS is a practical tool, highly sensitive in detecting response to treatment [25]. Minimal translation difficulties have led to an unknown number of cross-cultural adaptations [24]. Its major drawbacks are the need for marking and for being able to visualize and mark the line, which can make it impractical to use in an emergency situation. However, the VAS provides little practical advantage over VRS/VDS in routine patient care [19].

Moutte et al. published a trial on a prestructured questionnaire filled in by 75 emergency physicians in northern Europe [26]. The physicians stated that a Pain Scale with a VAS had been used by around 60% of physicians in young patients between 9 and 19 years of age, by 23% in children aged 3–8 years, and by 3% in children younger than 3 years of age. Emergency health practitioners reported a need for pain evaluation procedures in young patients. Olsen et al. performed a trial to estimate the effect of implementing a pain treatment algorithm in adult ICU patients expressing their pain [27]. The number of pain measurements was higher in the intervention group in comparison to the controls. Of note, the duration of ventilation and the length of ICU stay were reduced substantially in the intervention group compared to the control group. A number of outcome variables were significantly improved following the institution of the algorithm compared with the control group. Instruments for behavioral assessment are helpful in detecting the magnitude of pain and making treatment decisions.

(b) *The Numeric Rating Scale (NRS)* is a numeric scale composed of 11 points validated worldwide using various disease scenarios. Data obtained via NRS are easily documented and intuitively interpretable and meet regulatory requirements for pain assessment and documentation [28]. Evidence has demonstrated that a majority of acute care patients allow evaluation via a simple "0–10 scale" or NRS reliably with regard to their pain levels even in the prehospital phase [29]. Like the pain VAS, minimal language translation difficulties support the use of the NRS across cultures and languages [30].

Evidence indicated that patients prefer to give pain a number rather than simply state whether they need painkillers [31, 32]. The strengths of NRS over the VAS are its ability to be administered both verbally and in writing as well as its simplicity of scoring. However, similar to the VAS, the NRS is used to assess only one component of pain experience—pain intensity. It therefore does not capture the complexity and idiosyncratic nature of the pain experience or improvements stemming from fluctuations of the symptoms [24].

NRS is among the widely employed tools requesting the patient to rate his/her pain on a scale from 0 to 10, with 0 indicating no pain and 10 expressing the worst possible pain (Fig. 3.1b). It is also used in pediatric cases and illiterate individuals who can understand and verbalize numbers. The pain scores are stated as:

- 0 = no pain
- 1–3 = mild pain
- 4–6 = moderate pain
- 7–10 = severe pain

NRS can be used with most children above 8 years of age, and behavioral scales are reserved for those who cannot give a self-report [33]. The NRS is the most commonly utilized tool to estimate pain severity in cancer-related pain [34]. Goulet et al. studied adult patients to indicate the correlation of electronic medical record–based ratings of NRS with self-administered ones [35]. Although the correlation was high, the mean electronic medical record–based NRS score was significantly lower than the survey score ($p < 0.0001$).

(c) *Verbal Pain Scores (VPSs), Verbal Rating Scales (VRS), or Verbal Descriptor Scales are employed to* discern patients truly in pain but unable to express their situation, as well as influence the physician to inquire about the patient's pain.

VRS comprises a number of expressions to define increasing pain intensity (Fig. 3.1c). ED crowding was shown to lengthen the time to application of analgesic agents and increase mortality rate [36]. VPS usage under these conditions may be beneficial to detect and treat patients with an urgent need for intervention more expediently. Patients are asked to choose the word that best addresses their pain severity. The number of descriptors used has ranged from 4 (none, mild, moderate, and severe) to 15 [37]. These scales may prove difficult in usage, especially for cognitively impaired patients or those who have limited literacy, and they do not provide the number of choices available with the VAS or NRS, thus potentially limiting precision [38].

An example of the *Thermometer Pain Scale* is shown in Fig. 3.1d. The Pain Thermometer includes a thermometer alongside the words indicating different levels of pain intensity [39].

(d) *Nonverbal Scale*

The FACES Pain Scale—Revised (FPS-R) is a very popular visual scale to measure pain intensity, especially in young children [40]. As a self-report scale, it was adapted from the FPS to enable recording the intensity of pain on the 0–10 metric (Fig. 3.2) [41]. The scale consists of six *FACES* showing progressive pain intensities, beginning with a smiling face and ending with a crying face. The scale shows a close linear relationship with VAS between the ages of 4 and 16 years. FPS-R has been devised for children aged 3 years and above, and it is also used for the cognitively impaired elderly [31, 42].

Main advantages include the ease of application and a lack of additional requirements for usage except for the photocopied *FACES* and a marker to accomplish the task in the chaotic EDs. These scales are divided into two types: *pain behavior scales and pain behavior checklists*. Some of these scales are scored by identifying the number or intensity of behaviors. However, no research as yet confirms that a pain behavior score is a pain intensity score [43].

Pain Intensity

It is remarkable that pain behavior scores are not safe to be used as pain intensity scores. An example of a pain behavior scale is the Behavioral Pain Scale (BPS), developed for use in critically ill patients in the ICU [44].

It evaluates and scores three categories of behavior:

(a) Facial expression: Scores range from 1 for relaxed to 4 for grimacing.
(b) Upper-limb movement: Scores range from 1 for no movement to 4 for permanently retracted.
(c) Ventilator compliance: Scores range from 1 for tolerating ventilator to 4 for unable to control ventilation.

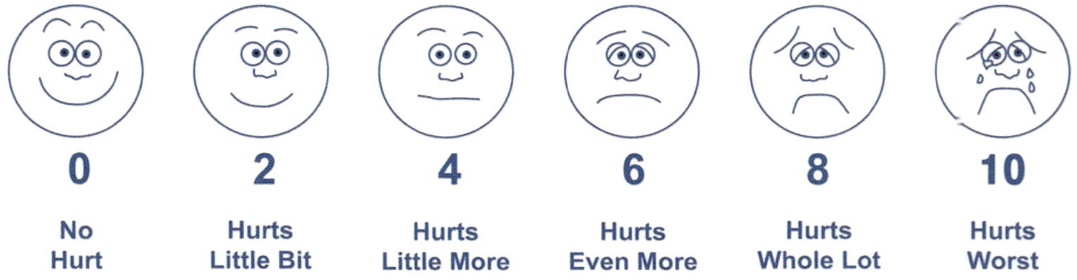

Fig. 3.2 FACES Pain Rating Scale, devised by Wong and Baker

A score above 3 represents the presence of pain, and the score can be used to assess the response to the intervention but cannot be interpreted to mean pain intensity. For a pain behavior scale to be useful, the patient must be able to respond in all categories of behavior. For example, the BPS would be useless in a patient who is receiving a neuromuscular blocking agent. *Brief Pain Inventory (BPI)* is a self-administered, validated questionnaire available in many languages and was originally used to assess pain intensity and location, as well as pain-related functional interference, among cancer patients (Fig. 3.3) [45].

The tool has been developed to capture two dimensions of pain: severity and interference. It was also intended to describe two components of interference—activity and affect (emotions). BPI was also translated and validated in different cultures and disease settings. Migliorini et al. recently used the scale to evaluate the efficacy of duloxetine in the management of fibromyalgia [46]. The authors compared the severity of pain with respect to different doses of the medication using the Multidimensional Pain Inventory (MPI), Fibromyalgia Impact Questionnaire (FIQ), and Clinical Global Impression (CGI). There were no significant differences between the scales in special regard to the assessments of pain and discomfort attributed to fibromyalgia (Table 3.3). The authors reported that the BPI-T also has good internal consistency (Cronbach's alpha coefficients: 0.76 and 0.85) in a trial performed on cardiac patients in Thailand [54].

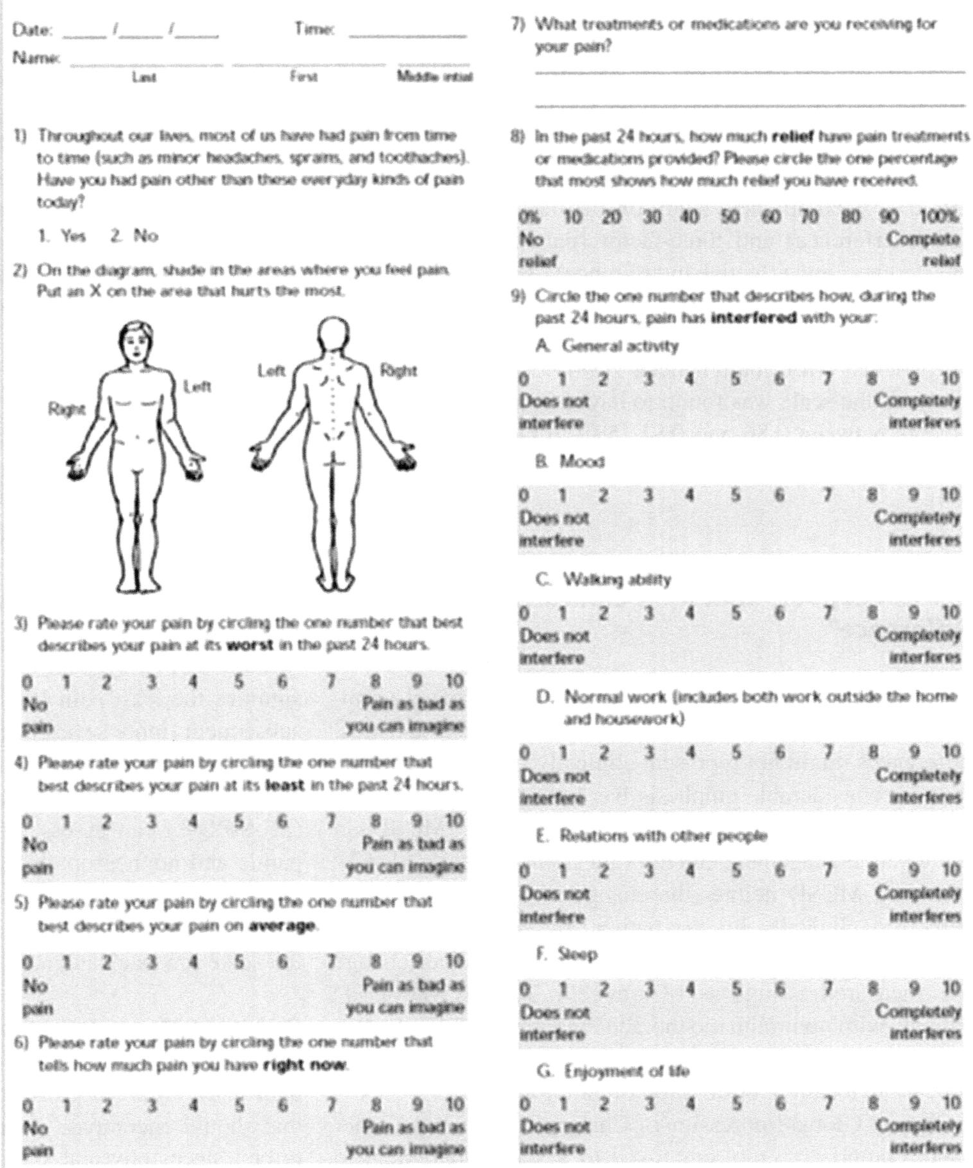
Date: ____/____/____ Time: ________

Name: ________ ________ ________
Last First Middle initial

1) Throughout our lives, most of us have had pain from time to time (such as minor headaches, sprains, and toothaches). Have you had pain other than these everyday kinds of pain today?

1. Yes 2. No

2) On the diagram, shade in the areas where you feel pain. Put an X on the area that hurts the most.

3) Please rate your pain by circling the one number that best describes your pain at its **worst** in the past 24 hours.

0 1 2 3 4 5 6 7 8 9 10
No pain — Pain as bad as you can imagine

4) Please rate your pain by circling the one number that best describes your pain at its **least** in the past 24 hours.

0 1 2 3 4 5 6 7 8 9 10
No pain — Pain as bad as you can imagine

5) Please rate your pain by circling the one number that best describes your pain on **average**.

0 1 2 3 4 5 6 7 8 9 10
No pain — Pain as bad as you can imagine

6) Please rate your pain by circling the one number that tells how much pain you have **right now**.

0 1 2 3 4 5 6 7 8 9 10
No pain — Pain as bad as you can imagine

7) What treatments or medications are you receiving for your pain?

8) In the past 24 hours, how much **relief** have pain treatments or medications provided? Please circle the one percentage that most shows how much relief you have received.

0% 10 20 30 40 50 60 70 80 90 100%
No relief — Complete relief

9) Circle the one number that describes how, during the past 24 hours, pain has **interfered** with your:

A. General activity

0 1 2 3 4 5 6 7 8 9 10
Does not interfere — Completely interferes

B. Mood

0 1 2 3 4 5 6 7 8 9 10
Does not interfere — Completely interferes

C. Walking ability

0 1 2 3 4 5 6 7 8 9 10
Does not interfere — Completely interferes

D. Normal work (includes both work outside the home and housework)

0 1 2 3 4 5 6 7 8 9 10
Does not interfere — Completely interferes

E. Relations with other people

0 1 2 3 4 5 6 7 8 9 10
Does not interfere — Completely interferes

F. Sleep

0 1 2 3 4 5 6 7 8 9 10
Does not interfere — Completely interferes

G. Enjoyment of life

0 1 2 3 4 5 6 7 8 9 10
Does not interfere — Completely interferes

Fig. 3.3 Brief Pain Inventory (BPI)

Table 3.3 Scales employed to evaluate pain Interference (pain-related disability) as pain-related outcome measures in the clinical setting

Generally applicable scales	Scales for site-specific pain interference
Pain Interference subscale of the BPI [47]	Roland Morris Disability Questionnaire (RMDQ) [48]
Pain Interference subscale of the Multidimensional Pain Inventory (MPI) [49]	Oswestry Disability Index (ODI) [50] for back
Pain Disability Index (PDI) [51]	Neck Disability Index (NDI) [52] for neck pain

Adapted from IASP [53]

The functional interference section of the BPI assesses the impact of pain on various aspects of daily functioning. Using a 0–10 scale (0 = does not interfere and 10 = completely interferes), the patient is asked to rate the degree to which pain has interfered with seven functions during the past 24 h: general activity, mood, walking ability, normal work, relations with other people, sleep, and enjoyment of life [55]. Human body drawings are provided for patients to mark the location of their pain.

The original BPI interference scale was modified to include recreational and social activities, as well as self-care [56, 57]. A comparison study on two-factor (pain intensity and interference) and three-factor (pain intensity, activity interference, and affective interference) representation of the modified BPI was published, and the researchers concluded that a two-factor representation of BPI gives the best results in patients with malignancies [58]. In a multinational analysis, the scale was found to have internal stability coefficients between 0.86 and 0.91 [59]. In Germany, the test–retest reliability at 30 min was shown as excellent ($r = 0.97$) [60].

The Concept of "Minimum Clinically Significant Difference"

Clinicians can overestimate the clinical effect of an unimportant difference in the scores. Since the recorded statistical differences might not represent clinically important changes in pain, considerable emphasis has been put on measuring the "minimum clinically significant difference" (MCSD) in acute pain management and relevant studies [22, 25, 61–63]. The term MCSD defines the change in pain needed to be perceived clinically by the patient and was measured as 13 mm on a 100-mm VAS, while physician-perceived change was measured as high as 18 mm [25]. The MCSD of ED patients with nontraumatic thoracoabdominal pain in Turkey is 24.2 mm, and it is not affected by gender, age, level of education, location, or duration of pain [64].

Patient Global Impression of Change Scales, on the other hand, comprises a tool employed to describe the extent to which the patient's condition has improved or deteriorated since a predefined time point, rather than a specific dimension of change determined by the clinician [65]. The scales emphasize the participants' rating of self-impressions of change between two fixed time points and between 7 and 15 points, via an NRS or a VAS [66].

Multidimensional Tools

Multidimensional tools allow a more comprehensive and complementary evaluation of pain. Various characteristics of pain, e.g., psychological, emotional, and behavioral aspects, are analyzed [67]. Most traditional methods of measurement (VAS, NRS, and VDS/VRS) evaluate pain as a unidimensional sensation.

When we use the term "pain," it generally encompasses many discrete qualities under a single term in the language, instead of a specific feeling that varies only in intensity. The McGill Pain Questionnaire (MPQ) is a multidimensional scale developed by Melzack and Torgerson to be used as a self-reported measure of pain, referring both to quality and quantity [68]. MPQ allows the clinician to estimate the quality of the experience by taking into account the severity, localization, and temporal and affective aspects of pain. To fulfill these tasks, the original MPQ was composed of 78 pain descriptors divided into four classes: the sensory, affective, evaluative, and miscellaneous quality of the pain experience (Fig. 3.4).

This tool also assesses pain severity via the Pain Rating Index (PRI) and the Present Pain Intensity (PPI). The PRI is based on a 1–5-intensity scale, and it includes a numerical grading of words descriptive of the sensory, affective, evaluative, and miscellaneous features of pain [69]. Patients are requested to select only those descriptors that accurately define their feelings at that moment. The word within each subclass that signifies the least pain is attributed a value of 1, followed by a value of 2 for the subsequent word, and so on. Within the PRI system, the word within each subclass that signifies the least pain is scored as 1, while 2 signifies the subsequent (more severe) description and so on [70]. On the other hand, the PPI score ranges from 1 (mild) to 5 (excruciating) [71]. The Short-form McGill Pain Questionnaire-2 (SF-MPQ-2) can assess the prominent findings of neuropathic and nonneuropathic pain to provide a valid, responsive, and efficient evaluation for relevant studies [72]. The authors pointed out that SF-MPQ-2 had excellent validity in the acute low back and radicular leg pain.

Outcome Measurements

The recommendations regarding *outcome measurements* for pain research are useful for making scheduled evaluations that should encompass an assessment of pain, fatigue, disturbed sleep, physical functioning, emotional functioning, global ratings of patient satisfaction, and quality of life

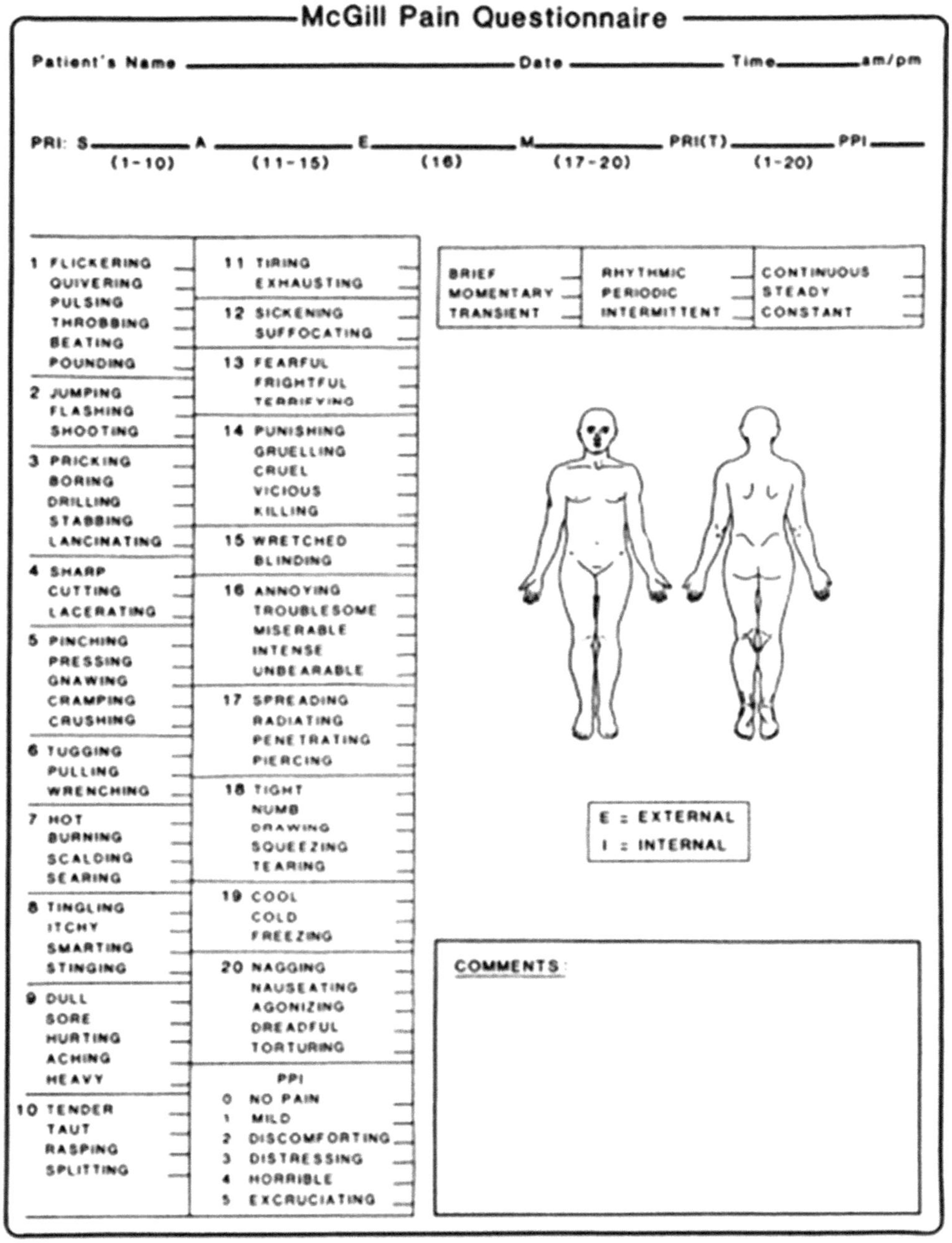
McGill Pain Questionnaire

Patient's Name ______ Date ______ Time ______ am/pm

PRI: S ______ (1-10) A ______ (11-15) E ______ (16) M ______ (17-20) PRI(T) ______ (1-20) PPI ______

1 FLICKERING, QUIVERING, PULSING, THROBBING, BEATING, POUNDING
2 JUMPING, FLASHING, SHOOTING
3 PRICKING, BORING, DRILLING, STABBING, LANCINATING
4 SHARP, CUTTING, LACERATING
5 PINCHING, PRESSING, GNAWING, CRAMPING, CRUSHING
6 TUGGING, PULLING, WRENCHING
7 HOT, BURNING, SCALDING, SEARING
8 TINGLING, ITCHY, SMARTING, STINGING
9 DULL, SORE, HURTING, ACHING, HEAVY
10 TENDER, TAUT, RASPING, SPLITTING
11 TIRING, EXHAUSTING
12 SICKENING, SUFFOCATING
13 FEARFUL, FRIGHTFUL, TERRIFYING
14 PUNISHING, GRUELLING, CRUEL, VICIOUS, KILLING
15 WRETCHED, BLINDING
16 ANNOYING, TROUBLESOME, MISERABLE, INTENSE, UNBEARABLE
17 SPREADING, RADIATING, PENETRATING, PIERCING
18 TIGHT, NUMB, DRAWING, SQUEEZING, TEARING
19 COOL, COLD, FREEZING
20 NAGGING, NAUSEATING, AGONIZING, DREADFUL, TORTURING

PPI
0 NO PAIN
1 MILD
2 DISCOMFORTING
3 DISTRESSING
4 HORRIBLE
5 EXCRUCIATING

BRIEF, MOMENTARY, TRANSIENT | RHYTHMIC, PERIODIC, INTERMITTENT | CONTINUOUS, STEADY, CONSTANT

E = EXTERNAL
I = INTERNAL

COMMENTS:

Fig. 3.4 The McGill Pain Questionnaire (MPQ): the sensitive (1–10), affective (11–15), evaluative (16), and miscellaneous (17–20) groups and their descriptors. The Pain Rating Index and the Present Pain Intensity

(QoL) [73]. There is still little agreement, and no unified approach has been devised in regard to measuring the various aspects of chronic pain.

Pain Reassessment

Herr et al. cited that pain reassessment can represent a collaborative process, although it is commonly neglected in routine practice [74]. Clinicians should not view a routine order for painkillers as a replacement for scheduled reassessments of pain. Of note, scheduled reassessments need to employ the same pain self-report tools and perform evaluations under similar situations [75].

Comparative Findings on Different Pain Measurement Tools

Pain is a multifaceted and subjective experience; thus, it is impossible to measure. Assessment of pain encompasses a multifaceted analysis of different aspects—sensorial, psychological, and experiential—in an objective way. The use of questionnaires and rating scales is viewed as the mainstay for the assessment of pain [68]. However, deciding on the best instrument for accurately recording self-reported pain is not straightforward. Researchers cited that there is a substantial discrepancy between NRS and VAS recordings, which indicates a need for clinical judgment to be incorporated into the measurement of actual levels of pain and suggests that relying on pain scales alone is not a comprehensive approach [76].

VAS, Color Analog Scale (CAS), and verbally administered NRS were found to have a strong correlation. The three scales can be interchangeably employed for acute pain evaluation in adults. Likewise, researchers published a comparative study of unidimensional pain scales as part of the work of the European Palliative Care Research Collaborative on pain assessment [77]. NRS showed better compliance in 15 of 19 studies reporting pain levels in comparison to the VAS and VRS, and thus, it was the instrument of choice in 11 studies based on higher compliance rates, better responsiveness and ease of use, and better applicability relative to VAS and/or VRS.

A systematic review published in 2018 provided important clues relevant to the use and practicability of the most widely employed pain scales [32]. Data collected for the review of the 19 clinical studies included in the analysis of the pain scales used in the acute setting were tabulated and summarized (Table 3.4). There were 12 (63%) moderate-quality (B) and seven (37%) low-quality (C) evidence derived from the studies, in regard to quality of evidence per Grading of Recommendations, Assessment, Development, and Evaluation (GRADE) guidelines.

Most of the studies in the analysis had a high correlation between VAS, VRS/VDS, and NRS, although some pointed out that there is a discrepancy in some situations. VDS and NRS have shown a strong correlation and can be used in practice depending on the preference. Older individuals preferred VDS to express their pain intensity [34, 35], including those with mild-to-moderate cognitive impairment. Accordingly, NRS was claimed to be the preferred scale in the cognitively intact group, while FPS-R was advocated in the cognitively impaired group [31].

Table 3.4 Summary of pain scale interpretation studies

Investigator(s), title, date, and Ref. #	Sample size and population	Quality of evidence (GRADE)[a]	Risk of bias[b]	Objectives	Findings	Notes and conclusions
McLean, et al. 2004 [29]	1227 prehospital patients >13 years old	C	H	To determine the feasibility of prehospital pain measurement among patients aged 13 years or older using a VRS and NRS	Prehospital pain assessment using a VRS and NRS was feasible in this patient population. Further studies are needed to confirm this in other settings	An 11-point scale is preferable for prehospital practice and could also be useful for research applications. Pain assessment using a VRS and NRS can be implemented with minimal paramedic training
Leigheb M, et al. 2017 [76]	137 adult ED patients	B	H	To evaluate the intensity and location of pain experienced by patients in the ED, the time to analgesic therapy in the ED, and the patient's satisfaction so as to identify potential interventions to improve management	The magnitude of NRS pain measurements was higher than VAS measurements	The discrepancy between NRS and VAS scores suggests that pain intensity cannot be determined accurately according to pain scale data alone but should also incorporate clinical judgment
Pereira et al. 2015 [78]	101 institutionalized elderly	C	U	Correlating two unidimensional scales for the measurement of self-reported pain intensity for the elderly and identifying a preference for one of the scales	There were moderate-to-strong, positive, and statistically significant associations between the scores of NRS and VDS: overall assessment ($r = 0.75$), the rest ($r = 0.92$), and movement ($r = 0.87$). Higher mean scores in NRS were associated with higher categories of pain intensity in VDS The association between the mean scores of NRS and the categories of VDS was significant, indicating convergent validity and a similar metric between the scales	Pain measurements among institutionalized elderly can be made by NRS and VDS; however, the preferred scale for the elderly was the VDS, regardless of gender

(continued)

Table 3.4 (continued)

Investigator(s), title, date, and Ref. #	Sample size and population	Quality of evidence (GRADE)[a]	Risk of bias[b]	Objectives	Findings	Notes and conclusions
Herr KA, et al. 2004 [74]	175: 86 younger (aged 25–55) and 89 older (>65) adults	B	U	To determine (1) the psychometric properties and utility of five types of commonly used pain rating scales when used with younger and older adults, (2) factors related to the failure to successfully use a pain rating scale, (3) pain rating scale preference, and (4) factors impacting scale preference	All five pain scales (VAS, FPS, VDS, 21-point NRS, and 11-point Verbal Numeric Scale (VNS)) were effective in discriminating different levels of pain sensation; however, the VDS was the most sensitive and reliable Failure rates for pain scale completion were minimal, except for the VAS The scale most preferred to represent pain intensity in both cohorts of subjects was the NRS, followed by the VDS	Although all five of the pain intensity rating scales were psychometrically sound when used with either age group, failures, internal consistency reliability, construct validity, scale sensitivity, and preference suggest that the VDS is the scale of choice for assessing pain intensity among older adults, including those with mild-to-moderate cognitive impairment
Ware LJ, et al. 2006 [31]	68 cognitively impaired minority sample	C	H	To determine the reliability and validity of selected pain intensity scales, including the FPS-R, VDS, NRS, and Iowa Pain Thermometer (IPT), with a cognitively impaired minority sample	Concurrent validity was supported with correlations ranging from 0.56 to 0.90. The lowest correlations were found between the FPS-R and the other scales, suggesting that the FPS-R may be measuring a broader construct incorporating pain	In terms of pain scale preference, the NRS (33%) was the preferred scale in the cognitively intact group, and the FPS-R (54%) was the preferred scale in the cognitively impaired group. African Americans and Hispanics preferred the FPS-R. Severely, moderately, and mildly impaired participants also preferred the FPS-R
Yazici et al. 2014 [79]	621 postoperative adult patients	B	L	To determine patient pain scale preferences and compare the level of agreement among pain scales commonly used during postoperative pain assessment	Patient preferences for pain scales were as follows: 97.4% FPS, 88.6% NRS, 84.1% VDS, 78.1% TPS, 60.1% SF-MPQ, 37.0% BPI, 11.4% VAS, and 10.5% MPQ. Education was an important factor in the preferences for all scales ($p < 0.000$). The level of pain determined by the VAS did not correlate with the level of pain identified by the NRS, TPS, FPS, and VDS ($p < 0.05$)	The NRS, TPS, FPS, and VDS were appropriate pain rating scales for the participants in this study, and the VAS should be used in combination with one of these scales
Bahreini M, et al. 2015 [80]	150 adult ED patients	C	H	To assess the agreement between VAS, Color Analog Scale (CAS), and NRS in the emergency setting	The three pain scales were strongly correlated at all time periods. The findings suggest that NRS, CAS, and VAS can be interchangeably applied for acute pain measurement in adult patients	Spearman correlation coefficients between NRS and CAS, NRS and VAS, and CAS and VAS were 0.95, 0.94, and 0.94, respectively ($p < 0.001$). On a scale of 0–10, the 95% limits of agreement between the paired NRS and VAS, VAS and CAS, and CAS and NRS ranged from −2.0 to 2.6, from −2.7 to 2.0, and from −2.1 to 2.0, respectively

(continued)

Table 3.4 (continued)

Investigator(s), title, date, and Ref. #	Sample size and population	Quality of evidence (GRADE)[a]	Risk of bias[b]	Objectives	Findings	Notes and conclusions
Aziato L, et al. 2015 [81]	150 postoperative patients	B	L	To select, develop, and validate context-appropriate unidimensional pain scales for pain assessment among adult postoperative patients	(Colour-Circle Pain Scale–[CCPS]) had higher scale preference than NRS and FPS. Convergent validity was very good and significant (0.70–0.75). Inter-rater reliability was high (0.923–0.928), and all the scales were sensitive to change in the intensity or level of pain experienced before and after analgesia	Using a valid tool for pain assessment gives the clinician an objective criterion for pain management. Due to the subjective nature of pain, consideration of sociocultural factors for the particular context ensures that the appropriate tool is used
Göransson KE, et al. 2015 [82]	217 adult ED patients	B	L	To compare correlations between values on the VAS and the NRS in patients in the ED and assess the patients' preference of scale	The pain scores generated from the NRS and the VAS were found to strongly correlate (mean difference: 0.41). Most patients found the NRS easier to use than the VAS (61% and 22%, respectively; $p < 0.001$)	A majority reported that the NRS reflected/described their pain better than the VAS (53% and 26% respectively; $p < 0.01$). NRS might be more appropriate to use in the ED
Edelen MO, et al. 2010 [83]	1960 elderly residents from 71 nursing homes	B	L	To compare VDS and NRS using item response theory (IRT) methods to identify the correspondence between the scales' response options by estimating item parameters for these and five additional pain items	The sample reported moderate amounts of pain on average. Examination of the IRT location parameters for the pain intensity items indicated the following approximate correspondence: VDS mild ≈ NRS 1–4, VDS moderate ≈ NRS 5–7, VDS severe ≈ NRS 8–9, and VDS very severe, horrible ≈ NRS 10	Either scale (VDS or NRS) can be used in practice depending on the preference of the clinician and the respondent
Pratici E, et al. 2017 [84]	97 women in labor	C	H	To determine the level of agreement between the calculated percentage pain reduction, derived from VAS or NRS, and patient-reported % pain reduction in patients having epidural analgesia	There was moderate agreement between the calculated percentage pain reduction from a VAS or NRS and patient-reported % pain reduction in epidural analgesia. The difference could range up to 30%	The concordance correlation coefficients with patient-reported percentage pain reduction were 0.76 and 0.77 for the VAS and NRS, respectively
Gagliese L, et al. 2005 [85]	504 postoperative adults	B	L	To compare the feasibility and validity of the NRS, VDS, and VAS (horizontal and vertical line orientation) for the assessment of pain intensity in younger and older surgical patients	Psychometric analyses suggested that the NRS was the preferred pain intensity scale. The VDS also had a favorable profile with low error rates and good face, convergent, and criterion validity	Difficulties with VAS use among the elderly were identified, including high rates of unscorable data and low face validity
Bijur PE, et al. 2003 [86]	108 adult ED patients	C	H	To assess the comparability of the NRS and VAS as measures of acute pain and identify the minimum clinically significant difference in pain that could be detected on the NRS	NRS scores were strongly correlated to VAS scores at all time periods ($r = 0.94$). The slope of the regression line was 1.01, and the y-intercept was −0.34	The verbally administered NRS can be substituted for the VAS in acute pain measurement

(continued)

Table 3.4 (continued)

Investigator(s), title, date, and Ref. #	Sample size and population	Quality of evidence (GRADE)[a]	Risk of bias[b]	Objectives	Findings	Notes and conclusions
Herr K, et al. 2007 [39]	97 adults with chronic joint pain	B	L	To compare the sensitivity and utility of the new IPT with four other pain scales: NRS, VNS, FPS, and VAS, using a naturally occurring pain condition and a controlled treatment with rheumatology patients	The IPT showed the lowest failure rate of all pain scales evaluated. Other scale failure rates were relatively low, except for the VNS and the VAS. No significant difference was noted in scale failure by age, gender, or education level, but cognitive impairment was significantly related to failure on the VAS and the NRS	All five pain scales were sensitive in detecting changes in pain intensity pre– and post–joint injection. All correlations between the scales were strong and significant; however, the intercorrelations for the older cohort were weaker. The scale most preferred in both cohorts of patients was the IPT, followed by the FPS
Taylor LJ, et al. 2005 [87]	66 cognitively impaired elderly	B	L	To determine the reliability and validity of selected pain intensity scales, such as the FPS, VDS, NRS, and the Iowa Pain Thermometer (IPT), to assess pain in cognitively impaired older adults	Concurrent validity of the VDS, NRS, and IPT was supported with Spearman's rank correlation coefficients ranging from 0.78 to 0.86 in the cognitively impaired group. The FPS, however, demonstrated weak correlations with other scales when used with the impaired group, ranging from 0.48 to 0.53. In the cognitively intact group, strong correlations ranging from 0.96 to 0.97 were found among all of the scales	When asked about scale preference, both the cognitively impaired and the intact groups preferred the IPT and the VDS. This study revealed that cognitive impairment did not inhibit participants' ability to use a variety of pain intensity scales, but the stability issue must be considered
Li L, et al. 2007 [88]	173 postoperative adults	B	U	To determine the psychometric properties and applicability of four pain scales in Chinese postoperative adults	All four pain intensity scales had good reliability and validity when used with Chinese adults. The intra-class correlation coefficients (ICCs) of the four scales across current, worst, least, and average pain on each postoperative day were consistently high (0.673–0.825), and all scales at each rating were strongly correlated ($r = 0.71–0.99$). Both the VDS and the FPS-R had low error rates. Nearly half of the participants (48.1%) preferred the FPS-R, followed by the NRS (24.4%), the VDS (23.1%), and the VAS (4.4%)	Although all four scales can be options for Chinese adults to report pain intensity, the FPS-R appears to be the best one. No significant differences were noted in terms of gender, age, or educational level
Li L, et al. 2009 [89]	180 postoperative elderly	B	U	To evaluate the reliability and validity of the FPS-R, NRS, and the Iowa Pain Thermometer (IPT) for pain assessment in Chinese elders who have had surgery	The intra-class correlation coefficients across current, worst, and least pain on each postoperative day were consistently high (0.949–0.965), and all scales at each rating were strongly correlated ($r = 0.833–0.962$). The scale mostly preferred was the IPT (54.7%), followed by the FPS-R (28.5%) and the NRS (15.6%). No significant differences were noted in participant preference by age or cognitive status, but preference for the IPT and the FPS-R were significantly related to gender and education level	Although all three scales show good reliability, validity, and sensitivity for assessing postoperative pain intensity in Chinese elders, the IPT appears to be a better choice based on patient preference

(continued)

Table 3.4 (continued)

Investigator(s), title, date, and Ref. #	Sample size and population	Quality of evidence (GRADE)[a]	Risk of bias[b]	Objectives	Findings	Notes and conclusions
Ismail AK, et al. 2015 [90]	133 ambulance patients	B	H	To evaluate the agreement between verbal NRS and VAS in measuring acute pain in the prehospital setting and identify the preference among paramedics and patients	VAS performs as well as VNRS in assessing acute pain in the prehospital setting. VAS and VNRS must not be used interchangeably to assess acute pain; either method should be used consistently	There was a strong correlation between VNRS and VAS at the scene ($r = 0.865$; $p < 0.001$), as well as on arrival at the hospital ($r = 0.933$; $p < 0.001$). Kappa values and analysis indicate good agreement between both scales for measuring acute pain
Akinpelu AO, et al. 2002 [91]	35 women with caesarean section	C	H	To evaluate the correlation of pain scores obtained on the VAS, the Box Numerical Scale (BNS), and the Verbal Rating Scale (VRS)	There was no significant difference between the pain scores obtained on the three pain rating scales. Significant correlations existed between pain scores obtained on the VAS and VRS ($r = 0.48$, $p = 0.003$); VAS and BNS ($r = 0.74$, $P = 0.000$); and BNS and VRS ($r = 0.74$, $P = 0.000$)	The three pain rating scales measure the same construct and could be used for pain measurement in obstetrically related conditions in this environment

Abbreviations: *FPS* FACES Pain Scale, *VAS* Visual Analog Scale, *NRS* Numeric Rating Scale, *VDS* Verbal Descriptor Scale, *TPS* Thermometer Pain Scale, *MPQ* McGill Pain Questionnaire, *SF-MPQ* Short-form McGill Pain Questionnaire, *BPI* Brief Pain Inventory

[a]Quality of evidence and definitions

(GRADE system) (GGHO)

Grade A: High level of evidence (The true effect lies close to our estimate of the effect)

Grade B: Moderate level of evidence (The true effect is likely to be close to our estimate of the effect, but there is a possibility that it is substantially different)

Grade C: Low level of evidence (The true effect may be substantially different from our estimate of the effect)

Grade D: Very low level of evidence (Our estimate of the effect is just a guess, and it is very likely that the true effect is substantially different from our estimate of the effect)

[b]Risk of bias: Studies were assessed for bias using the risk of bias criteria developed by Cochrane [22], which is based upon Cochrane's Risk of Bias Tool [23]. Studies were assessed with regard to selection bias, performance bias, detection bias, attrition bias, reporting bias, and other sources of bias. Studies were rated as "low risk of bias (L)," "high risk of bias (H)," or "unclear risk of bias (U)" on a general impression after evaluating all criteria

One of the first reviews on comparison of the three pain scales (VAS, VRS, and NRS) demonstrated that all three scales were valid, reliable, and appropriate for use, although the VAS had more practical difficulties than the others [92]. For general purposes, the NRS has good sensitivity and produces data that can be analyzed for audit purposes. Likewise, in a systematic review, authors investigated the use and performance of unidimensional pain scales and demonstrated that when compared with the VAS and VRS, NRS had better compliance in 15 of 19 studies reporting this and was the recommended tool in 11 studies [77]. Another recent study based on VAS and the Wong–Baker Faces Pain Rating Scale recorded the self-pain perception experienced by patients after a mini-implant placement [93]. The authors concluded that the maximum pain was recorded in the case of a palatal miniscrew (Table 3.5).

Geriatric Considerations

Advancing age increases the risk of persistent pain in the elderly due to multiple comorbidities and restricted physiological reserves. Around a decade ago, abdominal pain and fractures were found to be among the most common complaints prompting the elderly to present to the ED [94]. On the other hand, chronic diseases, acute injuries, and cancer contribute to the increasing prevalence of these referrals in the elderly. Therefore, assessment of both persistent and acute pain is an important part of preventative and palliative healthcare in this group [95].

Considerable difficulty was remarkable in some research with regard to the practical use of VAS, especially in older adults and disadvantaged populations. Yazici et al. reported that while the NRS, TPS, FPS, and VDS were used as practi-

Table 3.5 Comparisons between pain assessment tools

Name of the scale/tool	Ease of application	Pros and cons	Additional notes
Visual Analog Scale (VAS)	Easy	Needs the use of a pen and paper, no need for literacy	Practical to some extent
Numeric Rating Scale (NRS)	Easy	No need for the use of pen and paper, illiterate people can also verbalize numbers	Practical for illiterate and those with communication difficulties
Verbal Descriptor Scale (VDS)	Easy	The physician should have some time to explain the descriptors	Practical to some extent
The FACES Pain Scale (FPS)	Easy		Practical, especially for children, the illiterate, and those with communication difficulties
Thermometer Pain Scale (TPS)	Easy	No need for the use of pen and paper, illiterate people can also verbalize numbers	Practical for the illiterate and those with communication difficulties
McGill pain questionnaire (MPQ)	Difficult	Provides detailed information on both the quality and quantity of pain	The completion of the questionnaire can take a long time. May be cumbersome for the ED environment
Short-form McGill pain questionnaire (SF-MPQ)	Difficult		It can assess the major symptoms of both neuropathic and nonneuropathic pain
Brief pain Inventory (BPI)	Difficult	Designed to be used for adults, adaptable to computer use	Not validated for all pain conditions

Abbreviations: *FPS* FACES Pain Scale, *VAS* Visual Analog Scale, *NRS* Numeric Rating Scale, *VDS* Verbal Descriptor Scale, *TPS* Thermometer Pain Scale, *MPQ* McGill Pain Questionnaire, *SFMPQ* Short-form McGill Pain Questionnaire, *BPI* Brief Pain Inventory

cal pain rating tools, the VAS should be used in combination with one of these scales [79].

Quality of Life (QoL) as an Outcome Measure in the Elderly

In a recently published systematic review, Iking et al. analyzed the role of quality-of-life (QoL) assessments in elderly patients with proximal humeral fracture (PHF) [96]. They included studies describing the QoL or the level of pain of the patients with the EuroQoL-5 Dimension (EQ-5D) score or the VAS after the treatment of PHF, either nonoperatively (non-OP), with open-reduction and internal fixation using a Locking plate fixation (LPF), or with reverse total shoulder arthroplasty (RTSA). Although the mean VAS score across a great number of studies demonstrated a decreasing trend for all interventions, there are no clinically important differences between the QoL or pain in elderly patients with PHF after nonoperative treatment or surgical treatment with LPF or RTSA. On the other hand, the number of studies and level of evidence are rather low, and more advanced studies are necessary.

Patient-Reported Outcome Measures (PROMs) in the Management of Patients with Pain

Studies involving musculoskeletal procedures and conditions commonly employ *outcome measures related to* pain (e.g., functionality, patient satisfaction, QoL, and death rate) and individual and psychological symptoms (e.g., patient expectations, depression, anxiety, mental health, physiological stress, self-efficacy, coping, vitality, and emotion). *PROMs, on the other hand*, is the term to describe the information directly from the patient that can help clinicians and researchers understand the impact of disease, treatment, and health status directly as the patient perceives it [97]. PROMs are used to evaluate any given patient's health status at a point in time [98]. PROMs tools can be completed either during an illness or while treating a health condition. Some national bodies launched PROMs initiatives, including the Medical Outcomes Study (MOS), which paved the way to the development of the Short-Form-36 (SF-36) health survey. PROMs were developed for many different procedures and conditions. For example, these are used for joint replacement procedures since pain relief and improved function, among other aspects of health-related QoL, are primary objectives of a joint replacement surgery [99, 100].

In a recent analysis of the studies involving PROMs in patients presenting with neck pain to physical therapy, Ramirez et al. reported that many PROMs are used to evaluate the constructs of disability, pain intensity, psychosocial factors, and QoL [101]. The most frequently utilized PROMs were the Neck Disability Index (NDI), VAS, and NRS, while the most commonly used measures assessing the constructs of disability, pain intensity, QoL, and psychosocial functioning comprised the NDI, VAS, Short-Form-36 health survey, and Fear Avoidance Belief Questionnaire, respectively. The use of the NDI and the NRS or VAS was recommended to assess pain. The authors also noted that further research was necessary to recommend a QoL and psychosocial measure for patients presenting with neck pain.

Cross-Cultural and Sociodemographic Differences in Pain Assessment

Some research has suggested that *female patients* were often not asked about pain [102].

In 1995, Raftery et al. pointed out that women reported the severity of pain more commonly than men did and therefore received more pain medications [103]. Thus, the painful experience is a unique case for each individual, which warrants the use of different tools for assessment in routine practice. Of note, abnormalities in vital signs take priority over most interventions; for instance, patients with hypoxia and hypotension were less likely to be asked about their pain. Recent research provided substantial information abstracted from technological innovations in the evaluation and records of painful experience. An observational trial was performed using smartphones and tablets to score expressions in evaluations of fatigue, pain, anxiety, and QoL on an electronic VAS (eVAS) [104]. eVAS is reported to be a reliable and useful tool for people with multiple sclerosis to register their complaints.

A pilot study was performed on the tablet computer–based automated pain tracker (APT) to evaluate patient and nurse satisfaction with the device [105]. All patients reported that the APT was practical and easy to use, and a majority of them (93%) thought the APT should be used more frequently in the acute setting. The authors concluded that the iPad pain-tracking and reporting system provided higher patient satisfaction, improved pain care, operational efficiency, and better documentation of pain evaluation and management.

Key Themes

- Pain cannot be treated if it is not assessed. Correct and timely evaluation of pain and discomfort is the prerequisite to relieving suffering.
- Pain is a multifaceted and subjective experience; thus, it is difficult to measure. Assessment of pain encompasses a multifaceted analysis of different aspects—sensorial, psychological, and experiential—in an objective way.
- Clinicians should assess their patients' pain levels, regardless of the method or scale. The patient's self-report is the most accurate and reliable evidence of the existence of pain and its intensity.
- Pain should be assessed regularly and accurately to improve acute pain management.
- NRS and VAS are recommended to assess adults and children who can express their pain verbally.
- Each rating scale has pluses and minuses in practice. Research findings emphasize that most pain-rating scales are valid, reliable, and appropriate for use in the acute setting, while the VAS is more difficult for daily usage than the others.
- Special patient groups, including the elderly, minorities, and the cognitively impaired, have special needs in expressing their pain intensities. VDS and VRS have been found to be easier to use than others in rating pain levels. Pain in nonverbal adults and young children can be assessed via observational scales, including the Wong–Baker FACES scale, FLACC, and CRIES.
- Outcome assessments include validated and reliable measures as self-reports by patients in their own languages.

Conclusions

"Pain cannot be treated if it cannot be assessed." The most important principle is that clinicians should somehow assess their patients' pain levels, no matter which method or scale one uses to accomplish this task. The bulk of evidence published to date has demonstrated a gap for improvement to indicate pluses and minuses of each rating scale used for acute pain. The patient's self-report is the most accurate and reliable evidence of the existence of pain and its intensity in patients of all ages, irrespective of communication or cognitive deficits.

Pain is often underassessed, which may lead to inadequate management in the acute setting, including the prehospital setting. Timely evaluation of pain is not undertaken in almost one-half of cases, and when pain assessment is performed, many patients reporting moderate-to-severe pain do not receive analgesia. Barriers to adequate assessment and management of pain are multifactorial. These shortcomings include a lack of knowledge and training, reluctance to give opioids, and concerns about drug-seeking behavior or abuse. Choosing the most appropriate instrument for recording self-reported pain is not straightforward. Reports focus that although all pain-rating scales are valid, reliable, and appropriate for use in the ED and other acute settings, the VAS has somehow appeared to be more difficult than the others. Due to practical reasons, verbal descriptors or rating scales can be more useful to express the pain and discomfort of elderly patients, those with cognitive impairment and communication problems, children and minorities. Studies are going on in the field of pain management in acute illness and injury, and the usability of each tool should be studied on specific populations before reaching firm conclusions. PROMs are beneficial in the clinical setting to describe the impact of disease, treatment, and health status directly as the patient perceives it. Healthcare providers should adjust the pain management practices to improve PROMs to optimize the quality of life and other relevant outcomes at the individual and societal levels.

References

1. Li SF, Greenwald PW, Gennis P, Bijur PE, Gallagher EJ. Effect of age on acute pain perception of a standardized stimulus in the emergency department. Ann Emerg Med. 2001;38(6):644–7.
2. IASP Task Force on Taxonomy. Part III: pain terms, a current list with definitions and notes on usage. In: Merskey H, Bogduk N, editors. Classification of Chronic Pain. 2nd ed. Seattle: IASP Press; 1994. p. 209–14.
3. Lanser P, Gesell S. Pain management: the fifth vital sign. Healthc Benchmarks. 2001;8(6):68–70. PMID: 11474948.
4. Pain as the 5th vital sign toolkit. 2000. http://www.va.gov/pain-management/docs/toolkit.pdf. Accessed 11 Mar 2025.
5. American Pain Society. Principles of analgesic use in the treatment of acute pain and cancer pain. American Pain Society; 1999.
6. Lozner AW, Reisner A, Shear ML, et al. Pain severity is the key to emergency department patients' preferred frequency of pain assessment. Eur J Emerg Med. 2010;17(1):30–2.
7. The European Society for Emergency Medicine (EUSEM). Guidelines for the management of acute pain in emergency situations. 2020. Belgium www.eusem.org, URL: https://www.eusem.org/images/EUSEM_EPI_GUIDELINES_MARCH_2020.pdf.
8. Grant PS. Analgesia delivery in the ED. Am J Emerg Med. 2006;24(7):806–9.
9. Management of Pain in Adults. The Royal College of emergency medicine best practice guideline. London; 2021.
10. Mears L, Mears J. The pathophysiology, assessment, and management of acute pain. Br J Nurs. 2023;32(2):58–65. https://doi.org/10.12968/bjon.2023.32.2.58.
11. Becker J, Effraim PR, Dib-Hajj S, Rittner HL. Lessons learned in translating pain knowledge into practice. Pain Rep. 2023;8(6):e1100. https://doi.org/10.1097/PR9.0000000000001100.
12. Macintyre PE, Schug SA. Acute pain management, a practical guide. 5th ed. CRC Press; 2021. https://doi.org/10.1201/9780429295058.
13. Costigan M, Scholz J, Woolf CJ. Neuropathic pain: a maladaptive response of the nervous system to damage. Annu Rev Neurosci. 2009;32:1–32. https://doi.org/10.1146/annurev.neuro.051508.135531.
14. Fitzcharles MA, Cohen SP, Clauw DJ, Littlejohn G, Usui C, Häuser W. Nociplastic pain: towards an understanding of prevalent pain conditions. Lancet. 2021;397(10289):2098–110. https://doi.org/10.1016/S0140-6736(21)00392-5.
15. Freynhagen R, Parada HA, Calderon-Ospina CA, et al. Current understanding of the mixed pain concept: a brief narrative review. Curr Med Res Opin. 2019;35(6):1011–8. https://doi.org/10.1080/03007995.2018.1552042.
16. Schug SA, et al. Acute pain management: scientific evidence. 4th ed. Australian and New Zealand College of Anaesthetists and Faculty of Pain Medicine; 2015.
17. Agency for Health Care Policy and Research, Acute Pain Management Guideline Panel. Acute pain management: operative or medical procedures and trauma. In: Clinical practice guidelines. Rockville: U.S. Department of Health and Human Services; 1992.
18. Perry S, Heidrich G. Management of pain during debridement: a survey of US burn units. Pain. 1982;13(3):276–80.
19. Miner JR, Burton JH. Pain management. In: Walls R, Hockberger R, Gausche-Hill M, editors. Rosen's emergency medicine - concepts and clinical practice. 9th ed. Elsevier Canada. p. 34–51. Copyright 2018.
20. Crisman E, Appenzeller-Herzog C, Tabakovic S, Nickel CH, Minotti B. Multidimensional versus unidimensional pain scales for the assessment of analgesic requirement in the emergency department: a systematic review. Intern Emerg Med. 2024;19(5):1463–71. https://doi.org/10.1007/s11739-024-03608-5. Epub 2024 Apr 25. PMID: 38664325; PMCID: PMC11364591.
21. Ducharme J. Introduction and general approach to pain. In: Thomas SH, editor. Emergency department analgesia: an evidence based guide. Cambridge, UK: Cambridge University Press; 2008. p. 3–9.
22. Kelly AM. The minimum clinically significant difference in visual analogue scale pain score does not differ with severity of pain. Emerg Med J. 2001;18(3):205–7.
23. Jensen MP, Karoly P, Braver S. The measurement of clinical pain intensity: a comparison of six methods. Pain. 1986;27:117–26.
24. Hawker GA, Mian S, Kendzerska T, French M. Measures of adult pain: visual analog scale for pain (VAS pain), numeric rating scale for pain (NRS pain), McGill pain questionnaire (MPQ), short-form McGill pain questionnaire (SF-MPQ), chronic pain Grade scale (CPGS), short Form-36 bodily pain scale (SF-36 BPS), and measure of intermittent and constant osteoarthritis pain (ICOAP). Arthritis Care Res (Hoboken). 2011; 63(Suppl 11):S240–52.
25. Gallagher EJ, Liebman M, Bijur PE. Prospective validation of clinically important changes in pain severity measured on a visual analog scale. Ann Emerg Med. 2001;38(6):633–8.
26. Moutte SD, Brudvik C, Morken T. Physicians' use of pain scale and treatment procedures among children and youth in emergency primary care - a cross sectional study. BMC Emerg Med. 2015;15:33.
27. Olsen BF, Rustøen T, Sandvik L, Jacobsen M, Valeberg BT. Results of implementing a pain management algorithm in intensive care unit patients: the impact on pain assessment, length of stay, and duration of ventilation. J Crit Care. 2016;36:207–11.
28. Marco CA, Marco AP. Assessment of pain. In: Thomas SH, editor. Emergency department analgesia: an evidence based guide. Cambridge, UK: Cambridge University Press; 2008. p. 10–8.
29. McLean SA, Domeier RM, DeVore HK, Hill EM, Maio RF, Frederiksen SM. The feasibility of pain assessment in the prehospital setting. Prehosp Emerg Care. 2004;8(2):155–61.
30. Langley GB, Sheppeard H. The visual analogue scale: its use in pain measurement. Rheumatol Int. 1985;5:145–8.
31. Ware LJ, Epps CD, Herr K, Packard A. Evaluation of the revised faces pain scale, verbal descriptor scale, numeric rating scale, and Iowa pain thermometer in older minority adults. Pain Manag Nurs. 2006;7(3):117–25. https://doi.org/10.1016/j.pmn.2006.06.005. PMID: 16931417.
32. Karcioglu O, Topacoglu H, Dikme O, Dikme O. A systematic review of the pain scales in adults: which to use? Am J Emerg Med. 2018;36(4):707–14.
33. von Baeyer CL. Children's self-reports of pain intensity: scale selection, limitations and interpretation. Pain Res Manag. 2006;11(3):157–62.
34. Oldenmenger WH, van der Rijt CC. Feasibility of assessing patients' acceptable pain in a randomized controlled trial on a patient pain education program. Palliat Med. 2017;31(6):553–8.
35. Goulet JL, Brandt C, Crystal S, Fiellin DA, Gibert C, Gordon AJ, et al. Agreement between electronic medical record-based and self-administered pain numeric rating scale. Med Care. 2013;51(3):245–50.
36. Pines JM, Hollander JE. Emergency department crowding is associated with poor care for patients with severe pain. Ann Emerg Med. 2007;51(1):1–5.
37. Gracely RH, McGrath P, Dubner R. Ratio scales of sensory and affective verbal pain descriptors. Pain. 1978;5:5–18.
38. Ferraz MD, Quaresma MR, Aquino LRL, et al. Raliability of pain scales in the assessment of literate and illiterate patients with rheumatoid arthritis. J Rheumatol. 1990;17:1022–4.
39. Herr K, Spratt KF, Garand L, Li L. Evaluation of the Iowa pain thermometer and other selected pain intensity scales in younger

and older adult cohorts using controlled clinical pain: a preliminary study. Pain Med. 2007;8:585–600.
40. Hicks CL, von Baeyer CL, Spafford P, van Korlaar I, Goodenough B. The Faces Pain Scale - revised: toward a common metric in pediatric pain measurement. Pain. 2001;93(2):173–83.
41. Bieri D, Reeve R, Champion GD, Addicoat L, Ziegler J. The Faces Pain Scale for the self-assessment of the severity of pain experienced by children: development, initial validation and preliminary investigation for ratio scale properties. Pain. 1990;41(2):139–50.
42. McGrath PJ, Walco G, Turk DC, et al. Core outcome domains and measures for pediatric acute and chronic/recurrent pain clinical trials: PedIMMPACT recommendations. J Pain. 2008;9:771–83.
43. Pasero C, McCaffery M. No self-report means no pain-intensity rating. Am J Nurs. 2005;105(10):50–3.
44. Payen JF, Bru O, Bosson JL, et al. Assessing pain in critically ill sedated patients by using a behavioral pain scale. Crit Care Med. 2001;29(12):2258–63.
45. Cleeland CS, Ryan KM. Pain assessment: global use of the brief pain inventory. Ann Acad Med. 1994;23(2):129–38.
46. Migliorini F, Maffulli N, Eschweiler J, Baroncini A, Bell A, Colarossi G. Duloxetine for fibromyalgia syndrome: a systematic review and meta-analysis. J Orthop Surg Res. 2023;18(1):504. https://doi.org/10.1186/s13018-023-03995-z.
47. The University of Texas MD Anderson Cancer Center. The brief pain inventory. https://www.mdanderson.org/research/departments-labs-institutes/departments-divisions/symptom-research/symptom-assessment-tools/brief-pain-inventory.html.
48. Roland Morris Disability Questionnaire (RMDQ). URL: http://www.rmdq.org/.
49. Kerns RD, Turk DC, Rudy TE. The West Haven-Yale Multidimensional Pain Inventory (WHYMPI). Pain. 1985;23:345–56.
50. Fairbank JC, Couper J, Davies JB, O'Brien JP. The Oswestry low back pain disability questionnaire. Physiotherapy. 1980;66:271–3.
51. Tait RC, Chibnall JT, Krause S. The pain disability index: psychometric properties. Pain. 1990;40:171–82.
52. Vernon H, Mior S. The neck disability index: a study of reliability and validity. J Manipulative Physiol Ther. 1991;14:409–15.
53. IASP. International Association for the Study of Pain Multidisciplinary Pain Center Development Manual. IASP Multidisciplinary Pain Center Toolkit Advisory Group; 2021. URL: www.iasp-pain.org/MPCManual. Accessed: 02 Feb 2024.
54. Keawnantawat P, Thanasilp S, Preechawong S. Translation and validation of the Thai version of a modified brief pain inventory: a concise instrument for pain assessment in postoperative cardiac surgery. Pain Pract. 2017;17(6):763–73.
55. Cleeland CS. The Brief Pain Inventory User Guide; 2009. URL: https://www.mdanderson.org/documents/Departments-and-Divisions/Symptom-Research/BPI_UserGuide.pdf.
56. Tyler EJ, Jensen MP, Engel JM, Schwartz L. The reliability and validity of pain interference measures in persons with cerebral palsy. Arch Phys Med Rehabil. 2002;83(2):236–9.
57. Jensen MP, Ehde DM, Hoffman AJ, et al. Cognitions, coping and social environment predict adjustment to phantom limb pain. Pain. 2002;95(1–2):133–42.
58. Lapane KL, Quilliam BJ, Benson C, Chow W, Kim M. One, two, or three? Constructs of the brief pain inventory among patients with noncancer pain in the outpatient setting. J Pain Symptom Manag. 2014;47(2):325–33.
59. Serlin RC, Mendoza TR, Nakamura Y, Edwards KR, Cleeland CS. When is cancer pain mild, moderate or severe? Grading pain severity by its interference with function. Pain. 1995;61(2):277–84.
60. Radbruch L, Loick G, Kiencke P, et al. Validation of the German version of the brief pain inventory. J Pain Symptom Manag. 1999;18(3):180–7.
61. Bird SB, Dickson EW. Clinically significant changes in pain along the visual analog scale. Ann Emerg Med. 2001;38(6):639–43.
62. Todd KH, Funk KG, Funk JP, Bonacci R. Clinical significance of reported changes in pain severity. Ann Emerg Med. 1996;27(4):485–9.
63. Gallagher EJ, Bijur PE, Latimer C, Silver W. Reliability and validity of a visual analog scale for acute abdominal pain in the emergency department. Am J Emerg Med. 2002;20(4):287–90.
64. Degerli V, Karcioglu O, Larkin GL, Karaduman S, Korkmaz T, et al. The minimum clinically significant difference in acute nontraumatic thoracoabdominal pain in adult emergency department patients in Turkey. Hong Kong J Emerg Med. 2012;19(3):171–6.
65. Kamper SJ, Maher CG, Mackay G. Global rating of change scales: a review of strengths and weaknesses and considerations for design. J Man Manip Ther. 2009;17(3):163–70. https://doi.org/10.1179/jmt.2009.17.3.163.
66. Kamper SJ, Ostelo RW, Knol DL, Maher CG, de Vet HC, Hancock MJ. Global Perceived Effect scales provided reliable assessments of health transition in people with musculoskeletal disorders, but ratings are strongly influenced by current status. J Clin Epidemiol. 2010;63(7):760–766.e1. https://doi.org/10.1016/j.jclinepi.2009.09.009.
67. Duncan GH, Bushnell CM, Lavigne GJ. Comparison of verbal and visual analogue scales for measuring the intensity and unpleasantness of experimental pain. Pain. 1989;37:295–303.
68. Katz J, Melzack R. The McGill pain questionnaire: development, psychometric properties, and usefulness of the long form, short form, and short form-2. In: Turk DC, Melzack R, editors. Handbook of pain assessment. New York: The Guilford Press; 2011. p. 45–66.
69. Consuelo VM, Chiara F, Francesca SM, Patrizia D, Andrea S. The use of questionnaires in pain assessment during orthodontic treatments: a narrative review. Medicina (Kaunas). 2023;59(9):1681. https://doi.org/10.3390/medicina59091681.
70. Melzack R, Katz J. The McGill pain questionnaire: appraisal and current status. In: Turk DC, Melzack R, editors. Handbook of pain assessment. New York: Guilford Press; 1990. p. 152–68.
71. Shroff R, Dabholakar T. Mc gill pain questionnaire: a cross-cultural adaptation study in chronic neck pain. Int J Theor Phys. 2019;10:19–23.
72. Dworkin RH, Turk DC, Trudeau JJ, et al. Validation of the short-form McGill pain Questionnaire-2 (SF-MPQ-2) in acute low back pain. J Pain. 2015;16(4):357–66. https://doi.org/10.1016/j.jpain.2015.01.012.
73. Salaffi F, Ciapetti A, Carotti M. Pain assessment strategies in patients with musculoskeletal conditions. Reumatismo. 2012;64(4):216–29. https://doi.org/10.4081/reumatismo.2012.216.
74. Herr K, Titler M. Acute pain assessment and pharmacological management practices for the older adult with a hip fracture: a review of ED trends. J Emerg Nurs. 2009;35(4):312–20.
75. Hadjistavropoulos T, Fitzgerald TD, Marchildon GP. Practice guidelines for assessing pain in older persons with dementia residing in long-term care facilities. Physiother Can. 2010;62:104–13.
76. Leigheb M, Sabbatini M, Baldrighi M, Hasenboehler EA, Briacca L, Grassi F, et al. Prospective analysis of pain and pain management in an emergency department. Acta Biomed. 2017;88(Suppl 4):19–30.
77. Hjermstad MJ, Fayers PM, Haugen DF, et al. European palliative care research collaborative (EPCRC). Studies comparing numerical rating scales, verbal rating scales, and visual analogue scales for assessment of pain intensity in adults: a systematic literature review. J Pain Symptom Manag. 2011;41(6):1073–93
78. Pereira LV, Pereira Gde A, Moura LA, Fernandes RR. Pain intensity among institutionalized elderly: a comparison between

numerical scales and verbal descriptors. Rev Esc Enferm USP. 2015;49(5):804–10.

79. Yazici Sayin Y, Akyolcu N. Comparison of pain scale preferences and pain intensity according to pain scales among Turkish patients: a descriptive study. Pain Manag Nurs. 2014;15(1):156–64.
80. Bahreini M, Jalili M, Moradi-Lakeh M. A comparison of three self-report pain scales in adults with acute pain. J Emerg Med. 2015;48(1):10–8. https://doi.org/10.1016/j.jemermed.2014.07.039.
81. Aziato L, Dedey F, Marfo K, Asamani JA, Clegg-Lamptey JN. Validation of three pain scales among adult postoperative patients in Ghana. BMC Nurs. 2015;14:42. https://doi.org/10.1186/s12912-015-0094-6.
82. Göransson KE, Heilborn U, Selberg J, von Scheele S, Djärv T. Pain rating in the ED-a comparison between 2 scales in a Swedish hospital. Am J Emerg Med. 2015;33(3):419–22. https://doi.org/10.1016/j.ajem.2014.12.069.
83. Edelen MO, Saliba D. Correspondence of verbal descriptor and numeric rating scales for pain intensity: an item response theory calibration. J Gerontol A Biol Sci Med Sci. 2010;65(7):778–85. https://doi.org/10.1093/gerona/glp215.
84. Pratici E, Nebout S, Merbai N, Filippova J, Hajage D, Keita H. An observational study of agreement between percentage pain reduction calculated from visual analog or numerical rating scales versus that reported by parturients during labor epidural analgesia. Int J Obstet Anesth. 2017;30:39–43. https://doi.org/10.1016/j.ijoa.2017.02.001.
85. Gagliese L, Weizblit N, Ellis W, Chan VWS. The measurement of postoperative pain: a comparison of intensity scales in younger and older surgical patients. Pain. 2005;117(3):412–20. https://doi.org/10.1016/j.pain.2005.07.004.
86. Bijur PE, Latimer CT, Gallagher EJ. Validation of a verbally administered numerical rating scale of acute pain for use in the emergency department. Acad Emerg Med. 2003;10(4):390–2. https://doi.org/10.1111/j.1553-2712.2003.tb01355.x.
87. Taylor LJ, Harris J, Epps CD, Herr K. Psychometric evaluation of selected pain intensity scales for use with cognitively impaired and cognitively intact older adults. Rehabil Nurs. 2005;30(2):55–61. https://doi.org/10.1002/j.2048-7940.2005.tb00360.x.
88. Li L, Liu X, Herr K. Postoperative pain intensity assessment: a comparison of four scales in Chinese adults. Pain Med. 2007;8(3):223–34. https://doi.org/10.1111/j.1526-4637.2007.00296.x.
89. Li L, Herr K, Chen P. Postoperative pain assessment with three intensity scales in Chinese elders. J Nurs Scholarsh. 2009;41(3):241–9. https://doi.org/10.1111/j.1547-5069.2009.01280.x.
90. Ismail AK, Abdul Ghafar MA, Shamsuddin NS, Roslan NA, Kaharuddin H, Nik Muhamad NA. The assessment of acute pain in pre-hospital care using verbal numerical rating and visual analogue scales. J Emerg Med. 2015;49(3):287–93. https://doi.org/10.1016/j.jemermed.2015.02.043.
91. Akinpelu AO, Olowe OO. Correlative study of 3 pain rating scales among obstetric patients. Afr J Med Med Sci. 2002;31(2):123–6.
92. Williamson A, Hoggart B. Pain: a review of three commonly used pain rating scales. J Clin Nurs. 2005;14(7):798–804.
93. Sreenivasagan S, Subramanian AK, Selvaraj A, Marya A. Pain perception associated with mini-implants and interventions for pain management: a cross-sectional questionnaire-based survey. Biomed Res Int. 2021;29:4842865.
94. Hwang U, Belland LK, Handel DA, et al. Is all pain treated equally? A multicenter evaluation of acute pain care by age. Pain. 2014;155(12):2568–74.
95. Booker SQ, Herr KA. Assessment and measurement of pain in adults in later life. Clin Geriatr Med. 2016;32(4):677–92. https://doi.org/10.1016/j.cger.2016.06.012.
96. Iking J, Fischhuber K, Stolberg-Stolberg J, Raschke MJ, Katthagen JC, Köppe J. Quality of life and pain after proximal humeral fractures in the elderly: a systematic review. Medicina (Kaunas). 2023;59(10):1728. https://doi.org/10.3390/medicina59101728.
97. Weinfurt KP, Reeve BB. Patient-reported outcome measures in clinical research. JAMA. 2022;328:472–3.
98. Canadian Institute for Health Information (CIHI). PROMs Background Document. URL: https://www.cihi.ca/sites/default/files/proms_background_may21_en-web_0.pdf.
99. Rolfson O, Kärrholm J, Dahlberg LE, Garellick G. Patient-reported outcomes in the Swedish Hip Arthroplasty Register: results of a nationwide prospective observational study. J Bone Joint Surg Br. 2011;93(7):867–75. https://doi.org/10.1302/0301-620X.93B7.25737.
100. Peters RM, van Steenbergen LN, Stewart RE, Stevens M, Rijk PC, Bulstra SK, Zijlstra WP. Which patients improve most after total hip arthroplasty? Influence of patient characteristics on patient-reported outcome measures of 22,357 total hip arthroplasties in the Dutch Arthroplasty Register. Hip Int. 2021;31(5):593–602. https://doi.org/10.1177/1120700020913208.
101. Ramirez MM, Shepherd MH, Melnick SJ, et al. Patient-reported outcome measures in physical therapy practice for neck pain: an overview of reviews. J Patient Rep Outcomes. 2023;7(1):97. https://doi.org/10.1186/s41687-023-00637-0.
102. Dale J, Bjørnsen LP. Assessment of pain in a Norwegian emergency department. Scand J Trauma Resusc Emerg Med. 2015;23:86.
103. Raftery KA, Smith-Coggins R, Chen AH. Gender-associated differences in emergency department pain management. Ann Emerg Med. 1995;26(4):414–21. https://doi.org/10.1016/s0196-0644(95)70107-9.
104. Kos D, Raeymaekers J, Van Remoortel A, et al. Electronic visual analogue scales for pain, fatigue, anxiety and quality of life in people with multiple sclerosis using smartphone and tablet: a reliability and feasibility study. Clin Rehabil. 2017;31(9):1215–25.
105. Arthur AO, Whiteside S, Brown L, Minor C, Thomas SH. Patient use of tablet computers to facilitate emergency department pain assessment and documentation. ISRN Emerg Med. 2012;2012(1):254530.

4 Interprofessional Approach to Pain Management

Takova D. Wallace-Gay

Introduction

In the ever-changing landscape of healthcare, the management of pain is a pivotal challenge. As we navigate the complexities of pain and pain management, it becomes increasingly evident that a comprehensive and collaborative approach is essential for addressing the multifaceted nature of this issue. Often, pain management involves a siloed approach from healthcare practitioners, leaving room for improvement in management effectiveness and patient outcomes. Guidelines for pain treatment advocate an approach centered around the patient, emphasizing education and fostering interprofessional collaboration [6]. Additionally, interprofessional collaboration should be integrated into the education process to enhance clinician development and better prepare patients for complex issues such as pain management [8]. This may help practitioners and patients recognize that pain management is multifactorial and that optimal care includes a variety of professionals.

Understanding Pain

Pain presents in a myriad of forms and stands as a complex and intricate experience that transcends the confines of mere physical sensation. Its multifaceted nature encompasses not only the physiological aspects of nociception but also the psychological, social, and emotional dimensions. The traditional perception of pain as a straightforward sensory response to injury or illness has evolved, giving rise to a deeper understanding of the intricate interplay between biological, psychological, and sociocultural factors that contribute to its manifestation. The IASP's definition of pain underscores the subjective and psychological nature of pain and attempts to abstain from making the authenticity of pain dependent upon external, verifiable stimuli [3]. This holistic perspective is crucial in navigating the diverse landscape of pain experiences and forms the foundation upon which the necessity for an interprofessional approach to pain management is built.

The impact of pain on quality of life is profound and far-reaching. Beyond immediate discomfort, pain can permeate various facets of one's existence, influencing mood, relationships, and overall well-being. Specifically, chronic pain may significantly impact daily functioning. This impact has been documented in the literature and has been shown to significantly impair daily functioning, leading to reduced work capacity, social withdrawal, and other emotional challenges [10, 13]. It is imperative to recognize the intricate ways in which pain affects the lives of patients and the necessity of adopting a comprehensive approach that extends beyond conventional medical interventions. The need for comprehensive management arises from the limitations of traditional, unidimensional approaches. A recent review of the literature suggested that interventions characterized by interdisciplinarity, teamwork, and collaborative efforts enhance patient-reported pain outcomes compared to traditional approaches [4]. A singular focus of pain as a symptom may result in suboptimal outcomes, and the varying contributing factors that may be identifiable by a diverse healthcare team may be neglected. An interprofessional approach seeks to bridge these gaps by fostering collaboration among healthcare providers with different areas of expertise. This approach allows for a more nuanced approach to pain management that acknowledges the multifaceted nature of pain and aims to enhance the overall well-being of patients. The literature has described various groups who have provided distinct definitions for multidisciplinary pain management, most notably in neonatal and chronic non-cancer pain [2, 7] however, many of the previously described programs specialize in certain aspects of pain management [22]. Forthcoming interventions could

T. D. Wallace-Gay (✉)
The University of Texas at Tyler School of Medicine and Fisch College of Pharmacy, Tyler, TX, USA
e-mail: twallacegay@uttyler.edu

J. P. Reinert et al. (eds.), *Adjunctive Analgesic Strategies for the Bedside Clinician and Beyond*,
https://doi.org/10.1007/978-3-032-21675-5_4

emphasize the roles of all professional team members, including care managers, as well as establish mechanisms for patient follow-up, to effectively bridge the gap between clinical guidelines and the practical implementation of interprofessional, team-based pain care [4].

Roles and Responsibilities of Healthcare Professionals

Various healthcare professionals play integral roles in addressing the complexities of pain and contributing to comprehensive patient care. Multidisciplinary pain treatment facilities (MPTFs) have been described in the literature and are designed to provide patients with the resources to achieve necessary pain relief and improved psychological, behavioral, and physical functioning [15, 19].

Primary Care Practitioners

Primary care physicians (PCPs), physician associates, and nurse practitioners serve as the cornerstone of pain management, employing their medical expertise to diagnose and prescribe appropriate treatments. PCPs conduct thorough assessments, formulate treatment plans, and coordinate care to address both the physiological and psychological aspects of pain. Nurse practitioners and physician associates have an even more unique role because they play a vital role in patient education related to the diagnosis and ongoing monitoring, fostering a holistic approach to pain management [17].

Pharmacists

Pharmacists significantly contribute to pain management by ensuring safe and appropriate medication use. They collaborate with physicians to select the most suitable medications, educate patients on safe and appropriate use, and assist with monitoring for potential drug interactions and adverse events. The selection of medication requires close collaboration with the patient and other members of the team to identify pain severity, cost restraints, type of pain, and patient-specific characteristics [12]. This role is crucial for optimizing pain relief benefits while mitigating the risks of complex medication regimens.

Physical Therapists and Occupational Therapists

Physical and occupational therapists have unique roles in focusing on general physical function vs. improving the ability to perform activities of daily living. Both professionals focus on enhancing patients' functional abilities and quality of life. Through targeted exercises, physical therapists address musculoskeletal components of pain through the promotion of mobility and strength. Occupational therapists assist individuals in adapting to daily activities that will allow them to manage pain and improve overall well-being [20].

Psychologists and Psychiatrists

Psychologists and psychiatrists are essential in addressing the ever-present psychological aspects of pain management. Psychologists employ behavioral interventions, cognitive–behavioral therapy, and other treatment methods that assist with coping skills for pain-related stress, anxiety, and depression. Psychiatrists contribute by assisting in the diagnosis of mental health conditions and addressing those conditions that may exacerbate or complicate pain management [11, 17].

Nurses

Nurses play a crucial role as patient advocates and are involved in the day-to-day and initial assessments of pain management and pain symptoms, respectively. They provide hands-on care, administer medications, monitor patients for adverse events, and offer emotional support. Additionally, nurses are instrumental in providing care coordination and assisting patients with navigating the complexities of the healthcare system [16].

Social Workers

Social workers contribute by addressing any potential or known social determinants of health that impact pain management. They can identify resources, including financial and community support, for enhancing patients' overall treatment approach and benefits.

The patient also plays a vital role in the management of pain. Patients are active participants in their care, working collaboratively with healthcare professionals to communicate their pain experiences, preferences, and personal goals. Patients should be encouraged to adhere to their treatment plans, openly communicate with their team, and engage in self-management strategies.

The IASP recommends ongoing communication between team members, which will allow for many benefits, including [11, 17]:

- Multidimensional diagnosis of pain
- Rapid initiation of treatment plan
- Up-to-date, evidence-based treatment plans
- Faster return to work for patients
- Improved interdisciplinary knowledge
- Coordinated and individualized care plan

Other members of the team may include dieticians, community health workers, complementary and alternative providers (e.g., massage therapists, acupuncturists, etc.), and professionals from various subspecialties (e.g., anesthesiologists, neurologists, etc.). Although it may not be necessary or possible for all members of the team to be involved in the management of every chronic pain patient, identifying high-risk patients and employing a multidisciplinary team in their care are important.

Interprofessional Communication

Effective communication is a staple in the successful implementation of interprofessional collaboration in pain management. As diverse teams of healthcare professionals come together from their respective training to address the many aspects of a patient's pain experiences, it is imperative that everyone is able to communicate and understand care plans. The overall goal is to ensure that all members of the team, from physicians to nurses, pharmacists, therapists, and social workers, are well-informed and aligned in their approach to individualized patient care.

The benefits of collaborative communication in pain management are not focused solely on information exchange. A cohesive and communicative healthcare team fosters shared decision-making and shared understanding of the patient's unique profile and allows for a comprehensive and personalized approach to treatment. This level of teamwork and communication enhances the quality of care and contributes to improved patient outcomes.

Common communication strategies in interprofessional team management may include team meetings/huddles, case conferences, and electronic health record communication and information sharing. Fostering an environment of open communication and mutual respect among team members is crucial for creating an environment of free exchange of information.

To improve communication in pain management, formalized training programs may be employed to enhance communication skills, clearly delineate roles and responsibilities, and standardize communication tools. One such tool is Team Strategies & Tools to Enhance Performance & Patient Safety (TeamSTEPPS®). This strategy has been widely utilized as an evidence-based set of teamwork tools specifically aimed at improving communication and teamwork skills among healthcare teams [1]. The Comprehensive Pain Assessment Clinic (CoPAC) model was described by Glassburn et al. The authors described communication tools for effective teamwork, as follows (Fig. 4.1) [5]:

1. Pre-visit preparation: This strategy focuses on reducing duplication, increasing the efficiency of reviewing past medical history, and focusing on specific aspects of the history. For example, a physician may focus on diagnoses, medical treatments, and specialist evaluations, while a social work team focuses on reviewing social and mental health history, safety, and resource needs.
2. Pre-visit huddle and the huddle board: Here, team members are introduced to their specific roles as they relate to the patient's medical concerns and the clinical flow. Any notable items are placed on the huddle board under the discipline that will deliver that portion of the care plan.
3. Initial assessment of the patient: This is a subjective assessment that depends on the current moment vs. the overall progress of the patient. Typically, this procedure is performed by a nurse or medical assistant.
4. Coordination huddle and team handoff board: The team discusses the results of any initial assessment instruments and discusses barriers to care and other important care plan items. The team subsequently decides which team members need to meet with the patient and in which order.
5. Teamlet visit: Based on the prior strategic steps, key clinical areas are identified, and two-to-three-member teams collectively visit the patient. Occasionally, a practitioner will meet independently with the patient.
6. Care plan development: A shared care plan is developed.
7. Follow-up coordination: Most patients return to their primary care provider for ongoing follow-up; however, more complex patients may require follow-up with the entire team.
8. Post-clinical debriefs for continuous quality improvement (QI): The team discusses what went well, lessons learned, and other aspects of the QI process.

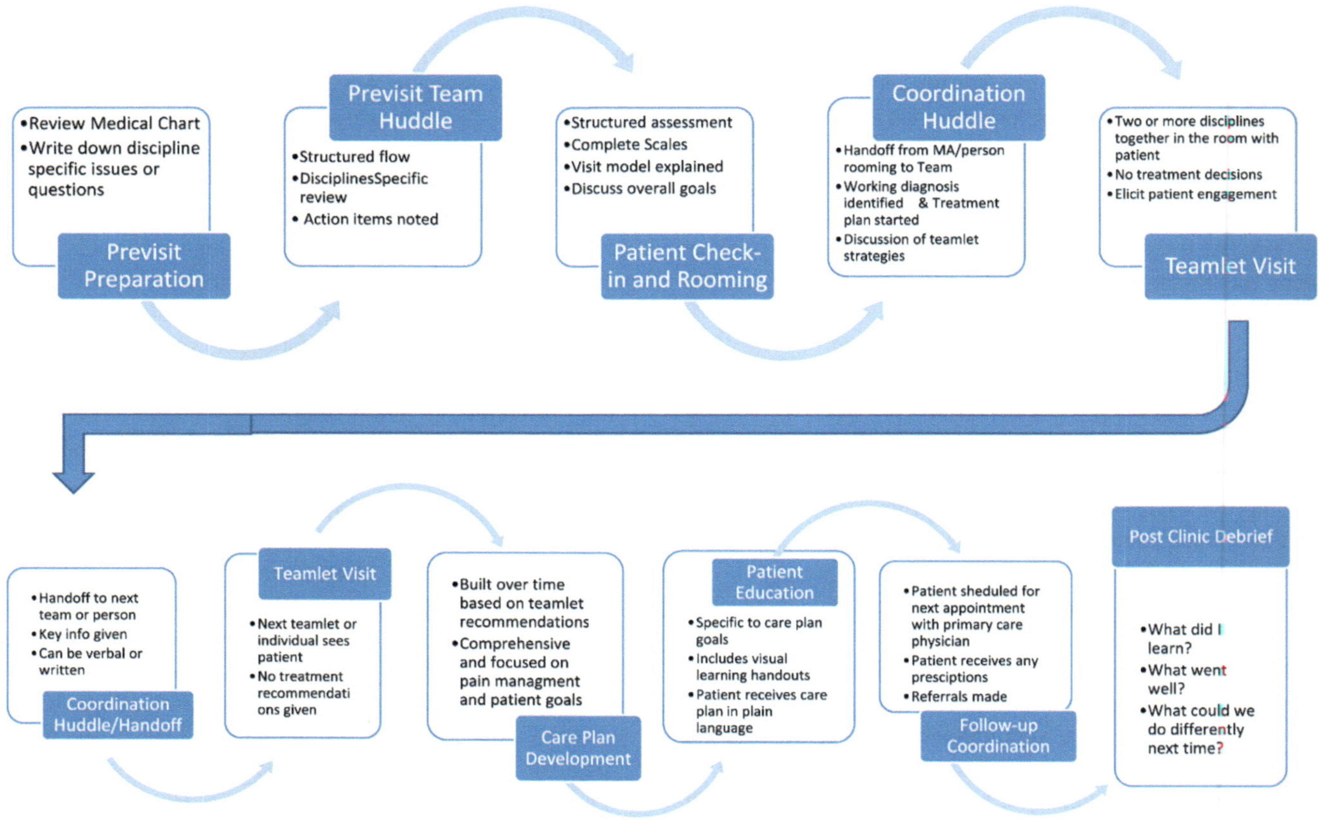

Fig. 4.1 The CoPAC model of clinic flow. (Reproduced with permission from the author. Glassburn et al. [5])

Although these strategies present a novel and ideal approach to pain management, notably, these strategies may not always be possible due to personnel and/or time constraints.

Collaborative Assessment, Diagnosis, Treatment, Planning, and Implementation

Interprofessional collaboration begins with a comprehensive pain assessment that involves input from different healthcare professionals. Physicians, nurses, physical therapists, psychologists, and other professionals collaboratively gather information to gain a comprehensive understanding of patients' pain experience. This interprofessional assessment considers not only the physical aspects of pain but also the psychological, social, and environmental factors influencing patient well-being. To address the fragmented delivery of chronic pain care, guidelines in pain management advocate for the implementation of integrated, interdisciplinary approaches.

Team-based diagnostic approaches are a hallmark of interprofessional collaboration in pain management. Physicians and nurse practitioners collaborate with specialists such as radiologists and neurologists to employ a multi-faceted diagnostic strategy. Imaging studies, diagnostic procedures, and thorough clinical examinations may be needed to accurately pinpoint the underlying causes of pain. The integration of various perspectives ensures a more nuanced diagnosis, leading to a more precise and effective treatment plan. Identifying the underlying causes of pain is crucial for developing individualized treatment plans. The collaborative efforts of healthcare professionals allow for a comprehensive exploration of potential contributors to pain, addressing not only symptoms but also the root causes. This approach is especially relevant in chronic pain cases, where a more holistic understanding of the patient's condition is paramount.

An integral aspect of interprofessional collaboration in pain management is the incorporation of the patient's perspective into the assessment process. Nurses, social workers, and psychologists work collaboratively to gather information about patients' pain experiences, preferences, and goals. This patient-centered approach ensures that the treatment plan aligns with the individual needs and values of the patient, promoting a more personalized and effective intervention.

Medication management involves physicians and pharmacists working together to prescribe and monitor the effectiveness and side effects of medications. Physical therapists and rehabilitation specialists contribute by designing tailored exercise regimens to address musculoskeletal components of pain and promoting mobility and function. Psychologists and behavioral therapists collaborate to implement psychological interventions addressing the emotional and cognitive aspects of pain. Complementary and alternative therapies, such as acupuncture or mindfulness practices, may also be integrated into the treatment plan, reflecting the collaborative consideration of diverse approaches.

Monitoring and adjusting treatment plans require ongoing collaboration among healthcare professionals. Regular team meetings allow for the review of patient progress and adjustments to the treatment plan based on the evolving needs of the individual. This iterative process ensures that the pain management plan remains responsive and adaptable to the dynamic nature of pain experiences [9, 21].

The utilization of fully developed interprofessional care strategies is still being developed in the literature; however, it is clear that incorporating multimodal interprofessional pain management may optimize overall patient care. As teams consider these shared decision-making approaches, they should recognize the underlying process of collaboration, including interpersonal and organizational aspects [14].

Application to Clinical Practice: Coordinated Care and Shared Decision-Making

In the realm of pain management, the translation of interprofessional collaboration into practical clinical applications is paramount. This section explores key models and approaches that embody the principles of coordinated care and shared decision-making, contributing to the effective treatment of pain.

The CoPAC Model

The CoPAC model serves as an exemplary framework for translating interprofessional collaboration into clinical practice. CoPAC strategically integrates various healthcare professionals, fostering a team-based approach to pain assessment and management. Pre-visit preparation, huddles, and coordinated team visits are fundamental components of the CoPAC model. This approach streamlines clinical flow, enhances efficiency, and ensures that each team member's expertise is harnessed effectively during patient encounters. The model emphasizes shared care plan development and post-clinical debriefs for continuous quality improvement, embodying the iterative and collaborative nature of interprofessional pain management [5].

Multidisciplinary Pain Treatment Facilities (MPTFs)

MPTFs represent dedicated spaces where healthcare professionals collaborate seamlessly to address the complex needs of individuals experiencing pain. These facilities, often designed around the principles of the CoPAC model, provide a comprehensive range of resources for pain relief, psychological support, and improved physical functioning. The multidisciplinary nature of MPTFs ensures that patients benefit from the combined expertise of physicians, nurses, therapists, and other specialists, creating an environment conducive to shared decision-making and patient-centered care [16].

Patient-Centered Medical Homes (PCMHs)

Patient-centered medical homes, characterized by a team-based approach and coordinated care, contribute significantly to effective pain management. In these settings, primary care physicians, nurse practitioners, and other healthcare professionals collaborate closely to address pain from a holistic perspective. Ensuring continuity of care is a key feature of promoting a seamless transition between different healthcare providers. Patient preferences are actively considered, fostering a shared decision-making process in which individuals actively participate in shaping their pain management plans [18].

A fundamental aspect of an interprofessional approach to pain management in clinical practice is addressing patient preferences. By actively involving patients in care decisions, healthcare teams can tailor interventions to align with individual needs and values. Ensuring continuity of care becomes essential, promoting a consistent and coordinated approach across various healthcare encounters. Treatment team visits offer a structured mechanism for multiple professionals to collaborate during patient appointments, facilitating comprehensive assessments and personalized care plans.

In essence, the application of an interprofessional approach to pain management in clinical practice involves adopting models such as CoPAC, leveraging the resources of multidisciplinary pain treatment facilities, and embracing patient-centered medical homes. By focusing on coordinated care and shared decision-making, healthcare professionals can provide more effective and patient-tailored interventions, ultimately enhancing the overall quality of pain management.

Interprofessional Education and Training

In the realm of pain management, the imperative for interprofessional education and training emerges as a cornerstone for fostering collaboration among diverse healthcare professionals. Recognizing the multidimensional nature of pain, cross-disciplinary training is crucial for breaking down silos and instilling shared language and understanding among healthcare teams. By engaging in joint educational experiences, physicians, nurses, pharmacists, therapists, and other professionals can gain insights into each other's roles, perspectives, and expertise, fostering a collaborative environment that transcends traditional disciplinary boundaries. The IASP outlines an objective curriculum designed to instill the knowledge and skills necessary in pain management as part of an interprofessional team. The main focus of this curriculum includes (1) recognizing and respecting roles and responsibilities and the competence of others and (2) knowing when, where, and how to involve other professionals [9]. Promoting interprofessional competencies is a fundamental objective of educational initiatives in pain management. These competencies extend beyond technical skills and encompass effective communication, teamwork, and shared decision-making. Training programs should aim to cultivate a deep appreciation for the contributions of each discipline, encouraging professionals to collaborate seamlessly in the assessment, diagnosis, and treatment of pain. Emphasizing these competencies allows healthcare teams to use tools to navigate the intricate landscape of pain management collaboratively, ensuring a more comprehensive and patient-centered approach. Core competencies for pain management are centered around meeting the needs of the person in pain and addressing fundamental concepts and complexities of pain (What is pain?), how pain is observed and assessed (How is pain recognized?), collaborative approaches to treatment options (How is pain relieved?), and the application of competencies across the life span in various settings, populations, and care models (How does context influence pain management?) [6].

Continuous education and skill development are essential components of sustaining effective interprofessional collaboration in pain management. As the field evolves with advancements in research, technology, and treatment modalities, healthcare professionals must stay abreast of the latest developments. Ongoing education ensures that interprofessional teams remain well-informed about emerging best practices, evidence-based interventions, and interdisciplinary approaches. By committing to lifelong learning, healthcare professionals can enhance their ability to adapt to changing patient needs and contribute to the ongoing improvement of pain management outcomes. In this way, interprofessional education and training serve as catalysts for creating a dynamic and responsive healthcare workforce capable of addressing the intricate challenges posed by pain. Interprofessional education is poised to yield significant advantages in actual clinical practice.

Conclusion

The significance of interprofessional collaboration in pain management cannot be overstated because it represents a paradigm shift toward a more comprehensive, patient-centered approach to addressing the complexities of pain. Through the collaborative efforts of healthcare professionals from diverse disciplines, a holistic understanding of pain can be achieved. The need for ongoing interprofessional collaboration in pain management is important since pain is a dynamic and evolving phenomenon, and its management requires continuous adaptation to the changing needs and circumstances of the patient. Additionally, the ever-expanding knowledge base in healthcare demands a collaborative effort to integrate the latest evidence, treatment approaches, and best practices. The synergy created through collaboration enhances communication, fosters a culture of mutual respect, and contributes to a more cohesive patient-centered approach to care. The enduring collaboration among healthcare professionals remains a staple for transformative patient outcomes.

References

1. Agency for Healthcare Research and Quality. Team strategies & tools to enhance performance & patient safety (TeamSTEPPS®) program. AHRQ; 2023. Retrieved June 16, 2025, from https://www.ahrq.gov/teamstepps-program/index.html.
2. Bapat R, Duran M, Piazza A, Pallotto EK, Joe P, Chuo J, Mingrone T, Hawes J, Powell M, Falciglia GH, Grover TR, Rintoul N, MacPherson MJ, Rose A, Brozanski B. A multicenter collaborative to improve postoperative pain management in the NICU. Pediatrics. 2023;152(2):e2022059860. https://doi.org/10.1542/peds.2022-059860.
3. Cole BE. Pain management: classifying, understanding, and treating pain. Hosp Physician. 2002;38:22–30.
4. Connell NB, Prathivadi P, Lorenz KA, Herman L, et al. Teaming in interdisciplinary chronic pain management interventions in primary care: a systematic review of randomized controlled trials. J Gen Intern Med. 2022;37:1501–12. https://doi.org/10.1007/s11606-021-07255-w.
5. Glassburn S, Delbridge E, Loghmani MT, Newton A, Binion K, Romito L, Willis D. Communication tools and strategies for interprofessional teamwork in a comprehensive pain assessment clinic in primary care. J Interprofessional Educ Pract. 2022;29:100541. https://doi.org/10.1016/j.xjep.2022.100541.
6. Gordon DB, Watt-Watson J, Hogans BB. Interprofessional pain education—with, from, and about competent, collaborative practice teams to transform pain care. Pain Rep. 2018;3(3):e663. https://doi.org/10.1097/PR9.0000000000000663.

7. Guzmán J, Esmail R, Karjalainen K, Malmivaara A, Irvin E, Bombardier C. Multidisciplinary rehabilitation for chronic low back pain: systematic review. BMJ. 2001;322(7301):1511–6. https://doi.org/10.1136/bmj.322.7301.1511.
8. Hunter J, Stinson P, Campbell J, Stevens F, Wagner B, Susan J. Simmons B, White M, van Wyk M. A novel pain interprofessional education strategy for trainees: assessing impact on interprofessional competencies and pediatric pain knowledge, pain research and management. 2015; 159580 (20):9. https://doi.org/10.1155/2015/159580.
9. International Association for the Study of Pain. (2018). IASP interprofessional pain curriculum outline. Retrieved June 16, 2025, from https://www.iasp-pain.org/education/curricula/iasp-interprofessional-pain-curriculum-outline/.
10. Latham J, Davis BD. The socioeconomic impact of chronic pain. Disabil Rehabil. 1994;16(1):39–44. https://doi.org/10.3109/09638289409166435.
11. Mavrocordatos P, Huygen F, Sichere P. Benefits of the multidisciplinary team for the patient. In: Toward a multidisciplinary approach in chronic pain management. Chronic Pain Europe; 2011. Retrieved June 16, 2025, from https://www.pae-eu.eu/wp-content/uploads/2013/12/Multidisciplinary-approach-in-chronic-pain-management.pdf.
12. Murphy L, Ng K, Isaac P, Swidrovich J, Zhang M, Sproule BA. The role of the pharmacist in the care of patients with chronic pain. Integr Pharm Res Pract. 2021;10:33–41. https://doi.org/10.2147/IPRP.S248699.
13. Niv D, Kreitler S. Pain and quality of life. Pain Pract. 2001;1(3):150–61. https://doi.org/10.1046/j.1533-2500.2001.01016.x.
14. Oncology Nursing Society. Multimodal interprofessional pain management offers relief with less opioids. ONS Voice; 2025. Retrieved from https://www.ons.org/publications-research/voice/news-views/02-2025/multimodal-interprofessional-pain-management-offers.
15. Ospina M, Harstall C. Multidisciplinary pain programs for chronic pain: evidence from systematic reviews. Alberta Heritage Foundation for Medical Research; 2023. [Report].
16. Peng P, Stinson JN, Choinière M, Dion D, Intrater H, LeFort S, Lynch M, Ong M, Rashiq S, Tkachuk G, Veillette Y. (STOPPAIN Investigators Group). Role of health care professionals in multidisciplinary pain treatment facilities in Canada. Pain Res Manag. 2008;13(6):484–88. https://doi.org/10.1155/2008/726804.
17. Physiopedia. Multidisciplinary care in pain management; 2023. Retrieved June 16, 2025, from https://www.physio-pedia.com/Multidisciplinary_Care_in_Pain_Management#cite_note-p6-7.
18. Pryzbylkowski P, Ashburn MA. The Pain Medical Home: A Patient-Centered Medical Home Model of Care for Patients with Chronic Pain. Anesthesiol Clin. 2015;33(4):785–793. https://doi.org/10.1016/j.anclin.2015.07.009.
19. International Association for the Study of Pain. Task force guidelines for desirable characteristics for pain treatment facilities; 2023. Retrieved June 16, 2025, from https://www.iasp-pain.org/advocacy/iasp-statements/desirable-characteristics-of-national-pain-strategies/.
20. Tsang A, Von Korff M, Lee S, Alonso J, Karam E, Angermeyer MC, Borges GL, Bromet EJ, Demyttenaere K, de Girolamo G, de Graaf R, Gureje O, Lepine JP, Haro JM, Levinson D, Oakley-Browne MA, Posada-Villa J, Seedat S, Watanabe M. Common chronic pain conditions in developed and developing countries: gender and age differences and comorbidity with depression-anxiety disorders. J Pain. 2008;9(10):883–91. https://doi.org/10.1016/j.jpain.2008.05.005.
21. van Dongen JJJ, van Bokhoven MA, Daniëls R, van der Weijden T, Emonts WW, Beurskens A. Developing interprofessional care plans in chronic care: a scoping review. BMC Fam Pract. 2016;17:137. https://doi.org/10.1186/s12875-016-0535-7.
22. Navani A, Manchikanti L, Albers SL, et al. Responsible, Safe, and Effective Use of Biologics in the Management of Low Back Pain: American Society of Interventional Pain Physicians (ASIPP) Guidelines. Pain Physician. 2019;22(1S):S1–74.

Part II

Adjunctive Analgesics

Acetaminophen

5

Justin P. Reinert

Definitions

Term	Definition
NNT	Number needed to treat, the average number of patients who need to be treated to achieve one additional beneficial outcome
Fixed-dose combination	A medication product combining two or more active ingredients at a fixed dose, such as acetaminophen with opioids or nonsteroidal anti-inflammatory drugs (NSAIDs)
NAPQI	N-acetyl-p-benzoquinone imine, the toxic metabolite of acetaminophen responsible for liver injury in overdose
NPO	Nothing by mouth
Photophobia	Sensitivity to light, a common symptom in migraine that acetaminophen monotherapy often fails to alleviate
Opioid sparing	Reduction in opioid use achieved by combining opioids with other analgesics like acetaminophen or NSAIDs
RCT	Reduction in opioid use achieved by combining opioids with other analgesics like acetaminophen or NSAIDs
VAS	Visual analog scale
EMS	Emergency medical services
ERAS	Enhanced recovery after surgery

Background

Acetaminophen was first synthesized in the late nineteenth century as a derivative of coal tar compounds during efforts to develop safer alternatives to acetanilide and phenacetin, analgesics known for their toxicity [1]. In 1877, Harmon Northrop Morse produced acetaminophen in a laboratory setting, but it was not until 1893 that Joseph von Mering recognized its analgesic and antipyretic properties in clinical use [1, 2]. Despite this early discovery, acetaminophen remained relatively obscure until phenacetin, once widely used, was withdrawn in the mid-twentieth century due to its nephrotoxic and carcinogenic effects [1]. This led to a resurgence of interest in acetaminophen, which was found to be a safer metabolite of phenacetin. In 1955, it was introduced to the US market as a prescription analgesic under the brand name Tylenol® and became available over the counter by 1959 [1–3].

Today, acetaminophen is among the most commonly used medications worldwide [4]. In the United States alone, it is estimated that over 50 million people use acetaminophen each week for pain relief or fever reduction, often in both prescription and nonprescription formulations. It is a component in more than 600 medications, including combination products for cold and flu, migraine, and musculoskeletal pain. The widespread availability and perceived safety of acetaminophen have contributed to its popularity but also to its risk of inadvertent overdose [5]. Acetaminophen-related hepatotoxicity remains a leading cause of acute liver failure in many developed countries, emphasizing the importance of patient education and regulatory strategies to mitigate unintentional misuse [5–7]. Regardless, acetaminophen remains a cornerstone of analgesic therapy in both ambulatory and institutional settings, valued for its efficacy, tolerability, and versatility across diverse patient populations.

The use of acetaminophen as an adjunctive analgesic is particularly prominent in perioperative, inpatient, and chronic pain management settings [8–11]. When combined with opioids, acetaminophen has been shown to provide additive or even synergistic analgesia, allowing for lower opioid requirements and a corresponding reduction in opioid-related adverse effects such as respiratory depression, constipation, and sedation [10, 11]. This opioid-sparing effect is a cornerstone of multimodal analgesia protocols, which aim to improve patient outcomes while addressing the challenges of

J. P. Reinert (✉)
Department of Pharmacy Practice, The University of Toledo College of Pharmacy and Pharmaceutical Sciences, Toledo, OH, USA
e-mail: Justin.reinert@Utoledo.edu

J. P. Reinert et al. (eds.), *Adjunctive Analgesic Strategies for the Bedside Clinician and Beyond*,
https://doi.org/10.1007/978-3-032-21675-5_5

opioid stewardship and minimizing risks associated with long-term opioid use.

In both acute and chronic settings, oral, rectal, and intravenous formulations of acetaminophen are available, each offering distinct advantages [10–12]. Intravenous acetaminophen achieves a more rapid onset and higher plasma concentrations compared to oral administration and may be especially beneficial in surgical patients or those unable to take medications enterally. Its incorporation into enhanced recovery after surgery (ERAS) protocols underscores its role in promoting early mobilization, reducing pain intensity, and shortening hospital stays [13].

Its widespread use and generally safe profile notwithstanding, the potential for hepatotoxicity remains a major limitation, particularly at doses exceeding 4 g per day or in patients with chronic alcohol use, malnutrition, or preexisting liver disease [6, 7]. Clinicians must balance efficacy and safety, considering patient-specific factors when selecting and dosing acetaminophen as part of an individualized pain management regimen.

Pharmacology, Pharmacokinetics, and Pharmacodynamics

Acetaminophen is a centrally acting analgesic and antipyretic agent with minimal anti-inflammatory properties [2, 14]. Its precise mechanism of action remains only partially elucidated, but it is believed to inhibit a variant of the cyclooxygenase enzyme (COX) in the central nervous system, leading to reduced synthesis of prostaglandins involved in pain and fever modulation [15]. Additionally, acetaminophen appears to influence serotonergic descending pain pathways and endocannabinoid signaling, contributing to its analgesic effect without the gastrointestinal, platelet, or renal side effects typically associated with nonsteroidal anti-inflammatory drugs (NSAIDs) [16].

Following oral administration, acetaminophen is rapidly and almost completely absorbed from the gastrointestinal tract, with peak plasma concentrations typically occurring within 30 min to 2 h [17]. It exhibits a bioavailability of approximately 60–90%, depending on formulation and gastric emptying time [17]. Acetaminophen undergoes extensive hepatic metabolism via three primary pathways: glucuronidation (~55%), sulfation (~30% to 35%), and oxidation (~5% to 10%) via the cytochrome P450 enzyme system, primarily CYP2E1 [18]. The oxidation pathway produces a reactive metabolite, N-acetyl-p-benzoquinone imine (NAPQI), which is normally detoxified by conjugation with glutathione. In overdose situations or when hepatic glutathione stores are depleted, NAPQI accumulation can result in hepatocellular injury [18].

The pharmacodynamic profile of acetaminophen reflects its central modulation of pain and thermoregulation [19, 20]. It effectively lowers febrile body temperature by acting on the hypothalamic heat-regulating center and provides mild-to-moderate analgesia, primarily for nociceptive pain. The onset of analgesia occurs within 30–60 min, and the duration of action generally ranges from 4 to 6 h, depending on the route of administration. Intravenous acetaminophen achieves higher and more consistent plasma concentrations than oral forms, which may translate into more effective and rapid pain control in acute care settings [19, 20].

Evidence of Efficacy

Primary Care and Internal Medicine

Acetaminophen remains a cornerstone analgesic in both primary care and hospital settings due to its favorable safety profile and broad applicability. In primary care, oral acetaminophen has demonstrated consistent, though modest, efficacy for the treatment of common acute pain conditions such as sore throat and headache [21]. Meta-analyses of randomized controlled trials (RCTs) have reported number-needed-to-treat (NNT) values around 4–5, indicating that acetaminophen provides clinically meaningful pain relief for a substantial proportion of patients compared to placebo [22]. These findings support its continued use as a first-line option for mild-to-moderate episodic pain management in outpatient settings, although evidence for other conditions like lower back pain is less robust.

Within the hospital environment, intravenous acetaminophen has been extensively studied as part of multimodal analgesia protocols, particularly in postoperative patients. Several randomized controlled trials demonstrate that IV acetaminophen can modestly reduce pain scores in the immediate postoperative period [23–25]. For example, in cardiac surgery patients undergoing sternotomy, administration of 1 g IV acetaminophen every 6 h resulted in statistically significant reductions in pain intensity, although this did not translate into meaningful opioid-sparing effects [23]. Similarly, in patients undergoing gastrectomy for gastric cancer, the addition of IV acetaminophen to thoracic epidural analgesia reduced the need for rescue analgesics and improved pain control during coughing episodes compared to epidural analgesia alone [24]. Broader data, including multiple surgical populations, confirm that IV acetaminophen reduces pain scores and is associated with a 30% decrease in opioid requirements within the first 4 h after surgery, with a number needed to treat of approximately four to achieve at least 50% pain relief [23–25].

However, evidence from large observational cohorts in general hospitalized populations offers a more nuanced picture [26]. Retrospective analyses involving tens of thousands of patients undergoing common surgeries such as joint arthroplasty and caesarean delivery found no significant improvements in total opioid consumption, length of hospital stay, or readmission rates attributable to IV acetaminophen use [27]. Some studies reported lower opioid use during the first 24 h postoperatively but paradoxically higher reported pain scores overall, suggesting that the analgesic benefits of IV acetaminophen may be context-dependent and influenced by factors such as surgical type, analgesic protocols, and patient characteristics [26–29].

When comparing oral and intravenous formulations in hospitalized patients, meta-analyses have found no clear superiority of IV acetaminophen over oral administration in terms of pain relief or opioid-sparing effects, particularly in orthopedic surgeries such as total hip and knee arthroplasty [30]. Given the higher cost and logistical challenges of IV administration, oral acetaminophen remains a cost-effective and practical alternative when patients can tolerate enteral medications.

Emergency Medicine

Randomized controlled trials comparing intravenous acetaminophen vs. morphine in adult renal colic consistently show equivalent pain relief at 30 min, with fewer adverse effects in the acetaminophen arms. In one double-blind study of 133 patients, 1 g IV acetaminophen achieved mean pain reductions of 63.7 mm vs. 56.6 mm for 0.1 mg/kg morphine on a 100-mm visual analog scale, with no statistically significant difference between the two (mean difference 7.1 mm, 95% CI −18 to 4) and fewer side effects reported in the acetaminophen group [31].

In prehospital or ambulance-based emergency care, a randomized trial conducted in Tehran compared 1 g IV acetaminophen vs. 30 mg IV ketorolac in patients with moderate-to-severe pain [32]. The Visual analog scale VAS reduction was clinically comparable between groups (14.9 ± 8.6 mm for acetaminophen vs. 16.0 ± 8.8 mm for ketorolac; $P = 0.429$), supporting IV acetaminophen as a viable non-NSAID option, especially where NSAIDs are contraindicated [32]. A retrospective Emergency medical services (EMS) data review similarly found no statistically significant difference in pain reduction when IV acetaminophen was used vs. ketorolac across traumatic and nontraumatic presentations [33].

For febrile or mild-to-moderate musculoskeletal injuries treated in the ED, the oral combination of 400 mg ibuprofen plus 1 g acetaminophen has been shown to provide analgesia equivalent to that of opioid–acetaminophen combinations. In a randomized clinical trial among 416 patients with extremity pain, pain reductions at 2 h were −4.3 for ibuprofen with acetaminophen vs. reductions of −4.4, −3.5, and −3.9 for oxycodone/APAP, hydrocodone/APAP, and codeine/APAP, respectively ($P = 0.053$). There were no clinically significant differences, suggesting non-opioid regimens may be effective in many cases [34].

Surgical and Perioperative Settings

Acetaminophen has become a cornerstone of multimodal analgesia in the surgical and perioperative care setting due to its opioid-sparing effects, favorable safety profile, and effectiveness in reducing mild-to-moderate postoperative pain. Its integration into Enhanced Recovery After Surgery (ERAS) protocols reflects its utility in improving patient outcomes by minimizing opioid requirements and facilitating early mobilization and discharge [13]. Numerous randomized controlled trials and meta-analyses support the use of acetaminophen in a variety of surgical procedures, including orthopedic, abdominal, and gynecologic surgeries [35].

Both oral and intravenous (IV) formulations of acetaminophen are used in surgical settings, each with distinct pharmacokinetic advantages. A Cochrane review found that oral acetaminophen, when administered preoperatively, reduced postoperative opioid consumption and improved pain scores when compared with placebo, although its effects were more modest than those observed with IV administration [36]. However, in the immediate postoperative period, especially in patients who are NPO or experiencing nausea, oral administration may be impractical or delayed.

In such scenarios, rectal acetaminophen serves as an alternative route. It is frequently used in pediatric surgery or when IV access is limited. Although rectal administration offers a useful noninvasive option, its pharmacokinetics are less predictable due to variable absorption and delayed onset of action. Peak plasma levels may not be reached until 2–3 h after administration, and bioavailability can range from 30% to 80% depending on the dose and formulation [17].

IV acetaminophen offers the most rapid onset and highest peak concentrations among the available formulations, with analgesic effects typically beginning within 15 min. It is especially beneficial in high-acuity surgical patients and those undergoing major procedures or when rapid, reliable pain relief is needed in the immediate postoperative phase. A multicenter, double-blind trial involving orthopedic surgery patients showed that IV acetaminophen significantly reduced pain intensity and delayed the time to first opioid administration compared to placebo [37]. However, its higher cost and similar long-term efficacy compared to oral administration often limit its use to specific clinical scenarios.

Special Populations

Acetaminophen is widely utilized in both geriatric and pediatric populations due to its generally favorable safety profile and broad availability in various formulations, and a detailed discussion of its use can be found in the geriatric and pediatric chapters of this textbook, respectively.

In geriatric patients, acetaminophen is typically considered the first-line agent for managing mild-to-moderate pain, particularly osteoarthritis and other musculoskeletal conditions, owing to its lower risk of gastrointestinal, renal, and cardiovascular adverse effects compared to nonsteroidal anti-inflammatory drugs (NSAIDs) [38]. Clinical guidelines, including those from the American Geriatrics Society, recommend acetaminophen as the initial pharmacologic therapy for chronic pain in older adults. However, age-related changes in hepatic metabolism and decreased hepatic reserve warrant caution with prolonged or high-dose use, especially in patients with multiple comorbidities or malnutrition, to minimize the risk of hepatotoxicity [39].

In the pediatric population, acetaminophen is one of the most frequently used medications for fever and pain management. It is approved for use in infants, children, and adolescents and is available in oral liquid, chewable, suppository, and intravenous formulations. When dosed correctly, acetaminophen is safe and effective for treating febrile illnesses, postoperative discomfort, teething, and minor injuries. The American Academy of Pediatrics supports its use as a first-line antipyretic and analgesic in children. However, accidental overdose remains a concern, especially when caregivers are unaware of the maximum daily dose or when multiple acetaminophen-containing products are used concurrently. Clear education on dosing and formulation differences is essential to ensure safety in pediatric care [40].

Evidence Not Supporting Routine Use

Dental Pain

Acetaminophen has been evaluated in postoperative dental pain, specifically after tooth extraction, and has been consistently shown to provide modest analgesia, although generally less effective than NSAIDs. A double-blind randomized trial of 30 orthodontic patients undergoing bilateral premolar extraction compared oral acetaminophen 500 mg three times daily against ibuprofen [41]. The groups reported similar pain control when surgical trauma was minimal, suggesting that acetaminophen may suffice in less invasive cases. [41] However, broader meta-analyses in dental extractions find NSAIDs and NSAID/acetaminophen combinations superior. For instance, systematic reviews demonstrate that standard doses of NSAIDs outperform acetaminophen with or without codeine for third molar extractions [42].

Sports-Related and Musculoskeletal Injury

Evidence on the use of acetaminophen for sports-related pain, such as delayed onset muscle soreness (DOMS), is limited and generally discouraging [43]. A large randomized controlled trial of marathon runners (n = 610) compared acetaminophen extended-release 1300 mg three times daily over 4 days to placebo [44]. While acetaminophen produced a statistically significant reduction in soreness on day one (mean −0.79 vs. −0.36 on a 0–10 scale) and improved sleep interference and treatment satisfaction, the absolute benefit was modest in magnitude. Expert commentaries emphasize that typical DOMS is self-limiting, and routine analgesic use may blunt necessary inflammation and risk masking serious conditions like rhabdomyolysis [43, 44].

Cancer Pain

Clinical trials in cancer populations do not consistently support acetaminophen as an effective adjunct in patients already receiving strong opioids. A randomized, double-blind, placebo-controlled crossover trial involving 30 patients with advanced cancer and high-dose opioid regimens found that adding oral acetaminophen (1 g every 4 h) produced a modest pain score improvement (mean difference ~0.4 VNS units; P = 0.03) and slight benefit in well-being but no reduction in opioid use [45]. A more recent RCT of 112 hospitalized cancer patients on strong opioids likewise found no significant benefit in pain reduction or reduction in morphine equivalent daily dose over 48 h when comparing regular acetaminophen to placebo (P = 0.37) [46]. Taken together, these data suggest limited utility for acetaminophen in moderate-to-severe cancer pain when opioids are already optimized.

Neuropathic and Nociplastic Pain

There is a paucity of randomized controlled trials evaluating acetaminophen for primary neuropathic or nociplastic pain conditions. Clinical guidelines and Cochrane reviews consistently report insufficient or no evidence supporting acetaminophen, even in combination with weak opioids like codeine, in disorders such as diabetic peripheral neuropathy or postherpetic neuralgia [47]. Moreover, fibromyalgia patients show minimal benefit from acetaminophen in clinical or mechanistic trials, failing to improve pain thresholds or functional outcomes to a clinically meaningful extent [47]. The data cumulatively suggest that acetaminophen lacks adequate efficacy in neuropathic/nociplastic syndromes and should not be relied upon as primary therapy.

Migraine and Severe Headache Syndromes

The efficacy of acetaminophen in moderate-to-severe migraine is limited compared to NSAIDs, triptans, or combination analgesics. In a randomized, double-blind, placebo-controlled trial involving 346 adults with moderate-to-severe episodic migraine, oral acetaminophen 1000 mg produced a significantly higher headache response rate at 2 h compared to placebo (52% vs. 32%; $P = 0.002$), as well as meaningful reductions in associated symptoms, such as nausea, photophobia, and functional disability [48]. While this establishes acetaminophen as statistically effective for some migraine attacks, its magnitude of effect with an NNT = 5 remains modest [48].

Current guidelines from the American Headache Society recommend acetaminophen only for mild, non-incapacitating migraine of slow onset; triptans and NSAIDs are preferred for moderate-to-severe attacks due to greater efficacy and consistency of response [49]. Acetaminophen monotherapy generally fails to alleviate the full spectrum of migraine features, such as photophobia or nausea, and offers limited functional improvement.

Additionally, acetaminophen is associated with risk of medication-overuse headache if taken frequently, defined as more than 15 headache days/month for ≥3 months, and must be used judiciously to avoid rebound headache and hepatotoxicity [49].

Applications to Clinical Practice

Opioid Synergy

Fixed-dose combination products like hydrocodone/acetaminophen and oxycodone/acetaminophen are widely prescribed for moderate-to–moderately severe acute pain, particularly in postoperative, dental, and musculoskeletal settings. Meta-analyses have demonstrated that these combinations provide superior analgesia compared to either component alone, particularly in the first hours following administration [50]. A Cochrane review found that a single dose of oxycodone 10 mg/acetaminophen 650 mg provided at least 50% pain relief in 70% of patients with acute postoperative pain, compared to approximately 30% with acetaminophen alone [51]. These findings support the clinical utility of combination therapy, particularly for short-term pain management.

NSAID Synergy

Extensive clinical experience and systematic reviews have demonstrated that combining acetaminophen with NSAIDs provides superior pain relief compared to either agent alone. In a qualitative systematic review of 21 randomized controlled trials ($n \approx 1900$) evaluating postoperative pain, over 80% of studies found that the acetaminophen/NSAID combination produced significantly greater analgesia, with a median pain reduction of ~35% and ~39% lower supplemental analgesic requirements, than monotherapy with either drug [52].

Muscle Relaxant Synergy

An open-label trial ($n = 183$) compared chlorzoxazone plus acetaminophen vs. each agent alone in patients with acute musculoskeletal low back conditions accompanied by spasms. The combination group reported faster symptom relief, achieving near-complete resolution by day 6, whereas approximately 40–50% of patients on acetaminophen alone still had pain or spasm at that time. The speed of onset was notably quicker (day 2 vs. day 4) in the combination group [51].

Gabapentinoid Synergy

Several randomized controlled trials and systematic reviews have examined perioperative pain management strategies combining acetaminophen and gabapentinoids, particularly pregabalin. A systematic review of 14 RCTs involving adult surgical patients found that nine out of 14 studies demonstrated significant reductions in both postoperative pain intensity and supplemental opioid use when gabapentinoids, mostly pregabalin, were included, often alongside acetaminophen and NSAIDs [54]. While gabapentin was evaluated in only two studies, pregabalin emerged as the primary agent associated with improved outcomes. These findings suggest that acetaminophen in combination with pregabalin can contribute to greater opioid sparing and improved analgesia in some perioperative settings [54].

However, the extent of benefit is modest and must be interpreted cautiously: A large meta-analysis, including 281 trials with approximately 24,700 patients, concluded that although gabapentinoids led to lower pain intensity scores at 6, 12, 24, and 48 h (mean differences ranging from −10 to −3/100), the reductions generally fell below the threshold for clinical relevance (<10/100), and there was no impact on subacute or chronic postoperative pain beyond 72 h [55]. The same analysis documented increased risks of dizziness, visual disturbance, and sedation, particularly when gabapentinoids were coadministered with opioids [55].

In an RCT of radical neck dissection patients, a preemptive analgesic protocol, including acetaminophen, naproxen, pregabalin, and dextromethorphan, significantly reduced postoperative pain and decreased total opioid use by approximately 54% compared to controls [56]. Yet despite these purported advantages, perioperative practices highlight controversy over the routine use of gabapentinoids: Although opioid consumption may decrease, clinical benefits in pain scores are inconsistent, and risks, particularly respiratory depression in high-risk patients, may outweigh modest gains.

Safety

Acetaminophen is widely regarded as a safe and effective analgesic and antipyretic when used within recommended dosing guidelines. Its safety profile is one of the primary reasons for its ubiquitous use across all age groups, including in vulnerable populations such as pediatrics, geriatrics, and pregnant individuals [38–40]. Unlike nonsteroidal anti-inflammatory drugs (NSAIDs), acetaminophen does not exert significant effects on platelet aggregation, gastrointestinal mucosa, or renal function, making it a preferred option for patients with bleeding risk, gastric ulcers, or renal impairment [2, 7]. The generally well-tolerated nature of acetaminophen, combined with its over-the-counter availability and multiple formulations, contributes to its widespread therapeutic application; however, acetaminophen is associated with significant safety concerns when dosing exceeds therapeutic thresholds. The most serious risk is dose-dependent hepatotoxicity, which can lead to acute liver failure, particularly when cumulative daily doses exceed 4000 mg in adults or 75 mg/kg/day in children [38, 39]. Hepatotoxicity is primarily mediated through the formation of a toxic metabolite, *N-acetyl-p-benzoquinone imine* (NAPQI), which overwhelms hepatic glutathione stores and causes oxidative injury [5]. Unintentional overdose can occur with polypharmacy, as many over-the-counter and prescription medications contain acetaminophen as a component. Additionally, patients with malnutrition, chronic alcohol use, or preexisting liver disease may have a lower threshold for toxicity [2]. Public health campaigns and regulatory interventions, such as limiting tablet strength and promoting clearer labeling, have aimed to mitigate these risks [7]. Overall, while acetaminophen remains a mainstay in pain and fever management, clinicians must maintain vigilance in dosing and patient education to ensure safe use.

Key Points

- Acetaminophen is widely used for mild-to-moderate pain and fever due to its favorable safety profile, minimal gastrointestinal and platelet effects, and broad availability.
- For moderate-to-severe migraine, acetaminophen shows limited efficacy compared to NSAIDs, triptans, and combination analgesics; it is generally recommended only for mild, non-incapacitating migraine.
- Combining acetaminophen with opioids or NSAIDs enhances analgesic efficacy through multimodal mechanisms, allowing for lower opioid doses and reduced side effects, with fixed-dose combinations commonly used for acute pain.
- Acetaminophen plus NSAID combinations consistently provide superior pain relief and opioid-sparing benefits in postoperative and acute pain settings without increasing adverse events.
- Limited evidence suggests that acetaminophen combined with muscle relaxants may improve outcomes in acute low back pain with muscle spasm, but more high-quality trials are needed.
- Perioperative use of acetaminophen combined with gabapentinoids can modestly reduce opioid use and pain intensity but may increase sedation and dizziness; clinical benefits remain debated.
- Hepatotoxicity is the most serious risk of acetaminophen overdose, especially above 4000 mg/day in adults or in vulnerable populations; careful dosing and patient education are essential to prevent liver injury.

Conclusions

Acetaminophen remains a cornerstone of analgesic and antipyretic therapy due to its favorable safety profile, broad accessibility, and versatility across diverse patient populations. Its unique pharmacologic properties, including central analgesic mechanisms and minimal gastrointestinal or platelet effects, make it an essential component of multimodal pain management strategies. While its efficacy is well-established for mild-to-moderate nociceptive pain, especially when combined with other agents such as opioids or select adjunctive medications, clinicians must be mindful of its limitations in certain pain syndromes and the critical importance of adhering to safe dosing guidelines to prevent hepatotoxicity. Ongoing research continues to refine the optimal use of acetaminophen, particularly in complex settings such as perioperative care and special populations. Ultimately, a thorough understanding of acetaminophen's pharmacology, clinical applications, and safety considerations enables healthcare providers to maximize its therapeutic benefits while minimizing risks, ensuring its continued role as a fundamental analgesic agent in contemporary practice.

References

1. Clissold SP. Paracetamol and phenacetin. Drugs. 1986;32(Supplement 4):46–59. Ayoub SS. Paracetamol (Acetaminophen): a familiar drug with an unexplained mechanism of action. Temperature (Austin). 2021;8(4):351–371.
2. Prescott LF. Paracetamol: past, present, and future. Am J Ther. 2000;7(2):143–7.
3. Paracetamol, digoxin, cisplatin. Curr Med Issues. 2018;16(3):110.
4. Kouznetsov VV. Exploring acetaminophen prodrugs and hybrids: a review. RSC Adv. 2024;14(14):9691–715.
5. Athersuch TJ, Antoine DJ, Boobis AR, et al. Paracetamol metabolism, hepatotoxicity, biomarkers and therapeutic interventions: a perspective. Toxicol Res. 2018;7(3):347–57.
6. Rubin JB, Hameed B, Gottfried M, Lee WM, Sarkar M. Acetaminophen-induced acute liver failure is more common and more severe in women. Clin Gastroenterol Hepatol. 2018;16(6):936–46.
7. Mitchell RA, Rathi S, Dahiya M, Zhu J, Hussaini T, Yoshida EM. Public awareness of acetaminophen and risks of drug induced liver injury: results of a large outpatient clinic survey. Strnad P, ed. PLoS One. 2020;15(3):e0229070.
8. Raiff D, Vaughan C, McGee A. Impact of intraoperative acetaminophen administration on postoperative opioid consumption in patients undergoing hip or knee replacement. Hosp Pharm. 2014;49(11):1022–32.
9. Brett K, Severn M. IV acetaminophen for acute pain in emergency departments: Cadth Health Technology review. Canadian Agency for Drugs and Technologies in Health; 2023.
10. Amaechi O, Human MM, Featherstone K. Pharmacologic therapy for acute pain. Am Fam Physician. 2021;104(1):63–72.
11. Patel A, Pai BHP, Diskina D, Reardon B, Lai YH. Comparison of clinical outcomes of acetaminophen IV vs PO in the perioperative setting for laparoscopic inguinal hernia repair surgeries: a triple-blinded, randomized controlled trial. J Clin Anesth. 2020;61:109628.
12. Hahn TW, Mogensen T, Lund C, Schouenborg L, Rasmussen M. High-dose rectal and oral acetaminophen in postoperative patients—serum and saliva concentrations. Acta Anaesthesiol Scand. 2000;44(3):302–6.
13. Sauro KM, Smith C, Ibadin S, et al. Enhanced recovery after surgery guidelines and hospital length of stay, readmission, complications, and mortality: a meta-analysis of randomized clinical trials. JAMA Netw Open. 2024;7(6):e2417310.
14. Graham GG, Scott KF. Mechanism of action of paracetamol. Am J Ther. 2005;12(1):46–55.
15. Esh CJ, Chrismas BCR, Mauger AR, Taylor L. Pharmacological hypotheses: is acetaminophen selective in its cyclooxygenase inhibition? Pharmacol Res Perspec. 2021;9(4):e00835.
16. Hamurtekin Y, Nouilati A, Demirbatir C, Hamurtekin E. The contribution of serotonergic receptors and nitric oxide systems in the analgesic effect of acetaminophen: an overview of the last decade. Turk J Pharm Sci. 2020;17(1):119–26.
17. Singla NK, Parulan C, Samson R, et al. Plasma and cerebrospinal fluid pharmacokinetic parameters after single-dose administration of intravenous, oral, or rectal acetaminophen. Pain Pract. 2012;12(7):523–32.
18. Mazaleuskaya LL, Sangkuhl K, Thorn CF, FitzGerald GA, Altman RB, Klein TE. PharmGKB summary: pathways of acetaminophen metabolism at the therapeutic versus toxic doses. Pharmacogenet Genomics. 2015;25(8):416–26.
19. Comstock GT, Halmo LS, Spyker DA. Pharmacokinetics and pharmacodynamics of acetaminophen. In: Acetaminophen toxicity. Elsevier; 2025. p. 221–73.
20. Ohashi N, Kohno T. Analgesic effect of acetaminophen: a review of known and novel mechanisms of action. Front Pharmacol. 2020;11:580289.
21. Gougain M, Moreau A, Boussageon R, Pickering G, Gueyffier F. Acute analgesic effect of paracetamol in primary care: incomplete evidence. Therapie. 2017;72(5):609–13.
22. Moore RA, Derry S, Aldington D, Wiffen PJ. Adverse events associated with single dose oral analgesics for acute postoperative pain in adults – an overview of Cochrane reviews. Cochrane Pain, Palliative and Supportive Care Group, ed. Cochrane Database of Systematic Reviews. Published online October 13, 2015.
23. Jelacic S, Bollag L, Bowdle A, Rivat C, Cain KC, Richebe P. Intravenous acetaminophen as an adjunct analgesic in cardiac surgery reduces opioid consumption but not opioid-related adverse effects: a randomized controlled trial. J Cardiothorac Vasc Anesth. 2016;30(4):997–1004.
24. Kinoshita J, Fushida S, et al. A randomized controlled trial of postoperative intravenous acetaminophen plus thoracic epidural analgesia vs. thoracic epidural analgesia alone after gastrectomy for gastric cancer. Gastric Cancer. 2019;22(2):392–402.
25. Ghaffarpasand F, Dadgostar E, Ilami G, et al. Intravenous acetaminophen (Paracetamol) for postcraniotomy pain: systematic review and meta-analysis of randomized controlled trials. World Neurosurg. 2020;134:569–76.
26. Mattern HP, Reichert JC, McConnell KJ. The effect of intravenous acetaminophen on patient outcomes within a large integrated delivery network. Pharmacotherapy. 2020;40(4):301–7.
27. Madere TC, Mendez JB, Nordmeyer ST, Heidel RE, Hamilton LA. Evaluation of intravenous acetaminophen on length of stay in abdominal surgery patients. Hosp Pharm. 2016;51(3):230–6.
28. Barrington J, Hansen R, Lovelace B, et al. Impact of intravenous acetaminophen on lengths of stay and discharge status after total knee arthroplasty. J Knee Surg. 2019;32(01):111–6.
29. Sun L, Zhu X, Zou J, Li Y, Han W. Comparison of intravenous and oral acetaminophen for pain control after total knee and hip arthroplasty: a systematic review and meta-analysis. Medicine. 2018;97(6):e9751.
30. Lu B, Tian AX, Fan ZR, et al. Effectiveness of oral vs intravenous acetaminophen on pain management following total joint arthroplasty: a systematic review and meta-analysis. World J Orthop. 2025;16(4):104452.
31. Sin B, Koop K, Liu M, Yeh JY, Thandi P. Intravenous acetaminophen for renal colic in the emergency department: where do we stand? Am J Ther. 2017;24(1):e12–9.
32. Mahshidfar B, Rezai M, Abbasi S, et al. Intravenous acetaminophen vs. ketorolac in terms of pain management in prehospital emergency services: a randomized clinical trial. Adv. J Emerg Med. 2019;3(4):e37.
33. McArthur R, Cash RE, Rafique Z, et al. Intravenous acetaminophen versus ketorolac for prehospital analgesia: a retrospective data review. J Emerg Med. 2024;67(3):e259–67.
34. Chang AK, Bijur PE, Esses D, Barnaby DP, Baer J. Effect of a single dose of oral opioid and nonopioid analgesics on acute extremity pain in the emergency department: a randomized clinical trial. JAMA. 2017;318(17):1661.
35. Wick EC, Grant MC, Wu CL. Postoperative multimodal analgesia pain management with nonopioid analgesics and techniques: a review. JAMA Surg. 2017;152(7):691.
36. Toms L, McQuay HJ, Derry S, Moore RA. Single dose oral paracetamol (Acetaminophen) for postoperative pain in adults. Cochrane Pain, Palliative and Supportive Care Group, ed. Cochrane Database of Systematic Reviews. 2008;2019(5).
37. Sinatra RS, Jahr JS, Reynolds LW, Viscusi ER, Groudine SB, Payen-Champenois C. Efficacy and safety of single and repeated administration of 1 gram intravenous acetaminophen injection

(Paracetamol) for pain management after major orthopedic surgery. Anesthesiology. 2005;102(4):822–31.
38. Rose VL. Guidelines from the American Geriatric Society target management of chronic pain in older persons. Am Fam Physician. 1998;58(5):1213–5.
39. Tan JL, Eastment JG, Poudel A, Hubbard RE. Age-related changes in hepatic function: an update on implications for drug therapy. Drugs Aging. 2015;32(12):999–1008.
40. Lee GY, Yamada J, Kyololo O, Shorkey A, Stevens B. Pediatric clinical practice guidelines for acute procedural pain: a systematic review. Pediatrics. 2014;133(3):500–15.
41. Deshpande A, Bhargava D, Gupta M. Analgesic efficacy of acetaminophen for controlling postextraction dental pain. Ann Maxillofac Surg. 2014;4(2):176–7.
42. Zahrowski JJ. Good evidence supports acetaminophen as an effective and safe reliever of acute postoperative pain. J Am Dent Assoc. 2010;141(4):455–6.
43. Mauger AR, Jones AM, Williams CA. Influence of acetaminophen on performance during time trial cycling. J Appl Physiol. 2010;108(1):98–104.
44. Prior MJ, Lavins BJ, Cooper K. A randomized, placebo-controlled trial of acetaminophen extended release for treatment of post-marathon muscle soreness. Clin J Pain. 2012;28(3):204–10.
45. Stockler M, Vardy J, Pillai A, Warr D. Acetaminophen (Paracetamol) improves pain and well-being in people with advanced cancer already receiving a strong opioid regimen: a randomized, double-blind, placebo-controlled cross-over trial. JCO. 2004;22(16):3389–94.
46. Leiva-Vásquez O, Letelier LM, Rojas L, et al. Is acetaminophen beneficial in patients with cancer pain who are on strong opioids? A randomized controlled trial. J Pain Symptom Manag. 2023;66(3):183–92.e1.
47. Wiffen PJ, Knaggs R, Derry S, Cole P, Phillips T, Moore RA. Paracetamol (Acetaminophen) with or without codeine or dihydrocodeine for neuropathic pain in adults. Cochrane Pain, Palliative and Supportive Care Group, ed. Cochrane Database of Systematic Reviews. 2016;2019(5).
48. Prior MJ, Codispoti JR, Fu M. A randomized, placebo-controlled trial of acetaminophen for treatment of migraine headache. Headache. 2010;50(5):819–33.
49. VanderPluym JH, Halker Singh RB, Urtecho M, et al. Acute treatments for episodic migraine in adults: a systematic review and meta-analysis. JAMA. 2021;325(23):2357.
50. Martinez V, Beloeil H, Marret E, Fletcher D, Ravaud P, Trinquart L. Non-opioid analgesics in adults after major surgery: systematic review with network meta-analysis of randomized trials. Br J Anaesth. 2017;118(1):22–31.
51. Gaskell H, Derry S, Moore RA, McQuay HJ. Single dose oral oxycodone and oxycodone plus paracetamol (Acetaminophen) for acute postoperative pain in adults. Cochrane Pain, Palliative and Supportive Care Group, ed. Cochrane Database of Systematic Reviews. 2009;2019(5).
52. Ong CK, Seymour RA, Lirk P, Merry AF. Combining Paracetamol (Acetaminophen) with nonsteroidal antiinflammatory drugs: a qualitative systematic review of analgesic efficacy for acute postoperative pain. Centre for Reviews and Dissemination (UK); 2010.
53. Patel HD, Uppin RB, Naidu AR, Rao YR, Khandarkar S, Garg A. Efficacy and safety of combination of nsaids and muscle relaxants in the management of acute low back pain. Pain Ther. 2019;8(1):121–32.
54. Gill C, Giuliano K. Gabapentinoids and acetaminophen as adjuvants for managing postoperative pain. AANA J. 2022;90(3):181–7.
55. Verret M, Lauzier F, Zarychanski R, et al. Perioperative use of gabapentinoids for the management of postoperative acute pain: a systematic review and meta-analysis. Anesthesiology. 2020;133(2):265–79.
56. Amiri HR, Mirzaei M, Beig Mohammadi MT, Tavakoli F. Multimodal preemptive analgesia with pregabalin, acetaminophen, naproxen, and dextromethorphan in radical neck dissection surgery: a randomized clinical trial. Anesth Pain Med. 2016;6(4):e33526.

Nonsteroidal Anti-inflammatory Drugs (NSAIDs)

6

Chelsea K. DiPasquale, Maya R. Chilbert, Stephanie Seyse, Jennifer S. Abeles, and Nicole E. Cieri-Hutcherson

Abbreviations

AA	Arachidonic acid
ACEi	Angiotensin-converting enzyme inhibitor
ACOG	American College of Obstetrics and Gynecologists
ACR	American College of Rheumatology
ADH	Antidiuretic hormone
AIN	Acute interstitial nephritis
AKI	Acute kidney injury
ARB	Angiotensin receptor blocker
CKD	Chronic kidney disease
COX	Cyclooxygenase
DRESS	Drug reaction with eosinophilia and systemic symptoms
FDA	Food and Drug Administration
GI	Gastrointestinal
GIB	Gastrointestinal bleeding
JIA	Juvenile idiopathic arthritis
LT	Liver test
MOS	Mitochondrial oxidative stress
NSAID	Nonsteroidal anti-inflammatory drug
OA	Osteoarthritis
PGI_1	Prostacyclin
RAAS	Renin–angiotensin–aldosterone system
SJS	Steven–Johnson Syndrome
SNRI	Serotonin norepinephrine reuptake inhibitor
SSRI	Selective serotonin reuptake inhibitor
TEN	Toxic epidermal necrolysis
TXA2	Thromboxane A2

Introduction

Opioids have traditionally been considered the foundation for pain management, but due to their addictive properties and adverse events, limiting their use is essential. Nonsteroidal anti-inflammatory drugs (NSAIDs) are a heterogeneous class of medications that are used to treat a variety of conditions commonly associated with inflammation and pain [1]. The NSAID class of medications inhibits both cyclooxygenase (COX)-1 and COX-2 or only COX-2, which can target inflammation and/or platelet aggregation. Due to their anti-inflammatory properties, NSAIDs are often used as an adjunct to additional pain management strategies and are considered part of a holistic pain approach [2]. These agents are easily accessible; some specific NSAIDs, including ibuprofen and naproxen, are available without a prescription. NSAIDs are not without side effects, some of which include the development of gastrointestinal (GI) ulcers, acute kidney injury (AKI), and fluid retention. Many of the beneficial and harmful impacts of NSAIDs can be linked to the degree of inhibition of COX-1 or COX-2 [1]. It has been determined that, though many of the traditional NSAIDs block both COX-1 and COX-2, most of the anti-inflammatory effects of NSAIDs are due to COX-2 inhibition [3]. This discovery led to the development of selective-COX-2 inhibitors, including celecoxib (Celebrex®) and rofecoxib (Vioxx®), which were later linked to an increase in cardiovascular events [4, 5]. Rofecoxib (Vioxx®) was subsequently removed from the market, and the Food and Drug Administration (FDA) requested a labeling change to warn of the risk of cardiovascular events [5]. This is likely due to a change in the natural balance of prothrombotic thromboxane A2 (TXA_2) and antithrombotic prostacyclin (PGI_1) [6–8]. COX-1 inhibition decreases the production of TXA_2, while COX-2 limits the production of PGI_1, which may result in nonselective NSAIDs providing more of a balance between pro- and antithrombotic events [3]. Individual patient risks and benefits need to be considered when selecting NSAIDs for pain management.

C. K. DiPasquale (✉) · S. Seyse
Kaleida Health, Buffalo General Medical Center, Buffalo, NY, USA

M. R. Chilbert · N. E. Cieri-Hutcherson
Department of Pharmacy Practice, University at Buffalo School of Pharmacy and Pharmaceutical Sciences, Wolters Kluwer Health, Buffalo, NY, USA

J. S. Abeles
Department of Medicine, Jacobs School of Medicine and Biomedical Sciences, Buffalo, NY, USA

J. P. Reinert et al. (eds.), *Adjunctive Analgesic Strategies for the Bedside Clinician and Beyond*,
https://doi.org/10.1007/978-3-032-21675-5_6

Pharmacology, Pharmacokinetics, and Pharmacodynamics

The mechanism of action of NSAIDs relates to their effects on arachidonic acid (AA) and, thus, the COX pathways [9, 10]. AA is produced from plasma membranes by phospholipids and is metabolized by three enzymatic pathways: COX, lipoxygenase, and cytochrome P-450. COX metabolism of AA produces prostaglandins D_2, E_2, F_{2a}, I_2, and TXA_2, which are synthesized in mast cells, blood vessels, endothelial cells, macrophages, platelets, and the lungs and kidneys [10]. The site of action of these prostaglandins varies but can include the cardiovascular system, lungs, gastrointestinal (GI) tract, kidneys, and other smooth muscles (Table 6.1) [9, 10].

Three COX enzymes have been identified, as they relate to the metabolism of AA [9–11]. COX-1 is constitutively expressed in most cells and is involved in gastric mucosal protection, regulation of acid secretion, renal hemodynamics, and platelet activation and vasoconstriction. COX-2 is induced by inflammatory stimuli, hormones, growth factors, and tumor promoters and is constitutively expressed in tissues of the central nervous system, lungs, and kidneys [9, 11–13]. Thus, COX-2 is known to result in inflammation, pain, and fever [14]. COX-3 is a slice variant of COX-1 and is selectively inhibited by analgesic and antipyretic drugs, such as acetaminophen [9–11].

NSAIDs produce their therapeutic effects mainly via reversible inhibition of prostanoid production, which includes prostaglandins and thromboxanes, thus preventing COX enzymes from metabolizing AA [9, 10]. The beneficial effects of NSAIDs (i.e., antipyretic, anti-inflammatory, and analgesic) are associated with the inhibition of COX-2, as opposed to the inhibition of COX-1 [12, 15]. NSAIDs that are more active against COX-1 generally result in more side effects, especially GI toxicity, than agents that have a higher potency for COX-2 and a better COX-2:COX-1 activity ratio. The use of nonselective NSAIDs (e.g., ibuprofen, indomethacin, and ketorolac) results in the inhibition of COX-2 owing to their therapeutic effects but also produces similar or, possibly, even greater amounts of COX-1 inhibition, thereby increasing the propensity for their deleterious adverse effects [15]. In general, increasing the doses of COX-2 selective agents could also lead to GI toxicity, as they have been shown to also inhibit COX-1. When COX-1 and COX-2 selectivity differ only slightly, additional variables (e.g., dose and half-life) may influence the potential for NSAID toxicity. The propensity for GI toxicity may be further magnified, as many NSAIDs also have a local irritant effect on GI mucosa, independent of their inhibition of COX, resulting from carboxylic acid or acidic enolic group compounds [12, 16]. Also independent of COX activity, NSAIDs can activate mitochondrial oxidative stress (MOS), leading to tissue inflammation and, eventually, the possibility for organ damage [9] (Fig. 6.1).

There had been an effort to design NSAIDs as prodrugs (e.g., sulindac, nabumetone, and salsalate) that would protect the GI tract from local irritation by masking the free acidic groups in NSAID molecules [16]. More recent research has developed several types of prodrugs that are designed to target a more specific activity (e.g., enhancing water solubility and dissolution, nitric oxide release, and hydrogen sulfide release) to diminish NSAID side effects or enhance therapeutic effects [9, 16]. Currently, there are numerous agents in various phases of testing.

NSAIDs are classified by their chemical structure and are more commonly classified based on their ability to inhibit COX-1 and COX-2, as these pathways provide a more general understanding of the safety and efficacy profile of the individual agent (Table 6.2) [9, 18].

NSAIDs are relatively lipid-soluble, weak acids that are highly protein-bound (greater than 90%), primarily to albumin, and widely distributed throughout the body [17, 19]. Any change in protein binding may increase the free drug fraction, thereby increasing the risk of adverse events [17]. NSAIDs mainly have high bioavailability and reach peak plasma concentrations within 2–3 h [9, 17, 19]. Absorption may be delayed by food intake and the utilization of antacids [17]. Topical NSAIDs can achieve high local tissue concentrations without systemic absorption, which results in local inhibition of COX enzymes without the associated adverse effects [14, 17]. NSAIDs are hepatically metabolized and subsequently eliminated in the urine or bile as inactive metabolites [9, 19]. NSAIDs are most commonly metabolized by the cytochrome P-450 system through CYP2C9 [9]. Clearance of NSAIDs in the elderly may be reduced due to changes in hepatic metabolism and may result in elevated plasma levels, especially when using agents with long half-lives [17]. Select NSAIDs, such as naproxen and ketoprofen, bypass the CYP system and are metabolized via glucuronidation or conjugation [9, 17]. There is the potential for metabolites of this metabolic pathway to hydrolyze back to the active form of the drug, thereby prolonging its elimination. NSAIDs have either a quick onset and short half-life (less than 6 h), such as diclofenac and ibuprofen, which are beneficial in acute pain, or a long half-life (greater than 10 h), such as naproxen and celecoxib, which may be more effective for chronic conditions [9, 19].

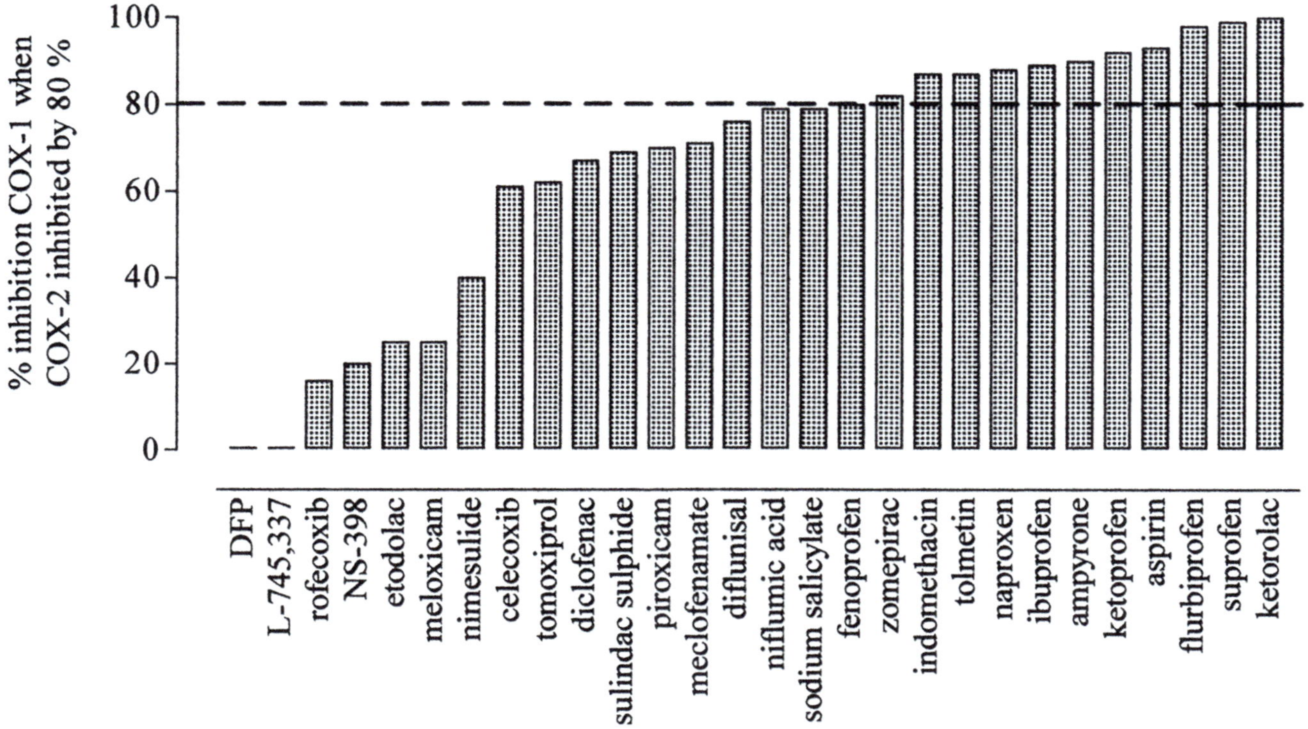

Fig. 6.1 Analysis of the percent inhibition of COX-1 seen when COX-2 human modified whole blood assay (WHMA) is inhibited by 80%. The dotted line indicates equiactivity, i.e., an 80% inhibition of COX-1 [17]

Table 6.1 Pharmacologic activity of prostaglandins produced by arachidonic acid [9, 10]

Prostaglandin	Cardiovascular system	Lungs	GI	Kidneys	Other
D_2	Vasodilator	Bronchoconstriction	–	–	Constricts the pulmonary artery
E_2	Vasodilator	Bronchodilation	Protects the gastric mucosa	Regulates glomerular filtration, renal blood flow, and diuresis in compromised kidneys	Contracts the uterine smooth muscle
F_{2a}		Bronchoconstriction	Protects the gastric mucosa	–	Contracts the uterine smooth muscle
I_2	Vasodilator	Bronchodilation	Protects the gastric mucosa	Regulates glomerular filtration, renal blood flow, and diuresis in compromised kidneys	Anticoagulant properties
TXA_2	Vasoconstrictor	Bronchoconstriction	–	–	Role in platelet aggregation

GI gastrointestinal, *TXA_2* thromboxane A2

Table 6.2 NSAID classification based on chemical structure [9, 18]

Chemical structure	NSAID examples
Salicylic acid derivatives	Aspirin Diflunisal
Propionic acids	Ibuprofen Naproxen
Enolic acids	Meloxicam Piroxicam
Acetic acid derivatives	Indomethacin Diclofenac Ketorolac
Anthranilic acid derivatives	Mefenamic acid
Diarylheterocyclics	Celecoxib

Evidence for Use

Efficacy

General Pain Management

Pain is a common symptom associated with inflammation [20]. The pathophysiologic response to tissue injury triggers the release of pro-inflammatory mediators from damaged cells, which activate primary afferent neurons and lead to a subsequent immune and inflammatory response [21]. This inflammatory response occurs when macrophages release various pro-inflammatory cytokines, resulting in subsequent activation and recruitment of leukocytes to the site of injury [22]. An inflammatory response may also result from different etiologies, which, for example, is observed in various forms of arthritis that result in inflammation of the joint and surrounding tissues [23]. Inflammation in rheumatoid arthritis (RA) occurs from underlying immune reactions, in osteoarthritis (OA) from overuse injury secondary to chronic low-grade inflammation (meta-inflammation), and in bacterial, viral, or fungal septic arthritis from increased cytokines present throughout the body [24]. Despite these differences, all inflammatory responses commonly result in the presence of nociceptive pain [21].

NSAIDs are beneficial in the management of nociceptive pain due to their COX inhibition and subsequent anti-inflammatory response [25]. NSAIDs can be used in both oral and topical formulations for nociceptive pain, with the choice in formulation dependent on the location and extent of the pain. According to a Cochrane Review, NSAIDs offer less substantial benefit in neuropathic pain, as the review failed to demonstrate a significant reduction in neuropathic pain and postherpetic neuralgia [26]. The risk of adverse events, especially with chronic use, coupled with the limited benefit in pain reduction, supports the lack of recommendation for use in this population [27]. In patients with cancer-related pain, NSAIDs have conflicting evidence for use [28]. A Cochrane Review of 11 trials that assessed the use of NSAIDs, with or without opioids, for at least a week in duration, demonstrated reductions in pain scores (i.e., moderate-to-severe-to-mild pain) in just four studies [29]. Further, a systematic review assessing NSAID use in approximately 3000 patients found that NSAIDs were more effective than placebo for pain control, but the addition of NSAIDs to an opioid agent demonstrated minimal improvement in pain scores when compared to either agent alone [30]. Thus, NSAIDs with or without opioids may be considered in mild-to-moderate pain, with a low threshold to stop these agents if adequate pain control is not achieved or adverse events occur [31].

Traditional and COX-2 selective NSAIDs are considered first-line agents in the management of many conditions that result in mild-to-moderate pain, such as musculoskeletal pain, headaches, dental pain, menstrual pain, and arthritis pain, given their availability over the counter and by prescription [25, 32]. In the treatment of non-low back pain, topical NSAIDs have demonstrated reductions in pain within 2 h of use, which were similar to topical anesthetics, oral NSAIDs, and acetaminophen, and also have the benefit of limiting systemic exposure [33]. In patients with more extensive injury or those who prefer to avoid topical therapy, oral NSAIDs with or without acetaminophen have demonstrated reductions in musculoskeletal pain and may also lead to improvements in physical function. NSAIDs alone or as part of a multimodal approach are also recommended as the initial management for dental pain, including that related to surgical tooth extraction [34]. A meta-analysis that assessed pain management after tooth extraction found that NSAIDs were among the most effective agents for reducing pain [35]. Pain-related outcomes were better in the groups receiving NSAIDs with or without acetaminophen when compared to a regimen that utilized opioids. The benefit of NSAIDs for the management of primary dysmenorrhea is substantial, likely related to the withdrawal of progesterone during menstruation, leading to COX-2 activation and a decrease in hydroxyprostaglandin dehydrogenase [32, 36]. Their benefit is supported by a Cochrane Review that showed more substantial reductions in pain with NSAIDs when compared to acetaminophen [37]. While hormonal contraceptives may help with dysmenorrhea, the data and, thus, the indication for use in primary dysmenorrhea are weaker than NSAIDs [36]. They are often reserved for patients who desire concomitant contraception or those with dysmenorrhea caused by endometriosis, in which hormonal contraceptive therapy is first-line.

NSAIDs are commonly used and effective for managing tension-type headaches and migraines of mild-to-moderate severity [38, 39]. Their role in treating tension-type headaches is well-established, with many studies demonstrating significant improvements in pain and quicker time to pain relief when compared to acetaminophen [40]. In migraine management, NSAIDs have demonstrated the greatest benefit and are first-line therapy for those of mild-to-moderate intensity, with migraine-specific agents reserved for more severe or refractory migraines [39, 41, 42]. A Cochrane Review that compared various NSAIDs to placebo showed significant improvements in migraine severity and complete pain relief at 2 h with a number needed to treat of three and seven, respectively [42]. However, not all patients respond adequately to first-line treatments for acute migraine attacks [32, 38]. As a result, many individuals require the addition of a migraine-specific agent to achieve better symptom relief [32, 38].

NSAIDs play a key role in both the acute and chronic management of OA due to its persistent inflammatory state, with higher doses often providing greater relief [43]. To reduce systemic exposure, topical NSAIDs are recommended as the initial management for knee and hand OA, as they have demonstrated similar benefit in pain when compared to oral formulations [44, 45]. In patients where topical NSAIDs are impractical, such as hand OA requiring frequent hand washing or in joints that are too deep below the surface to confer benefit (e.g., the hip), oral NSAIDs may be used and confer a strong recommendation [44]. Incorporation of NSAIDs into a multimodal approach, often in combination with acetaminophen and/or intra-articular injections, has demonstrated significant improvements in pain and functionality [32]. The chronicity of arthritis symptoms in a progressively aging population increases the need for vigilant monitoring of adverse events associated with NSAIDs, with the choice of traditional NSAID or COX-2 inhibitor based on the known side effect profiles [43, 46]. RA is also associated with a chronic state of inflammation; however, NSAIDs are not recommended in the American College of Rheumatology (ACR) guidelines, as they do not modify disease progression, which is a goal of therapy in this disease state [47]. Despite this, several NSAIDs have an FDA-labeled indication for the management of pain in RA, primarily due to their ability to inhibit pro-inflammatory enzymes, which, in turn, leads to the suppression of prostaglandin production [48]. Short-term use for symptomatic management may be considered, but long-term use is not supported, given the risk of adverse effects, most notably GI toxicity [48].

Patients with sickle cell disease have a genetic mutation in the beta-globulin gene on chromosome 11, which results in the formation of a sickled hemoglobin, or hemoglobin S [49]. During an acute pain crisis, also known as a vaso-occlusive event, the deoxygenated sickled hemoglobin obstructs blood flow in small capillaries, causing downstream ischemia and pain. While opioids are commonly used to manage these crises, the addition of a short course of NSAIDs (i.e., 5–7 days) may be considered to reduce pain scores and minimize opioid exposure [49, 50].

The use of NSAIDs in patients experiencing chronic pain from avascular necrosis, a complication often associated with blood disorders and autoimmune diseases like sickle cell disease and RA, remains less well-defined [51]. Celecoxib has demonstrated reductions in pain and improvements in overall functional mobility when compared to placebo; however, long-term use has been associated with an increased risk of gastrointestinal toxicity [52]. Thus, NSAIDs are not recommended for monotherapy in this population but may be incorporated into a comprehensive pain management plan if the benefits outweigh the risks [51].

Perioperative Pain Management

Enhanced Recovery After Surgery (ERAS) is a society that has created various surgical guidelines that aim to address and mitigate perioperative complications through the utilization of multiple pre-, intra-, and postoperative interventions [53, 54]. One such complication includes postoperative pain, which is often multifactorial and has historically been managed with opioids [55–57]. The risk of misuse and dependence, coupled with the undesirable dose-related side effects, supports minimizing the use of these agents in the postoperative setting [57, 58]. As a result, a key component of the ERAS protocols is the implementation of a multimodal, opioid-sparing pain management plan [53, 59–61]. This approach utilizes multiple agents and techniques targeting different pain pathways to create a synergistic approach for pain management in an effort to improve postoperative pain control while reducing opioid consumption [55, 60]. NSAIDs are among the drug classes commonly utilized in the perioperative setting to achieve these goals [55, 62].

Recommendations for preoperative, as opposed to postoperative, NSAID use are not observed as frequently in the ERAS guidelines, given the ongoing debate regarding their efficacy [59, 63]. Many studies have demonstrated the benefits of preoperative traditional NSAID and COX-2 inhibitor use, often in combination with gabapentinoids and acetaminophen, in the reduction in pain scores, opioid use, time to medication redosing, and, in some cases, hospital length of stay [56, 63–70]. In contrast, a systematic review and meta-analysis of 80 randomized trials, 20 of which included NSAIDs, demonstrated that preemptive analgesia use leads to improvements in postoperative pain in just 24 trials [71]. These findings, coupled with the concern for postoperative acute kidney injury (AKI), may be factors limiting preoperative NSAID use [66, 68]. If utilized, the choice of NSAID and dosage should consider patient-specific factors, including comorbidities and a risk for adverse effects, with COX-2 inhibitors generally conferring a lower bleeding risk [56, 60, 61, 72]. Benefits of administration include ease of administration and cost-effectiveness, as they are given as a one-time preoperative dose [56, 59, 63].

Traditional and COX-2 selective NSAIDs are becoming one of the cornerstone medication classes used postoperatively [58]. NSAIDs have demonstrated superiority when compared to acetaminophen monotherapy in reducing pain scores and time to re-medication, with the benefits even more pronounced when given in combination with other non-opioid pain medications as part of a multimodal pain approach [73, 74]. While no specific NSAID regimen has been universally established, the choice of NSAID, route of administration, timing of initiation, and frequency of administration (i.e., scheduled or as needed) should be tailored to patient- and procedure-related factors [75, 76]. Procedure-related considerations include the type of surgery and its associated risks, while patient-related factors include the ability to tolerate oral medications and the presence of comorbidities that increase the risk of AKI, gastrointestinal bleeding (GIB), or surgical site bleeding [59, 64, 68, 77]. In high-risk patients, such as the elderly, those with preexisting kidney disease, prior significant bleeding, and hypovolemic patients, delaying NSAID initiation until it has been determined that renal function is not impaired may be preferred [64, 77]. Outside of these high-risk groups, initiation of NSAIDs can be done as soon as 6 h postoperatively, with many scheduled regimens started by postoperative day one [58, 78, 79]. In general, the use of scheduled NSAIDs, barring any contraindications, may be the preferred regimen, given the beneficial opioid-sparing and pain-reducing effects [54, 64, 80].

Bleeding risk is a potential concern with NSAID use, but in the perioperative setting, short-term administration is generally well-accepted [81, 82]. Delaying NSAID initiation out of concern for bleeding is not routinely recommended [60, 62, 77, 83]. Further, the risk of anastomotic leakage with NSAID use in gastrointestinal-related surgeries has not been supported in recent literature [81, 82]. If bleeding is a concern, COX-2 inhibitors may be preferred as they have no effect on platelet aggregation and, therefore, confer a lower bleeding risk when compared to traditional NSAIDs. However, this benefit should be weighed against the potential risk of serious cardiovascular thrombotic events in patients with preexisting cardiovascular disease [55, 56, 72, 74].

While newer ERAS guidelines support the use of NSAIDs in the perioperative setting, patient- and procedure-related factors should be considered [75, 76]. Many guidelines either do not address or do not support the use of NSAIDs in the perioperative setting due to medication-related concerns; however, clinical implications for these agents are increasing [53, 65, 84, 85]. Literature supporting the use of NSAIDs perioperatively is ever-evolving, with future ERAS guidelines being subject to change based on these findings. The implications for short-term use of NSAIDs can be substantial and provide benefit to both the patient and health system, especially with appropriate patient selection [60, 61, 80].

Safety

Though NSAIDs have been shown to decrease pain scores and opioid consumption, consideration for patient safety is also imperative.

Bleeding

NSAIDs increase the risk of gastrointestinal bleeding (GIB), particularly upper GIB, due to their local irritant effects on the mucosa and inhibition of COX-1 [16, 86]. This inhibition reduces protective prostaglandin E2 and prostacyclin I2, which normally help by decreasing gastric acid secretion, enhancing mucosal blood flow, and promoting the release of viscous mucus [16, 86]. There is an increased risk of upper GIB with all NSAIDs, but nonselective NSAIDs have a higher incidence risk ratio compared to COX-2 selective NSAIDs. The risk of upper GIB increases substantially with combinations of medications, the highest being with corticosteroids, aldosterone antagonists, and anticoagulants [87]. A variety of gastroprotective agents can be used to decrease the risk of bleeding while using NSAIDs [88, 89]. These include proton pump inhibitors, histamine-2-receptor antagonists, and misoprostol. These agents should be considered as adjunctive therapy in patients who have a history of upper GIB while on an NSAID or who are at high risk for bleeding.

Cardiovascular Risk

The cardiovascular impact of NSAIDs may be based on the balance of COX-1 and COX-2 inhibition, though all NSAIDs carry a risk [3, 90]. COX-1 is constitutively expressed on platelets and leads to the formation of TXA_2, which leads to platelet aggregation [1]. The inhibition of COX-1 prevents the formation of TXA_2 and decreases platelet aggregation, which is the primary utilization of aspirin in patients with cardiovascular disease [3]. On the other hand, COX-2 catalyzes the production of PGI2, which is anti-aggregatory and vasodilatory, and thus, the inhibition of COX-2 can lead to a prothrombotic state and vasoconstriction. It has been clearly shown that there is a link between COX-2 inhibition and an increase in cardiovascular risk, which was the reason that rofecoxib (Vioxx®) was taken off the market [6–8]. The data for nonselective NSAIDs is not as robust, but all NSAIDs do carry the labeled warning of cardiovascular events, and it is prudent to avoid NSAIDs in patients at risk for or with cardiovascular disease [7, 91–94]. A meta-analysis including 446,763 patients receiving celecoxib, diclofenac, ibuprofen, celecoxib, and rofecoxib determined that all NSAIDs are associated with a risk of acute myocardial infarction despite their specificity and that the risk is greatest for those taking higher doses and within 1 month of therapy [90].

Acute Kidney Injury

COX-1 and COX-2 are constitutively expressed in the kidneys and help modulate renal blood flow, inhibit sodium reabsorption, promote diuresis through blunting of antidiuretic hormone (ADH), and stimulate renin release [95–98]. Inhibition of COX, by either traditional NSAIDs or COX-2 selective inhibitors, can thereby increase the risk of developing a hemodynamically mediated AKI and the associated fluid and electrolyte abnormalities [99–101]. Through similar mechanisms, NSAIDs may also increase the risk of acute interstitial nephritis (AIN); however, the absolute risk is quite low and most commonly occurs weeks to months after the initial NSAID exposure [102, 103]. Patients deemed to be at the highest risk of such complications include those with exposure to high cumulative doses and use of interacting medications such as renin–angiotensin–aldosterone system (RAAS) inhibitors, diuretics, or concurrent vasoconstrictors (i.e., calcineurin inhibitors) and the elderly due to predisposition to electrolyte abnormalities and advancement in chronic kidney disease (CKD) from loss of renal reserve [99, 104–106]. Depletion in true and effective circulating blood volume may also be a predisposing factor, which can be observed in those with excessive volume loss or poor oral intake, nephrotic syndrome, cirrhosis, congestive heart failure, or hypoalbuminemia.

The possible life-threatening risks associated with an NSAID-induced AKI are related to volume overload and electrolyte abnormalities [99]. Hypervolemia and hyponatremia occur as a result of inhibition of the natriuretic effects of prostaglandins and amplification of ADH and RAAS activation, especially in those prone to fluid retention and with advanced CKD [107–109]. Sodium and fluid retention, coupled by a decrease in NSAID-associated renin production, increases blood pressure by an average of 3–6 mmHg and may render some antihypertensive classes less effective, including thiazide diuretics, angiotensin-converting enzyme inhibitors (ACEi), and angiotensin receptor blockers (ARBs) [99, 110–112]. Hyperkalemia results from a deficiency in prostaglandin-mediated renin release, resulting in hypoaldosteronism and, therefore, a reduction in potassium excretion [99, 113]. Given these risks, NSAIDs should be used with caution in patients with CKD [99].

In the early stages of CKD, short- and long-term NSAIDs use can be considered in the absence of risk factors for complications [99]. Patients with Stage 4 and 5 CKD, in the absence of kidney replacement therapy, are at a greater risk of NSAID-related complications, especially hyperkalemia, and use should be considered with great caution. Topical NSAID use may mitigate the risk of NSAID-related renal complications; however, increased monitoring is still necessary [99, 114].

Hypersensitivity Reactions

NSAIDs are a common cause of medication-induced hypersensitivity reactions, classified based on timing (early vs. delayed), type (respiratory, cutaneous, or urticaria/angioedema), and phenotype (single- vs. multiple-NSAID-induced) [115, 116]. Due to this variability, managing NSAID hypersensitivity is complex and requires a structured, stepwise approach [115].

Aspirin is linked to hypersensitivity in patients with upper and lower respiratory conditions, known as aspirin-exacerbated respiratory disease (AERD) [115]. This reaction is primarily due to COX-1 inhibition and, thus, a reduction in prostaglandins [115, 116]. Symptoms typically occur within 30–120 min, with higher risk in individuals with respiratory diseases, high NSAID doses, or the use of strong COX-1 inhibitors (2011, 2019). In contrast, weaker COX-1 inhibitors and COX-2 selective agents have a lower risk and are often well-tolerated in patients with single- and multiple-NSAID-induced reactions [115, 116]. Patients with hypersensitivity to a COX-1 selective NSAID should avoid other strong COX-1 inhibitors and those with a similar chemical structure, while COX-2 inhibitors or alternative medications may be trialed under careful monitoring [115, 116]. If strong COX-1 inhibitors are necessary, desensitization is recommended [115].

NSAID-induced urticaria and angioedema can appear within minutes to 24 h after ingestion, with urticaria more common in adults and angioedema in children [116]. Owing to a similar proposed mechanism for reaction, management follows the same approach as respiratory reactions [115]. If NSAID-induced urticaria/angioedema is suspected but not definitive, skin testing is advised before reintroducing agents with a similar chemical structure and COX-1 potency [116]. Anaphylactic reactions, though rare, are usually linked to a single NSAID and are thought to be Immunoglubulin E (IgE)-mediated [115, 116]. NSAIDs with similar chemical structures should be avoided [115]. Non-cross-reactivity can be confirmed by administering aspirin or an unrelated NSAID at a reduced dose under close surveillance [116].

Delayed reactions to NSAIDs, occurring over 24 h after exposure, range from cutaneous to systemic reactions (e.g., fixed drug eruptions, severe bullous reactions, maculopapular drug eruptions, aseptic meningitis, pneumonitis, nephritis, and contact dermatitis) [115, 117]. These type IV, T-cell-mediated reactions can occur with both COX-1 and COX-2 inhibitors [117]. Due to structural differences, aspirin may be a viable alternative if clinically indicated [117]. However, due to limited evidence, avoiding all NSAIDs is recommended regardless of the initial agent's chemical structure or COX selectivity [117].

Other Adverse Effects

Elevations in liver tests (LTs) can occur with NSAID use as a result of idiosyncratic mitochondrial dysfunction, with diclofenac and sulindac carrying the greatest risk [118]. In rare cases, severe and sometimes fatal cases of hepatic injury have occurred, including fulminant hepatitis, liver necrosis, and hepatic failure [94, 118]. Periodic assessment of LTs is warranted with chronic NSAID use, with cessation of therapy once LTs reach three times the upper limit of normal [118].

NSAID-related hypersensitivity reactions are uncommon and are thought to result from prostaglandin inhibition and the subsequent production of mast cells, basophils, and eosinophils [119, 120]. In patients with aspirin-sensitive asthma, there is a risk of cross-reactivity with NSAIDs, and therefore, their use may trigger possibly fatal bronchospasms [7, 94, 120]. Other hypersensitivity reactions may include rash and urticaria, as well as IgE-mediated reactions such as erythema multiforme, exfoliative dermatitis, Stevens–Johnson syndrome (SJS), toxic epidermal necrolysis (TEN), and drug reaction with eosinophilia and systemic symptoms

(DRESS) [7, 94, 119]. Patients who develop such reactions should not be rechallenged with any NSAID, given the risk of cross-reactivity [7, 94, 119, 120].

Special Populations

Pregnancy

There is limited data demonstrating the safety and tolerability of NSAIDs in pregnant women, with a majority of data coming from animal studies. Animal studies have demonstrated negative implications of supratherapeutic doses of NSAIDs on organogenesis; however, these effects have not been reproducible at therapeutic or subtherapeutic doses [94, 116]. NSAIDs may result in low amniotic fluid starting at 20 weeks' gestation, which resulted in the FDA issuing a warning surrounding their use [121]. Starting at 30 weeks' gestation, NSAIDs may increase the risk of premature closure of the fetal ductus arteriosus, significantly limiting their utility during this time period [116]. The use of NSAIDs up to 20 weeks' gestation should be considered only if the benefits outweigh risks, with use avoided thereafter, given the risk of fetal toxicity.

Postpartum

NSAIDs are often utilized as part of a multimodal pain management approach in postpartum care following vaginal and caesarean delivery [122]. The American College of Obstetrics and Gynecologists (ACOG) recommended scheduled use of acetaminophen and ibuprofen for pain management, independent of the route of delivery. Prior recommendations to avoid NSAIDs in patients with postpartum hypertension are no longer supported, as recent studies have failed to demonstrate a clear correlation between NSAID exposure and persistent hypertension [123, 124].

Breastfeeding

NSAIDs may be found in breast milk bound to milk proteins at low concentrations [122]. The relative infant dose (RID) of NSAIDs is often less than 1%, suggesting that infant exposure is low [125]. Despite their presence in breast milk, the ACOG recommends ibuprofen as one of the first-line analgesics for breastfeeding women [122, 126]. In the immediate postoperative period, oral or parenteral ketorolac may also be considered [122, 127, 128]. These recommendations should always be coupled with an assessment of the benefit of using these agents against the potential harm to the breastfeeding infant [7, 122].

Pediatrics

NSAIDs are commonly utilized in the pediatric population for acute conditions, given their beneficial effects in reducing pain, inflammation, and fever [129]. Additionally, children with juvenile idiopathic arthritis (JIA) may benefit from NSAID use; however, the ACR recommends only a short trial as initial monotherapy based on a low level of evidence, given that only a small portion of patients will respond to their use [130, 131]. Routine use in patients with JIA who are less than 2 years of age is not routinely recommended, given a lack of safety data [91, 94].

Despite their widespread use for acute and chronic conditions, clinical trial data evaluating the short- and long-term safety and tolerability is limited [132]. Traditional NSAIDs still carry the risk of renal, gastrointestinal, cardiovascular, and hematologic adverse effects, with COX-2 inhibitors carrying an even greater risk of cardiotoxicity. Additionally, salicylate use is not recommended due to the potential risk of Reye's syndrome, a rare but serious and potentially fatal condition. To minimize risks, NSAID treatment should always start at the lowest age- and weight-appropriate dose and be used for the shortest duration necessary [129]. If chronic therapy is warranted, frequent monitoring for adverse events is necessary.

Advanced Age

NSAIDs are commonly used in geriatric patients for the acute and chronic management of pain and inflammation [133]. Physiologic changes related to aging, coupled with drug interactions and the patient's comorbid conditions, may predispose geriatric patients to a greater risk of NSAID-related adverse events, most notably renal, gastrointestinal, and cardiovascular toxicities [134, 135]. The loss of renal reserve, advancement of CKD, and decreased circulating blood volume increase the risk of AKI and its subsequent volume- and electrolyte-related complications [99, 134]. Gastrointestinal toxicities increase in severity and frequency as patients age, with the risk often being related to cumulative exposure [134, 135]. The labeled warning for cardiovascular events applies to all patient populations; however, a history of cardiovascular or cerebrovascular events is more common in the geriatric population, thereby predisposing patients to further events [7, 91–94, 134, 135]. Other complications related to NSAID use include an increased risk of falls and psychiatric events, including psychosis, agitation, delirium, and hallucinations, likely related to alterations in prostaglandin presence in the central nervous system [135]. It is imperative to consider these factors and weigh the benefits and risks of use when selecting a traditional NSAID or COX-2 inhibitor. All NSAIDs should be used at the lowest effective dose and for the shortest duration possible, with careful monitoring for toxicities [134, 135].

Drug Interactions

NSAIDs interact with many commonly used medications as a result of both pharmacokinetic and pharmacodynamic interactions [136]. Celecoxib is a substrate of CYP2C9 and an inhibitor of CYP2D6 [137]. Close monitoring of inducers, inhibitors, and substrates of these pathways is warranted with concomitant administration.

Concomitant use of NSAIDs with other medications that alter hemostasis, such as anticoagulants, antiplatelets, selective serotonin reuptake inhibitors (SSRIs), and serotonin norepinephrine reuptake inhibitors (SNRIs), can predispose patients to bleeding [136]. Concomitant aspirin use may not only increase bleeding risk, but use with certain NSAIDs, such as ibuprofen, can block the antiplatelet effects of aspirin [136, 138]. If patients require the use of aspirin for cardiovascular protection, concomitant ibuprofen or COX-2 inhibitor use is not recommended [139].

The therapeutic effects of many antihypertensive drug classes, including thiazide diuretics, ACEi, and ARBs, may be diminished with concomitant NSAID use, given the sodium and fluid retention, coupled with increased renin production [99, 136]. Close monitoring of blood pressure and renal function is warranted if used concomitantly, especially in patients with a predisposition to renal injury [136].

The risk of GI toxicities may be increased and, therefore, warrants close monitoring when NSAIDs and COX-2 inhibitors are used in combination with salicylates, corticosteroids, and alcohol [136, 140]. Other serious drug interactions include lithium, methotrexate, cyclosporine, pemetrexed, and digoxin [136]. Increased concentrations and/or decreased clearance of these agents may result in drug toxicities related to the specific agent being utilized. The risk of toxicities is greater with prescription-strength NSAIDs; however, close monitoring for toxicities with all doses is still necessary.

Applications to Clinical Practice

Traditional NSAIDs and COX-2 inhibitors, in both systemic and topical formulations, are indicated for many acute and chronic conditions that result in pain [25, 32]. Their place in therapy, whether it be first- or second-line or as monotherapy or part of an adjunctive analgesia approach, depends on the indication in which it is being utilized (Table 6.3) [28, 31, 34, 36, 39, 41, 44, 51, 141–146]. In addition to their role in general pain management, NSAIDs are becoming key components in the perioperative setting, often used in combination with other non-opioid analgesics (Table 6.4) [58]. Surgery-specific ERAS guidelines highlight the nuances for use in both the pre- and postoperative setting. In general, most guidelines do not delineate a specific NSAID that is preferred for acute and/or chronic pain management [147]. Thus, the choice of NSAID

Table 6.3 NSAID's place in therapy based on condition [27, 28, 31, 34, 36, 39, 41, 44, 47, 51, 141–146]

Condition	Place in therapy
Musculoskeletal pain	Topical NSAIDs, with or without menthol gel, should be used as first-line therapy for adults with acute pain from non–low back, musculoskeletal injuries Oral NSAIDs may be considered as alternative options for pharmacologic treatment for adults with acute pain from non–low back, musculoskeletal injuries
Low back pain	Oral NSAIDs are the first-line pharmacologic therapy for patients with acute and chronic low back pain
Dysmenorrhea	Oral NSAIDs are the first-line pharmacologic therapy for dysmenorrhea not associated with endometriosis. Use is recommended on a fixed schedule, starting 1–2 days before the anticipated onset of menses and continued for 2–3 days
Dental pain	Oral NSAIDs, with or without concomitant APAP, are recommended first-line for dental pain and pain associated with surgical tooth extraction
Neuropathic pain	Not included in guideline recommendations
Headaches	NSAIDs are one of the many first-line agents for the acute treatment of mild-to-moderate migraines. NSAIDs with the greatest efficacy include celecoxib, diclofenac, ibuprofen, and naproxen Parenteral NSAIDs may be considered for migraines refractory to a triptan NSAIDs, specifically ibuprofen, are one of the first-line treatments for acute tension-type headaches
Osteoarthritis	Topical NSAIDs are strongly recommended as the first-line pharmacological approach for knee OA and conditionally recommended for hand OA, and use should be considered prior to oral NSAIDs Oral NSAIDs are strongly recommended as a first-line pharmacologic approach for hand, knee, and hip OA
Rheumatoid arthritis	Not included in guideline recommendations
Sickle cell disease	For acute pain, guidelines suggest a short course (i.e., 5–7 days) of NSAIDs, in addition to opioids, for acute pain management as a low-level recommendation For chronic pain due to sickle cell disease–related avascular necrosis of bone, guidelines offer a low-level recommendation for using NSAIDs as a management option for adults within a comprehensive disease and pain management plan. No recommendation is provided for children
Cancer-related pain	NSAIDs may be considered one of the first-line agents for mild-to-moderate pain, either as monotherapy or in addition to adjuvant analgesics or opioids, after considering the risks associated with their use and patient comorbidities
Perioperative pain	See individual guidelines for specific recommendations. NSAIDs are often incorporated as part of a multimodal, opioid-sparing pain approach

NSAID nonsteroidal anti-inflammatory drug, *APAP* acetaminophen, *OA* osteoarthritis, *SCD* sickle cell disease

Table 6.4 ERAS guideline recommendations for NSAID utilization in the perioperative setting [53, 54, 56, 59–69, 75–77, 80, 83–85, 141, 147, 164–168]

ERAS guideline	Preoperative recommendation(s)	Postoperative recommendation(s)	Considerations for use
Guidelines supporting NSAID utilization			
Gastrointestinal surgery Bariatric surgery Breast reconstitution Elective colorectal surgery Cytoreductive surgery Emergency laparotomy Gynecologic oncology Vulvar and vaginal surgery Major head and neck cancer surgery with free flap reconstitution Liver surgery Elective abdominal and pelvic surgery Lumbar spinal fusion Caesarean delivery Esophagectomy Total hip and knee Replacement surgery Pancreatoduodenectomy Lung surgery Radical cystectomy for Bladder cancer Lower-extremity vascular bypasses Open aortic vascular surgery	One-time dose of an NSAID or COX-2i as part of a multimodal approach may be considered in select surgeries NSAIDs are not recommended in emergency laparotomy or liver surgery, given the risk of kidney injury	Initiate a multimodal approach that includes NSAIDs, either IV or PO Limited recommendations exist on the preferred frequency of administration (i.e., scheduled or as needed) In select surgeries (e.g., emergency laparotomy, esophagectomy, and pancreatoduodenectomy), consider delaying NSAID initiation until it has been determined that renal function is not impaired and the risk of bleeding has passed	COX-2i may reduce the risk of surgical site and GI bleeding; however, caution should be exercised in those with a history of CV events Avoid inappropriate use in patients with preexisting kidney disease or a predisposition to bleeding events The literature is inconclusive on avoiding NSAIDs, given the risk of anastomotic leakage after GI surgeries. Risk of anastomotic leakage is the greatest with diclofenac and nonselective NSAIDs and a duration of use of ≥3 days
Guidelines not supporting/recognizing NSAID utilization			
Cardiac surgery Gastrectomy Liver transplantation Neonatal intestinal surgery	No recommendations provided regarding NSAID use	No recommendations provided regarding NSAID use, given the associated risk	RCTs and retrospective studies exist to support NSAID use in select patients (e.g., cardiac surgery). If utilized, consider the risk profile of the individual agent

NSAIDs nonsteroidal anti-inflammatory drugs, *COX-2i* cyclooxygenase-2 inhibitors, *IV* intravenous, *PO* oral, *CV* cardiovascular, *GI* gastrointestinal, *HIPEC* hyperthermic intraperitoneal chemotherapy, *RCT* randomized controlled trial

should be based on patient- and disease-specific considerations as well as the known adverse effect profile of the NSAID, which is attributed to its COX selectivity [25].

The availability of NSAIDs, whether over the counter or by prescription, varies depending on the specific drug, as well as its dosage and formulation (Table 6.5) [148, 149]. Dosing of NSAIDs, for both initial and maintenance doses, should always occur at the lowest effective dose needed to maintain effective pain control [129]. Many indications for which NSAIDs may be used do not outline specific dosing recommendations, and therefore, dosing should follow that outlined in the package insert for the individual agent (Table 6.5) [7, 91–94, 150–162]. NSAIDs have a well-documented ceiling effect [163]. This is a dose at which the maximal analgesic effect is achieved, and increasing the dose beyond this level does not achieve additional analgesic benefit but can increase the risk of adverse effects [163]. Most literature documenting the ceiling effect of NSAIDs is found in acute pain management in the emergency department using ketorolac and ibuprofen [163]. Compared to other NSAIDs, ketorolac has the highest dose-related adverse effect profile [163]. This is due in part to the fact that ketorolac has the highest COX-1 selectivity of any NSAID, increasing its likelihood of toxicity to the gastrointestinal mucosa by fivefold [163]. Comparative studies suggest that low-dose ketorolac (10–15 mg of parenteral ketorolac) is as effective as higher doses such as 30 mg [163]. As such, the American Academy of Emergency Medicine recommends NSAID administration at the lowest effective dose [163].

Drug interactions, as well as an individual patient's propensity for adverse effects, should always be considered when selecting and dosing these agents, both for general and perioperative pain [75]. Higher cumulative doses, advanced age, and decreased effective circulating blood volume are all conditions that should necessitate lower starting doses and vigilant monitoring for NSAID-related adverse effects, both with acute and chronic use. Utilizing NSAIDs as part of an opioid-sparing, multimodal approach may have the ability to maximize pain relief while minimizing adverse effects from individual agents [99, 104–106]. These considerations, in addition to the benefits and risks of use, should always be discussed with the patient before initiating therapy.

Table 6.5 NSAID dosing considerations [7, 91–94, 148–162]

NSAID	Prescription status	Dosing[a]	Clinical pearls
Nonselective			
Diclofenac	Systemic products available by prescription only Topical products available by prescription and OTC	Systemic: Diclofenac potassium or sodium formulations. *Acute pain/OA/RA*: 100–150 mg per day given in two to four divided doses. MDD: 150 mg. Diclofenac acid: *OA*: 18–35 mg three times daily. MDD: 105 mg. Topical: *Acute pain.* Patch 1.3%: Apply one patch once (Licart®) or twice (Flector®) daily to the most painful area. *OA (lower extremity).* Gel: Apply 4 g to each affected area up to four times daily. Maximum dose per joint: 16 g/day; maximum total body dose (all combined joints): 32 g/day. Solution 1.5%: Apply 40 drops to each affected knee up to four times daily. Solution 2%: Apply 40 mg (two pump actuations) to each affected knee up to twice daily. *OA (upper extremity).* Gel: Apply 2 g to each affected area up to four times daily; maximum dose per joint: 8 g/day; maximum total body dose (all combined joints): 32 g/day.	Available as topical and systemic preparations Monotherapy or adjunctive agent for acute pain Solution application: Apply ten drops at a time, rub in evenly, then apply ten more drops until a total of 40 drops has been applied Oral: Metabolized via CYP2C9
Diflunisal	Prescription-only	*OA/RA/mild-to-moderate pain*: 500–1000 mg every 12 h MDD: 1500 mg	Utilized for acute and chronic pain Tablets should not be crushed
Etodolac	Prescription-only	*OA/RA*: 400 mg twice daily, 300 mg two or three times daily, or 500 mg twice daily *Acute pain*: 200–400 mg every 6–8 h MDD: 1000 mg	Utilized for acute and chronic pain Available as extended release
Fenoprofen	Prescription-only	*Mild-to-moderate pain*: 200 mg every 4–6 h *OA/RA*: 400–600 mg three or four times daily MDD: 3200 mg	Utilized for acute and chronic pain
Flurbiprofen	Prescription-only	*Acute pain*: 150–300 mg per day in three or four divided doses *OA/RA*: 200–300 mg per day in two to four divided doses Maximum dose: 100 mg per dose	Available as an ophthalmic solution for intraoperative miosis prevention Utilized for acute and chronic pain
Ibuprofen	Available OTC, also available in alternative prescription-only strengths	*Acute/chronic pain*: 200–400 mg every 4–6 h as needed or 600–800 mg every 6–8 h as needed *Migraine (acute)*: 400–600 mg once *Dysmenorrhea*: 400 mg every 4 h as needed or 600–800 mg every 6–8 h as needed MDD: 3200 mg initially; 2400 mg with chronic use	Limit to less than or equal to 14 days per month for migraine treatment to avoid medication-overuse headache OTC MDD is 1200 mg per day; use for >10 days is not recommended unless directed by a healthcare provider
Indomethacin	Prescription-only	*Acute pain*: 20 mg three times daily or 40 mg two or three times daily *OA/RA*: IR: 25 mg two or three times daily, may be increased at weekly intervals. ER: 75 mg once daily. MDD: 100–200 mg, depending on indication	Several other indications for use, such as pericarditis, ankylosing spondylitis, and tendonitis Utilized for acute and chronic pain

(continued)

Table 6.5 (continued)

NSAID	Prescription status	Dosing[a]	Clinical pearls
Ketorolac	Prescription-only	*Pain*: ≥50 kg and <65 years of age: IV: 30 mg once or 15–30 mg every 6 h as needed. IM: 30–60 mg once or 15–30 mg every 6 h as needed. Oral: 20 mg once, followed by 10 mg every 4–6 h as needed. <50 kg or ≥65 years of age: IV: 15 mg once or 15 mg every 6 h as needed. IM: 30 mg once or 15 mg every 6 h as needed. Oral: 10 mg every 4–6 h as needed. *Migraine (acute):* ≥50 kg and <65 years of age: IV: 30 mg once. IM: 60 mg once. <50 kg or ≥65 years of age: IV: 15 mg once. IM: 30 mg once. MDD: IV/IM: 120 mg unless weight <50 kg or age ≥65, then 60 mg daily. Oral: 40 mg.	Maximum of 5 days of combined treatment (IV/IM/PO) Available parenterally for IV or IM administration Weight- and age-based dose adjustments are recommended Oral formulation is not an indication for minor or chronic conditions
Mefenamic acid	Prescription-only	*Pain or primary dysmenorrhea*: 500 mg initially, then 250 mg every 6 h as needed *Dysmenorrhea:* 500 mg three times daily MDD: 1500 mg	Not to exceed 3 days for dysmenorrhea or 7 days for mild-to-moderate pain Not recommended for use in patients less than 14 years of age
Meloxicam	Prescription-only	*OA/RA*: Capsule (OA only): 5 mg once daily; may increase to 10 mg once daily. Suspension: 7.5 mg once daily; may increase to 15 mg once daily. Tablet: 7.5 mg once daily; may increase to 15 mg once daily. *Acute pain*: 30 mg IV daily MDD (oral): 10–15 mg depending on formulation	Utilized for acute and chronic pain
Naproxen	Available OTC, also available in alternative prescription-only strengths	*Acute/chronic pain*: IR: 500 mg once, then 250–500 mg every 12 h as needed or 250 mg every 6–8 h as needed. ER: 1000 mg once daily. OTC: 200–400 mg once, then 200 mg every 8–12 h as needed. *Migraine (acute):* IR: 500–750 mg once. *Dysmenorrhea:* IR: 500 mg once beginning at menses onset or 1–2 days prior, then 500 mg every 12 h or 250 mg every 6–8 h as needed. ER: 1000 mg once daily as needed. MDD: IR: 1250 mg on day 1, then 1000 mg on subsequent days. ER: 1500 mg. OTC: 400 mg in any 8–12-h period or 600 mg in a 24-h period.	Limit to less than or equal to 14 days per month for migraine treatment to avoid medication-overuse headache Utilized for acute and chronic pain
Oxaprozin	Prescription-only	*OA/RA*: 1200 mg (to 1800 mg for tablets) once daily MDD: <50 kg: 1200 mg ≥to 50 kg: 1200 mg (capsules) to 1800 mg (tablets)	Utilized for acute and chronic pain

(continued)

Table 6.5 (continued)

NSAID	Prescription status	Dosing[a]	Clinical pearls
Piroxicam	Prescription-only	*OA/RA*: 20 mg once daily MDD: 20 mg	Utilized for acute and chronic pain
Sulindac	Prescription-only	*OA/RA*: 150 mg twice daily MDD: 400 mg	Utilized for acute and chronic pain Utilized for other indications, including gout, tendonitis, and ankylosing spondylitis
Tolmetin	Prescription-only	*OA/RA*: 400 mg three times daily, may increase to 600 mg three times daily MDD: 1800 mg	Utilized for acute and chronic pain
Selective			
Celecoxib	Prescription-only	*Migraine (acute)*: 120 mg once *OA*: 200 mg per day in one or two divided doses, may increase to 400 mg per day *Pain (acute)*: 400 mg followed by 200 mg 12 h later, then 200 mg twice daily as needed *Pain (chronic)*: 200 mg once daily or 100–200 mg twice daily as needed MDD: Migraine: 120 mg. OA/pain: 400 mg.	Limit to less than or equal to 14 days per month for migraine treatment to avoid medication-overuse headache

NSAID nonsteroidal anti-inflammatory drug, *OTC* over the counter, *OA* osteoarthritis, *RA* rheumatoid arthritis, *MDD* maximum daily dose, *IR* immediate release, *ER* extended release, *IV* intravenous, *IM* intramuscular, *PO* oral

[a]Off-label dosing for pain indications is not included

Key Themes

- NSAIDs reduce pain and inflammation, making them suitable agents for common pain-related disease states, with their use also becoming more prevalent in the perioperative setting, given their opioid-sparing effects.
- NSAIDs are first-line for many types of pain and should be used with adjunctive analgesics, when possible, as part of a multimodal pain approach with an overall goal of reducing pain and opioid exposure.
- The beneficial effects of NSAIDs on inflammation are a result of cyclooxygenase (COX) inhibition; however, the COX selectivity can also predict possible adverse effects with nonselective inhibitors owing to a greater risk of GI bleeding and acute kidney injury and COX-2 inhibitors owing to a greater risk of cardiovascular events.
- The starting and maintenance doses of NSAIDs should always consider the patient's age, comorbidities, and organ dysfunction while also using the lowest dose needed for effective pain control to minimize the risk of adverse events associated with their use.
- All NSAIDs have a ceiling effect at which increasing the dose does not achieve additional analgesic benefit but can increase the risk of adverse effects.

Conclusions

NSAIDs are a heterogeneous class of medications that have implications in the management of many acute and chronic pain-related conditions. Their benefit in reducing pain and inflammation relates to their inhibition of COX-1 and/or COX-2; however, the selectivity of the agent may also be useful in predicting possible adverse effects, such as acute renal failure and gastrointestinal bleeding, with more nonselective agents and cardiovascular events with more COX-2 selective agents. The role of both traditional NSAIDs and COX-2 inhibitors in the management of general pain, such as musculoskeletal pain, dysmenorrhea, osteoarthritis, headaches, and dental pain, has been well-defined in literature. In the perioperative setting, NSAIDs are being utilized at an increasing frequency, both pre- and postoperatively, given their beneficial effects on reducing pain intensity and opioid utilization. Utilization of NSAIDs as part of a holistic, multimodal approach to pain management could have the benefits of maximizing pain relief while minimizing risks associated with the individual agents. The choice of agent and dose utilized, regardless of pain indication, should take into consideration the adverse effect profile of the NSAID, as it relates to the COX selectivity as well as patient- and indication-specific considerations that may increase the propensity for adverse effects. Therefore, it is imperative to consider the risks and benefits any time an NSAID is utilized for pain or inflammation related to an acute or chronic condition in an effort to increase patient satisfaction regarding their pain.

References

1. Schaffer D, Florin T, Eagle C, et al. Risk of serious NSAID-related gastrointestinal events during long-term exposure: a systematic review. Med J Aust. 2006;185:501–6. https://doi.org/10.5694/j.1326-5377.2006.tb00665.x.
2. Tamblyn R, Berkson L, Dauphinee WD, et al. Unnecessary prescribing of NSAIDs and the management of NSAID-related gastropathy in medical practice. Ann Intern Med. 1997;127:429–38. https://doi.org/10.7326/0003-4819-127-6-199709150-00003.
3. Vane JR, Bakhle YS, Botting RM. Cyclooxygenases 1 and 2. Annu Rev Pharmacol Toxicol. 1998;38:97–120. https://doi.org/10.1146/annurev.pharmtox.38.1.97.
4. Penning TD, Talley JJ, Bertenshaw SR, et al. Synthesis and biological evaluation of the 1, 5-diarylpyrazole class of cyclooxygenase-2 inhibitors: identification of 4-[5-(4-methylphenyl)-3-(trifluoromethyl)-1 H-pyrazol-1-yl] benzenesulfonamide (SC-58635, celecoxib). J Med Chem. 1997;40:1347–65. https://doi.org/10.1021/jm960803q.
5. Prasit P, Wang Z, Brideau C, et al. The discovery of rofecoxib, [MK 966, VIOXX®, 4-(4′-methylsulfonylphenyl)-3-phenyl-2 (5H)-furanone], an orally active cyclooxygenase-2 inhibitor. Bioorg Med Chem Lett. 1999;9:1773–8. https://doi.org/10.1016/s0960-894x(99)00288-7.
6. Solomon DH, Schneeweiss S, Glynn RJ, et al. Relationship between selective cyclooxygenase-2 inhibitors and acute myocardial infarction in older adults. Circulation. 2004;109:2068–73. https://doi.org/10.1161/01.CIR.0000127578.21885.3E.
7. Bresalier RS, Sandler RS, Quan H, et al. Cardiovascular events associated with rofecoxib in a colorectal adenoma chemoprevention trial. N Engl J Med. 2005;352:1092–102. https://doi.org/10.1056/NEJMoa050493.
8. Solomon SD, McMurray JJ, Pfeffer MA, et al. Cardiovascular risk associated with celecoxib in a clinical trial for colorectal adenoma prevention. N Engl J Med. 2005;352:1071–80. https://doi.org/10.1056/NEJMoa050405.
9. Atkinson T, Fudin J. Nonsteroidal anti-inflammatory drugs for acute and chronic pain. Phys Med Rehabil Clin N Am. 2020;31:219–31. https://doi.org/10.1016/j.pmr.2020.01.002.
10. Bindu S, Mazumder S, Bandyopadhyay U. Non-steroidal anti-inflammatory drugs (NSAIDs) and organ damage: a current perspective. Biochem Pharmacol. 2020;180:114147. https://doi.org/10.1016/j.bcp.2020.114147.
11. Chaiamnuay S, Allison J, Curtis J. Risk versus benefits of cyclooxygenase-2-selective non steroidal anti-inflammatory drugs. Am J Health Syst Pharm. 2006;63:1837–51. https://doi.org/10.2146/ajhp050519.
12. Grosser T, Ricciotti E, FitzGerald G. Nonsteroidal anti-inflammatory drugs. In: Goodman & Gilman's: the pharmacological basis of therapeutics. 14th ed. McGraw Hill; 2024.
13. Conaghan P. A turbulent decade for NSAIDs: update on current concepts of classification, epidemiology, comparative efficacy, and toxicity. Rheumatol Int. 2012;32:1491–502. https://doi.org/10.1007/s00296-011-2263-6.
14. Cook J, Geisel J, Halushka P, et al. Prostaglandins, thromboxane, leukotrienes, and cytochrome P-450 metabolites of arachidonic acid. New Horiz. 1993;1(1):60–9.
15. Patrignani P, Patrono C. Cyclooxygenase inhibitors: from pharmacology to clinical read-outs. Biochim Biophys Acta. 2015;1851:422–32. https://doi.org/10.1016/j.bbalip.2014.09.016.
16. Qandil A. Prodrugs of non steroidal anti-inflammatory drugs (NSAIDs), more than meets the eye: a critical review. Int J Mol Sci. 2012;13:17244–74. https://doi.org/10.3390/ijms131217244.
17. Warner T, Giuliano F, Vojnovic I, et al. Nonsteroid drug selectivities for cyclo-oxygenase-1 rather than cyclo-oxygenase-2 are associated with human gastrointestinal toxicity: a full in vitro analysis. Proc Natl Acad Sci USA. 1999;96:7563–8. https://doi.org/10.1073/pnas.96.13.7563.
18. Vane J, Botting R. Mechanism of action of nonsteroidal anti-inflammatory drugs. Am J Med. 1998;104(3A):2S–8S. https://doi.org/10.1016/s0002-9343(97)00203-9.
19. Wang B, Wu L, Chen J, et al. Metabolism pathways of arachidonic acids: mechanisms and potential therapeutic targets. Signal Transduct Target Ther. 2021;6:94. https://doi.org/10.1038/s41392-020-00443-w.
20. Lee MC, Abrahams M. Pain and analgesics. In: Clinical pharmacology. 12th ed. Amsterdam: Elsevier; 2019. p. 288–307.
21. Amaya F, Izumi Y, Matsuda M, et al. Tissue injury and related mediators of pain exacerbation. Curr Neuropharmacol. 2013;6:592–7. https://doi.org/10.2174/1570159X11311060003.
22. Zhang JM, An J. Cytokines, inflammation, and pain. Int Anesthesiol Clin. 2007;45(2):27–37. https://doi.org/10.1097/AIA.0b013e318034194e.
23. Arthritis. Chicago: Encyclopedia Britannica; 2024. https://www.britannica.com/science/dislocation. Accessed 19 Mar 2024.
24. Sun AR, Udduttula A, Li J, et al. Cartilage tissue engineering for obesity-induced osteoarthritis: physiology, challenges, and future prospects. J Orthop Translat. 2021;26:3–15. https://doi.org/10.1016/j.jot.2020.07.004.
25. Machado GC, Abdel-Shaheed C, Underwood M, et al. Non-steroidal anti-inflammatory drugs (NSAIDs) for musculoskeletal pain. BMJ. 2021;372:n104. https://doi.org/10.1136/bmj.n104.
26. Moore RA, Chi CC, Wiffen PJ, et al. Oral nonsteroidal anti-inflammatory drugs for neuropathic pain. Cochrane Database Syst Rev. 2015;10:CD010902. https://doi.org/10.1002/14651858.cd010902.pub2.
27. Bates D, Schultheis BC, Hanes MC, et al. A comprehensive algorithm for management of neuropathic pain. Pain Med. 2019;20:S2–S12. https://doi.org/10.1093/pm/pnz075.
28. Scarborough BM, Smith CB. Optimal pain management for patients with cancer in the modern era. CA Cancer J Clin. 2018;68(3):182–96. https://doi.org/10.3322/caac.21453.
29. Derry S, Wiffen PJ, Moore RA, et al. Oral nonsteroidal anti-inflammatory drugs (NSAIDs) for cancer pain in adults. Cochrane Database Syst Rev. 2017;7:CD012638. https://doi.org/10.1002/14651858.CD012638.pub2.
30. McNicol E, Strassels S, Goudas L, et al. Nonsteroidal anti-inflammatory drugs, alone or combined with opioids, for cancer pain: a systematic review. J Clin Oncol. 2004;22(10):1975–92. https://doi.org/10.1200/JCO.2004.10.524.
31. Swarm RA, Paice JA, Anghelescu DL, et al. Adult cancer pain, version 3.2019, NCCN clinical practice guidelines in oncology. J Natl Compr Cancer Netw. 2019;17(8):977–1007. https://doi.org/10.6004/jnccn.2019.0038.
32. D'Arcy Y, McCarberg B. Managing patient pain: a focus on NSAID OTC formulations for relief of musculoskeletal and other common sources pain. J Fam Pract. 2018;67(8):S67–72.
33. Busse JW, Sadeghirad B, Oparin Y, et al. Management of acute pain from non–low back, musculoskeletal injuries: a systematic

review and network meta-analysis of randomized trials. Ann Inter Med. 2020;173(9):730–8. https://doi.org/10.7326/M19-3601.
34. Carrasco-Labra A, Polk DE, Urquhart O, et al. Evidence-based clinical practice guideline for the pharmacologic management of acute dental pain in adolescents, adults, and older adults: a report from the American Dental Association Science and Research Institute, the University of Pittsburgh, and the University of Pennsylvania. J Am Dent Assoc. 2024;155(2):102–117.e9. https://doi.org/10.1016/j.adaj.2023.10.009.
35. Miroshnyhenko A, Ibrahim S, Azab M, et al. Acute postoperative pain due to dental extraction in the adult population: a systematic review and network meta-analysis. J Dent Res. 2023;102(4):391–401. https://doi.org/10.1177/00220345221139230.
36. Osayande AS, Mehulic S. Diagnosis and initial management of dysmenorrhea. Am Fam Physician. 2014;89(5):341–6.
37. Majoribanks J, Ayeleke RO, Farquhar C, et al. Nonsteroidal anti-inflammatory drugs for dysmenorrhoea. Cochrane Database Syst Rev. 2015;1:CD001751. https://doi.org/10.1002/14651858.CD001751.pub3.
38. Affaitati G, Martelletti P, Lopopolo M, et al. Use of nonsteroidal anti-inflammatory drugs for symptomatic treatment of episodic headache. Pain Pract. 2017;17:392–401. https://doi.org/10.1111/papr.12461.
39. Ailani J, Burch RC, Robbins MS, et al. The American headache society consensus statement: update on integrating new migraine treatments into clinical practice. Headache. 2021;61:1021–39. https://doi.org/10.1111/head.14153.
40. Schachtel BP, Furey SA, Thoden WR. Nonprescription ibuprofen and acetaminophen in the treatment of tension-type headache. J Clin Pharmacol. 1996;36:1120–5.
41. Mayans L, Walling A. Acute migraine headache: treatment strategies. Am Fam Physician. 2018;97(4):243–51.
42. Rabbie R, Derry S, Moore RA. Ibuprofen with or without an antiemetic for acute migraine headaches in adults. Cochrane Database Syst Rev. 2013;4:CD008039. https://doi.org/10.1002/14651858.CD008039.pub3.
43. Argoff CE. Recent developments in the treatment of osteoarthritis with NSAIDs. Curr Med Res Opin. 2011;27(7):1315–27. https://doi.org/10.1185/03007995.2011.568058.
44. Kolasinski SL, Neogi T, Hochberg MC, et al. 2019 American College of Rheumatology/Arthritis Foundation guideline for the management of osteoarthritis of the hand, hip, and knee. Arthritis Care Res. 2020;72:149–62. https://doi.org/10.1002/art.41142.
45. Rannou F, Pelletier JP, Martel-Pelletier J. Efficacy and safety of topical NSAIDs in the management of osteoarthritis: evidence from real-life setting trials and surveys. Semin Arthritis Rheum. 2016;45:S18–21. https://doi.org/10.1016/j.semarthrit.2015.11.007.
46. Nissen SE, Yeomans ND, Solomon DH, et al. Cardiovascular safety of celecoxib, naproxen, or ibuprofen for arthritis. N Engl J Med. 2016;375(26):2519–29. https://doi.org/10.1056/NEJMoa1611593.
47. Fraenkel L, Bathon JM, England BR, et al. 2021 American College of Rheumatology guideline for the treatment of rheumatoid arthritis. Arthritis Care Res. 2021;73:924–39. https://doi.org/10.1002/acr.24596.
48. Ong CKS, Lirk P, Tan CH, et al. An evidence-based update on nonsteroidal anti-inflammatory drugs. Clin Med Res. 2007;5(1):19–34. https://doi.org/10.3121/cmr.2007.698.
49. Benzon H, Raja SN, Fishman SM, et al. Essentials of pain medicine. 4th ed. Amsterdam: Elsevier; 2018.
50. Perlin E, Finke H, Castro O, et al. Enhancement of pain control with ketorolac tromethamine in patients with sickle cell vaso-occlusive crisis. Am J Hematol. 1994;46(1):43–7. https://doi.org/10.1002/ajh.2830460108.
51. Brandow AM, Carroll P, Creary S, et al. American Society of Hematology 2020 guidelines for sickle cell disease: management of acute and chronic pain. Blood Adv. 2020;4(12):2656–701. https://doi.org/10.1182/bloodadvances.2020001851.
52. Xu C, Gu K, Yasen Y, et al. Efficacy and safety of celecoxib therapy in osteoarthritis: a meta-analysis of randomized controlled trials. Medicine. 2016;95(20):e3585. https://doi.org/10.1097/MD.0000000000003585.
53. Engelman DT, Ali WB, Williams JB, et al. Guidelines for perioperative care in cardiac surgery enhanced recovery after surgery society recommendations. JAMA Surg. 2019;154(8):755–76.
54. Thorell A, MacCormick AD, Awad S, et al. Guidelines for perioperative care in bariatric surgery: Enhanced Recovery After Surgery (ERAS) society recommendations. World J Surg. 2016;40:2065–83.
55. Barr LF, Boss MJ, Mazzeffi MA, et al. Postoperative multimodal analgesia in cardiac surgery. Crit Care Clin. 2020;36(4):631–51.
56. Debono B, Wainwright TW, Wang MY, et al. Consensus statement for perioperative care in lumbar spinal fusion: Enhanced Recovery After Surgery (ERAS) society recommendations. Spine J. 2021;21(5):729–52.
57. Wick EC, Grant MC, Wu CL. Postoperative multimodal analgesia pain management with nonopioid analgesics and techniques. JAMA Surg. 2017;152(7):691–7.
58. Rafiq S, Steinbruchel AD, Wanscher MJ, et al. Multimodal analgesia versus traditional opiate based analgesia after cardiac surgery, a randomized controlled trial. J Card Surg. 2014;9:52.
59. Gustafsson UO, Scott MJ, Hubner M, et al. Guidelines for perioperative Care in Elective Colorectal Surgery: Enhanced Recovery After Surgery (ERAS) society recommendations: 2018. World J Surg. 2018;43:659–95.
60. McGingle KL, Spangler EL, Pichel AC, et al. Perioperative care in open aortic vascular surgery: a consensus statement by the Enhanced Recovery After Surgery (ERAS) society and Society for Vascular Surgery. J Vasc Surg. 2022;75(6):1796–820.
61. McGingle KL, Spangler EL, Ayyash K, et al. A framework for perioperative care for lower extremity vascular bypasses: a consensus statement by the Enhanced Recovery after Surgery (ERAS) society and society for vascular surgery. J Vasc Surg. 2023;77(5):1295–315.
62. Wainwright TW, Gill M, McDonald DA, et al. Consensus statement for perioperative care in total hip replacement and total knee replacement surgery: Enhanced Recovery After Surgery (ERAS) society recommendations. Acta Orthop. 2020;91(1):3–19.
63. Temple-Oberle C, Shea-Budgell MA, Tan M, et al. Consensus review of optimal perioperative Care in Breast Reconstruction: Enhanced Recovery after Surgery (ERAS) society recommendations. Plast Reconstr Surg. 2017;139(5):1056–71.
64. Batchelor TJP, Rasburn NJ, Abdelnour-Berchtold E, et al. Guidelines for enhanced recovery after lung surgery: recommendations of the Enhanced Recovery After Surgery (ERAS) society and the European Society of Thoracic Surgeons (ESTS). Eur J Cardiothorac Surg. 2019;55(1):91–115.
65. Mortensen K, Nilsson M, Slim K, et al. Consensus guidelines for enhanced recovery after gastrectomy Enhanced Recovery After Surgery (ERAS) society recommendations. Br J Surg. 2014;101(10):1209–29.
66. Joliat GR, Kobayashi K, Hasegawa K, et al. Guidelines for perioperative care for liver surgery: Enhanced Recovery After Surgery (ERAS) society recommendations 2022. World J Surg. 2023;47:11–34.
67. Peden CJ, Aggarwal G, Aitken RJ. Guidelines for perioperative care for emergency laparotomy Enhanced Recovery After Surgery (ERAS) society recommendations: part 1—preoperative: diagnosis, rapid assessment and optimization. World J Surg. 2021;45:1272–90.

68. Melloul E, Lassen K, Roulin D, et al. Guidelines for perioperative care for pancreatoduodenectomy: enhanced recovery after surgery (ERAS) recommendations 2019. World J Surg. 2020;44:2056–84.
69. Dort JC, Farwell G, Findlay M, et al. Optimal perioperative care in major head and neck cancer surgery with free flap reconstruction. A consensus review and recommendations from the enhanced recovery after surgery society. JAMA Otolaryngol Head Neck Surg. 2017;143(3):292–303.
70. Priya V, Divatia JV, Sareen R, et al. Efficacy of intravenous ketoprofen for pre-emptive analgesia. J Postgrad Med. 2002;48(2):109–12.
71. Møiniche S, Kehlet H, Dahl JB, et al. A qualitative and quantitative systematic review of preemptive analgesia for postoperative pain relief: the role of timing of analgesia. Anesthesiology. 2002;96:725–41.
72. Meunier A, Lisander B, Good L. Effects of celecoxib on blood loss, pain, and recovery of function after total knee replacement: a randomized placebo-controlled trial. Acta Orthop. 2007;78(5):661–7.
73. Derry CJ, Derry S, Moore RA. Single dose oral ibuprofen plus paracetamol (acetaminophen) for acute postoperative pain. Cochrane Database Syst Rev. 2013;6:CD010210.
74. Elia N, Lysakowski C, Tramer MR, et al. Does multimodal analgesia with acetaminophen, nonsteroidal antiinflammatory drugs, or selective cyclooxygenase-2 inhibitors and patient-controlled analgesia morphine offer advantages over morphine alone? Meta-analyses of randomized trials. Anesthesiology. 2005;103:1296–304.
75. Nelson G, Fofopoulou C, Taylor J, et al. Enhanced Recovery After Surgery (ERAS) society guidelines for gynecologic oncology: addressing implementation challenges - 2023 update. Gynecol Oncol. 2023;173:58–67.
76. Hübner M, Kusamura S, Villeneuve L, et al. Guidelines for perioperative care in cytoreductive surgery (CRS) with or without hyperthermic IntraPEritoneal chemotherapy (HIPEC): Enhanced Recovery After Surgery (ERAS) society recommendations part I: preoperative and intraoperative management. Eur J Surg Oncol. 2020;46(12):2292–310.
77. Low DE, Allum W, De Mazoni G, et al. Guidelines for perioperative care in esophagectomy: Enhanced Recovery After Surgery (ERAS) society recommendations. World J Surg. 2019;43:299–330.
78. Ong CKS, Seymour RA, Lirk P, et al. Combining paracetamol (acetaminophen) with nonsteroidal antiinflammatory drugs: a qualitative systematic review of analgesic efficacy for acute postoperative pain. Anesth Analg. 2010;110(4):1170–9.
79. Sekiguchi H, Inoue G, Nakazawa T, et al. Loxoprofen sodium and celecoxib for postoperative pain in patients after spinal surgery: a randomized comparative study. J Orthop Sci. 2015;20:617–23.
80. Feldheiser A, Aziz O, Baldini G, et al. Enhanced Recovery After Surgery (ERAS) for gastrointestinal surgery, part 2: consensus statement for anaesthesia practice. Acta Anaesthesiol Scand. 2016;60(3):289–334.
81. Cata JP, Nguyen LT, Ifeanyi-Pillettea IC, et al. An assessment of the survival impact of multimodal anesthesia/analgesia technique in adults undergoing cytoreductive surgery with hyperthermic intraperitoneal chemotherapy: a propensity score matched analysis. Int J Hyperth. 2019;36(1):369–75.
82. Arron M, Lier E, de Wilt J, et al. Postoperative administration of non-steroidal anti-inflammatory drugs in colorectal cancer surgery does not increase anastomotic leak rate; a systematic review and meta-analysis. Eur J Surg Oncol. 2020;46(12):2167–73.
83. Scott MJ, Aggarwal G, Aitken RJ, et al. Consensus guidelines for perioperative care for emergency laparotomy Enhanced Recovery After Surgery (ERAS) society recommendations part 2—emergency laparotomy: intra-and postoperative care. World J Surg. 2023;47:1850–80.
84. Brustia R, Monsel A, Skurzak S, et al. Guidelines for perioperative care for liver transplantation: Enhanced Recovery After Surgery (ERAS) recommendations. Transplantation. 2022;106(3):552–61. https://doi.org/10.1097/TP.0000000000003808.
85. Brindle ME, McDiarmid C, Short K, et al. Consensus guidelines for perioperative care in neonatal intestinal surgery: Enhanced Recovery After Surgery (ERAS) society recommendations. World J Surg. 2020;44:2482–92.
86. Rao P, Knaus EE. Evolution of nonsteroidal anti-inflammatory drugs (NSAIDs): cyclooxygenase (COX) inhibition and beyond. J Pharm Pharm Sci. 2008;11:81s–110s. https://doi.org/10.18433/j3t886.
87. Masclee GM, Valkhoff VE, Coloma PM, et al. Risk of upper gastrointestinal bleeding from different drug combinations. Gastroenterology. 2014;147:784–92. https://doi.org/10.1053/j.gastro.2014.06.007.
88. Lanza FL, Chan FK, Quigley EM, et al. Guidelines for prevention of NSAID-related ulcer complications. Am J Gastroenterol. 2009;104:728–38. https://doi.org/10.1038/ajg.2009.115.
89. Kim TJ, Kim ER, Hong SN, et al. Effectiveness of acid suppressants and other mucoprotective agents in reducing the risk of occult gastrointestinal bleeding in nonsteroidal anti-inflammatory drug users. Sci Rep. 2019;9:11696. https://doi.org/10.18433/j3t886.
90. Bally M, Dendukuri N, Rich B, et al. Risk of acute myocardial infarction with NSAIDs in real world use: bayesian meta-analysis of individual patient data. BMJ. 2017;357:j1909. https://doi.org/10.1136/bmj.j1909.
91. FDA. Access FDA: Motrin ® (ibuprofen). Silver Spring: U.S Food and Drug Administration; 2007. https://www.accessdata.fda.gov/drugsatfda_docs/label/2007/017463s105lbl.pdf. Accessed 19 Mar 2024.
92. FDA. Access FDA: Naprelan ® (naproxen sodium). Silver Spring: U.S Food and Drug Administration; 2017. https://www.accessdata.fda.gov/drugsatfda_docs/label/2017/020353s034lbl.pdf. Accessed 19 Mar 2024.
93. FDA. Access FDA: Voltaren ® (diclofenac sodium). Silver Spring: U.S Food and Drug Administration; 2021. https://www.accessdata.fda.gov/drugsatfda_docs/label/2021/019201s048lbl.pdf. Accessed 19 Mar 2024.
94. FDA. Access FDA: Mobic ® (meloxicam). Silver Spring: U.S Food and Drug Administration; 2012. https://accessdata.fda.gov/drugsatfda_docs/label/2012/020938s022lbl.pdf. Access 19 Mar 2024.
95. FDA. Access FDA: Celebrex ® (celecoxib). Silver Spring: U.S Food and Drug Administration; 2018. https://www.accessdata.fda.gov/drugsatfda_docs/label/2018/020998s050lbl.pdf. Accessed 19 Mar 2024.
96. Eras J, Perazella MA. NSAIDs and the kidney revisited: are selective cyclooxygenase-2 inhibitors safe? Am J Med Sci. 2001;321:181–90. https://doi.org/10.1097/00000441-200103000-00005.
97. Cooper C, Chapurlat R, Al-Daghari N, et al. Safety of oral non-selective non-steroidal anti-inflammatory drugs in osteoarthritis: what does the literature say? Drugs Aging. 2019;36:15–24. https://doi.org/10.1007/s40266-019-00660-1.
98. Clive DM, Stoff JS. Renal syndromes associated with nonsteroidal antiinflammatory drugs. N Engl J Med. 1984;310:563–72. https://doi.org/10.1056/NEJM198403013100905.
99. Smith WL. Prostanoid biosynthesis and mechanisms of action. Am J Phys. 1992;263:F181–91. https://doi.org/10.1152/ajprenal.1992.263.2.F181.
100. Baker M, Perazella MA. NSAIDs in CKD: are they safe? Am J Kidney Dis. 2020;76(4):546–57. https://doi.org/10.1053/j.ajkd.2020.03.023.
101. Gambaro G, Perazella MA. Adverse renal effects of anti-inflammatory agents: evaluation of selective and nonselective

cyclooxygenase inhibitors. J Intern Med. 2003;253:643–52. https://doi.org/10.1046/j.1365-2796.2003.01146.x.
102. Brewater UC, Perazella MA. Acute tubulointerstitial nephritis associated with celecoxib. Nephrol Dial Transplant. 2004;19(4):1017–918. https://doi.org/10.1093/ndt/gfh033.
103. Whelton A. Nephrotoxicity of nonsteroidal anti-inflammatory drugs: physiologic foundations and clinical implications. Am J Med. 1999;106(5B):13S–24S. https://doi.org/10.1016/s0002-9343(99)00113-8.
104. Leonard CE, Freeman CP, Newcomb CW, et al. Proton pump inhibitors and traditional nonsteroidal anti-inflammatory drugs and the risk of acute interstitial nephritis and acute kidney injury. Pharmacoepidemiol Drug Saf. 2012;21:1155–72. https://doi.org/10.1002/pds.3329.
105. Nath KA, Chmielewski DH, Hostetter TH. Regulatory role of prostanoids in glomerular microcirculation of remnant nephrons. Am J Phys. 1987;252:F829–37. https://doi.org/10.1152/ajprenal.1987.252.5.F829.
106. Lipman GS, Shea K, Christensen M, et al. Ibuprofen versus placebo effect on acute kidney injury in ultramarathons: a randomised controlled trial. Emerg Med J. 2017;34:637–42. https://doi.org/10.1136/emermed-2016-206353.
107. Blackshear JL, Davidman M, Stillman MT. Identification of risk for renal insufficiency from nonsteroidal anti-inflammatory drugs. Arch Intern Med. 1983;143:1130–4. https://doi.org/10.1001/archinte.1983.00350060052007.
108. Sriperumbuduri S, Hiremath S. The case for cautious consumption: NSAIDs in chronic kidney disease. Curr Opin Nephrol Hypertens. 2019;28:163–70. https://doi.org/10.1097/MNH.0000000000000473.
109. Soi V, Yee J. Sodium homeostasis in chronic kidney disease. Adv Chronic Kidney Dis. 2017;24:325–31. https://doi.org/10.1053/j.ackd.2017.08.001.
110. Perazella MA. COX-2 selective inhibitors: analysis of the renal effects. Expert Opin Drug Saf. 2002;1:53–64. https://doi.org/10.1517/14740338.1.1.53.
111. Pope JE, Anderson JJ, Felson DT. A meta-analysis of the effects of nonsteroidal anti-inflammatory drugs on blood pressure. Arch Intern Med. 1993;153:477–84. https://doi.org/10.1001/archinte.1993.00410040045007.
112. Johnson AG, Nguyen TV, Day RO. Do nonsteroidal anti-inflammatory drugs affect blood pressure? A meta-analysis. Ann Intern Med. 1994;121(4):289–300. https://doi.org/10.7326/0003-4819-121-4-199408150-00011.
113. Kalafutova S, Juraskova B, Vlcek J. The impact of combinations of non-steroidal anti-inflammatory drugs and anti-hypertensive agents on blood pressure. Adv Clin Exp Med. 2014;23:993–1000. https://doi.org/10.17219/acem/37357.
114. Perazella MA. Drug-induced hyperkalemia: old culprits and new offenders. Am J Med. 2000;109:307–14. https://doi.org/10.1016/s0002-9343(00)00496-4.
115. Kowalski ML, Makowska JS, Blanca M, et al. Hypersensitivity to nonsteroidal anti-inflammatory drugs (NSAIDs)—classification, diagnosis and management: review of the EAACI/ENDA and GA2LEN/HANNA. Allergy. 2011;66:818–29. https://doi.org/10.1111/j.1398-9995.2011.02557.x.
116. Doña I, Pérez-Sànchez N, Eguiluz-Gracia I, et al. Progress in understanding hypersensitivity reactions to nonsteroidal anti-inflammatory drugs. Allergy. 2020;75:561–75. https://doi.org/10.1111/all.14032.
117. Laidlaw TM, Cahill KN. Current knowledge and management of hypersensitivity to aspirin and NSAIDs. J Allergy Clin Immunol Pract. 2017;5(3):537–45. https://doi.org/10.1016/j.jaip.2016.10.021.
118. McPherson ML, Cimino NM. Topical NSAID formulations. Pain Med. 2013;14(1):S35–9. https://doi.org/10.1111/pme.12288.
119. Meunier L, Larrey D. Recent advances in hepatotoxicity of non steroidal anti-inflammatory drugs. Ann Hepatol. 2018;17(2):187–91. https://doi.org/10.5604/01.3001.0010.8633.
120. Blanca-Lopez N, Soriano V, Garcia-Martin E, et al. NSAID-induced reactions: classification, prevalence, impact, and management strategies. J Asthma Allergy. 2019;12:217–33. https://doi.org/10.2147/JAA.S164806.
121. Antonucci R, Zaffanello M, Puxeddu E, et al. Use of non-steroidal anti-inflammatory drugs in pregnancy: impact on the fetus. Curr Drug Metab. 2012;13(4):474–90. https://doi.org/10.2174/138920012800166607.
122. U.S. Food and Drug Administration (2023) FDA recommends avoiding use of NSAIDs in pregnancy at 20 weeks or later because they can result in low amniotic fluid. https://www.fda.gov/drugs/drug-safety-and-availability/fda-recommends-avoiding-use-nsaids-pregnancy-20-weeks-or-later-because-they-can-result-low-amniotic. Accessed 11 Mar 2023.
123. Bryant A, Miller RS. Pharmacologic stepwise multimodal approach for postpartum pain management: ACOG clinical consensus no. 1. Obstet Gynecol. 2021;138(3):507–17.
124. Vigil-De Gracia P, Solis V, Ortega N. Ibuprofen versus acetaminophen as a post-partum analgesic for women with severe pre-eclampsia: randomized clinical study. J Matern Fetal Neonatal Med. 2017;30:1279–82. https://doi.org/10.1080/14767058.2016.1210599.
125. Blue NR, Murray-Krezan C, Drake-Lavelle S, et al. Effect of ibuprofen vs acetaminophen on postpartum hypertension in pre-eclampsia with severe features: a double-masked, randomized controlled trial. Am J Obstet Gynecol. 2018;218(6):616.e1–8. https://doi.org/10.1016/j.ajog.2018.02.016.
126. Lactmed ®. Bethesda: National Institute of Child Health and Human Development; 2006. https://www.ncbi.nlm.nih.gov/books/NBK500986/. Accessed 27 Mar 2024.
127. National Library of Medicine: Ibuprofen. Bethesda: Drugs and Lactation Database; 2021. https://www.ncbi.nlm.nih.gov/books/NBK500986/. Accessed 11 Mar 2024.
128. National Library of Medicine: Ketorolac. Bethesda: Drugs and Lactation Database; 2021. https://www.ncbi.nlm.nih.gov/books/NBK500998/. Accessed 11 Mar 2024.
129. Wischnik A, Manth SM, Lloyd J, et al. The excretion of ketorolac tromethamine into breast milk after multiple oral dosing. Eur J Clin Pharmacol. 1989;36:521–4. https://doi.org/10.1007/BF00558080.
130. Cooney MF. Pain management in children: NSAID use in the perioperative and emergency department settings. Paediatr Drugs. 2021;23(4):361–72. https://doi.org/10.1007/s40272-021-00449-z.
131. Sura A, Failing C, Sturza J, et al. Patient characteristics associated with response to NSAID monotherapy in children with systemic juvenile idiopathic arthritis. Pediatr Rheumatol Online J. 2018;16:2. https://doi.org/10.1186/s12969-017-0219-4.
132. Onel KB, Horton DB, Lovell DJ, et al. 2021 American College of Rheumatology guidelines for the treatment of juvenile idiopathic arthritis: therapeutic approaches for Oligoarthritis, temporomandibular joint arthritis, and systemic juvenile idiopathic arthritis. Arthritis Care Res. 2022;74(4):521–37. https://doi.org/10.1002/acr.24853.
133. Ziesenitz VC, Welzel T, Van Dyk M, et al. Efficacy and safety of NSAIDs in infants: a comprehensive review of the literature of the past 20 years. Paediatr Drugs. 2022;24(6):603–55. https://doi.org/10.1007/s40272-022-00514-.
134. Buffum M, Buffum JC. Nonsteroidal anti-inflammatory drugs in the elderly. Pain Manag Nurs. 2000;1(2):40–50. https://doi.org/10.1053/jpmn.2000.777.
135. McCarberg BH. NSAIDs in the older patient: balancing benefits and harms. Pain Med. 2013;14:S43–4. https://doi.org/10.1111/pme.12253.

136. Wongrakpanich S, Wongrakpanich A, Melhado K, et al. A comprehensive review of non-steroidal anti-inflammatory drug use in the elderly. Aging Dis. 2018;9(1):143–50. https://doi.org/10.14336/AD.2017.0306.
137. Moore N, Pollack C, Butkerait P. Adverse drug reactions and drug–drug interactions with over-the-counter NSAIDs. Ther Clin Risk Manag. 2015;11:1061–75. https://doi.org/10.2147/TCRM.S79135.
138. Gong L, Thorn CF, Bertagnolli MM, et al. Celecoxib pathways: pharmacokinetics and pharmacodynamics. Pharmacogenet Genomics. 2012;22(4):310–8. https://doi.org/10.1097/FPC.0b013e32834f94cb.
139. Derry S, Loke YK. Risk of gastrointestinal haemorrhage with long term use of aspirin: meta-analysis. BMJ. 2000;321(7270):1183–7. https://doi.org/10.1136/bmj.321.7270.1183.
140. Hochberg MC, Altman RD, April KT, et al. American College of Rheumatology 2012 recommendations for the use of nonpharmacologic and pharmacologic therapies in osteoarthritis of the hand, hip, and knee. Arthritis Care Res. 2012;64(4):465–74. https://doi.org/10.1002/acr.21596.
141. Fries JF, Bruce B. Rates of serious gastrointestinal events from low dose use of acetylsalicylic acid, acetaminophen, and ibuprofen in patients with osteoarthritis and rheumatoid arthritis. J Rheumatol. 2003;30(10):2226–33.
142. Scott MJ, Baldini G, Fearon KCH, et al. Enhanced Recovery After Surgery (ERAS) for gastrointestinal surgery, part 1: pathophysiological considerations. Acta Anaesthesiol Scand. 2015;59:1212–31.
143. Qaseem A, McLean RM, O'Gurek D, et al. Nonpharmacologic and pharmacologic management of acute pain from non-low back, musculoskeletal injuries in adults: a clinical guideline from the American College of Physicians and American Academy of Family Physicians. Ann Intern Med. 2020;173(9):739–48. https://doi.org/10.7326/M19-3602.
144. Qaseem A, Wilt TJ, McLean RM, et al. Noninvasive treatments for acute, subacute, and chronic low back pain: a clinical practice guideline from the American College of Physicians. Ann Intern Med. 2017;166(7):514–30. https://doi.org/10.7326/M16-2367.
145. Dowell D, Ragan KR, Jones CM, et al. CDC clinical practice guideline for prescribing opioids for pain - United States. Ctr Dis Control Prev. 2022;71(3):1–95.
146. Ford B, Dore M, Harris E. Outpatient primary care management of headaches: guidelines from the VA/DoD. Am Fam Physician. 2021;104:316–20.
147. United States Department of Health and Human Services (2014) Evidence-based management of sickle cell disease, expert panel report. Available via National Heart Lung, and Blood Institute. https://www.nhlbi.nih.gov/sites/default/files/media/docs/sickle-cell-disease-report%20020816_0.pdf. Accessed 21 Mar 2024.
148. Macones GA, Caughey AB, Wood SL, et al. Guidelines for postoperative care in cesarean delivery: Enhanced Recovery After Surgery (ERAS) society recommendations (part 3). Am J Obstet Gynecol. 2019;221(3):247.e1–9.
149. UpToDate ® Lexidrug. Netherlands: Wolters Kluwer; 2024. https://www.wolterskluwer.com/en/solutions/uptodate/pro/lexidrug. Accessed 23 Mar 2024.
150. Micromedex. Ann Arbor: Merative; 2023. https://www.micromedexsolutions.com/home/dispatch/. Accessed 23 Mar 2024.
151. FDA. Access FDA: Dolobid ® (diflunisal). Silver Spring: U.S Food and Drug Administration; 2007. https://www.accessdata.fda.gov/drugsatfda_docs/label/2017/020353s034lbl.pdf. Accessed 19 Mar 2024.
152. FDA. Access FDA: Lodine ® (etodolac). Silver Spring: U.S Food and Drug Administration; 2005. https://www.accessdata.fda.gov/drugsatfda_docs/label/2006/018922s022,020584s009lbl.pdf. Accessed 19 Mar 2024.
153. FDA. Access FDA: Nalfon ® (fenoprofen calcium). Silver Spring: U.S Food and Drug Administration; 2016. https://www.accessdata.fda.gov/drugsatfda_docs/label/2016/017604s046lbl.pdf. Accessed 19 Mar 2024.
154. FDA. Access FDA: Ansaid ® (flurbiprofen). Silver Spring: U.S Food and Drug Administration; 2016. https://www.accessdata.fda.gov/drugsatfda_docs/label/2016/018766s020lbl.pdf. Accessed 19 Mar 2024.
155. FDA. Access FDA: Indocin ® (indomethacin). Silver Spring: U.S Food and Drug Administration; 2019. https://www.accessdata.fda.gov/drugsatfda_docs/label/2019/016059s100lbl.pdf. Accessed 19 Mar 2024.
156. FDA. Access FDA: Toradol ® (Ketorolac tromethamine injection). Silver Spring: U.S Food and Drug Administration; 2022. https://labeling.pfizer.com/ShowLabeling.aspx?format=PDF&id=4487. Accessed 19 Mar 2024.
157. FDA. Access FDA: Toradol ® (ketorolac tromethamine tablets). Silver Spring: U.S Food and Drug Administration; 2013. https://www.accessdata.fda.gov/drugsatfda_docs/label/2013/019645s019lbl.pdf. Accessed 19 Mar 2024.
158. FDA. Access FDA: Ponstel ® (mefenamic acid). Silver Spring: U.S Food and Drug Administration; 2021. https://www.accessdata.fda.gov/drugsatfda_docs/label/2021/015034s045lbl.pdf. Accessed 19 Mar 2024.
159. FDA. Access FDA: Daypro ® (oxaprozin). Silver Spring: U.S Food and Drug Administration; 2016. https://www.accessdata.fda.gov/drugsatfda_docs/label/2016/018841s028lbl.pdf. Accessed 19 Mar 2024.
160. FDA. Access FDA: Feldene ® (piroxicam). Silver Spring: U.S Food and Drug Administration; 2015. https://www.accessdata.fda.gov/drugsatfda_docs/label/2015/018147s033s038s039s040s042lbl.pdf. Accessed 19 Mar 2024.
161. FDA. Access FDA: Clinoril ® (sulindac). Silver Spring: U.S Food and Drug Administration; 2010. https://www.accessdata.fda.gov/drugsatfda_docs/label/2010/017911s074lbl.pdf. Accessed 19 Mar 2024.
162. FDA. Access FDA: Tolectin ® (tolmetin sodium). Silver Spring: U.S Food and Drug Administration; 2007. https://www.accessdata.fda.gov/drugsatfda_docs/label/2008/018084s052s017628s068lbl.pdf. Accessed 19 Mar 2024.
163. Jaglal R, Nemec EC 2nd. What is the analgesic ceiling dose of ketorolac for treating acute pain in the ED? JAAPA. 2023;36:43–4. https://doi.org/10.1097/01.JAA.0000923576.90074.2a.
164. Motov S, Masoudi A, Drapkin J, et al. Comparison of oral Ibuprofen at three single-dose regimens for treating acute pain in the emergency department: a randomized controlled trial. Ann Emerg Med. 2019;74:530–7. https://doi.org/10.1016/j.annemergmed.2019.05.037.
165. Cerantola Y, Valerio M, Persson B, et al. Guidelines for perioperative care after radical cystectomy for bladder cancer: Enhanced Recovery After Surgery (ERAS) society recommendations. Clin Nutr. 2013;32(6):879–87.
166. Oodit R, Biccard BM, Panieri E, et al. Guidelines for perioperative care in elective abdominal and pelvic surgery at primary and secondary hospitals in low– middle-income countries (LMIC's): Enhanced Recovery After Surgery (ERAS) society recommendation. World J Surg. 2022;46:1826–43.
167. Altman AD, Robert M, Armbrust R, et al. Guidelines for vulvar and vaginal surgery: enhanced recovery after surgery society recommendations. Am J Obstet Gynecol. 2020;223(4):475–85.
168. Hübner M, Kusamura S, Villeneuve L, et al. Guidelines for Perioperative Care in Cytoreductive Surgery (CRS) with or without hyperthermic IntraPEritoneal chemotherapy (HIPEC): Enhanced Recovery After Surgery (ERAS) Society Recommendations - Part II: Postoperative management and special considerations. Eur J Surg Oncol. 2020;46(12):2311–23.

Gabapentin/Pregabalin

7

Mojdeh S. Heavner, Grace Erdman, Marie C. Ziesat, and Faith M. Armstrong

Abbreviations

AE	Adverse event
CNS	Central nervous system
CLBP	Chronic low back pain
DPN	Diabetic peripheral neuropathy
ERAS	Enhanced Recovery After Surgery
FDA	Food and Drug Administration
GABA	Gamma-aminobutyric acid
GBS	Guillain–Barré syndrome
HIV	Human immunodeficiency virus
ICU	Intensive care unit
LAT	L-amino acid transporters
NeuPSIG	Neuropathic Pain Special Interest Group
RCTs	Randomized controlled trials
PACU	Postanesthesia care unit
PHN	Postherpetic neuralgia
SCI	Spinal cord injury
TDD	Total daily dose

Key Themes

- Interest in gabapentinoid medications, gabapentin and pregabalin, has increased over the past few decades, for a variety of approved and off-label indications.
- Evidence supporting their use in neuropathic pain conditions suggests that about half of the patients experience adequate effectiveness, but many patients require discontinuation of therapy due to adverse effects.
- Despite Enhanced Recovery After Surgery (ERAS) protocols including gabapentinoids as a standard of care for many indications, the most consistently robust evidence to support this practice is found only in the setting of spinal surgery.
- Gabapentinoids represent a viable alternative to opioids for analgesia, but further study is needed to justify broad utilization.

Background

The gabapentinoid medications, gabapentin and pregabalin, have gained increasing popularity for a variety of conditions over the past few decades. Gabapentin was first approved in 1993 by the US Food and Drug Administration (FDA) under the trade name Neurontin®, as an adjunctive agent for treatment of partial seizures. In 2000, Neurontin® gained FDA approval for the treatment of partial seizures in children aged 3 and older and then in 2002 for the treatment of postherpetic neuralgia (PHN). A once-daily formulation of gabapentin (Gralise®) was approved by the FDA for postherpetic neuralgia in 2011, followed by a gabapentin prodrug (gabapentin enacarbil: brand name Horizant®) for restless leg syndrome and postherpetic neuralgia in 2012 [79]. Pregabalin (only available in the United States under the trade name Lyrica®) was approved by the FDA in 2004 for seizures, postherpetic neuralgia (PHN), and diabetic peripheral neuropathy (DPN); in 2007 for fibromyalgia; and in 2012 for pain associated with spinal cord injury (SCI) [29].

Gabapentin use has increased dramatically. In 2021, gabapentin was ranked the tenth most prescribed medication in the United States, with 47,125,973 prescriptions for 10,697,239 patients [29]. Annual sales in 1995 were reported at $98 million and grew to $3 billion in 2004, when the drug became available as a generic [79]. The vast majority of its use is likely for unapproved indications, with estimates of around 80% off-label use reported previously [29]. Pregabalin was in the top 100 most prescribed

M. S. Heavner (✉)
Department of Practice, Sciences, and Health Outcomes Research, University of Maryland School of Pharmacy, Baltimore, MD, USA
e-mail: mheavner@rx.umaryland.edu

G. Erdman
University of Maryland Medical Center, Baltimore, MD, USA

M. C. Ziesat · F. M. Armstrong
University of Maryland Baltimore Washington Medical Center, Glen Burnie, MD, USA

J. P. Reinert et al. (eds.), *Adjunctive Analgesic Strategies for the Bedside Clinician and Beyond*,
https://doi.org/10.1007/978-3-032-21675-5_7

drugs, with 8,996,019 prescriptions for 1,687,032 patients [42]. A study of the Medical Expenditure Panel Survey (MEPS) reported that the number of individuals using gabapentinoids tripled between 2002 and 2015 in the United States. Similar rates of growth have been reported in other countries [40]. US ambulatory care visits involving gabapentinoids have increased from 7.4 million in 2003 to 27 million in 2016. Notably, these data are primarily driven by gabapentin utilization, with pregabalin data remaining largely stable over time. Individuals who are more likely to require gabapentinoids are those who are younger than 65 years of age and white and have governmental insurance and multiple chronic conditions. Approximately one-third (32.9%) of the ambulatory care visits involving gabapentinoids also involve opioids. Gabapentinoids are most prescribed by primary care providers (45.8%), with a minority prescribed by neurologists (8.2%), surgeons (6.2%), and psychiatrists (4.8%). Due to concerns of overprescribing, initiatives to curb gabapentinoid use include mandatory reporting of gabapentin prescriptions to drug monitoring programs in certain states (e.g., MA, OH, and VA), classifying gabapentin and pregabalin as a Schedule V Controlled Substance, and limiting prescribing quantity (e.g., KY), as well as prior authorization and step therapy for pregabalin [19, 86].

This chapter provides a focused review of gabapentinoid pharmacology and examines the evidence supporting their use in neuropathic, chronic, and perioperative pain, with a brief description of their role in critically ill patients. The latter half provides applications to clinical practice, highlighting risk–benefit considerations, dosing strategies, and the importance of an interprofessional approach to patient management.

Pharmacology: Pharmacokinetics and Pharmacodynamics

Pharmacokinetics

Table 7.1 highlights and compares pharmacokinetic parameters for both gabapentinoid drugs. Pregabalin exhibits more rapid and complete absorption compared to gabapentin, with peak serum concentrations seen at 1 and 3 h, respectively. Pregabalin also has an oral bioavailability of over 90% compared to the 30–60% bioavailability of gabapentin, which results in 2.4–2.8 times more potency than that of gabapentin [7]. This discrepancy is explained by the anatomical site of absorption for each medication. Gabapentin is absorbed in the small intestine where L-amino acid transporters (LAT) facilitate drug transport on an intracellular level and can become saturated. As a result, analgesic response can plateau at doses of 3600 mg per day [14]. In contrast, pregabalin absorption occurs in the small intestine and proximal colon, which allows other transport carriers to supplement the LAT activity. This presents as non-saturable kinetics, with analgesic responses seen in doses up to 450 mg/day. Administration of food with gabapentinoids does not affect their bioavailability, so coadministration is not considered a clinically significant interaction [7].

Table 7.1 Summary of pharmacokinetic properties of gabapentinoids

Pharmacokinetic parameter	Gabapentin	Pregabalin
Peak serum concentration	3 h	1 h
Oral bioavailability	30–60%	90%
Site of absorption	Small intestine	Small intestine and proximal colon
Volume of distribution	0.8 L/kg	0.5 L/kg
Renal excretion	100% unchanged	92–99%
Elimination half-life	5–7 h	5.5–6.7 h

Bockbrader et al. [7], Chincholkar [14], Takahashi et al. [72]

Both gabapentin and pregabalin are highly water-soluble, with a volume of distribution of 0.8 and 0.5 L/kg, respectively [7]. Plasma protein binding is negligible for both agents, so they can readily cross the blood-brain barrier through active transport of LAT [72]. Gabapentinoids are not metabolized and are excreted unchanged in the urine, with an approximate elimination half-life of 6 h [7].

Pharmacodynamics

While gabapentin and pregabalin share structural similarity to gamma-aminobutyric acid (GABA), they do not bind to GABA receptors. The gabapentinoids have a high affinity for the α2δ-1 subunit of voltage-gated calcium channels that play a role in modulating neurotransmitter release [27]. While the exact mechanism of gabapentinoids in analgesia is not fully delineated, there are several theories that attempt to explain the clinical response [14].

In response to painful stimuli or damage to the somatosensory system, α2δ-1 subunit levels become elevated, particularly in the dorsal horn of the spinal cord, which manifests as neuropathic pain [4, 75]. The major proposed mechanism of analgesic effect is through gabapentinoid inhibition of the activity of the α2δ-1 subunit of voltage-gated calcium channels that are present throughout the central nervous system (CNS) [4, 85]. Through the modulation of neurotransmitter release, gabapentinoids work within the somatosensory cortex to dampen the sensory signaling associated with conditions like neuropathic pain [47]. Gabapentinoids also block the binding of thrombospondin to the α2δ-1 subunit to inhibit the formation of new excitatory synapses that can potentiate the pain and

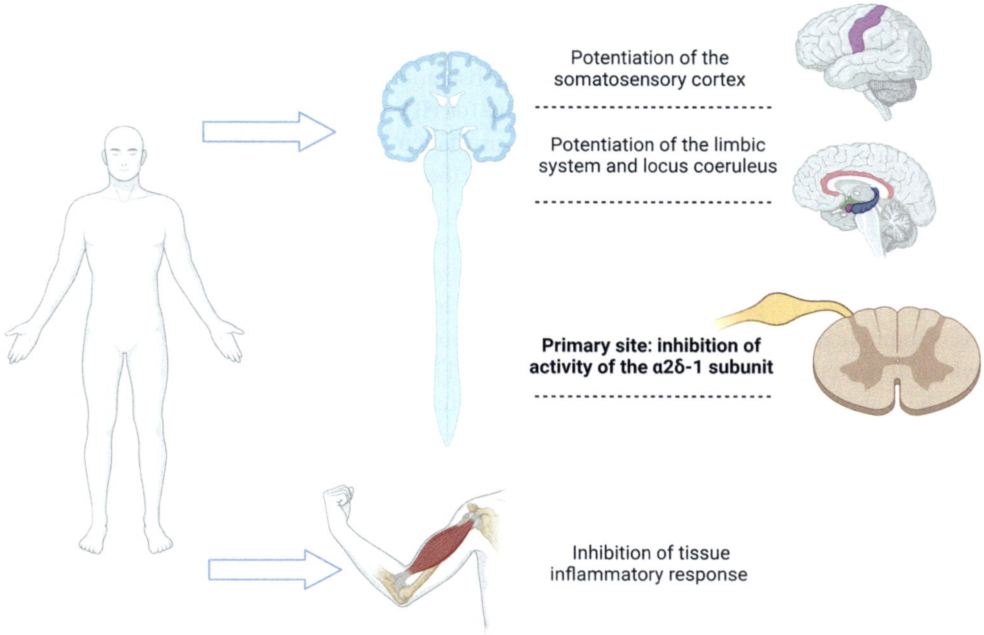

Fig. 7.1 Proposed sites of analgesic activity by gabapentinoids

inflammatory response [23, 58]. Blocking neurotransmitter release at the dorsal horn can also inhibit the release of serotonin and norepinephrine as part of endogenous pain pathways to elicit an analgesic effect, in addition to influencing locus coeruleus activity [14, 70]. Beyond this, there are also effects on the limbic system through changes in inhibitory and excitatory neurotransmission [47]. Figure 7.1 provides a visual representation of several proposed sites of analgesic action by gabapentinoids.

Neuropathic and Chronic Pain

The Neuropathic Pain Special Interest Group (NeuPSIG) of the International Association for the Study of Pain updated its guidelines in 2015 based on the results of a large systematic review and meta-analysis and recommended gabapentinoids as first-line therapies for most forms of neuropathic pain [25]. However, the strongest evidence for their use is for the treatment of PHN [22, 26, 65, 77], DPN [26, 45, 64, 73], neuropathic pain after spinal cord injury (SCI) [16, 32, 49, 73], and pain related to fibromyalgia [68]. Use of gabapentinoids for other chronic pain syndromes, such as chronic low back pain (CLBP), cancer-related pain, and human immunodeficiency virus (HIV)–related neuropathy is not consistently supported by available data.

In 2017, a Cochrane review by Wiffen et al. evaluated the efficacy of gabapentin for chronic neuropathic pain across 37 randomized, double-blind trials with over 5900 patients. In all of these trials, gabapentin was compared with either placebo or other active treatments for neuropathic pain, and primary outcomes were the percentage of patients who experienced moderate (at least 30% pain relief over baseline) to substantial (at least 50% pain relief over baseline) analgesia. The outcome of substantial pain relief was regarded as the most important, as this level of pain reduction is usually associated with improvement in other areas of life, such as sleep interference, fatigue, and depression. The total daily dose (TDD) of gabapentin in the reviewed studies ranged from 1800 to 3600 mg. For PHN and DPN, approximately 32% and 38% of patients, respectively, experienced at least a 50% reduction in pain with gabapentin when compared to placebo. However, adverse events (AEs) were more common in the gabapentin groups across all conditions, with 63% of patients experiencing at least one AE. The most common AEs were dizziness, somnolence, gait disturbances, and the development of peripheral edema [81].

In 2019, a Cochrane review by Derry et al. evaluated the efficacy of pregabalin for chronic neuropathic pain across 45 randomized, double-blinded trials with more than 11,900 patients. They compared pregabalin (TDD: 150, 300, and 600 mg) with placebo or other active treatments for neuropathic pain (85% of patients had PHN, DPN, and mixed neuropathic pain) and considered primary outcomes of moderate-to-substantial pain relief over baseline with the indices described in the review by Wiffen. With TDDs of 300 and 600 mg, substantial pain relief was noted in 32% and 41%, respectively, in patients with PHN, and in 31% and 41%, respectively, in patients with DPN. More patients in the pregabalin groups experienced a moderate level of pain relief across both conditions, and results suggest a dose-dependent effect. In those experiencing mixed or traumatic neuropathic pain, a TDD of 600 mg was associated with substantial pain relief in 26% of patients. The use of pregabalin for HIV neuropathy was not supported, and there was insufficient evidence to support the use of pregabalin for those with neuropathic cancer pain or for neuropathic pain related to sciatica or CLBP. Like the results in Wiffen's review, those in the pregabalin groups experienced more AEs, with approximately 60% of patients experiencing at least one AE. Somnolence and dizziness were the most reported AEs, which appeared to correlate with increasing dose [17].

The gabapentinoids have been extensively studied and recommended as first-line therapies for neuropathic pain due to SCI, although the exact mechanism behind this type of neuropathic pain remains unclear [32, 49, 73]. In the post-SCI patient population, inadequate pain control has been suggested to weaken or slow the effectiveness of rehabilitation treatments and community reintegration, making analgesia a vital aspect of a patient's recovery [21]. While only pregabalin is FDA-approved for the treatment of post-SCI neuropathic pain, gabapentin is still used widely off-label for this indication.

A 2020 systematic review and meta-analysis of eight studies evaluated the efficacy of gabapentin and pregabalin for the treatment of neuropathic pain due to SCI and was the first meta-analysis to compare the two gabapentinoids head-to-head [16]. When comparing pregabalin (TDD: 150–600 mg) to placebo, three randomized controlled trials (RCTs) with a total of 377 patients showed that pregabalin had a significant effect on the reduction of pain scores (and was also more effective than placebo for anxiety, depression, and sleep interference). Gabapentin (TDD: 100–3600 mg) was compared to placebo in three studies with a total of 65 patients. In two studies, gabapentin was more effective for pain relief when compared to placebo but showed no substantial benefit in the third study. Notably, the latter study used diphenhydramine as an active placebo, the dose range for gabapentin was quite wide (TDD: 100–1200 mg), and there was some concern over attrition bias. When compared head-to-head, two crossover studies including 40 patients were reviewed. The TDD ranges for gabapentin and pregabalin were 300–3600 mg and 150–600 mg, respectively. No significant difference was noted in pain scores between the two groups. Except in one study, more AEs were noted in the gabapentinoid groups, with somnolence, dizziness, and peripheral edema being common in the pregabalin groups. Similar AEs were noted in the gabapentin groups (one study did not show a significant difference in AEs in the gabapentin group vs. placebo) [16]. The results of this meta-analysis, among the other studies considered, suggest the benefit of gabapentinoids for the treatment of SCI as long as their AE profile can be tolerated by the patient [32, 49].

Outside of those indications specified by the NeuPSIG, a 2016 Cochrane review examined the efficacy of pregabalin across eight studies with over 3200 patients with fibromyalgia. Patients were administered a TDD of 150, 300, 450, or 600 mg. No significant benefit was conferred with pregabalin 150 mg daily. The most favorable outcomes were observed in those receiving pregabalin at doses between 300 and 600 mg. More AEs were reported with escalating doses of pregabalin, with somnolence, dizziness, weight gain, and edema being more common and affecting up to 90% of those in the pregabalin groups (though AEs were reported in about 75% of the placebo groups) [18].

CLBP has a lifetime prevalence of up to 23% and an unspecified etiology in up to 85% of patients [1, 68]. Assessing whether there is a true neuropathic component to a patient's CLBP is difficult, and data for the use of gabapentinoids in these cases are inconsistent. A 2017 review of eight studies with over 900 patients aimed to evaluate the efficacy and safety of gabapentinoid use for nonspecific CLBP. The TDD ranged from 300 to 3600 mg for gabapentin and from 100 to 600 mg for pregabalin [68]. Overall, no substantial benefit was noted with the use of gabapentin vs. placebo, pregabalin vs. other analgesia, or pregabalin as an adjunct to existing pain regimens. Dizziness, fatigue, and difficulties with mentation were more common in the gabapentinoid groups. Given the AE profile of gabapentinoids, along with a lack of sufficient evidence of efficacy, the authors of the review recommended avoiding gabapentinoids for the treatment of CLBP. In studies where pregabalin has been shown to have a significant effect on pain control, it was often used in conjunction with other analgesics [52, 71]. A 2021 pooled analysis of two multicenter observational studies in Japan including 700 patients with CLBP or chronic cervical pain associated with radiating lower- and upper-extremity limb pain, respectively, suggested the effectiveness of pregabalin treatment from a patient perspective. However, a significant limitation in this study was the fact that most of the patients in the pregabalin groups received concomitant analgesia with other agents (at least 91% of those in the CLBP group and at least 72% of those in the cervical spine pain group) [71]. Most patients with chronic pain are generally using more than one analgesic agent; therefore, the efficacy of pregabalin alone remains unclear.

In conclusion, while gabapentinoids are recommended in patients with neuropathic pain due to PHN, DPN, and post-SCI, their actual efficacy in these patients can vary. The Cochrane review by Wiffen suggests that about three or four out of ten patients will achieve high levels of analgesia with gabapentin, but over half will not, and they are likely to experience AEs [81]. While some patients will experience substantial analgesia with pregabalin, many will have no benefit or discontinue treatment due to AEs [17]. In post-SCI patients and those with fibromyalgia, the gabapentinoids seem to have a good analgesic effect if their AE profile can be tolerated. Given the high incidence of AEs, as noted throughout the above review, along with the risk of respiratory depression when used with opioids, cautious administration of gabapentinoids for analgesia in select patient populations is recommended. Despite their frequent off-label use, there is no adequate evidence to support the administration of gabapentinoids for other types of chronic pain, such as CLBP, HIV neuropathy, or cancer-related neuropathy.

Perioperative and Postoperative Use of Gabapentinoids

As the surgical community shifts away from opioids, interest in gabapentinoids as an adjunct to multimodal surgical pain regimens has grown. Studies have focused on pain reduction and, more specifically, on a reduction in opioid use with the addition of gabapentin and pregabalin to pre- and postoperative pain treatment regimens. Enhanced Recovery After Surgery (ERAS) protocols, with the aim of minimizing opioid usage and limiting hospital stays, now routinely include gabapentinoids. AEs such as respiratory depression, delirium, and increased postanesthesia recovery stays have been described. The data across surgical subspecialties regarding the effectiveness of these medications vary, but most literature favors gabapentinoids as a tool to reduce pain, postoperative nausea and vomiting, and opioid consumption.

Studies investigating the impact of gabapentin and pregabalin on opioid consumption in the initial postoperative period show a generally favorable, although modest, reduction. Some studies report a significant reduction in opioid use following gabapentinoid administration, particularly within the first 24–48 h after surgery [31, 43]. Meta-analyses on specific surgical procedures like total knee arthroplasty and total hip arthroplasty also support this opioid-sparing effect [34, 84]. However, other studies, including a meta-analysis on general postoperative pain management, did not find a clinically significant reduction in opioid use [80].

Most trials only examined opioid consumption in the immediate postoperative period within the first 24 h. One randomized controlled trial examining 410 patients across multiple surgical specialties showed no effect on chronic opioid use, measured at 6 months and 1 year, after perioperative gabapentin administration [33].

As opioids commonly result in postoperative nausea and vomiting, the reduction in opioids would presumably lessen this AE. A meta-analysis of 281 trials and 24,682 patients examining perioperative gabapentinoids vs. placebo showed a decrease in postoperative nausea and vomiting in the gabapentinoid group [78].

The evidence regarding gabapentinoids' impact on length of hospital stay is inconclusive. While some studies suggest a potential benefit [24], others did not report a statistically significant effect [51]. Gabapentin and pregabalin might prolong stay in the postanesthesia care unit (PACU) due to sedation [69]. However, nearly all patients are also receiving opioids of varying degrees during these procedures, which confounds these studies.

Gabapentinoids are generally well-tolerated, but drowsiness and dizziness are common AEs. Pregabalin was associated with more dizziness and visual disturbances than gabapentin [78]. Some studies suggest a potential link between perioperative gabapentin use and delirium in elderly patients [57], but a meta-analysis showed no statistically significant effect of gabapentinoids on respiratory failure, ataxia/falls, or delirium [78].

ERAS protocols employed in multiple surgical subspecialties emphasize multimodal pain management strategies, including regional anesthesia, nonsteroidal anti-inflammatory drugs, acetaminophen, antiemetics, improved oral and intravenous hydration, and gabapentinoids. Studies evaluating ERAS pathways incorporating gabapentin for surgeries like total mastectomy [15], colorectal surgery [30], and live donor nephrectomy [11] demonstrate improved pain control and reduced opioid consumption. Gabapentinoids are used in conjunction with multimodal therapy during these protocols, so the effects of gabapentin and pregabalin are not typically studied in isolation in these populations.

Both gabapentin and pregabalin show some efficacy in reducing postoperative pain across various surgical specialties. However, the degree of effectiveness, dosages used, and duration of therapy vary widely. Preoperative doses ranging between 100 and 1200 mg of gabapentin and 150 and 300 mg of pregabalin were described in these studies. Duration ranged from a single preoperative dose to continuation of therapy for 24–48 h postoperatively.

Spinal surgery has the most robust evidence for perioperative gabapentinoid use. Some data suggest that pregabalin might be more effective than gabapentin for pain control after spinal surgeries [2, 34, 76]. Gabapentin shows some benefit in reducing pain after total knee and hip arthroplasty [34, 84]. Studies investigating pregabalin or gabapentin during breast cancer surgery show that both drugs may reduce acute and chronic pain, but the evidence is not conclusive [61, 69]. Thoracic surgery has employed ERAS protocols using gabapentinoids, but the data are limited because they, again, do not examine the independent effects of these drugs but only the multimodal therapy [87]. Limited data suggest that gabapentin might be effective for pain control in pediatric thoracic surgery [74]. Urologic and transplant data show promising results for both penile implants and kidney transplants [11, 48]. Studies support the use of gabapentin and pregabalin for pain management after head and neck surgeries [46, 67]. No studies specifically evaluate gabapentin or pregabalin for pain control in gynecologic or obstetric surgery; however, several studies suggest that ERAS protocols including these medications can reduce opioid use after gynecological surgeries, including C-sections [3, 24, 44, 51].

Limited data on specific procedures like colectomy, cholecystectomy, and hernia repair suggest some benefit of gabapentin and pregabalin for pain management. Although gabapentinoids are used frequently for chronic neuropathic pain in the setting of nerve injury after inguinal hernia repair, there are no studies to support the benefit of routine perioperative use of gabapentinoids for hernia surgery [5].

In summary, heterogeneity in study designs, surgical procedures, medication protocols, and follow-up periods limits drawing definitive conclusions about overall gabapentinoid efficacy. Gabapentin and pregabalin may be beneficial additions to multimodal pain management strategies, particularly for specific surgical procedures, most notably spinal surgery. While evidence suggests a potential for reducing opioid use and postoperative nausea and vomiting, the effect varies. Further research is needed to determine the optimal role of gabapentin and pregabalin in different surgical specialties. This includes investigating dosage optimization for each surgical procedure, patient selection, and long-term effects to evaluate the impact on chronic pain development.

Role of Gabapentinoids in Critically Ill Patients

In the critically ill patient population, providing adequate analgesia is an essential component of intensive care unit (ICU) care. Multiple studies have demonstrated that many ICU patients experience pain both at rest and during procedures [12, 60], and inadequate analgesia can lead to detrimental long-term effects, including post-traumatic stress disorder and chronic pain [35, 54]. The myriad of physiologic responses to pain in a critically ill patient includes delirium, increased myocardial oxygen demand, hormonal imbalances, and various respiratory complications that can contribute to increased duration of mechanical ventilation [63]. Opioids have long been the mainstay of pain control in the ICU but can contribute to hemodynamic instability and oversedation. The use of gabapentinoids as adjuncts for analgesia in critically ill patients has been a hopeful avenue in minimizing opiate use in the ICU.

Evidence for the use of gabapentinoids in ICU patients is discussed in the pain, agitation–sedation, delirium, immobility, and sleep clinical practice guidelines published by the Society of Critical Care Medicine and focuses on a multimodal approach to pain control with the goal of minimizing opioids. A total of four RCTs were included in these guidelines, two of which evaluated gabapentin use in ICU patients with Guillain–Barré syndrome (GBS) [20]. The first demonstrated that a dose of 15 mg/kg/d of gabapentin led to a significant decrease in fentanyl requirements over days 1–7 of ICU admission in 18 patients with GBS [55]. The second, including 36 patients with GBS admitted to the ICU, demonstrated significantly lower numeric pain scores reported by patients receiving gabapentin 300 mg TID when compared to those who received either carbamazepine 100 mg TID or placebo [56]. The remaining two RCTs evaluated the use of pregabalin (150 mg before the procedure and then daily) vs. placebo for decreasing opioid requirements in post–cardiac surgery ICU patients [41, 59]. Although both trials demonstrated decreased opioid requirements in the postoperative period, there was no difference in the length of ICU stay or time on mechanical ventilation. Additionally, concerns were raised regarding bias and imprecision in the latter study.

The evidence for the use of gabapentinoids as adjuncts for analgesia in the general ICU population, exclusive of postoperative cardiac surgery patients or those with GBS, is limited. A randomized, double-blind, placebo-controlled trial performed by Salarian et al. evaluated the use of gabapentin 300 mg TID vs. placebo in 43 mechanically ventilated ICU patients receiving concomitant fentanyl and midazolam infusions. They found that the target level of sedation (Ramsay sedation scale score 2–3) was reached in both groups, with the gabapentin group requiring significantly less fentanyl and midazolam compared to placebo. Patients in the gabapentin group also experienced less delirium. Additionally, the duration of mechanical ventilation and the length of ICU stay were shorter in the gabapentin group, but these results were not statistically significant. No significant differences in the frequency of hypotension, bradycardia, or respiratory depression were noted between the two groups [66].

However, evidence supporting the use of gabapentinoids in general ICU populations remains limited and less conclusive. In a 2021 retrospective review of 1147 mechanically ventilated patients receiving fentanyl infusions, 275 patients were found to have received gabapentin at any point in their hospital stay. Although fentanyl utilization did not decrease, patients who had received gabapentin utilized less midazolam [82]. It is unclear whether the use of less midazolam would encourage the initiation of gabapentin on a broader scale, as the standard of care is moving away from deep sedation practices, except in select clinical scenarios.

A randomized, double-blind, controlled trial of gabapentin 300 mg TID vs. placebo as part of a multimodal analgesic regimen for traumatic rib fractures in critically ill patients showed no benefit in pain scores, opioid consumption, or pulmonary mechanics in the gabapentin group. Forty patients were included and well-matched based on the median RibScore, degree of pulmonary contusion, and severity of injury score. The length of neither hospital nor ICU stay differed between groups, and there was no significant improvement in acute outcomes over 1 month [53].

Outside of analgesia, an interesting potential role for gabapentinoids in the ICU relates to sedation and propofol use. A study involving ten healthy volunteers found that the administration of gabapentin 400 mg prior to propofol induction significantly decreased the target propofol blood concentration necessary to achieve adequate sedation levels when compared to propofol alone [38]. Similarly, a study including 40 patients undergoing total mastectomy demonstrated that preoperative administration of gabapentin 600 mg decreased intraoperative propofol requirements after anesthesia was induced and reduced the amount of postoperative morphine required for pain control [6]. No significant adverse cardiopulmonary effects were noted in patients receiving gabapentin in either study. Though the sample sizes in both studies were small, this raises the question of whether gabapentin administration could be evaluated for use in patients with difficulty weaning from propofol and could be a target of future studies.

In short, the evidence for gabapentinoid use in the general ICU population as an opioid-sparing agent exclusive of neuropathic pain is not robust. Results from Salarian et al. are promising, and the trend toward decreased duration of mechanical ventilation and length of ICU stay will hopefully prompt future research. However, clinicians must consider the limitations of gabapentinoid administration in the ICU, a substantial one being the varying degrees of renal dysfunction exhibited by many critically ill patients. In such patients, although gabapentinoids could be utilized at reduced doses, it is unclear if their efficacy would be maintained. Additionally, many ICU patients exhibit encephalopathy in the setting of their critical illness, underlying comorbidities, and/or polypharmacy. Initiation of gabapentinoids in these patients may have the potential of contributing to or worsening encephalopathy, given their known adverse effects of somnolence and dizziness, which most often occur during the initiation of treatment. Therefore, it is the opinion of these authors that gabapentinoids should be used for analgesia with extreme caution and only in select ICU patient populations pending additional, larger studies.

Applications to Clinical Practice

Dosing Considerations

Due to the renal elimination of gabapentinoids, there is a risk of drug accumulation in patients with kidney injury or failure, which can lead to encephalopathy, falls, and injuries secondary to those falls [39]. Table 7.2 outlines recommended dose adjustments according to the severity of renal impairment. Patients with renal failure also have an increased risk of respiratory depression when gabapentinoids are used in combination with other agents that affect the central nervous system (CNS). Providers should also take caution when prescribing these medications in elderly patients, as the American Geriatrics Society considers gabapentinoids to be potentially inappropriate when used with opioids [9]. A cohort study examining falls among over 12,000 elderly patients determined that patients were at a greater risk of falls when gabapentinoids were added to an existing opioid regimen, compared to the initiation of both agents simultaneously [13]. To mitigate the central effects of gabapentinoids in both elderly patients and those with renal impairment, it is recommended to initiate the medications at lower doses and titrate slowly over the course of several weeks. There are also benefits to scheduling doses at bedtime so that any sedating effects will not interfere with daytime activities.

Table 7.2 Maximum gabapentinoid dosing recommendations in renal dysfunction

Creatinine clearance threshold	Gabapentin	Pregabalin
30–59 mL/min	700 mg twice daily	150 mg twice daily
15–29 mL/min	700 mg once daily	75 mg twice daily
<15 mL/min	300 mg daily	75 mg daily
Post-hemodialysis supplement	300 mg after hemodialysis	150 mg after hemodialysis

Raouf et al. [62]

Gabapentin and pregabalin are available in multiple formulations, making them accessible to a wide range of patient groups. Both medications are traditionally dispensed as capsules but are also manufactured as oral solutions, which are convenient for patients with difficulty swallowing or who may need to administer medications through a feeding tube. If hospitals, facilities, or insurance cannot supply the oral solution, gabapentinoid capsules can be opened and mixed with water or sprinkled on food, if needed [28]. For patients who prefer fewer medication administrations throughout the day, gabapentin extended-release tablets or controlled-release pregabalin capsules can be considered to maximize adherence and convenience for the patient.

Safety Considerations

Beyond their role in neuropathic pain and off-label uses, gabapentinoids possess several benefits in clinical practice, one of which is their minimal risk of drug–drug interactions due to their lack of metabolism and protein binding. They are also leveraged to spare opioids in several populations such as critically ill and postoperative patients, though there can be a risk of enhanced respiratory and neurologic depression among patients who use concomitant CNS depressants [8].

The primary risks associated with gabapentin and pregabalin are derived from their AE profiles, mainly those relating to the central nervous system. Both can cause dizziness, somnolence, and fatigue, and most adverse drug effects involving higher cortical function are observed at higher doses [83]. Abdominal distension, dry mouth, and nausea have been reported, and these generally occur at the time of initiation and diminish over the course of subsequent weeks. Weight gain can be observed but is associated with higher doses and prolonged durations of treatment, while peripheral edema can affect up to 17% of patients at any point during therapy [10]. There have been some case reports noting an association with pregabalin and new-onset heart failure, but larger studies have not found an increased risk of heart failure in these patients compared to those taking gabapentin [37].

There is some risk of medication abuse and addiction with the use of gabapentin and pregabalin. Pregabalin is considered to have a higher abuse potential due to its increased potency and more favorable pharmacokinetics [8]. While the risk of fatal overdose with gabapentinoids alone is low, they can be lethal when combined with other psychoactive medications. For this reason, gabapentinoids should be avoided in patients with a history of substance use disorder or administered cautiously with strict therapeutic and prescription monitoring [8].

Interdisciplinary Considerations in Practice

When prescribing gabapentinoids, it is critical to consider each patient's unique needs, comorbidities, and past medical history. Patients who are elderly or have a history of kidney disease may be at a greater risk of falls due to the risk of drug accumulation. This risk can become more profound if the patient is also taking an anticoagulant or has a history of osteopenia or osteoporosis, introducing the risk of catastrophic bleeds or debilitating fractures.

Providers should aim to avoid prescribing gabapentinoids to patients with a history of substance use disorder and take caution when considering their use for patients who are also prescribed opioids due to the risk of CNS and respiratory depression. In these cases, patients should visit their provider at least annually to assess the ongoing efficacy of the medication and the risk of potential misuse [14].

Both patients and providers should be aware of the need to titrate the dose of pregabalin and gabapentin to effect and recognize that it can take weeks to achieve the target dose. Gabapentinoids must be administered on a scheduled basis as opposed to "as needed"; otherwise, adequate inhibition of the calcium channels will not be achieved [36]. Beyond this, if patients do not experience improvement in pain after their designated trial period, the medication should be discontinued. If patients must transition from one agent to another, there is no evidence-based dose conversion guide; however, a pharmacokinetic simulation suggested two possible strategies that used a 6:1 ratio of gabapentin to pregabalin [7]. One option involves discontinuing one agent and initiating the other at the time of the next scheduled dose. The second strategy consists of coadministering both medications at 50% of their desired doses for 4 days before fully transitioning to a singular agent [7].

In some clinical situations, particularly in the acute setting, providers may prefer to withhold home medications like gabapentinoids to avoid potential sedative effects and allow for a more comprehensive neurologic exam. It is important to recognize, however, that abrupt discontinuation of gabapentinoids can precipitate withdrawal and manifest as seizures, even if the patient is not taking the prescription for an indication related to epilepsy. Withdrawal symptoms generally appear between 24 and 48 h after medication cessation but can appear as early as 12 h after a missed dose and up to 7 days afterward [50]. For this reason, the best practice is to gradually taper the medication over at least 1 week to avoid precipitating withdrawal. If this is not feasible in the acute setting, providers can consider resuming a partial dose of a patient's gabapentinoid to mitigate the risk of withdrawal.

Conclusions

Gabapentinoids have FDA approval for a variety of conditions, and off-label uses are quite common, leading to widespread prescribing, especially for gabapentin. These agents are a viable option when considering a multimodal or opioid-sparing approach for analgesia. Gabapentin and pregabalin have been shown to improve outcomes with perioperative use in select surgical populations, and there is robust evidence to support their effectiveness in neuropathic pain management. Data on critically ill patients are limited, but this patient group might present an opportunity for future research, especially as an opioid-sparing strategy. These agents have largely favorable pharmacokinetics, but thoughtful consideration of age and renal function is important to avoid adverse effects. Therefore, a multidisciplinary and collaborative approach to care is needed to ensure optimal outcomes and maximize the risk–benefit balance.

References

1. Balagué F, Mannion AF, Pellisé F, Cedraschi C. Non-specific low back pain. Lancet. 2012;379:482–91. https://doi.org/10.1016/S0140-6736(11)60610-7.
2. Baloch SR, Hashmi IA, Rafi MS, Wasim A, Mazar S, Malick N, Tayyab B, Riaz H. Role of pregabalin to decrease postoperative pain in microdiscectomy: a randomized clinical trial. Cureus. 2021;13:e12870. https://doi.org/10.7759/cureus.12870.

3. Bauchat JR, Habib AS. Evidence-based anesthesia for major gynecologic surgery. Anesthesiol Clin. 2015;33:173–207. https://doi.org/10.1016/j.anclin.2014.11.011.
4. Bauer CS, Rahman W, Tran-Van-Minh A, Lujan R, Dickenson AH, Dolphin AC. The anti-allodynic α2δ ligand pregabalin inhibits the trafficking of the calcium channel α2δ-1 subunit to presynaptic terminals *in vivo*. Biochem Soc Trans. 2010;38:525–8. https://doi.org/10.1042/BST0380525.
5. Bekawi MS, El Wakeel LM, Al Taher WMA, Mageed WMA. Clinical study evaluating pregabalin efficacy and tolerability for pain management in patients undergoing laparoscopic cholecystectomy. Clin J Pain. 2014;30:944–52. https://doi.org/10.1097/AJP.0000000000000060.
6. Bharti N, Bala I, Narayan V, Singh G. Effect of gabapentin pretreatment on propofol consumption, hemodynamic variables, and postoperative pain relief in breast cancer surgery. Acta Anaesthesiol Taiwanica. 2013;51:10–3. https://doi.org/10.1016/j.aat.2013.03.009.
7. Bockbrader HN, Wesche D, Miller R, Chapel S, Janiczek N, Burger P. A comparison of the pharmacokinetics and pharmacodynamics of pregabalin and gabapentin. Clin Pharmacokinet. 2010;49:661–9. https://doi.org/10.2165/11536200-000000000-00000.
8. Bonnet U, Scherbaum N. How addictive are gabapentin and pregabalin? A systematic review. Eur Neuropsychopharmacol. 2017;27:1185–215. https://doi.org/10.1016/j.euroneuro.2017.08.430.
9. By the 2019 American Geriatrics Society Beers Criteria® Update Expert Panel. American Geriatrics Society 2019 updated AGS beers criteria® for potentially inappropriate medication use in older adults. J Am Geriatr Soc. 2019;67:674–94. https://doi.org/10.1111/jgs.15767.
10. Calkins A, Shurman J, Jaros M, Kim R, Shang G. Peripheral edema and weight gain in adult patients with painful diabetic peripheral neuropathy (DPN) receiving gabapentin enacarbil (GEn) or pregabalin enrolled in a randomized phase 2 trial (I6-1.004). Neurology. 2014;82:I6–1.004. https://doi.org/10.1212/WNL.82.10_supplement.I6-1.004.
11. Campsen J, Call T, Allen CM, Presson AP, Martinez E, Rofaiel G, Kim RD. Prospective, double-blind, randomized clinical trial comparing an ERAS pathway with ketorolac and pregabalin versus standard of care plus placebo during live donor nephrectomy for kidney transplant. Am J Transplant. 2019;19:1777–81. https://doi.org/10.1111/ajt.15242.
12. Chanques G, Sebbane M, Barbotte E, Viel E, Eledjam J-J, Jaber S. A prospective study of pain at rest: incidence and characteristics of an unrecognized symptom in surgical and trauma *versus* medical intensive care unit patients. Anesthesiology. 2007;107:858–60. https://doi.org/10.1097/01.anes.0000287211.98642.51.
13. Chen C, Winterstein AG, Lo-Ciganic W-H, Tighe PJ, Wei Y-JJ. Concurrent use of prescription gabapentinoids with opioids and risk for fall-related injury among older US Medicare beneficiaries with chronic noncancer pain: a population-based cohort study. PLoS Med. 2022;19:e1003921. https://doi.org/10.1371/journal.pmed.1003921.
14. Chincholkar M. Gabapentinoids: pharmacokinetics, pharmacodynamics and considerations for clinical practice. Br J Pain. 2020;14:104–14. https://doi.org/10.1177/2049463720912496.
15. Chiu C, Aleshi P, Esserman LJ, Inglis-Arkell C, Yap E, Whitlock EL, Harbell MW. Improved analgesia and reduced post-operative nausea and vomiting after implementation of an enhanced recovery after surgery (ERAS) pathway for total mastectomy. BMC Anesthesiol. 2018;18:41. https://doi.org/10.1186/s12871-018-0505-9.
16. Davari M, Amani B, Amani B, Khanijahani A, Akbarzadeh A, Shabestan R. Pregabalin and gabapentin in neuropathic pain management after spinal cord injury: a systematic review and meta-analysis. Korean J Pain. 2020;33:3–12. https://doi.org/10.3344/kjp.2020.33.1.3.
17. Derry S, Bell RF, Straube S, Wiffen PJ, Aldington D, Moore RA. Pregabalin for neuropathic pain in adults. Cochrane Database Syst Rev. 2019;1(1):CD007076. https://doi.org/10.1002/14651858.CD007076.pub3.
18. Derry S, Cording M, Wiffen PJ, Law S, Phillips T, Moore RA. Pregabalin for pain in fibromyalgia in adults. Cochrane Database Syst Rev. 2016;1(1):CD007076. https://doi.org/10.1002/14651858.CD011790.pub2.
19. Drug Enforcement Administration, Department of Justice. Schedules of controlled substances: placement of pregabalin into schedule V. Final rule. Fed Regist. 2005;70(144):43633–5.
20. Devlin JW, Skrobik Y, Gélinas C, Needham DM, Slooter AJC, Pandharipande PP, Watson PL, Weinhouse GL, Nunnally ME, Rochwerg B, Balas MC, van den Boogaard M, Bosma KJ, Brummel NE, Chanques G, Denehy L, Drouot X, Fraser GL, Harris JE, Joffe AM, Kho ME, Kress JP, Lanphere JA, McKinley S, Neufeld KJ, Pisani MA, Payen J-F, Pun BT, Puntillo KA, Riker RR, Robinson BRH, Shehabi Y, Szumita PM, Winkelman C, Centofanti JE, Price C, Nikayin S, Misak CJ, Flood PD, Kiedrowski K, Alhazzani W. Clinical practice guidelines for the prevention and management of pain, agitation/sedation, delirium, immobility, and sleep disruption in adult patients in the ICU. Crit Care Med. 2018;46:e825–73. https://doi.org/10.1097/CCM.0000000000003299.
21. Donnelly C, Eng JJ. Pain following spinal cord injury: the impact on community reintegration. Spinal Cord. 2005;43:278–82. https://doi.org/10.1038/sj.sc.3101702.
22. Dworkin RH, Corbin AE, Young JP, Sharma U, LaMoreaux L, Bockbrader H, Garofalo EA, Poole RM. Pregabalin for the treatment of postherpetic neuralgia: a randomized, placebo-controlled trial. Neurology. 2003;60:1274–83. https://doi.org/10.1212/01.WNL.0000055433.55136.55.
23. Eroglu Ç, Allen NJ, Susman MW, O'Rourke NA, Park CY, Özkan E, Chakraborty C, Mulinyawe SB, Annis DS, Huberman AD, Green EM, Lawler J, Dolmetsch R, Garcia KC, Smith SJ, Luo ZD, Rosenthal A, Mosher DF, Barres BA. Gabapentin receptor α2δ-1 is a neuronal thrombospondin receptor responsible for excitatory CNS synaptogenesis. Cell. 2009;139:380–92. https://doi.org/10.1016/j.cell.2009.09.025.
24. Felder L, Saccone G, Scuotto S, Monks DT, Carvalho JCA, Zullo F, Berghella V. Perioperative gabapentin and post cesarean pain control: a systematic review and meta-analysis of randomized controlled trials. Eur J Obstet Gynecol Reprod Biol. 2019;233:98–106. https://doi.org/10.1016/j.ejogrb.2018.11.026.
25. Finnerup NB, Attal N, Haroutounian S, McNicol E, Baron R, Dworkin RH, Gilron I, Haanpää M, Hansson P, Jensen TS, Kamerman PR, Lund K, Moore A, Raja SN, Rice ASC, Rowbotham M, Sena E, Siddall P, Smith BH, Wallace M. Pharmacotherapy for neuropathic pain in adults: a systematic review and meta-analysis. Lancet Neurol. 2015;14:162–73. https://doi.org/10.1016/S1474-4422(14)70251-0.
26. Freynhagen R, Strojek K, Griesing T, Whalen E, Balkenohl M. Efficacy of pregabalin in neuropathic pain evaluated in a 12-week, randomised, double-blind, multicentre, placebo-controlled trial of flexible- and fixed-dose regimens. Pain. 2005;115:254–63. https://doi.org/10.1016/j.pain.2005.02.032.
27. Gee NS, Brown JP, Dissanayake VUK, Offord J, Thurlow R, Woodruff GN. The novel anticonvulsant drug, gabapentin (Neurontin), binds to the α2δ subunit of a Calcium Channel. J Biol Chem. 1996;271:5768–76. https://doi.org/10.1074/jbc.271.10.5768.
28. Gidal BE, Maly MM, Kowalski JW, Rutecki PA, Pitterle ME, Cook DE. Gabapentin absorption: effect of mixing with foods of varying

macronutrient composition. Ann Pharmacother. 1998;32:405–9. https://doi.org/10.1345/aph.17281.
29. Goodman CW, Brett AS. A clinical overview of off-label use of gabapentinoid drugs. JAMA Intern Med. 2019;179:695. https://doi.org/10.1001/jamainternmed.2019.0086.
30. Gustafsson UO, Scott MJ, Hubner M, Nygren J, Demartines N, Francis N, Rockall TA, Young-Fadok TM, Hill AG, Soop M, De Boer HD, Urman RD, Chang GJ, Fichera A, Kessler H, Grass F, Whang EE, Fawcett WJ, Carli F, Lobo DN, Rollins KE, Balfour A, Baldini G, Riedel B, Ljungqvist O. Guidelines for perioperative care in elective colorectal surgery: enhanced recovery after surgery (ERAS ®) society recommendations: 2018. World J Surg. 2019;43:659–95. https://doi.org/10.1007/s00268-018-4844-y.
31. Haffner M, Saiz AM, Nathe R, Hwang J, Migdal C, Klineberg E, Roberto R. Preoperative multimodal analgesia decreases 24-hour postoperative narcotic consumption in elective spinal fusion patients. Spine J. 2019;19:1753–63. https://doi.org/10.1016/j.spinee.2019.07.005.
32. Hagen EM, Rekand T. Management of neuropathic pain associated with spinal cord injury. Pain Ther. 2015;4:51–65. https://doi.org/10.1007/s40122-015-0033-y.
33. Hah J, Mackey SC, Schmidt P, McCue R, Humphreys K, Trafton J, Efron B, Clay D, Sharifzadeh Y, Ruchelli G, Goodman S, Huddleston J, Maloney WJ, Dirbas FM, Shrager J, Costouros JG, Curtin C, Carroll I. Effect of perioperative gabapentin on postoperative pain resolution and opioid cessation in a mixed surgical cohort: a randomized clinical trial. JAMA Surg. 2018;153:303–11. https://doi.org/10.1001/jamasurg.2017.4915.
34. Han C, Li X, Jiang H, Ma J, Ma X. The use of gabapentin in the management of postoperative pain after total hip arthroplasty: a meta-analysis of randomised controlled trials. J Orthop Surg Res. 2016;11:79. https://doi.org/10.1186/s13018-016-0412-z.
35. Hayhurst CJ, Jackson JC, Archer KR, Thompson JL, Chandrasekhar R, Hughes CG. Pain and its long-term interference of daily life after critical illness. Anesth Analg. 2018;127:690–7. https://doi.org/10.1213/ANE.0000000000003358.
36. Heblich F, Tran-Van-Minh A, Hendrich J, Watschinger K, Dolphin AC. Time course and specificity of the pharmacological disruption of the trafficking of voltage-gated calcium channels by gabapentin. Channels. 2008;2:4–9. https://doi.org/10.4161/chan.2.1.6045.
37. Ho JM-W, Macdonald EM, Luo J, Gomes T, Antoniou T, Mamdani MM, Juurlink DN. Pregabalin and heart failure: A population-based study. Pharmacoepidemiol Drug Saf. 2017;26:1087–92. https://doi.org/10.1002/pds.4239.
38. Hosokawa R, Ito S, Hirokawa J, Oshima Y, Yokoyama T. Effectiveness of preanesthetic administration of gabapentin on sedative action during intravenous sedation with propofol. J Anesth. 2018;32:813–21. https://doi.org/10.1007/s00540-018-2559-8.
39. Ishida JH, McCulloch CE, Steinman MA, Grimes BA, Johansen KL. Gabapentin and pregabalin use and association with adverse outcomes among hemodialysis patients. J Am Soc Nephrol. 2018;29:1970–8. https://doi.org/10.1681/ASN.2018010096.
40. Johansen ME. Gabapentinoid use in the United States 2002 through 2015. JAMA Intern Med. 2018;178:292. https://doi.org/10.1001/jamainternmed.2017.7856.
41. Joshi S, Jagadeesh A. Efficacy of perioperative pregabalin in acute and chronic post-operative pain after off-pump coronary artery bypass surgery: a randomized, double-blind placebo controlled trial. Ann Card Anaesth. 2013;16:180. https://doi.org/10.4103/0971-9784.114239.
42. Kane SP. The top 200 of 2021, ClinCalc DrugStats database, version 2024.01. ClinCalc; 2024.
43. Ladich EM, Zhou KQ, Spence DL, Moore CB. Opioid-sparing anesthesia: gabapentin and postoperative pain. J Perianesth Nurs. 2022;37:966–70. https://doi.org/10.1016/j.jopan.2022.04.008.
44. Lasala J, Mena GE, Iniesta MD, Cata J, Pitcher B, Wendell W, Zorrilla-Vaca A, Cain K, Basabe M, Suki T, Meyer LA, Ramirez PT. Impact of anesthesia technique on post-operative opioid use in open gynecologic surgery in an enhanced recovery after surgery pathway. Int J Gynecol Cancer. 2021;31:569–74. https://doi.org/10.1136/ijgc-2020-002004.
45. Lesser H, Sharma U, LaMoreaux L, Poole RM. Pregabalin relieves symptoms of painful diabetic neuropathy: a randomized controlled trial. Neurology. 2004;63:2104–10. https://doi.org/10.1212/01.WNL.0000145767.36287.A1.
46. Liébana-Hermoso S, Manzano-Moreno FJ, Vallecillo-Capilla MF, Olmedo-Gaya MV. Oral pregabalin for acute pain relief after cervicofacial surgery: a systematic review. Clin Oral Investig. 2018;22:119–29. https://doi.org/10.1007/s00784-017-2272-2.
47. Lin H-C, Huang Y-H, Chao T-HH, Lin W-Y, Sun W-Z, Yen C-T. Gabapentin reverses central hypersensitivity and suppresses medial prefrontal cortical glucose metabolism in rats with neuropathic pain. Mol Pain. 2014;10:63. https://doi.org/10.1186/1744-8069-10-63.
48. Lucas J, Gross M, Yafi F, DeLay K, Christianson S, El-Khatib FM, Osman M, Simhan J. A multi-institutional assessment of multimodal analgesia in penile implant recipients demonstrates dramatic reduction in pain scores and narcotic usage. J Sex Med. 2020;17:518–25. https://doi.org/10.1016/j.jsxm.2019.11.267.
49. Mehta S, McIntyre A, Dijkers M, Loh E, Teasell RW. Gabapentinoids are effective in decreasing neuropathic pain and other secondary outcomes after spinal cord injury: a meta-analysis. Arch Phys Med Rehabil. 2014;95:2180–6. https://doi.org/10.1016/j.apmr.2014.06.010.
50. Mersfelder TL, Nichols WH. Gabapentin: abuse, dependence, and withdrawal. Ann Pharmacother. 2016;50:229–33. https://doi.org/10.1177/1060028015620800.
51. Monks DT, Hoppe DW, Downey K, Shah V, Bernstein P, Carvalho JCA. A perioperative course of gabapentin does not produce a clinically meaningful improvement in analgesia after cesarean delivery. Anesthesiology. 2015;123:320–6. https://doi.org/10.1097/ALN.0000000000000722.
52. Morlion B. Pharmacotherapy of low back pain: targeting nociceptive and neuropathic pain components. Curr Med Res Opin. 2011;27:11–33. https://doi.org/10.1185/03007995.2010.534446.
53. Moskowitz EE, Garabedian L, Harden K, Perkins-Pride E, Asfaw M, Preslaski C, Liasia KN, Lawless R, Burlew CC, Pieracci F. Corrigendum to “A double-blind, randomized controlled trial of gabapentin vs. placebo for acute pain management in critically ill patients with rib fractures”. Injury. 2019;50:1406. https://doi.org/10.1016/j.injury.2019.05.026. [Injury 49 (9) (2018) 1693–1698].
54. Myhren H, Ekeberg Ø, Tøien K, Karlsson S, Stokland O. Posttraumatic stress, anxiety and depression symptoms in patients during the first year post intensive care unit discharge. Crit Care. 2010;14:R14. https://doi.org/10.1186/cc8870.
55. Pandey CK, Bose N, Garg G, Singh N, Baronia A, Agarwal A, Singh PK, Singh U. Gabapentin for the treatment of pain in Guillain-Barré syndrome: a double-blinded, placebo-controlled, crossover study. Anesth Analg. 2002;95:1719–23. https://doi.org/10.1097/00000539-200212000-00046.
56. Pandey CK, Raza M, Tripathi M, Navkar DV, Kumar A, Singh UK. The comparative evaluation of gabapentin and carbamazepine for pain management in Guillain-Barr?? syndrome patients in the intensive care unit. Anesth Analg. 2005;101:220–5. https://doi.org/10.1213/01.ANE.0000152186.89020.36.
57. Park CM, Inouye SK, Marcantonio ER, Metzger E, Bateman BT, Lie JJ, Lee SB, Levin R, Kim DH. Perioperative gabapentin use and in-hospital adverse clinical events among older adults after

major surgery. JAMA Intern Med. 2022;182:1117. https://doi.org/10.1001/jamainternmed.2022.3680.

58. Park J, Yu YP, Zhou C-Y, Li K-W, Wang D, Chang E, Kim D-S, Vo B, Zhang X, Gong N, Sharp K, Steward O, Vitko I, Perez-Reyes E, Eroglu C, Barres B, Zaucke F, Feng G, Luo ZD. Central mechanisms mediating thrombospondin-4-induced pain states. J Biol Chem. 2016;291:13335–48. https://doi.org/10.1074/jbc.M116.723478.
59. Pesonen A, Suojaranta-Ylinen R, Hammarén E, Kontinen VK, Raivio P, Tarkkila P, Rosenberg PH. Pregabalin has an opioid-sparing effect in elderly patients after cardiac surgery: a randomized placebo-controlled trial. Br J Anaesth. 2011;106:873–81. https://doi.org/10.1093/bja/aer083.
60. Puntillo KA, Max A, Timsit J-F, Vignoud L, Chanques G, Robleda G, Roche-Campo F, Mancebo J, Divatia JV, Soares M, Ionescu DC, Grintescu IM, Vasiliu IL, Maggiore SM, Rusinova K, Owczuk R, Egerod I, Papathanassoglou EDE, Kyranou M, Joynt GM, Burghi G, Freebairn RC, Ho KM, Kaarlola A, Gerritsen RT, Kesecioglu J, Sulaj MMS, Norrenberg M, Benoit DD, Seha MSG, Hennein A, Periera FJ, Benbenishty JS, Abroug F, Aquilina A, Monte JRC, An Y, Azoulay E. Determinants of procedural pain intensity in the intensive care unit. The Europain® study. Am J Respir Crit Care Med. 2014;189:39–47. https://doi.org/10.1164/rccm.201306-1174OC.
61. Rai AS, Khan JS, Dhaliwal J, Busse JW, Choi S, Devereaux PJ, Clarke H. Preoperative pregabalin or gabapentin for acute and chronic postoperative pain among patients undergoing breast cancer surgery: a systematic review and meta-analysis of randomized controlled trials. J Plast Reconstr Aesthet Surg. 2017;70:1317–28. https://doi.org/10.1016/j.bjps.2017.05.054.
62. Raouf M, Atkinson T, Crumb M, Fudin J. Rational dosing of gabapentin and pregabalin in chronic kidney disease. J Pain Res. 2017;10:275–8. https://doi.org/10.2147/JPR.S130942.
63. Rawal G, Kumar R, Yadav S, Sujana R. Pain management in intensive care unit: a brief review. Med Res Chronicles. 2019;6:302. https://doi.org/10.26838/MEDRECH.2019.6.6.544.
64. Rosenstock J, Tuchman M, LaMoreaux L, Sharma U. Pregabalin for the treatment of painful diabetic peripheral neuropathy: a double-blind, placebo-controlled trial. Pain. 2004;110:628–38. https://doi.org/10.1016/j.pain.2004.05.001.
65. Sabatowski R, Gálvez R, Cherry DA, Jacquot F, Vincent E, Maisonobe P, Versavel M. Pregabalin reduces pain and improves sleep and mood disturbances in patients with post-herpetic neuralgia: results of a randomised, placebo-controlled clinical trial. Pain. 2004;109:26–35. https://doi.org/10.1016/j.pain.2004.01.001.
66. Salarian S, Memary E, Taheri F, Bagher B. Gabapentin as add-on to fentanyl and midazolam in patients receiving mechanical ventilation: a randomized, blinded study. Turk J Anaesthesiol Reanim. 2022;50:101–6. https://doi.org/10.5152/TJAR.2022.21366.
67. Sanders JG, Dawes PJD. Gabapentin for perioperative analgesia in otorhinolaryngology-head and neck surgery: systematic review. Otolaryngol Head Neck Surg. 2016;155:893–903. https://doi.org/10.1177/0194599816659042.
68. Shanthanna H, Gilron I, Rajarathinam M, AlAmri R, Kamath S, Thabane L, Devereaux PJ, Bhandari M. Benefits and safety of gabapentinoids in chronic low back pain: a systematic review and meta-analysis of randomized controlled trials. PLoS Med. 2017;14:e1002369. https://doi.org/10.1371/journal.pmed.1002369.
69. Siddiqui NT, Yousefzadeh A, Yousuf M, Kumar D, Choudhry FK, Friedman Z. The effect of gabapentin on delayed discharge from the postanesthesia care unit: a retrospective analysis. Pain Pract. 2018;18:18–22. https://doi.org/10.1111/papr.12575.
70. Suto T, Severino AL, Eisenach JC, Hayashida K. Gabapentin increases extracellular glutamatergic level in the locus coeruleus via astroglial glutamate transporter-dependent mechanisms. Neuropharmacology. 2014;81:95–100. https://doi.org/10.1016/j.neuropharm.2014.01.040.
71. Taguchi T, Nakano S, Nozawa K. Effectiveness of pregabalin treatment for neuropathic pain in patients with spine diseases: a pooled analysis of two multicenter observational studies in Japan. J Pain Res. 2021;14:757–71. https://doi.org/10.2147/JPR.S293556.
72. Takahashi Y, Nishimura T, Higuchi K, Noguchi S, Tega Y, Kurosawa T, Deguchi Y, Tomi M. Transport of pregabalin via L-type amino acid transporter 1 (SLC7A5) in human brain capillary endothelial cell line. Pharm Res. 2018;35:246. https://doi.org/10.1007/s11095-018-2532-0.
73. Teasell RW, Mehta S, Aubut J-AL, Foulon B, Wolfe DL, Hsieh JTC, Townson AF, Short C. A systematic review of pharmacologic treatments of pain after spinal cord injury. Arch Phys Med Rehabil. 2010;91:816–31. https://doi.org/10.1016/j.apmr.2010.01.022.
74. Tomaszek L, Fenikowski D, Maciejewski P, Komotajtys H, Gawron D. Perioperative gabapentin in pediatric thoracic surgery patients—randomized, placebo-controlled, phase 4 trial. Pain Med. 2020;21:1562–71. https://doi.org/10.1093/pm/pnz207.
75. Treede R-D, Jensen TS, Campbell JN, Cruccu G, Dostrovsky JO, Griffin JW, Hansson P, Hughes R, Nurmikko T, Serra J. Neuropathic pain: redefinition and a grading system for clinical and research purposes. Neurology. 2008;70:1630–5. https://doi.org/10.1212/01.wnl.0000282763.29778.59.
76. Tsai SHL, Hu C-W, El Sammak S, Durrani S, Ghaith AK, Lin CCJ, Krzyż EZ, Bydon M, Fu TS, Lin TY. Different gabapentin and pregabalin dosages for perioperative pain control in patients undergoing spine surgery: a systematic review and network meta-analysis. JAMA Netw Open. 2023;6:e2328121. https://doi.org/10.1001/jamanetworkopen.2023.28121.
77. Van Seventer R, Feister HA, Young JP, Stoker M, Versavel M, Rigaudy L. Efficacy and tolerability of twice-daily pregabalin for treating pain and related sleep interference in postherpetic neuralgia: a 13-week, randomized trial. Curr Med Res Opin. 2006;22:375–84. https://doi.org/10.1185/030079906X80404.
78. Verret M, Lauzier F, Zarychanski R, Perron C, Savard X, Pinard AM, Leblanc G, Cossi MJ, Neveu X, Turgeon AF, the Canadian Perioperative Anesthesia Clinical Trials (PACT) Group. Perioperative use of gabapentinoids for the management of postoperative acute pain. Anesthesiology. 2020;133:265–79. https://doi.org/10.1097/ALN.0000000000003428.
79. Wallach JD, Ross JS. Gabapentin approvals, off-label use, and lessons for postmarketing evaluation efforts. JAMA. 2018;319:776. https://doi.org/10.1001/jama.2017.21897.
80. Wick EC, Grant MC, Wu CL. Postoperative multimodal analgesia pain management with nonopioid analgesics and techniques: a review. JAMA Surg. 2017;152:691. https://doi.org/10.1001/jamasurg.2017.0898.
81. Wiffen PJ, Derry S, Bell RF, Rice AS, Tölle TR, Phillips T, Moore RA. Gabapentin for chronic neuropathic pain in adults. Cochrane Database Syst Rev. 2017;6(6):CD007938. https://doi.org/10.1002/14651858.CD007938.pub4.
82. Yeary J, Juang P, Lashinsky J, Owen E. 810: the use of gabapentin for pain and outcomes in intensive care unit patients. Crit Care Med. 2021;49:401. https://doi.org/10.1097/01.ccm.0000729128.07639.08.
83. Zaccara G, Gangemi P, Perucca P, Specchio L. The adverse event profile of pregabalin: a systematic review and meta-analysis of randomized controlled trials. Epilepsia. 2011;52:826–36. https://doi.org/10.1111/j.1528-1167.2010.02966.x.
84. Zhai L, Song Z, Liu K. The effect of gabapentin on acute postoperative pain in patients undergoing Total knee arthroplasty: a meta-analysis. Medicine. 2016;95:e3673. https://doi.org/10.1097/MD.0000000000003673.

85. Zhou C, Luo ZD. Electrophysiological characterization of spinal neuron sensitization by elevated calcium channel alpha-2-delta-1 subunit protein. Eur J Pain. 2014;18:649–58. https://doi.org/10.1002/j.1532-2149.2013.00416.x.
86. Zhou L, Bhattacharjee S, Kwoh CK, Tighe PJ, Malone DC, Slack M, Wilson DL, Brown JD, Lo-Ciganic W-H. Trends, patient and prescriber characteristics in gabapentinoid use in a sample of United States ambulatory care visits from 2003 to 2016. J Clin Med. 2019;9:83. https://doi.org/10.3390/jcm9010083.
87. Zorrilla-Vaca A, Rice D, Brown JK, Antonoff M, Sepesi B, Hofstetter W, Swisher S, Walsh G, Vaporciyan A, Mehran R, Hagberg C, Mena GE. Sustained reduction of discharge opioid prescriptions in an enhanced recovery after thoracic surgery program: a multilevel generalized linear model. Surgery. 2022;171:504–10. https://doi.org/10.1016/j.surg.2021.08.039.

Antidepressants

8

Denver Shipman

Abbreviations

CBC	Complete blood count
CDC	Centers for Disease Control
CMP	Comprehensive metabolic panel
CNS	Central nervous system
COMT	Catechol-O-methyltransferase
CYP	Cytochrome P450
DA	Dopamine
DAT	Dopamine transporter
DSM	*Diagnostic and Statistical Manual of Mental Disorders*
FDA	Food And Drug Administration
GABA	Gamma amino butyric acid
GAD	Generalized anxiety disorder
H	Histamine
IM	Intramuscular
IR	Immediate release
IV	Intravenous
LFT	Liver function test
MAOI	Monoamine oxidase inhibitor
NE	Norepinephrine
NET	Norepinephrine transporter
NSAID	Nonsteroidal anti-inflammatory drug
SAMHSA	Substance Abuse and Mental Health Services Administration
SERT	Serotonin transporter
SNRI	Serotonin and norepinephrine reuptake inhibitor
SQ	Subcutaneous
SR	Sustained release
SSRI	Selective serotonin reuptake inhibitor
TCA	Tricyclic antidepressant
TSH	Thyroid-stimulating hormone
UDS	Urine drug screen
ER	Extended release
5–HT	Serotonin

Background/Introduction

The Substance Abuse and Mental Health Services Administration (SAMHSA) estimates that 22.8% of US adults experienced mental illness in 2021 [1]. During the same year, the Centers for Disease Control (CDC) estimated that 20.9% of US adults experienced chronic pain [2]. The concurrence of psychiatric disorders and pain has been shown to worsen each condition's complexity, severity, and outcomes [3, 4]. Comorbid depression has been shown to increase the physical disability and economic burden caused by pain [5–7]. The presence of pain is also known to worsen psychiatric outcomes, with individuals experiencing pain having a 51% higher risk of experiencing suicidal behavior in one large 10-year-duration study [8].

With available data on the efficacy of antidepressants for pain, whether as monotherapy or as adjunctive therapy, antidepressants should be considered for patients experiencing pain. Although psychiatric disorders and comorbid pain are often encountered in the clinical setting, antidepressants may often be overlooked as an option for patients solely experi-

D. Shipman (✉)
Robert J Dole VA Medical Center, Wichita, KS, USA

J. P. Reinert et al. (eds.), *Adjunctive Analgesic Strategies for the Bedside Clinician and Beyond*,
https://doi.org/10.1007/978-3-032-21675-5_8

encing pain. Antidepressants may also be useful for patients where abuse potential is a concern, as they are much less likely to be abused or become addictive, especially in comparison to opioids [9].

Although less commonly discussed when compared to opioids, antidepressants do have the potential to cause withdrawal symptoms if abruptly stopped [10, 11]. These withdrawal symptoms commonly include anxiety, flu-like symptoms, insomnia, nausea, dizziness, electrical sensations, muscle spasms, and headache [10].

Pharmacology, Pharmacokinetics, and Pharmacodynamics

Antidepressants are a class of medications with a wide array of mechanisms of action. All antidepressants discussed in this chapter affect the presynaptic neuron to inhibit the reuptake of neurotransmitters. Many other antidepressants are available and have many other mechanisms of action, but this chapter will focus on the antidepressants that are used for the management of pain.

Receptor Systems

Serotonin

Serotonin, also known as 5-hydroxytryptamine or 5-HT, is a monoamine neurotransmitter with many biological functions. Serotonin is involved in the regulation of numerous organs and aspects of homeostasis. All antidepressant classes discussed in this chapter have some degree of action on the serotonergic nervous system. These antidepressants act on the presynaptic serotonin transporter (SERT), which normally returns serotonin from the synaptic cleft back into the presynaptic neuron. Antidepressants block the effect of SERT, thereby allowing serotonin more time to carry out its intended biological functions, such as binding with postsynaptic 5-HT receptors. There are seven subfamilies of 5-HT receptors, with some subfamilies being divided further into 15 subtypes. The role that any given 5-HT receptor subtype plays in pain regulation has not been reviewed comprehensively, and the role of individual serotonin receptor subtypes in pain transmission continues to be investigated [12]. Clinical trials studying antidepressants solely affecting the 5-HT system, such as selective serotonin reuptake inhibitors (SSRIs), have produced mixed results [13].

After 5-HT is released into the synaptic cleft, it is free to bind to any available 5-HT receptor. 5-HT receptors are present throughout the body and may be involved in regulating numerous functions even within a single organ system or neuronal pathway. Because of this, medications increasing 5-HT have a wide range of side effects involving multiple organ systems. In extreme cases, excessive accumulation of serotonin may lead to severe acute illnesses such as serotonin syndrome, a life-threatening illness characterized by hypotension; tachycardia; hyperreflexia; tremor; diaphoresis; diarrhea; and changes in cognition. 5-HT is cleared from the central nervous system (CNS) by being degraded by various synaptic enzymes such as monoamine oxidase (MAO) and catechol-O-methyltransferase (COMT). Medications that inhibit the action of these enzymes may potentiate the rise in levels of serotonin and lead to further risk of serotonin syndrome that would be present then if antidepressants were used alone.

Norepinephrine

Norepinephrine, often abbreviated as NE and formerly known as noradrenaline, is another monoamine neurotransmitter. The structure of norepinephrine is very similar to epinephrine; it is present in many of the same neurotransmitter pathways as epinephrine and causes many similar effects. Norepinephrine is responsible for pain reduction through its inhibitory actions on the neuronal pathways involved in pain transmission [14, 15]. Serotonin and norepinephrine reuptake inhibitor (SNRI) and tricyclic antidepressant (TCA) families of antidepressants act on the presynaptic norepinephrine transporter (NET) to block the reuptake of norepinephrine back into the presynaptic neuron. Inhibition of NET results in norepinephrine being present in the postsynaptic cleft for a longer duration, thereby allowing it more chance to bind to receptors. NET is also partly responsible for the reuptake of the neurotransmitter dopamine (DA) [16].

After NE is released into the synaptic cleft, it is free to bind to adrenergic nervous system receptors such as α_1, α_2, β_1, β_2, and β_3. The effects of NE binding to these receptors are highly variable and dependent on the specific receptor subtype and organ system in which it is present. Notable mechanisms of action and pain management involving these receptors include α_1 agonism, resulting in vasoconstriction, and α_2 agonism, resulting in sedative and anesthetic effects [17, 18]. The antidepressants discussed in this chapter do not result in a significant enough increase in NE to cause the degree of response seen from full adrenergic agonists and vasodilators, but their mild effect on these pathways is thought to contribute to their functions and pain management [19].

Dopamine

Dopamine (DA) is another monoamine neurotransmitter close in structure to NE and epinephrine. DA is thought to play a significant role in addiction by being released after pleasurable activities or substances, which reinforces the association of pleasure with these stimuli [20]. The serotonin and norepinephrine reuptake inhibitor (SNRI) and tricyclic antidepressant (TCA) families of antidepressants act on the presynaptic dopamine transporter (DAT) to block the reuptake of dopamine back into the presynaptic neuron. DA is also removed from the synaptic cleft by NET [16]. Inhibition of DAT allows DA to be present in the synaptic cleft for longer periods and a greater chance for DA to bind to its target receptors. There are five major dopamine receptors, D_1–D_5, but dopamine is also able to bind to α and β receptors [20, 21].

DA plays several roles in pain management. Its release after the use of opioids reinforces their use by causing feelings of euphoria or pleasure. The chronic use of opioids reinforces this association and increases the likelihood of addiction [22]. Agonism of DA receptors can result in a reduction in pain by decreasing nociception signaling [23].

Histamine

Histamine (H) is a molecule involved in immune response, inflammation, regulation of sleep, vasodilation, digestion, and many other physiological functions. There are four histamine receptors, H_1–H_4.

The TCA class of antidepressants are antagonists of histamine receptors, and their antagonism of H_1 receptors in particular results in many of their side effects. These side effects include sedation, blurred vision, tinnitus, weight gain, changes in mood and cognition, and many others. TCAs are used less frequently in the treatment of depression than SSRIs and SNRIs due to their high frequency of side effects, many of which are due to their antihistamine effect. There are benefits to TCAs having an antihistamine effect, as they may reduce the effects of allergies and inflammation.

Muscarinic

Muscarinic receptors are widely present throughout the body. There are five muscarinic receptors, M_1–M_5, each facilitating major roles throughout the body.

The TCA class of antidepressants are antagonists of muscarinic receptors, often having an anticholinergic effect due to these receptors being in the cholinergic nervous system. The anticholinergic side effects of TCAs result in them being used less frequently than SSRIs or SNRIs. The anticholinergic effects of TCAs are not thought to have a role in pain modulation but do cause side effects that can be severe and life-threatening and may include bradycardia, cognitive changes, pupil dilation, dry mouth, changes in vision, urinary retention, constipation, and hyperthermia.

Medications

SSRIs

Medication	Dosage range	Half-life (hours)	Main metabolic pathways	Special notes
Citalopram	10–40 mg daily	35	Hepatic: CYP3A4, CYP2C19	Max dose of 20 mg daily in patients >60 years Greatest potential for QT prolongation of any SSRI
Escitalopram	5–20 mg daily	27–32	Hepatic: CYP3A4, CYP2C19	S-enantiomer of citalopram Less potential for QT prolongation than citalopram [24]
Fluoxetine	10–80 mg daily	96–144	Hepatic: CYP2D6	Longest half-life of any SSRI Strong CYP2D6 inhibitor [25]
Fluvoxamine	25–300 mg daily	16	Hepatic: Non-CYP pathways	Inhibits CYP1A2, CYP2C9, CYP2C19, CYP2D6, and CYP3A4
Paroxetine	ER: 12.5–62.5 mg daily IR: 10–50 mg daily	15–21	Hepatic: CYP2D6	Shortest half-life of any SSRI
Sertraline	25–200 mg daily	24–26	Hepatic: non-CYP pathways	CYP2D6 inhibitor

SNRIs

Medication	Dosage range	Half-life (hours)	Main metabolic pathways	Special notes
Desvenlafaxine	50–200 mg daily	10–11	Hepatic: UGT, CYP3A4	Metabolite of venlafaxine CYP2D6 inhibitor
Duloxetine	20–120 mg daily	12	Hepatic: CYP1A2, CYP2D6	Food and Drug Administration (FDA) approvals for fibromyalgia, chronic musculoskeletal pain, and neuropathy due to diabetes mellitus
Levomilnacipran	20–120 mg daily	12	Hepatic: CYP3A4	L-enantiomer of milnacipran
Milnacipran	12.5 mg daily–100 mg twice daily	6–8	Hepatic: Non-CYP pathways	FDA approval for fibromyalgia
Venlafaxine	ER: 37.5–225 mg daily IR: 75 mg/day–225 mg/day divided into two or three doses	5	Hepatic: CYP2D6	

TCAs

Medication	Dosage range	Half-life (hours)	Main metabolic pathways	Special notes
Amitriptyline	25–150 mg daily	9–35	Hepatic: CYP3A4, CYP2C9, CYP2D6	
Amoxapine	25–300 mg daily	8	Hepatic: CYP2D6	
Clomipramine	25–250 mg daily	32	Hepatic: CYP2C19, CYP3A4, CYP1A2	
Desipramine	25–200 mg divided into one or two doses	17	Hepatic: CYP2D6, CYP1A2	Metabolite of imipramine
Doxepin	10–150 mg daily	15	Hepatic: CYP2C19, CYP2D6	Also available as a topical cream
Imipramine	25–200 mg divided into one or two doses	6–18	Hepatic: CYP2C19	
Nortriptyline	25–150 mg daily	15–39	Hepatic: CYP2D6	Metabolite of amitriptyline
Protriptyline	5–60 mg divided into 3–4 doses	54–198	Hepatic: CYP2D6	Longest half-life of any TCA
Trimipramine	25–200 mg divided into one to three doses	23	Hepatic: CYP2D6	

Evidence for Use

Efficacy

Of all available antidepressants, only duloxetine and milnacipran have FDA approval for pain management. Duloxetine is approved for neuropathic pain, fibromyalgia, chronic musculoskeletal pain, and diabetic peripheral neuropathic pain. Milnacipran is approved for fibromyalgia. Post-marketing studies and literature reviews have shown the efficacy of antidepressants in treating pain, including specific analyses of fibromyalgia, headache, diabetic neuropathy, and cancer pain [3]. The 2022 CDC guidelines for the treatment of pain include recommendations on the use of duloxetine and milnacipran, as well as TCAs and SNRIs as a class [71]. Many studies reveal that improvement in either pain or depression is associated with improvement in the other.

Evidence for TCAs

TCAs had been shown to be effective for the treatment of pain well before the availability of newer medications such as SSRIs and SNRIs. Administration of amitriptyline, imipramine, desipramine, and doxepin at doses of 150–300 mg/day has been shown to result in statistically significant pain relief [26].

Imipramine was studied for the treatment of chronic low back pain in a sample of 50 patients, the majority of whom did not experience depression, and was found to result in statistically significant improvement in pain symptoms, and a linear relationship between serum drug levels was also observed [27]. While the effects of the studies did not reach statistical significance, the effects it has as an active metabolite could contribute to the efficacy of imipramine. Studies of imipramine for neuropathy report some level of response, with most patients receiving doses between 100 and 150 mg/day [32–36]. Desipramine is a metabolite of imipramine and has also been studied for pain management, with some smaller studies targeting a 150–250-mg daily dose for neuropathy [28–31].

Amitriptyline and its metabolite nortriptyline have also been used in pain management. Studies of the effect of amitriptyline on fibromyalgia have generally reported positive results, with doses ranging between 5 and 50 mg/day [37]. A study of the effect of amitriptyline supplemented with pregabalin for the treatment of diabetic peripheral neuropathy showed significant pain reduction, and patients randomized to amitriptyline monotherapy in the 6 weeks leading up to combination therapy also experienced pain reduction [38]. Another study showed that amitriptyline 25 mg/day led to a reduction in disability from chronic low back pain at 3 months of treatment but that the improvement became nonsignificant at 6 months, with authors speculating that a larger trial may be needed to show sustained significance [39]. Nortriptyline has been similarly studied in neuropathic pain, with doses usually ranging from 25 to 100 mg/day, with most studies showing a reduction in pain but some specific subtypes of pain, such as paresthesia, showing no difference between nortriptyline and placebo [40–45]. In one other study of treatment for knee pain due to osteoarthritis, no significant difference was found between nortriptyline and placebo [46].

A trial of topical doxepin cream as monotherapy and as a combined doxepin/capsaicin cream over 4 weeks showed a significant reduction in neuropathic pain [47]. A combination product containing both ingredients is not commercially available, but products exist with each individual component. Other TCAs do not have robust evidence for their use in pain management, but due to the similarities to other TCAs, they may be of clinical utility in certain patients.

Evidence for SSRIs

SSRIs are often used as first-line therapy for many mood and anxiety disorders, but these medications also have evidence for use in pain. SSRIs are generally better tolerated than TCAs, having fewer side effects and less risk of toxicity and overdose.

Sertraline has been studied in noncardiac chest pain and was found to cause a significant improvement in pain intensity and unpleasantness, but there were no significant changes in mood between sertraline and placebo. [48, 49] Another study showed improvement in pain outcomes in males with chronic pelvic pain syndrome, but it was not significantly different when compared to placebo [50]. A study in women with chronic pelvic pain reported significant improvement in mood but no significant effect on pain [51].

Paroxetine was also studied in noncardiac chest pain in patients without panic disorder or major depression. Patients treated with paroxetine had a greater improvement on the Clinical Global Impressions Scale than with placebo, but similar rates of improvement were seen on self-rated pain measures between paroxetine and placebo [52]. Paroxetine was studied in chronic low back pain, with doses up to 30 mg/day, and compared to maprotiline and placebo, with patients with major depression excluded from the study. The study found that paroxetine had a lower effect on chronic back pain than placebo and a significantly lower effect than maprotiline [53]. Paroxetine was also found to be effective at a fixed dose of 40 mg/day for the treatment of diabetic neuropathy but less effective than imipramine [33].

A study of fluoxetine for the treatment of diabetic neuropathy found that fluoxetine was only effective in patients with depression [30]. Other trials of fluoxetine have shown positive results in treating fibromyalgia symptoms, persistent somatoform pain disorder, low back pain, whiplash-associated cervical pain, and chronic prostatitis/chronic pelvic pain syndrome [54–58].

Fluvoxamine has not achieved as much popularity or frequency of prescribing as other SSRIs, and due to this, it may have less post-marketing data and is less likely to be studied for pain [59]. Fluvoxamine was shown to significantly reduce pain intensity and improve urinary flow rates in the treatment of prostatodynia using doses of 50–300 mg daily and reduce central poststroke pain at doses of 25–125 mg daily [60, 61].

Citalopram was shown to have a significant effect in treating diabetic neuropathy and somatoform pain disorder at doses of 40 mg/day [62, 63]. It was not effective in treating chronic pelvic pain and fibromyalgia [64, 65]. Escitalopram 20 mg/day has been shown to be effective for the treatment of polyneuropathy and chronic low back pain and at doses of 10–20 mg/day for the treatment of multisomatoform disorder [66–69].

Despite positive findings in many smaller studies, SSRIs generally do not have robust large trial data supporting their use in pain management when compared to TCAs and SNRIs and are used less frequently for pain management in clinical practice. SSRIs may best fit into an individual patient's treatment when comorbid depression or anxiety is present and when SNRIs or TCAs cannot be prescribed.

Evidence for SNRIs

Duloxetine has the most evidence for use of any antidepressant in the treatment of pain. It has FDA-approved indications for the treatment of fibromyalgia, chronic musculoskeletal pain, and diabetic neuropathy. Usual starting doses are 20–30 mg daily, and although the maximum dose is

120 mg daily, there is no greater effect with doses higher than 60 mg for all labeled indications [68]. Duloxetine has been studied in combination with pregabalin for diabetic peripheral neuropathy and has been found to be more effective than monotherapy with either medication [38].

Venlafaxine has similarly been studied for pain and has been found effective in many trials but does not carry FDA indications for pain. The full SNRI effect of venlafaxine is not achieved unless using doses >150 mg/day, with lower doses only inhibiting serotonin reuptake due to the medication's preferential binding for SERT [72]. Because of this, when used in pain management, venlafaxine is often prescribed at doses ≥150 mg/day [35, 38, 70, 73]. Desvenlafaxine is more recently approved and has less data for use in pain management, but doses of 200–400 mg/day have been shown to be effective in the treatment of diabetic neuropathy [74].

Milnacipran is FDA-approved for the treatment of fibromyalgia but not approved for the treatment of depression, for which it is used off label. Milnacipran was studied in chronic low back pain but was found to have no difference in response compared to placebo [75]. Another study found no difference between milnacipran and placebo in treating rheumatoid arthritis pain [76]. Levomilnacipran is the most recently FDA-approved SNRI and does not have data on its use and pain. Its enantiomer, levomilnacipran, is only approved for depression.

Safety

Due to the use for the treatment of depression, patients using antidepressants as adjuncts for pain management should be screened for suicidal ideation. Management of risk of overdose includes adequate screening of access to lethal means, such as large supplies of medication, especially opioids and TCAs, due to their lethality in overdose. Use of opioids and TCAs in the treatment of pain with comorbid depression is not contraindicated, and so these medications should be considered if appropriate for the individual patient.

TCAs should be used with caution in elderly and frail patients due to their risks of anticholinergic effects, increased risks of falls, and adverse cardiac effects. TCAs are included in the American Geriatrics Society 2023 Beers Criteria, a list of medications that may pose greater risks in elderly patients [77]. While all antidepressant medications have the potential to prolong the QT interval, TCAs and citalopram carry a greater risk compared to other options.

All antidepressants should be avoided in patients receiving monoamine oxidase inhibitors (MAOIs). The concurrent use of MAOIs and antidepressants increases the risk of neurotoxicity, seizures, and serotonin syndrome. If a patient is to start an antidepressant after treatment with an MAOI, a minimum of 14 days should elapse before the initiation of antidepressants. If a patient is switching from an antidepressant to an MAOI, a washout period of at least five half-lives of the antidepressant should occur before starting the MAOI. Due to the variability of antidepressant half-lives, this may be as short as 5 days or as long as 5 weeks.

Applications to Clinical Practice

Dosing Considerations

Doses of antidepressants that have been shown to be effective in the treatment of pain may not overlap with doses effective for the treatment of their psychiatric indications. If antidepressants are to be started, consideration should be given to what the target dosage range will be when treating comorbid pain. In some cases, such as desvenlafaxine, the treatment dose used for pain may be many times higher than the treatment dose used for depression. In other cases, such as duloxetine, it is known that no greater effect is achieved after reaching a certain dose, although higher doses have been approved for use by the FDA. In other instances, the dose used for the treatment of pain is much lower than the dose for the treatment of depression, such as amitriptyline, which is shown to be most effective for depression at doses of at least 150 mg/day but is effective for pain at much lower doses [75]. TCAs may be tolerable in lower doses used for pain, but in their higher treatment doses for depression, they may become less favorable due to their increasing side effects.

When used in the treatment of psychiatric disorders, antidepressants generally take 6–8 weeks to reach their maximum effect and are often maintained at treatment doses for months to years, if not indefinitely. In the treatment of pain, antidepressants may take effect more quickly and may not need to be used for as long if the sources of pain are addressed.

Key Themes

- Addressing comorbid conditions is an important component in pain management.
- Antidepressants are a safe and effective treatment for pain, but the effectiveness varies between individual medications.

- TCAs and SNRIs have the most robust data for use in pain, with the most support being for neuropathic pain and fibromyalgia.

Conclusions

Antidepressants are a beneficial addition to pain management regimens for many patients. A thorough review of comorbidities and specific pain subtypes may aid in identifying patients who would benefit from treatment with antidepressants. Multiple studies support the idea that an improvement in symptoms of pain or depression has an impact on improving the other, that SNRIs and TCAs may be the most effective antidepressants for pain, and that treatment options such as antidepressants may reduce overall medication burden by the avoidance of using multiple medications to treat each condition separately.

References

1. Substance Abuse and Mental Health Services Administration. Key substance use and mental health indicators in the United States: results from the 2021 National Survey on Drug Use and Health, HHS Publication No. PEP22-07-01-005, NSDUH Series H-57. Center for Behavioral Health Statistics and Quality, Substance Abuse and Mental Health Services Administration; 2022. https://www.samhsa.gov/data/report/2021-nsduh-annual-national-report
2. Rikard SM, Strahan AE, Schmit KM, Guy GP Jr. Chronic pain among adults—United States, 2019–2021. MMWR Morb Mortal Wkly Rep. 2023;72:379–85. https://doi.org/10.15585/mmwr.mm7215a1.
3. Bair MJ, Robinson RL, Katon W, Kroenke K. Depression and pain comorbidity: a literature review. Arch Intern Med. 2003;163(20):2433–45. https://doi.org/10.1001/archinte.163.20.2433.
4. Johnston KJA, Huckins LM. Chronic pain and psychiatric conditions. Complex Psychiatry. 2023;9(1–4):24–43. https://doi.org/10.1159/000527041.
5. Ericsson M, Poston WS, Linder J, Taylor JE, Haddock CK, Foreyt JP. Depression predicts disability in long-term chronic pain patients. Disabil Rehabil. 2002;24:334–40.
6. Greenberg PE, Leong SA, Birnbaum HG, Robinson RL. The economic burden of depression with painful symptoms. J Clin Psychiatry. 2003;64(Suppl 7):17–23. PMID: 12755648.
7. Engel CC, von Korff M, Katon WJ. Back pain in primary care: predictors of high health-care costs. Pain. 1996;65(2–3):197–204. https://doi.org/10.1016/0304-3959(95)00164-6. PMID: 8826507.
8. Chen C, Pettersson E, Summit AG, Boersma K, Chang Z, Kuja-Halkola R, Lichtenstein P, Quinn PD. Chronic pain conditions and risk of suicidal behavior: a 10-year longitudinal co-twin control study. BMC Med. 2023;21(1):9. https://doi.org/10.1186/s12916-022-02703-8. PMID: 36600296; PMCID: PMC9814420.
9. Evans EA, Sullivan MA. Abuse and misuse of antidepressants. Subst Abus Rehabil. 2014;(5):107–20. https://doi.org/10.2147/SAR.S37917. PMID: 25187753; PMCID: PMC4140701.
10. Davies J, Read J. A systematic review into the incidence, severity and duration of antidepressant withdrawal effects: are guidelines evidence-based? Addict Behav. 2019;97:111–21. https://doi.org/10.1016/j.addbeh.2018.08.027. Epub 2018 Sep 4. PMID: 30292574.
11. Jauhar S, Hayes J, Goodwin GM, Baldwin DS, Cowen PJ, Nutt DJ. Antidepressants, withdrawal, and addiction; where are we now? J Psychopharmacol. 2019;33(6):655–9. https://doi.org/10.1177/0269881119845799. Epub 2019 May 21. PMID: 31111764; PMCID: PMC7613097.
12. Liu QQ, Yao XX, Gao SH, Li R, Li BJ, Yang W, Cui RJ. Role of 5-HT receptors in neuropathic pain: potential therapeutic implications. Pharmacol Res. 2020;159:104949. https://doi.org/10.1016/j.phrs.2020.104949. Epub 2020 May 25. PMID: 32464329.
13. Patetsos E, Horjales-Araujo E. Treating chronic pain with SSRIs: what do we know? Pain Res Manag. 2016;2016:2020915. https://doi.org/10.1155/2016/2020915. Epub 2016 Jul 3. PMID: 27445601; PMCID: PMC4947493.
14. Taylor BK, Westlund KN. The noradrenergic locus coeruleus as a chronic pain generator. J Neurosci Res. 2017;95(6):1336–46. https://doi.org/10.1002/jnr.23956. Epub 2016 Sep 29. PMID: 27685982; PMCID: PMC5374049.
15. Marks DM, Shah MJ, Patkar AA, Masand PS, Park GY, Pae CU. Serotonin-norepinephrine reuptake inhibitors for pain control: premise and promise. Curr Neuropharmacol. 2009;7(4):331–6. https://doi.org/10.2174/157015909790031201. PMID: 20514212; PMCID: PMC2811866.
16. Morón JA, Brockington A, Wise RA, Rocha BA, Hope BT. Dopamine uptake through the norepinephrine transporter in brain regions with low levels of the dopamine transporter: evidence from knock-out mouse lines. J Neurosci. 2002;22(2):389–95. https://doi.org/10.1523/JNEUROSCI.22-02-00389.2002. PMID: 11784783; PMCID: PMC6758674.
17. Piascik MT, Perez DM. Alpha1-adrenergic receptors: new insights and directions. J Pharmacol Exp Ther. 2001;298(2):403–10. PMID: 11454900.
18. Khan ZP, Ferguson CN, Jones RM. Alpha-2 and imidazoline receptor agonists their pharmacology and therapeutic role. Anaesthesia. 1999;54:146–65. https://doi.org/10.1046/j.1365-2044.1999.00659.x.
19. Micó JA, Ardid D, Berrocoso E, Eschalier A. Antidepressants and pain. Trends Pharmacol Sci. 2006;27(7):348–54. https://doi.org/10.1016/j.tips.2006.05.004. Epub 2006 Jun 9. PMID: 16762426.
20. Solinas M, Belujon P, Fernagut PO, Jaber M, Thiriet N. Dopamine and addiction: what have we learned from 40 years of research. J Neural Transm (Vienna). 2019;126(4):481–516. https://doi.org/10.1007/s00702-018-1957-2. Epub 2018 Dec 19. PMID: 30569209.
21. De Backer D, Biston P, Devriendt J, Madl C, Chochrad D, Aldecoa C, Brasseur A, Defrance P, Gottignies P, Vincent JL, SOAP II Investigators. Comparison of dopamine and norepinephrine in the treatment of shock. N Engl J Med. 2010;362(9):779–89. https://doi.org/10.1056/NEJMoa0907118. PMID: 20200382.
22. Diana M. The dopamine hypothesis of drug addiction and its potential therapeutic value. Front Psych. 2011;(2):64. https://doi.org/10.3389/fpsyt.2011.00064. PMID: 22144966; PMCID: PMC3225760.

23. Li C, Liu S, Lu X, Tao F. Role of descending dopaminergic pathways in pain modulation. Curr Neuropharmacol. 2019;17(12):1176–82. https://doi.org/10.2174/1570159X17666190430102531. PMID: 31182003; PMCID: PMC7057207.
24. Hasnain M, Howland RH, Vieweg WV. Escitalopram and QTc prolongation. J Psychiatry Neurosci. 2013;38(4):E11. https://doi.org/10.1503/jpn.130055. PMID: 23791140; PMCID: PMC3692726.
25. Sager JE, Lutz JD, Foti RS, Davis C, Kunze KL, Isoherranen N. Fluoxetine- and norfluoxetine-mediated complex drug-drug interactions: in vitro to in vivo correlation of effects on CYP2D6, CYP2C19, and CYP3A4. Clin Pharmacol Ther. 2014;95(6):653–62. https://doi.org/10.1038/clpt.2014.50. Epub 2014 Feb 25. PMID: 24569517; PMCID: PMC4029899
26. Lindsay PG, Wyckoff M. The depression-pain syndrome and its response to antidepressants. Psychosomatics. 1981;22(7):571–3, 576–7. https://doi.org/10.1016/S0033-3182(81)73478-9. PMID: 7267947.
27. Alcoff J, Jones E, Rust P, Newman R. Controlled trial of imipramine for chronic low back pain. J Fam Pract. 1982;14(5):841–6. PMID: 6210751.
28. Kishore-Kumar R, Max MB, Schafer SC, Gaughan AM, Smoller B, Gracely RH, Dubner R. Desipramine relieves postherpetic neuralgia. Clin Pharmacol Ther. 1990;47(3):305–12.
29. Max MB, Kishore-Kumar R, Schafer SC, Meister B, Gracely RH, Smoller B, Dubner R. Efficacy of desipramine in painful diabetic neuropathy: a placebo-controlled trial. Pain. 1991;45:3–9.
30. Max MB, Lynch SA, Muir J, Shoaf SE, Smoller B, Dubner R. Effects of desipramine, amitriptyline, and fluoxetine on pain in diabetic neuropathy. N Engl J Med. 1992;326(19):1250–6.
31. Rowbotham MC, Reisner LA, Davies PS, Fields HL. Treatment response in antidepressant-naïve postherpetic neuralgia patients: double-blind, randomized trial. J Pain. 2005;6(11):741–6.
32. Kvinesdal B, Molin J, Froland A, Gram LF. Imipramine in the treatment of painful diabetic neuropathy of the extremities [Imipramin ved behandling af smerter ved diabetisk ekstremitetsneuropati]. Ugeskr Laeger. 1983;145(39):3018–9.
33. Sindrup SH, Gram LF, Brosen K, Eshoj O, Mogensen EF. The selective serotonin reuptake inhibitor paroxetine is effective in the treatment of diabetic neuropathy symptoms. Pain. 1990;42:135–44.
34. Sindrup SH, Tuxen C, Gram LF, Grodum E, Skjold T, Brosen K, Beck-Nielsen H. Lack of effect of mianserin on the symptoms of diabetic neuropathy. Eur J Clin Pharmacol. 1992;43:251–5.
35. Sindrup SH, Bach FW, Madsen C, et al. Venlafaxine versus imipramine in painful polyneuropathy: a randomized, controlled trial. Neurology. 2003;60:1284–9.
36. Turkington RW. Depression masquerading as diabetic neuropathy. J Am Med Assoc. 1980;243(11):1147–50.
37. O'Malley PG, Balden E, Tomkins G, Santoro J, Kroenke K, Jackson JL. Treatment of fibromyalgia with antidepressants: a meta-analysis. J Gen Intern Med. 2000;15(9):659–66. https://doi.org/10.1046/j.1525-1497.2000.06279.x. PMID: 11029681; PMCID: PMC1495596.
38. Tesfaye S, Sloan G, Petrie J, White D, Bradburn M, Julious S, Rajbhandari S, Sharma S, Rayman G, Gouni R, Alam U, Cooper C, Loban A, Sutherland K, Glover R, Waterhouse S, Turton E, Horspool M, Gandhi R, Maguire D, Jude EB, Ahmed SH, Vas P, Hariman C, McDougall C, Devers M, Tsatlidis V, Johnson M, Rice ASC, Bouhassira D, Bennett DL, Selvarajah D, OPTION-DM trial group. Comparison of amitriptyline supplemented with pregabalin, pregabalin supplemented with amitriptyline, and duloxetine supplemented with pregabalin for the treatment of diabetic peripheral neuropathic pain (OPTION-DM): a multicentre, double-blind, randomised crossover trial. Lancet. 2022;400(10353):680–90. https://doi.org/10.1016/S0140-6736(22)01472-6. Epub 2022 Aug 22. Erratum in: Lancet. 2022 Sep 10;400(10355):810. PMID: 36007534; PMCID: PMC9418415.
39. Urquhart DM, Wluka AE, van Tulder M, Heritier S, Forbes A, Fong C, Wang Y, Sim MR, Gibson SJ, Arnold C, Cicuttini FM. Efficacy of low-dose amitriptyline for chronic low back pain: A randomized clinical trial. JAMA Intern Med. 2018;178(11):1474–1481. https://doi.org/10.1001/jamainternmed.2018.4222. Erratum in: JAMA Intern Med. 2019 Mar 1;179(3):457. PMID: 30285054; PMCID: PMC6248203.
40. Chandra K, Shafiq N, Pandhi P, Gupta S, Malhotra S. Gabapentin versus nortriptyline in post-herpetic neuralgia patients: a randomized, double-blind clinical trial–the GONIP Trial. Int J Clin Pharmacol Ther. 2006;44(8):358–63. [PUBMED: 16961166].
41. Gilron I, Bailey JM, Tu D, Holden RR, Jackson AC, Houlden R. Nortriptyline and gabapentin, alone and in combination for neuropathic pain: a double-blind, randomised controlled crossover trial. Lancet. 2009;374(9697):1252–61. https://doi.org/10.1016/S0140-6736(09)61081-3.
42. Hammack JE, Michalak JC, Loprinzi CL, Sloan JA, Novotny PJ, Soori GS, et al. Phase III evaluation of nortriptyline for alleviation of symptoms of cis-platinum-induced peripheral neuropathy. Pain. 2002;98(1–2):195–203. https://doi.org/10.1016/S0304-3959(02)00047-7.
43. Khoromi S, Cui L, Nackers L, Max MB. Morphine, nortriptyline and their combination vs. placebo in patients with chronic lumbar root pain. Pain. 2007;130(1–2):66–75. https://doi.org/10.1016/j.pain.2006.10.029.
44. Panerai AE, Monza G, Movilia P, Bianchi M, Francucci BM, Tiengo M. A randomized, within-patient, cross-over, placebo-controlled trial on the efficacy and tolerability of the tricyclic antidepressants chlorimipramine and nortriptyline in central pain. Acta Neurol Scand. 1990;82(1):34–8. [PUBMED: 2239134]
45. Watson CP, Vernich L, Chipman M, Reed K. Nortriptyline versus amitriptyline in postherpetic neuralgia: a randomized trial. Neurology. 1998;51(4):1166–71. [PUBMED: 9781549]
46. Hudson B, Williman JA, Stamp LK, Alchin JS, Hooper GJ, Mangin D, Thompson BFL, Toop L. Nortriptyline for pain in knee osteoarthritis: a double-blind randomised controlled trial in New Zealand general practice. Br J Gen Pract. 2021;71(708):e538–46. https://doi.org/10.3399/BJGP.2020.0797. PMID: 33571950; PMCID: PMC8177953.
47. McCleane G. Topical application of doxepin hydrochloride, capsaicin and a combination of both produces analgesia in chronic human neuropathic pain: a randomized, double-blind, placebo-controlled study. Br J Clin Pharmacol. 2000;49(6):574–9. https://doi.org/10.1046/j.1365-2125.2000.00200.x. PMID: 10848721; PMCID: PMC2015036.
48. Keefe FJ, Shelby RA, Somers TJ, et al. Effects of coping skills training and sertraline in patients with non-cardiac chest pain: a randomized controlled study. Pain. 2011;152(4):730–41. https://doi.org/10.1016/j.pain.2010.08.040.
49. Varia I, Logue E, O'Connor C, et al. Randomized trial of sertraline in patients with unexplained chest pain of noncardiac origin. Am Heart J. 2000;140(3):367–72. https://doi.org/10.1067/mhj.2000.108514.
50. Lee RA, West RM, Wilson JD. The response to sertraline in men with chronic pelvic pain syndrome. Sex Transm Infect. 2005;81(2):147–9. https://doi.org/10.1136/sti.2004.010868.
51. Engel CC Jr, Walker EA, Engel AL, Bullis J, Armstrong A. A randomized, double-blind crossover trial of sertraline in women with chronic pelvic pain. J Psychosom Res. 1998;44(2):203–7. https://doi.org/10.1016/S0022-3999(97)00215-8.
52. Doraiswamy PM, Varia I, Hellegers C, et al. A randomized controlled trial of paroxetine for noncardiac chest pain. Psychopharmacol Bull. 2006;39(1):15–24.

53. Atkinson JH, Slater MA, Wahlgren DR, Williams RA, Zisook S, Pruitt SD, Epping-Jordan JE, Patterson TL, Grant I, Abramson I, Garfin SR. Effects of noradrenergic and serotonergic antidepressants on chronic low back pain intensity. Pain. 1999;83(2):137–45. https://doi.org/10.1016/s0304-3959(99)00082-2. PMID: 10534584.
54. Arnold LM, Hess EV, Hudson JI, Welge JA, Berno SE, Keck PE Jr. A randomized, placebo-controlled, double-blind, flexible-dose study of fluoxetine in the treatment of women with fibromyalgia. Am J Med. 2002;112(3):191–7. https://doi.org/10.1016/s0002-9343(01)01089-0. PMID: 11893345.
55. Goldenberg D, Mayskiy M, Mossey C, Ruthazer R, Schmid C. A randomized, double-blind crossover trial of fluoxetine and amitriptyline in the treatment of fibromyalgia. Arthritis Rheum. 1996;39(11):1852–9. https://doi.org/10.1002/art.1780391111. PMID: 8912507.
56. Luo YL, Zhang MY, Wu WY, Li CB, Lu Z, Li QW. A randomized double-blind clinical trial on analgesic efficacy of fluoxetine for persistent somatoform pain disorder. Prog Neuro-Psychopharmacol Biol Psychiatry. 2009;33(8):1522–5. https://doi.org/10.1016/j.pnpbp.2009.08.013. Epub 2009 Sep 4. PMID: 19733606.
57. Schreiber S, Vinokur S, Shavelzon V, Pick CG, Zahavi E, Shir Y. A randomized trial of fluoxetine versus amitriptyline in musculo-skeletal pain. Isr J Psychiatry Relat Sci. 2001;38(2):88–94. PMID: 11475920.
58. Xia D, Wang P, Chen J, Wang S, Jiang H. Fluoxetine ameliorates symptoms of refractory chronic prostatitis/chronic pelvic pain syndrome. Chin Med J. 2011;124(14):2158–61. PMID: 21933619.
59. Kane SP. The Top 200 of 2020, ClinCalc DrugStats database, Version 202208 ClinCalc: https://clincalccom/DrugStats/Top200Drugsaspx Updated August 24, 2022. Accessed 30 Dec 2023.
60. Turkington D, Grant JB, Ferrier IN, Rao NS, Linsley KR, Young AH. A randomized controlled trial of fluvoxamine in prostatodynia, a male somatoform pain disorder. J Clin Psychiatry. 2002;63(9):778–81. https://doi.org/10.4088/jcp.v63n0905. PMID: 12363117.
61. Shimodozono M, Kawahira K, Kamishita T, Ogata A, Tohgo S, Tanaka N. Reduction of central poststroke pain with the selective serotonin reuptake inhibitor fluvoxamine. Int J Neurosci. 2002;112(10):1173–81. https://doi.org/10.1080/00207450290026139. PMID: 12587520.
62. Aragona M, Bancheri L, Perinelli D, et al. Randomized double-blind comparison of serotonergic (citalopram) versus noradrenergic (Reboxetine) reuptake inhibitors in outpatients with somatoform, DSM-IV-TR pain disorder. Eur J Pain. 2005;9(1):33–8. https://doi.org/10.1016/j.ejpain.2004.03.003.
63. Sindrup SH, Bjerre U, Dejgaard A, Brøsen K, Aaes-Jørgensen T, Gram LF. The selective serotonin reuptake inhibitor citalopram relieves the symptoms of diabetic neuropathy. Clin Pharmacol Ther. 1992;52(5):547–52. https://doi.org/10.1038/clpt.1992.183.
64. Brown CS, Franks AS, Wan J, Ling FW. Citalopram in the treatment of women with chronic pelvic pain: an open-label trial. J Reprod Med. 2008;53(3):191–5.
65. Nørregaard J, Volkmann H, Danneskiold-Samsøe B. A randomized controlled trial of citalopram in the treatment of fibromyalgia. Pain. 1995;61(3):445–9. https://doi.org/10.1016/0304-3959(94)00218-4.
66. Mazza M, Mazza O, Pazzaglia C, Padua L, Mazza S. Escitalopram 20 mg versus duloxetine 60 mg for the treatment of chronic low back pain. Expert Opin Pharmacother. 2010;11(7):1049–52. https://doi.org/10.1517/14656561003730413. PMID: 20402551.
67. Otto M, Bach FW, Jensen TS, Brøsen K, Sindrup SH. Escitalopram in painful polyneuropathy: a randomized, placebo-controlled, cross-over trial. Pain. 2008;139(2):275–83. https://doi.org/10.1016/j.pain.2008.04.012. Epub 2008 Jun 10. PMID: 18547727.
68. Muller JE, Wentzel I, Koen L, Niehaus DJ, Seedat S, Stein DJ. Escitalopram in the treatment of multisomatoform disorder: a double-blind, placebo-controlled trial. Int Clin Psychopharmacol. 2008;23(1):43–8. https://doi.org/10.1097/YIC.0b013e32825ea301. PMID: 18090507.
69. Product Information: CYMBALTA(R) oral delayed-release capsules, duloxetine oral delayed-release capsules. Lilly USA LLC (per FDA), Indianapolis, IN, 2020.
70. Finnerup NB, Attal N, Haroutounian S, McNicol E, Baron R, Dworkin RH, Gilron I, Haanpää M, Hansson P, Jensen TS, Kamerman PR, Lund K, Moore A, Raja SN, Rice AS, Rowbotham M, Sena E, Siddall P, Smith BH, Wallace M. Pharmacotherapy for neuropathic pain in adults: a systematic review and meta-analysis. Lancet Neurol. 2015;14(2):162–73. https://doi.org/10.1016/S1474-4422(14)70251-0. Epub 2015 Jan 7. PMID: 25575710; PMCID: PMC4493167
71. Dowell D, Ragan KR, Jones CM, Baldwin GT, Chou R. CDC clinical practice guideline for prescribing opioids for pain—United States, 2022. MMWR Recomm Rep 2022;71(No. RR-3):1–95. https://doi.org/10.15585/mmwr.rr7103a1
72. Bymaster FP, Dreshfield-Ahmad LJ, Threlkeld PG, Shaw JL, Thompson L, Nelson DL, Hemrick-Luecke SK, Wong DT. Comparative affinity of duloxetine and venlafaxine for serotonin and norepinephrine transporters in vitro and in vivo, human serotonin receptor subtypes, and other neuronal receptors. Neuropsychopharmacology. 2001;25(6):871–80. https://doi.org/10.1016/S0893-133X(01)00298-6. PMID: 11750180.
73. Price R, Smith D, Franklin G, Gronseth G, Pignone M, David WS, Armon C, Perkins BA, Bril V, Rae-Grant A, Halperin J, Licking N, O'Brien MD, Wessels SR, MacGregor LC, Fink K, Harkless LB, Colbert L, Callaghan BC. Oral and topical treatment of painful diabetic polyneuropathy: practice guideline update summary: report of the AAN guideline subcommittee. Neurology. 2022;98(1):31–43. https://doi.org/10.1212/WNL.0000000000013038. PMID: 34965987.
74. Allen R, Sharma U, Barlas S. Clinical experience with desvenlafaxine in treatment of pain associated with diabetic peripheral neuropathy. J Pain Res. 2014;(7):339–51. https://doi.org/10.2147/JPR.S55682. PMID: 25018648; PMCID: PMC4075949.
75. Derry S, Phillips T, Moore RA, Wiffen PJ. Milnacipran for neuropathic pain in adults. Cochrane Database Syst Rev. 2015;2015(7):CD011789. https://doi.org/10.1002/14651858.CD011789. PMID: 26148202; PMCID: PMC6485877.
76. Lee YC, Massarotti E, Edwards RR, Lu B, Liu C, Lo Y, Wohlfahrt A, Kim ND, Clauw DJ, Solomon DH. Effect of Milnacipran on pain in patients with rheumatoid arthritis with widespread pain: a randomized blinded crossover trial. J Rheumatol. 2016;43(1):38–45. https://doi.org/10.3899/jrheum.150550. Epub 2015 Dec 1. PMID: 26628607; PMCID: PMC4698221.
77. By the 2023. American Geriatrics Society Beers Criteria® Update Expert Panel. American Geriatrics Society 2023 updated AGS Beers Criteria® for potentially inappropriate medication use in older adults. J Am Geriatr Soc. 2023;71(7):2052–81. https://doi.org/10.1111/jgs.18372. Epub 2023 May 4. PMID: 37139824.

Alpha$_2$ Agonists

9

J. Cole Wilder, Aliya Abdulla, and Matthew A. Wanat

Abbreviations

ASAM	American Society of Addiction Medicine
CI	Confidence interval
CNS	Central nervous system
CrCl	Creatinine clearance
CYP	Cytochrome P
FDA	Food and Drug Administration
ICU	Intensive care unit
PO	By mouth
RR	Relative risk

Introduction

Adrenergic receptors can be classified into two groups, alpha and beta, based on the inhibition or excitation of effector cells and the location of the receptors [2]. The alpha-receptor agonists are then differentiated into alpha$_1$ and alpha$_2$, where the latter was discovered to have effects within the central and peripheral nervous system. These receptor effects were discovered by utilizing a selective alpha$_2$ antagonist, yohimbine, to determine whether there were multiple alpha-adrenergic receptors [64].

J. C. Wilder
Department of Foundational Sciences, John Shufeldt School of Medicine and Medical Engineering, Tempe, AZ, USA

A. Abdulla
Department of Pharmacy, Houston Methodist Hospital, Houston, TX, USA

M. A. Wanat (✉)
Department of Pharmacy Practice and Translational Research, The University of Houston College of Pharmacy, Houston, TX, USA

Department of Pharmacy, Houston Methodist Hospital, Houston, TX, USA
e-mail: MAWanat@uh.edu

Under the alpha$_2$ agonist umbrella, there are three subtypes: alpha$_{2A}$, alpha$_{2B}$, and alpha$_{2C}$. All three subtypes inhibit adenylyl cyclase, which then reduces the levels of cyclic adenosine monophosphate and causes hyperpolarization of noradrenergic neurons in the medial dorsal pons, such as the locus coeruleus, the center for sympathetic outflow to the forebrain [59]. This process facilitates the suppression of neural firing by inhibiting calcium ions from entering the nerve terminal, which inevitably inhibits the release of endogenous agonists, such as norepinephrine, and results in sedative effects [11]. Figure 9.1 details the mechanism of alpha$_2$ receptors. Subsequent effects on the vasomotor centers of the rostral ventrolateral medulla can be propagated by this negative feedback loop and cause bradycardia and hypotension, which can increase activity in the parasympathetic neurons. Stimulation of alpha$_2$ receptors in the dorsal horn of the spine is thought to be the primary mechanism of the analgesic effect of this drug class [23, 34].

The alpha$_{2B}$ receptors are found primarily on the vascular smooth muscle and facilitate vasopressor effects and trigger anti-shivering mechanisms, whereas alpha$_{2A}$ and alpha$_{2C}$ receptor subtypes are found in the central nervous system (CNS). These receptors play a key role in analgosedative effects. Alpha$_{2C}$ receptors, in particular, produce a startle response that allows for the contraction of muscles as well as blood pressure and breathing variation [8, 23, 54].

While there are several alpha$_2$ agonists within this class, the most utilized agents are clonidine, tizanidine, and dexmedetomidine.

Pharmacology, Pharmacokinetics, and Pharmacodynamics

Clonidine

Clonidine is lipid-soluble, with a volume of distribution of 2.9 L/kg in adult patients, making extravascular site distribu-

J. P. Reinert et al. (eds.), *Adjunctive Analgesic Strategies for the Bedside Clinician and Beyond*,
https://doi.org/10.1007/978-3-032-21675-5_9

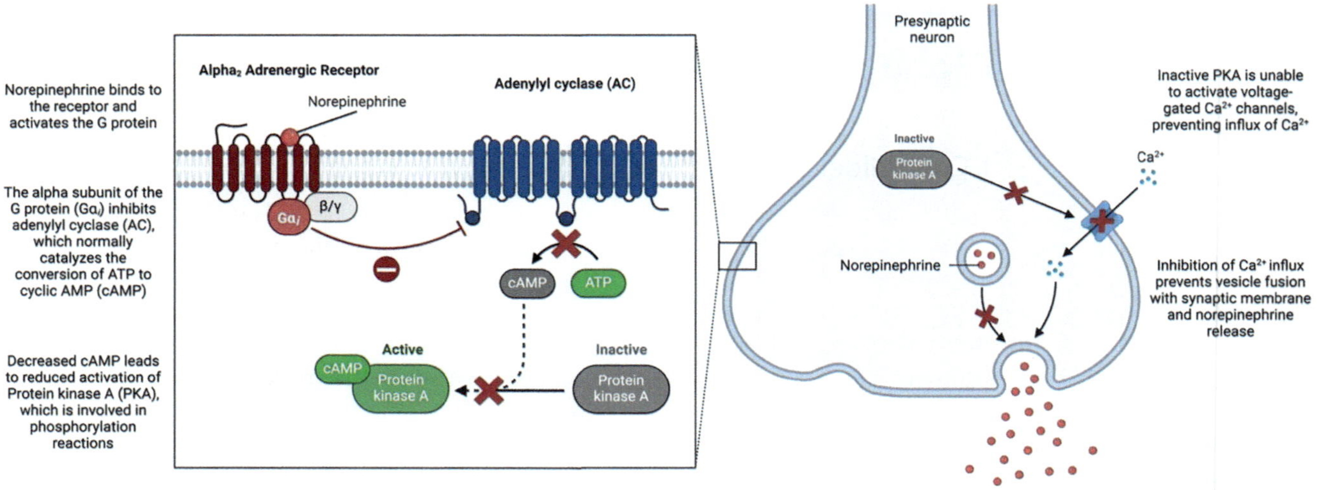

Fig. 9.1 Alpha$_2$ adrenergic receptor mechanism

tion excellent. Clonidine is commercially available as an immediate-release oral tablet, extended-release oral tablet, or topical patch. Clonidine epidural solution is commercially available for epidural therapies but is not commonly used for perioperative or intensive care unit (ICU) pain management. Clonidine is anywhere from 75% to 90% bioavailable, with 20–40% being protein-bound and reaching peak concentrations within 60–90 min. Specifically, its antihypertensive effects are seen within 1 h. However, as a transdermal patch, antihypertensive effects may take 48–72 h to occur. Clonidine is metabolized hepatically through conversion to inactive metabolites, which are ultimately excreted in the urine, 50% unchanged. The clearance of the drug is age-dependent, where the half-life in neonates is 44–72 h, in children 8–12 h, and in adults 12–16 h. Alternatively, after patch removal, the half-life of the drug is 20 h [23, 54].

Clonidine is best known for its use as an antihypertensive; however, like other agents within this class, it has notable effects on analgosedation as an adjunct agent through stimulating alpha$_2$ adrenoreceptors located in the spinal cord's dorsal horn. It has a stronger affinity for alpha$_2$ versus alpha$_1$ receptors at a ratio of 200:1 and primarily acts on centrally located alpha$_2$ receptors. Clonidine's ability to stimulate central brain stem adrenergic receptors and decrease sympathetic nervous system activity triggers a lowering of systemic blood pressure by peripheral vasodilation. However, due to its ability to maintain controlled hypotension, there is a severe risk of rebound hypertension if patients abruptly discontinue this agent. This can occur up to 20 h after the dose was last taken [23].

Clonidine has also been utilized in the pediatric population for pretreatment anxiety to decrease anesthetic requirements for patients by up to 50% [69]. Additionally, hyperactivity disorders or attention-deficit issues have been addressed with the utilization of clonidine. The behavior can be mitigated by decreasing the firing of the presynaptic neurons that release norepinephrine [53]. Insomnia in pediatric patients can be addressed by the effects of clonidine on serotonin and gamma-aminobutyric acid receptors [56]. Within the kidneys, clonidine can decrease plasma catecholamines and renin, which may promote diuresis [23].

Specifically, within the realm of analgesia, clonidine works through a different mechanism than other agents, such as opioids, to provide its effects. It has minimal effects on respiratory depression or tolerance, making it an ideal agent for analgosedation. It can be used topically, with local effects on receptors without significant CNS adverse effects, or systemically for analgesia and has good success with diabetic neuropathy. Clonidine has been used to enhance the effects of anti-inflammatory agents along with opioids to decrease total opioid use [3]. Additionally, clonidine can decrease the minimum alveolar concentration requirements of inhaled anesthetic agents such as sevoflurane [76].

Some safety considerations to consider with the use of this medication are common adverse drug events such as drowsiness, orthostatic and rebound hypertension, and bradycardia. Hyperglycemia may also occur due to clonidine's inhibition of insulin release. In patients with hypovolemia, spontaneous bradycardia, a prolonged PR interval, or atrioventricular block, the use of clonidine is contraindicated and should be avoided [54].

Tizanidine

Tizanidine, another oral alpha$_2$ agonist, produces similar effects to clonidine, with centrally acting effects near the central nervous system. It has a peak effect at 1–2 h and a duration of action of 3–6 h. Both tablets and capsules have a bioavailability of 40% under fasting conditions; however, with food, the peak plasma concentration is increased by 30% with tablets and decreased by 20% with capsules. Tizanidine is 30% protein-bound and metabolized hepatically via CYP1A2 to inactive metabolites. It has a volume of distribution of 2.4 L/kg and is excreted 60% via the urine and 20% via feces [72].

It is used as an adjunct agent due to its analgosedative and anxiolytic properties. However, it may be favored over clonidine because of its decreased side effect profile, resulting in less hypotension and bradycardia than clonidine. With its shorter half-life of 2.5 h, it can be used for acute analgosedation scenarios and has allowed for a reduction in postoperative shivering. Additionally, it has been shown to decrease spasticity in patients due to its presynaptic inhibition and is used for myofascial pain and muscle tone [72].

Dexmedetomidine

Dexmedetomidine is a highly selective alpha$_2$ agonist, specifically alpha$_{2A}$, with the greatest affinity for this receptor compared to clonidine and tizanidine. Its specificity ratio is 1620:1 for alpha$_2$: alpha$_1$. First approved in 1999, dexmedetomidine was brought to the market as an analgosedation agent for less-than-24-h periods in the ICU patient population [21]. This approval was changed in 2008 to include sedation in the preoperative period and for procedures. In today's practice, dexmedetomidine is used very commonly, both alone and in conjunction with other agents, to produce sedative, analgesic, anxiolytic, and sympatholytic effects on patients [37].

This lipophilic agent is highly protein-bound, with a volume of distribution of approximately 118 L, which results in quick redistribution to peripheral tissues. Its onset is in 2–10 min intravenously (IV), with a peak effect at 15–60 min. The half-life is variable, ranging from 4 min after a 10-min infusion to 4 h after an 8-h infusion; this provides a rapid onset of the drug but a short duration of action. Dexmedetomidine displays linear kinetics in those with normal renal and hepatic function. Its metabolism is through both glucuronidation and biotransformation by CYP2A6 hepatically. Ultimately, the drug is excreted in the urine and a small amount in the feces [37, 54]. While widely used in its intravenous formulation, dexmedetomidine has various other routes of administration, including being given orally, sublingually, intranasally, and intramuscularly.

The alpha$_2$ receptors that dexmedetomidine focuses its effects on are primarily located in the brain and spinal cord. Those located within the pons and medulla of the brain stem act on the sympathetic activity of the peripheral nervous system. The impacts of dexmedetomidine differ based on the site of action. Presynaptic activity will decrease norepinephrine release to the autonomic nervous system; however, postsynaptic activity of the alpha$_2$ receptors will hyperpolarize the neuronal membranes. These mechanisms are further explained in Table 9.1 [21, 78].

A key benefit to the usage of this agent in comparison to other analgosedatives is that it allows for light sedation when used alone, has a rapid onset, and is easily titratable. As with other alpha$_2$ agonists, it causes minimal respiratory depression, and its use can allow patients to wean off analgosedation altogether. Dexmedetomidine is used primarily for prolonged sedation and procedural analgosedation. When adding dexmedetomidine to other agents, it has been shown to decrease the use of opioids by 50–75% and decrease benzodiazepine use by 80% [78]. Additionally, the rapid distribution half-life allows for quicker recovery. Like other alpha$_2$ agonists, dexmedetomidine may be used for postoperative shivering and has also been used as part of peripheral nerve blocks. In those with a history of emergence delirium, this agent can be used as a premedication before procedures or as a bolus intraoperatively [30].

However, it is important to keep in mind the risks that accompany the utilization of the drug. Key considerations are the impacts on the cardiovascular system. When dexmedetomidine is used as an IV bolus or rapidly administered, it loses its alpha$_2$ receptor selectivity, which can result in a rise in blood pressure and a decrease in heart rate for a brief period of time. Hypertension is a risk due to the transient activation of peripheral alpha$_{2B}$ receptors during a bolus administration and the opposing effects of the central alpha$_{2A}$ receptors. Due to this bradycardic effect, dexmedetomidine is contraindicated in patients with significant heart block or bradyarrhythmia. Those who have cardiac valvular stenosis or extreme hypovolemia should also avoid this drug due to its vasodilatory properties.

Table 9.1 Alpha$_2$ agonist activity by dexmedetomidine

Location of action	Impacts of dexmedetomidine
Local coeruleus	Norepinephrine synthesis in the pontine center causes sedation and hypnosis A negative feedback loop is produced presynaptically to guide norepinephrine release. This will inhibit the descending medullospinal noradrenergic pathways
Rostral ventrolateral medulla	Dexmedetomidine inhibits the presynaptic neuronal pathway and activates the parasympathetic neurons in the nucleus ambiguous, resulting in bradycardia and hypotension
Dorsal horn	Dexmedetomidine will cause a decrease in glutamate and substance P within the dorsal horn, which will reduce ascending spinal pathways and contribute to analgesic effects

Evidence for Use

Efficacy

Clonidine

The effectiveness of clonidine in the treatment of acute pain has been well-documented, with most studies evaluating its utility in the perioperative setting. Oral administration of clonidine has been shown to both prolong the analgesic effects of opioids and reduce dose requirements postoperatively [24, 52, 57]. Oral formulations of clonidine have also been shown to reduce pain scores and opioid analgesic agent dose requirements in patients with acute pain associated with various conditions [16, 63]. When administered neuraxially, clonidine has been shown to improve analgesic quality and duration and reduce the requirement for opioid analgesics after surgery. Additionally, clonidine exerts an immunomodulatory effect, reducing pro-inflammatory cytokines and substance P concentrations. When combined with local anesthetic agents and administered neuraxially or perineurally, clonidine demonstrates a synergistic effect, minimizing the dose requirements of both agents [52].

The effectiveness of clonidine has also been evaluated for the management of chronic pain syndromes. Neuraxial clonidine administration via an intrathecal catheter was shown to be effective in the treatment of chronic, intractable cancer-related pain, with nearly half of the study population successfully maintained with adequate long-term pain control requiring minimal dose escalation. Likewise, a small retrospective review demonstrated significant relief of chronic pain for up to 24 months with either a single administration or a continuous intrathecal infusion of clonidine with or without adjunctive opioid analgesics. Epidural administration of clonidine has also been evaluated in several studies; however, intravenous administration may be superior in efficacy, with similar adverse effects.

Additionally, data from randomized controlled trials has demonstrated the effectiveness of topical administration of clonidine for the treatment of chronic pain associated with diabetic neuropathy, particularly when the quality of pain is described as sharp or stabbing [39].

Clonidine occupies a significant role in the management of opioid withdrawal and is recommended as a therapeutic option in the most recent treatment guidelines published by the American Society of Addiction Medicine (ASAM). Many of the clinical manifestations of opioid withdrawal, such as hypertension, tachycardia, agitation, anxiety, insomnia, and tremor, are the result of central noradrenergic hyperactivity in the locus coeruleus. The alpha$_2$ adrenergic receptor–mediated sympatholytic effects of clonidine mitigate the symptoms associated with opioid withdrawal [71]. Although it lacks the Food and Drug Administration (FDA) approval, clonidine has been successfully used off label for the management of opioid withdrawal for over two decades. However, it has been found to be less effective than buprenorphine and methadone in the management of opioid withdrawal–related symptom management [71]. Clonidine may also play a similar role in the reduction of autonomic hyperactivity associated with alcohol withdrawal syndrome, in combination with benzodiazepines [51].

Tizanidine

Tizanidine is primarily utilized as a skeletal muscle relaxant, exhibiting both antispastic and antispasmodic pharmacologic activity, indicated for the management of several conditions associated with acute musculoskeletal pain [45, 77, 86]. Evidence also supports the incorporation of tizanidine as a component of multimodal analgesic strategies for patients in the perioperative setting. A review article published by Zhu and colleagues summarizes data from several well-designed studies that describes the benefits of tizanidine when administered 60–90 min prior to surgery. Findings include a significant reduction in postoperative pain scores and a decrease in perioperative analgesic consumption. Notably, the beneficial effects of preemptive analgesia with tizanidine were consistently observed across a variety of spinal, abdominal, and maxillofacial surgical procedures [86]. Premedication with tizanidine also resulted in a significant reduction (approximately 25%) in the dose of propofol required for the maintenance of general anesthesia during surgery [72]. Studies have also shown improvement in other patient outcomes after surgery, including a decreased incidence of postoperative shivering and a statistically significant reduction in the length of postanesthesia care unit stay [72, 73].

In addition to its preemptive analgesic and opioid-sparing effects, tizanidine has also been shown to limit variations in blood pressure and heart rate due to the sympathetic nervous system response associated with laryngoscopy and anesthesia induction. Such hemodynamic alterations may be ameliorated by the alpha$_2$ adrenergic receptor–mediated sympatholytic effects of tizanidine [72]. Tizanidine has also demonstrated some clinical utility in the treatment of chronic pain disorders. Preliminary clinical studies with limited sample sizes have demonstrated the beneficial effects of tizanidine on myofascial pain syndrome, which included improvements in clinically assessed pain criteria and a statistically significant decrease in the intensity of pain and pain-associated functional limitations [45, 46].

Tizanidine has also demonstrated clinical utility in headache disorders, including for the management of tension-type headaches [18]. Tizanidine has also been shown to reduce headache frequency, intensity, severity, and duration of pain in patients with both migraine and tension-type headaches when used daily as prophylactic therapy [66]. A systematic review conducted by Oldfield et al. [55] highlighted additional evidence supporting the use of tizanidine for chronic pain associated with headache disorders as well as with fibromyalgia. Findings from small cohort studies show reduced pain intensity associated with fibromyalgia compared to patients receiving a placebo, with the beneficial effects lasting for the duration of tizanidine use, after which the pain returned.

Tizanidine holds promise as a potential therapeutic option for the treatment of neuropathic pain conditions. Data from animal models suggests a beneficial effect of tizanidine in neuropathic pain, mediated through the inhibition of proinflammatory cytokine production [60]. A small open-label study conducted by Semenchuk and Sherman evaluated the effectiveness of tizanidine for the management of patients with neuropathic pain. Of the 23 patients enrolled, 15 endorsed an improvement in pain levels after 8 weeks of tizanidine therapy, with two of these patients achieving complete pain relief. A statistically significant reduction in the average weekly pain scores from baseline was observed, as well as a reduction in neuropathic pain quality and an improvement in the quality of life [67]. Such findings warrant further investigation with randomized controlled trials to further elucidate the therapeutic utility of tizanidine in neuropathic pain.

Dexmedetomidine

Dexmedetomidine is a commonly used pharmacologic agent in the intensive care and perioperative settings, with FDA-approved indications for use in sedation of mechanically ventilated patients, procedural sedation in non-mechanically ventilated patients, general anesthesia. Its sedative, hypnotic, and anxiolytic properties are well-documented, as is its safety, especially with regard to the preservation of respiratory function. Dexmedetomidine has also demonstrated modest independent analgesic activity, postulated to be the result of altered pain perception via its sedative and anxiolytic actions [13]. Despite its limited analgesic activity when used as monotherapy, the primary role of dexmedetomidine in the management of pain is off-label use as an adjuvant agent to improve the effectiveness and prolong the duration of local and regional anesthesia and reduce the need for opioid analgesic agents in the perioperative setting.

Several well-designed clinical trials and data from systematic reviews have demonstrated the effectiveness of dexmedetomidine as an adjunctive agent for perineural coadministration with local anesthetic agents in peripheral nerve blockade. Adjunctive dexmedetomidine was found to reduce dose requirements for both local anesthetics and opioids, in addition to improving the quality and increasing the duration of analgesia in adult patients undergoing surgical procedures. Studies have evaluated dexmedetomidine as an adjunct to peripheral nerve block administered at doses between 0.5 and 2 mcg/kg, with a dose of 1 mcg/kg determined to be optimal and with higher doses resulting in a greater frequency of adverse effects [12]. A systematic review and meta-analysis conducted by Wu and colleagues also examined the efficacy and safety of dexmedetomidine as an adjuvant agent for neuraxial administration. Although the studies were heterogeneous, neuraxial dexmedetomidine demonstrated a reduction in 24-h postoperative pain and an increase in the duration of both analgesic effects and sensorimotor blockade. Additionally, the onset of action for coadministered local anesthesia was significantly reduced [83].

Despite the abundance of evidence supporting the neuraxial and perineural administration of dexmedetomidine, widespread clinical use remains limited. This may be because dexmedetomidine currently lacks FDA-approved indications for use as an adjunct to locoregional anesthesia, as well as a result of pharmaceutical concerns related to dexmedetomidine formulations appropriate for intrathecal administration. Additionally, optimal dosing strategies remain to be elucidated, and the risk of adverse effects such as hypotension and bradycardia must be carefully considered [70].

Intravenous administration of dexmedetomidine has also been shown to yield comparable outcomes to those seen with spinal and perineural administration. Abdallah et al. [1] conducted a systematic review and meta-analysis that found that intravenous dexmedetomidine resulted in a clinically significant prolongation of the duration of neuraxial anesthesia, as well as a delay in the time to the first postoperative analgesic dose by more than 50%. Adverse effects were similar to those seen with locoregional administration of dexmedetomidine, with bradycardia occurring more frequently than hypotension. Intravenous administration, with its proven safety profile and well-documented efficacy, may limit the necessity for neuraxial and perineural dexmedetomidine administration in the future [1].

As described previously, dexmedetomidine is beneficial in reducing perioperative opioid requirements. In the preoperative setting, data suggests that intravenous dexmedetomidine reduces the amount of opioid analgesics and volatile anesthetics required for maintenance of general anesthesia. When administered intraoperatively, dexmedetomidine was found to reduce the total required dose of opioids during the first 24 h postoperatively despite the drug possessing a terminal half-life of approximately 2 h [74].

A retrospective analysis conducted by Venn et al. [78] found that opioid requirements were reduced by more than half with dexmedetomidine administration compared to placebo in the postoperative care setting. In a recent Cochrane review, dexmedetomidine was quantified as exhibiting a distinct opioid-sparing effect, decreasing the amount of opioid consumption by approximately 25% during a period of 24 h after abdominal surgery, with no appreciable difference in postoperative pain [35]. Importantly, the opioid-sparing effect demonstrated by dexmedetomidine resulted in a corresponding reduction in opioid-related adverse effects. A recent retrospective study performed by Ke et al. [38] showed a significant reduction in the incidence of postoperative nausea and vomiting (PONV), constipation, pruritus, and respiratory depression with the administration of dexmedetomidine compared with patients receiving opioids alone.

Beyond those described previously, several other, though less well-defined, roles of dexmedetomidine have been described. The utility of dexmedetomidine to treat neuropathic pain has been demonstrated in preclinical animal models, but clinical data with human subjects is limited primarily to case reports [85]. Likewise, data supporting the feasibility of dexmedetomidine therapy for chronic pain management is also limited [25]. Dexmedetomidine is also an effective therapeutic option for the prevention and treatment of opioid-induced hyperalgesia, potentially through restoring normal physiologic nociceptive and antinociceptive responses [40, 61]. In a case series published by Belgrade and Hall [4], dexmedetomidine administration resulted in a significant reduction in opioid doses required for analgesia in 64% of patients. Further studies are warranted to firmly define the role of dexmedetomidine as an analgesic agent in these clinical scenarios.

Safety

Clonidine

As the utilization of clonidine as a therapeutic agent has spanned nearly five decades, its adverse effect profile is well-documented. Due to its alpha$_2$ adrenergic receptor–mediated inhibitory actions on central catecholamine release, clonidine may cause hypotension and bradycardia, resulting in a reduction in cardiac output by decreasing the heart rate, as well as a reduction in blood pressure due to peripheral vasodilation. Caution should be utilized when administering clonidine to patients with preexisting atrioventricular nodal conduction delays and those with a prolonged PR interval, as symptomatic bradycardia may result [84]. Dose-related excess sedation has also been well-documented as an adverse effect [52]. Simulation of alpha$_2$ receptors within pancreatic beta cells results in an inhibition of insulin secretion and subsequent hyperglycemia. Additionally, clonidine has demonstrated an antisialagogue effect, resulting in xerostomia [3].

Due to the sympatholytic effects of clonidine, abrupt discontinuation may precipitate a withdrawal syndrome characterized by rebound catecholamine excess, resulting in clinical manifestations of hypertension, tachycardia, altered mental status, diaphoresis, and tremor, with symptom onset occurring within 4–8 h after the last dose. The severity of the withdrawal syndrome is thought to be a dose-dependent phenomenon, although cases of withdrawal have been documented in patients receiving therapeutic doses of clonidine [36]. However, several infrequent case reports of withdrawal syndrome have been documented with oral, transdermal, and neuraxial clonidine administration [22, 41, 48].

To reduce the risk of potentiating withdrawal, clonidine should not be administered as a once-daily regimen or on an as-needed basis. Doses should be tapered prior to discontinuation, especially in patients with prolonged durations of clonidine therapy and those receiving concurrent beta-adrenergic receptor blocker therapy or non-dihydropyridine calcium channel blockers [79]. Strategies for the management of clonidine withdrawal syndrome include mixed-acting antihypertensive agents with both alpha- and beta-adrenergic receptor antagonism, such as labetalol, or a direct vasodilator, such as hydralazine. Additionally, clonidine therapy may be reinitiated [68].

Tizanidine

Due to its pharmacologic similarity with clonidine, tizanidine exhibits a similar adverse effect profile, including xerostomia, sedation, potential for rebound symptoms with abrupt discontinuation, and concerns for hypotension and bradycardia. However, compared to clonidine, tizanidine's alpha$_2$ adrenergic receptor–mediated effects on blood pressure and heart rate are considerably reduced due to its pharmacokinetic properties, including a short duration of action, relatively brief elimination half-life, and limited oral bioavailability [23, 86]. Other common adverse effects include asthenia and dizziness [80].

Tizanidine use may result in transient and asymptomatic elevations in hepatic aminotransferase enzymes, and case reports of hepatotoxicity have been described [14]. Tizanidine undergoes extensive phase I metabolism via CYP1A2, leading to an increased risk of adverse effects when tizanidine is combined with other pharmacologic agents that inhibit the CYP1A2 enzyme. The concomitant administration of tizanidine with ciprofloxacin or fluvoxamine is contraindicated, resulting in a sevenfold and 12-fold increase, respectively, in tizanidine serum concentrations, leading to profound hypotension and sedation [26, 27, 80]. Additionally, caution should be used when tizanidine is administered in combination with other CNS depressants, including opioid analgesics and benzodiazepines, as these agents may compound the sedative effects of tizanidine.

Dexmedetomidine

Respiratory depression is the major safety concern when administering agents for analgosedation—particularly opioid analgesics and benzodiazepines. However, dexmedetomidine has minimal effect on respiratory function. In a crossover trial conducted using healthy volunteers, dexmedetomidine was found to elicit no clinically significant detrimental effects on patients' oxygenation or ventilation—even at supramaximal doses of up to 2.1 mcg/kg/h [32]. Nevertheless, caution should be exercised with dexmedetomidine use in patients of advanced age or when administered concomitantly with respiratory depressant agents [31].

Although the incidence of respiratory depression associated with dexmedetomidine is negligible, instances of clinically relevant upper airway obstruction have been demonstrated in small crossover trials conducted using healthy volunteers. The pharyngeal muscle tone, which contributes to the maintenance of airway patency during wakefulness, is diminished as a result of the anesthetic effects of dexmedetomidine [44, 50]. Continuous monitoring of respiratory function, including capnography to assess ventilatory status, as well as the use of pulse oximetry, is warranted with the administration of dexmedetomidine in non-mechanically ventilated patients.

The adverse effect profile of dexmedetomidine is primarily related to its effects on hemodynamics. The most common adverse effects associated with dexmedetomidine are hypotension and bradycardia, produced by the sympatholytic effects of central alpha$_{2A}$ receptor activation. However, a dose-dependent biphasic blood pressure response, which initially manifests as transient hypertension and reflex bradycardia resulting from the vasoconstrictive effects mediated via the stimulation of alpha$_{2B}$ receptors in the peripheral vasculature, has also been demonstrated with rapid intravenous infusion rates and intravenous bolus administration of dexmedetomidine loading doses [42, 81]. Increased caution should be exercised with dexmedetomidine use in patients with baseline hypotension, hypovolemia, heart failure, and coronary artery disease and those of advanced age [20, 33]. A published case series describes a potential concern, although remote, for cardiac arrest secondary to severe bradycardia with dexmedetomidine use [5]. Patients with underlying cardiac conduction delays or ventricular dysfunction may be at a greater risk of poor outcomes. Continuous electrocardiographic (ECG) monitoring is recommended, particularly in patients with known cardiac conduction disturbances.

According to the manufacturer's labeling, the maximum therapeutic duration of dexmedetomidine is 24 h. However, the safety of prolonged dexmedetomidine administration is well-evidenced [28]. Data from randomized controlled trials suggests that dexmedetomidine may be used safely for up to 30 days in mechanically ventilated patients [62].

Discontinuation of clonidine and tizanidine may result in a withdrawal syndrome. Due to their shared pharmacologic action, abrupt cessation of dexmedetomidine may likewise result in a clonidine-like withdrawal syndrome. Based on the data derived from recent retrospective studies, rebound hypertension, tachycardia, and delirium, consistent with withdrawal syndrome, were observed in approximately one-third of adult and pediatric patients receiving dexmedetomidine [9, 29, 58]. Predisposing risk factors for dexmedetomidine withdrawal syndrome include a prior history of hypertension, duration of therapy greater than 24 h, higher maximum and/or cumulative doses, and abrupt discontinuation of therapy [65]. To mitigate the risk of withdrawal, dexmedetomidine should be tapered prior to discontinuation, particularly in patients with concomitant hypertension or those receiving prolonged infusions of dexmedetomidine [17, 49]. Additionally, the administration of an oral clonidine taper regimen may be beneficial in preventing dexmedetomidine withdrawal syndrome while allowing for more rapid weaning [6, 7].

Applications in Clinical Practice

The use of alpha$_2$ agonists for pain management has been studied in a variety of different patient populations and settings. Multimodal pain management with alpha$_2$ agonists can be beneficial for a variety of patients, particularly in situations where a combination of analgesic strategies is required to achieve target pain control. Although these agents primarily exhibit their effects through sedative and anxiolytic properties, alpha$_2$ agonists have been shown to exhibit opioid-sparing effects and are primarily used as adjunct agents. There is a compelling amount of evidence demonstrating both the efficacy and safety of alpha$_2$ agonists when used in a variety of clinical settings and patient populations. These trials include well-designed prospective and retrospective clinical trials and systematic reviews demonstrating the effectiveness of these agents.

Clinical scenarios and patient populations that may benefit from multimodal pain management with alpha$_2$ agonists are highlighted in Table 9.2. Dexmedetomidine is a preferred sedative agent in critically ill patients because of its minimal effect on respiration and limited side effect profile, as per the Society of Critical Care Medicine guidelines [15]. In addition to its sedative properties, dexmedetomidine provides analgesia and opioid-sparing effects through the modulation of nociceptive pathways and inhibition of catecholamine release [81]. Because of its minimal effect on respiratory drive, dexmedetomidine can be used during extubation and after extubation for sedation and pain control where propofol and continuous infusion opioids are not appropriate. Dexmedetomidine has also been shown to improve pain and decrease the risk of delirium in cardiac surgery patients [43]. Additionally, dexmedetomidine reduces the amount of opioid and inhaled anesthetic gases needed during surgery and has been shown to decrease opioid needs by as much as 50% in the postoperative setting. Several studies have also shown effectiveness in transitioning patients from intravenous dexmedetomidine to enteral cloni-

Table 9.2 Scenarios where alpha$_2$ agonists may be used in practice for pain management

Clinical scenario or patient population	Description of scenario (summary)	Alpha$_2$ agonists studied in this scenario
Critically ill patients	Alpha$_2$ agonists, particularly dexmedetomidine, are commonly used in the intensive care setting for sedation and analgesia. The sedative and analgesic properties of these agents can help manage pain in critically ill patients while minimizing the need for higher doses of opioids. Intravenous dexmedetomidine can be transitioned to enteral clonidine around extubation as adjunct pain management	Clonidine Dexmedetomidine
Postoperative pain management	Patients undergoing surgery (cardiac, orthopedic, general surgery) associated with moderate to severe postoperative pain may benefit from multimodal pain management that includes alpha$_2$ agonists. Tizanidine is beneficial for concurrent muscle spasm or related pain	Clonidine Dexmedetomidine Tizanidine
Procedural sedation/pain control	Alpha$_2$ agonists can be used for procedural sedation, particularly in settings where minimizing respiratory depression is important. In situations where minimal sedation is desired, such as outpatient procedures or diagnostic tests, alpha$_2$ agonists may be preferred over traditional sedatives due to their unique sedative and analgesic properties with minimal impact on respiratory function	Dexmedetomidine
Chronic or complex pain conditions	Patients with complex pain scenarios, involving a combination of nociceptive and neuropathic pain components, may benefit from the multimodal approach provided by alpha$_2$ agonists in conjunction with other analgesics targeting different pain pathways. This includes musculoskeletal pain, neuropathic pain, or pain causing anxiety or sleep disturbances	Clonidine Dexmedetomidine Tizanidine
Prevention of opioid-induced hyperalgesia	Alpha$_2$ agonists may be considered to help prevent opioid-induced hyperalgesia, a clinical scenario where prolonged opioid use leads to increased pain sensitivity and worsened pain control. Utilizing alpha$_2$ agonists can decrease the overall opioid requirement	Clonidine Dexmedetomidine Tizanidine
Treatment of opioid withdrawal	Alpha$_2$ agonists can be used to manage withdrawal symptoms in patients on opioids, alcohol, or other substances. They provide analgesic effects while managing withdrawal symptoms such as agitation, anxiety, muscle spasms, insomnia, and overactive sympathetic nervous system functions	Clonidine

dine for pain control [19, 75]. However, dexmedetomidine has a much higher affinity for alpha$_2$ receptors and provides more sedative effects than clonidine.

Alpha$_2$ agonists may be utilized for pain management in patients requiring procedural sedation. In situations where minimal sedation is desired, such as short outpatient procedures or diagnostic tests, alpha$_2$ agonists may be preferred over traditional sedatives due to their unique sedative and analgesic properties with nominal impact on respiratory function. In addition to the minimal impact on respiratory function, alpha$_2$ agonists have rapid distribution half-lives, allowing for quicker recovery when used in procedural scenarios [23, 54, 72].

Patients with complex pain scenarios involving a combination of nociceptive and neuropathic pain may benefit from a multimodal approach using alpha$_2$ agonists in conjunction with other analgesics. Alpha$_2$ agonists are commonly prescribed with opioids to provide pain relief and minimize side effects and the risk of opioid dependence and tolerance. Dexmedetomidine, as an intravenous agent, may be useful when these patients are acutely ill in the hospital setting, while clonidine and tizanidine may be used as oral agents for chronic therapy. Topical clonidine may also be used for localized pain relief in patients with chronic pain conditions, such as diabetic neuropathy [82]. Patients on chronic opioids are at an increased risk of opioid-induced hyperalgesia, a clinical syndrome where prolonged opioid use leads to increased pain sensitivity and impaired pain control. Alpha$_2$ agonists can decrease the overall opioid requirements and potentially prevent this side effect [39]. For patients with a chronic neuropathic pain component or fibromyalgia, alpha$_2$ agonists have been shown to reduce the perception of pain and provide pain relief through central pain pathways and pain signals in the spinal cord. For pain with a strong musculoskeletal component, tizanidine is most effective and provides muscle relaxation effects [77]. Because of their sedative effects, clonidine and tizanidine may be useful for pain relief for patients with concurrent anxiety or sleep disturbances. Clonidine or tizanidine may also be used in combination with non-opioid agents like nonsteroidal anti-inflammatory drugs or acetaminophen to manage musculoskeletal pain.

Table 9.3 provides common dosing regimens of alpha$_2$ agonists when used for adjunct pain control or other indications. Dexmedetomidine is available as an intravenous product and comes in vials that can be reconstituted in dextrose or normal saline or as a premixed intravenous bag. A sublingual film dosage form of dexmedetomidine is FDA-approved for agitation associated with bipolar disorder; however, this dosage form has not been studied for pain management. Clonidine is available as an immediate-release oral tablet, extended-release oral tablet, topical patch, and compounded topical gel. Clonidine epidural solution is commercially available for epidural therapies but is not commonly used for perioperative or ICU pain management. Tizanidine is only available in an oral dosage form and comes as capsules and tablets.

Factors to Consider When Starting Therapy

The selection of an alpha$_2$ agonist for pain management should be individualized, taking into consideration the patient-specific characteristics and the type of pain experienced. The patient's medical history and current clinical status should be evaluated, specifically considering any history of cardiovascular disease and current hemodynamic status. These agents can all cause severe bradycardia, heart block, and hypotension. These effects can be potentiated in elderly patients, potentially due to decreased clearance of medication, resulting in a longer duration of effect [10]. Patients with low body weight or patients with existing bradycardia or hypotension are also at risk of side effects [28, 33]. Concurrent medications the patient is receiving should also be evaluated, with close attention paid to medications that may impact atrioventricular node function, such as beta-blockers or non-dihydropyridine calcium channel blockers, or other sympatholytic agents, as additive bradycardia and hypotension can occur. An assessment of baseline mental status and cognition should be performed, as alpha$_2$ agonists can all cause varying levels of CNS depression [23, 26].

The kidneys and liver are responsible for the metabolism and excretion of these medications. Routine monitoring of renal and hepatic function should be performed to determine if dose adjustments are needed and minimize adverse effects. Dexmedetomidine does not require renal or hepatic dose adjustments, but clonidine should be started at a low dose and titrated slowly in patients with a glomerular filtration rate less than 30 ml/min/1.73m^2. Tizanidine is primarily renally cleared and requires the most significant dose adjustment, with renal clearance reduced by as much as 50% in patients with a creatinine clearance (CrCl) <25 ml/min. Tizanidine should be started and titrated cautiously in patients with hepatic impairment.

Individual responses to alpha$_2$ agonists can vary widely and should be monitored when starting therapy [15]. Therapy should be initiated at the lowest dose and titrated slowly to the desired pain control. These medications should not be abruptly discontinued due to the risk of withdrawal symp-

Table 9.3 Dosing considerations with alpha$_2$ agonists

Medication	Dose	Duration	Additional considerations
Clonidine	ICU sedation, transition from dexmedetomidine: 0.1–0.3 mg PO every 6–8 h; decrease dexmedetomidine by 25% after each clonidine dose Pain: 0.1–0.3 mg PO every 6–8 h; 0.1–0.3 mg/day transdermal patch every 7 days	Short-term (days) to long-term therapy (months/years)	Taper therapy; do not abruptly discontinue, as it can cause rebound symptoms and hypertensive crises
Dexmedetomidine	ICU sedation/analgesia: 0.2–1.5 mcg/kg/hr. IV infusion Procedural sedation/analgesia: 0.5–1 mcg/kg IV bolus, then 0.2–1 mcg/kg/hr. IV infusion	Short-term (hours to days)	Bolus doses can worsen hemodynamic effects. Taper therapy; do not abruptly discontinue
Tizanidine	Pain (musculoskeletal): 2–4 mg PO q 8–12 h, as needed	Short-term (days) preferred, may be used long-term	Taper therapy; do not abruptly discontinue, as it can cause rebound symptoms and hypertensive crises

toms and significant rebound hypertension, especially with clonidine. Alpha$_2$ agonists should be used for the shortest duration of therapy as warranted and closely monitored if being used for long-term therapy in patients with chronic pain syndromes.

Monitoring of Therapy

Regular monitoring and adjustment of pain management therapy are essential for optimizing outcomes and minimizing potential adverse effects when using alpha$_2$ agonists. Commercially available drug levels for alpha$_2$ agonist agents are not routinely available in clinical practice and are not commonly used. Clonidine levels can be measured, but levels have not correlated well to toxicity and are not recommended to guide adjustment of therapy [47]. Monitoring for efficacy and toxicity should be done via patient assessment of vital signs, pain and sedation scores, and laboratory monitoring, such as renal and liver function.

Alpha$_2$ agonists should be used with caution in hemodynamically unstable patients or those with preexisting cardiovascular disease. Major hemodynamic side effects seen with alpha$_2$ agonists, especially dexmedetomidine and clonidine, include bradycardia and hypotension. These side effects are less pronounced with the use of tizanidine compared to other agents. Hemodynamic effects from alpha$_2$ agonists can be seen within 4 h of starting therapy. Risk factors for hypotension and/or bradycardia include low baseline blood pressure or heart rate, increased age, giving a loading dose (dexmedetomidine), history of coronary artery disease, and prolonged infusion times [28, 33]. Patients receiving these agents should have close hemodynamic monitoring performed.

Patients on alpha$_2$ agonists should not have therapy abruptly discontinued for the risk of withdrawal and rebound symptoms. Common withdrawal symptoms to monitor patients for include hypertension, tachycardia, diaphoresis, and altered mental status. Prolonged use of agents, especially dexmedetomidine, may lead to tolerance and tachyphylaxis, which can cause loss of sedation and pain control and lead to withdrawal-like symptoms.

Several clinically significant drug–drug interactions may be present with the alpha$_2$ agonist agents and should be managed. Dexmedetomidine is a minor CYP2A6 substrate and does not have many direct drug interactions that impair metabolism or elimination. Caution should be used with concurrent medications that can decrease heart rate or blood pressure, however. Clonidine does not have any known metabolism or transport effects, but caution should be used with medications that can worsen bradycardia or hypotension or medications that can cause central nervous system depression. Tizanidine is a major substrate of CYP1A2, so it should not be used in combination with medications that are strong CYP1A2 inhibitors, such as ciprofloxacin or cimetidine, and should be used with caution with other medications that cause bradycardia or CNS depression.

Key Themes

- Alpha$_2$ agonists enhance the effectiveness and prolong the duration of local anesthetic agents when coadministered neuraxially and perineurally or when administered intravenously.
- Alpha$_2$ agonists have been used as adjunct pain medications in a variety of clinical settings, including in critically ill patients, for postoperative and procedural pain management, and in chronic or complex pain disorders.
- Alpha$_2$ agonists exhibit an opioid-sparing effect and allow for additive analgesic and sedative effects that may facilitate opioid and benzodiazepine weaning without the increased risk of respiratory depression.
- Adverse effects of concern with alpha$_2$ agonists include bradycardia and hypotension, as well as the potential for withdrawal syndrome with abrupt discontinuation.
- Alpha$_2$ agonists have minimal impact on respiratory function, which is a benefit compared to opioid medications.

Conclusions

Alpha$_2$ agonists have been used in a variety of clinical settings and patient populations to provide analgesic effects. They can be given via a wide range of administration routes, including orally, intravenously, or neuraxially, to provide analgesic effects and prolong the duration of local anesthetic agents. Alpha$_2$ agonists also provide opioid-sparing effects, minimizing potential opioid-related adverse effects and the risk of opioid-induced hyperalgesia. Alpha$_2$ agonists cause minimal respiratory depression, making them an ideal agent to facilitate weaning of other medications such as opioids or benzodiazepines. Common side effects of alpha$_2$ agonists include bradycardia and hypotension, and close monitoring should be implemented when using these agents. Abrupt discontinuation should also be avoided to decrease the risk of withdrawal syndromes.

References

1. Abdallah FW, Abrishami A, Brull R. The facilitatory effects of intravenous dexmedetomidine on the duration of spinal anesthesia: a systematic review and meta-analysis. Anesth Analg. 2013;117(1):271–8.

2. Ahlquist RP. A study of the adrenotropic receptors. Am J Phys. 1948;153(3):586–600. https://doi.org/10.1152/ajplegacy.1948.153.3.586.
3. Basker S, Singh G, Jacob R. Clonidine in paediatrics—a review. Indian J Anaesth. 2009;53(3):270–80.
4. Belgrade M, Hall S. Dexmedetomidine infusion for the management of opioid-induced hyperalgesia. Pain Med. 2010;11(12):1819–26. https://doi.org/10.1111/j.1526-4637.2010.00973.x.
5. Bharati S, Pal A, Biswas C, Biswas R. Incidence of cardiac arrest increases with the indiscriminate use of dexmedetomidine: a case series and review of published case reports. Acta Anaesthesiol Taiwanica. 2011;49(4):165–7.
6. Bhatt K, Thompson Quan A, Baumgartner L, Jia S, Croci R, Puntillo K, et al. Effects of a clonidine taper on dexmedetomidine use and withdrawal in adult critically ill patients—a pilot study. Crit Care Explor. 2020;2(11):e0245.
7. Bouajram RH, Bhatt K, Croci R, Baumgartner L, Puntillo K, Ramsay J, et al. Incidence of dexmedetomidine withdrawal in adult critically ill patients: a pilot study. Crit Care Explor. 2019;1(8):e0035.
8. Buerkle H, Yaksh TL. Pharmacological evidence for different alpha 2-adrenergic receptor sites mediating analgesia and sedation in the rat. Br J Anaesth. 1998;81(2):208–15. https://doi.org/10.1093/bja/81.2.208.
9. Burbano NH, Otero AV, Berry DE, Orr RA, Munoz RA. Discontinuation of prolonged infusions of dexmedetomidine in critically ill children with heart disease. Intensive Care Med. 2012;38(2):300–7.
10. By the 2023 American Geriatrics Society Beers Criteria® Update Expert Panel. American Geriatrics Society 2023 updated AGS Beers Criteria® for potentially inappropriate medication use in older adults. J Am Geriatr Soc. 2023;71(7):2052–81. https://doi.org/10.1111/jgs.18372.
11. Carollo DS, Nossaman BD, Ramadhyani U. Dexmedetomidine: a review of clinical applications. Curr Opin Anaesthesiol. 2008;21(4):457–61. https://doi.org/10.1097/ACO.0b013e328305e3ef.
12. Chen Z, Liu Z, Feng C, Jin Y, Zhao X. Dexmedetomidine as an adjuvant in peripheral nerve block. DDDT. 2023;17:1463–84.
13. Cortinez LI, Hsu YW, Sum-Ping ST, Young C, Keifer JC, MacLeod D, et al. Dexmedetomidine pharmacodynamics: part II. Anesthesiology. 2004;101(5):1077–83.
14. De Graaf EM, Oosterveld M, Tjabbes T, Stricker BHC. A case of tizanidine-induced hepatic injury. J Hepatol. 1996;25(5):772–3. https://doi.org/10.1016/s0168-8278(96)80252-2.
15. Devlin JW, Skrobik Y, Gelinas C, et al. Clinical practice guidelines for the prevention and management of pain, agitation/sedation, delirium, immobility, and sleep disruption in adult patients in the ICU. Crit Care Med. 2018;46(9):e825–73. https://doi.org/10.1097/CCM.0000000000003299.
16. Esmailian M, Golshani K, Tavakolifard N, Amiri A. Effects of adding oral clonidine to standard treatments on pain intensity of patients with acute renal colic: a randomized clinical trial. Adv Biomed Res. 2022;11(1):28.
17. Flieller LA, Alaniz C, Pleva MR, Miller JT. Incidence of rebound hypertension after discontinuation of dexmedetomidine. Pharmacotherapy. 2019;39(10):970–4.
18. Fogelholm R, Murros K. Tizanidine in chronic tension-type headache: a placebo controlled double-blind cross-over study. Headache J Head Face Pain. 1992;32(10):509–13. https://doi.org/10.1111/j.1526-4610.1992.hed3210509.x.
19. Gagnon DJ, Riker RR, Glisic EK, Kelner A, Perrey HM, Fraser GL. Transition from dexmedetomidine to enteral clonidine for ICU sedation: an observational pilot study. Pharmacotherapy. 2015;35(3):251–9. https://doi.org/10.1002/phar.1559.
20. Gerlach A, Blais D, Gm J, Burcham P, Stawicki S, Cook C, et al. Predictors of dexmedetomidine-associated hypotension in critically ill patients. Int J Crit Illn Inj Sci. 2016;6(3):109.
21. Gertler R, Brown HC, Mitchell DH, Silvius EN. Dexmedetomidine: a novel sedative-analgesic agent. Proc Bayl Univ Med Cent. 2001;14(1):13–21.
22. Geyskes G, Boer P, Mees DE, Clonidine withdrawal. Mechanism and frequency of rebound hypertension. Brit J Clin Pharma. 1979;7(1):55–62.
23. Giovannitti JA, Thoms SM, Crawford JJ. Alpha-2 adrenergic receptor agonists: a review of current clinical applications. Anesth Prog. 2015;62(1):31–8. https://doi.org/10.2344/0003-3006-62.1.31.
24. Goyagi T, Tanaka M, Nishikawa T. Oral clonidine premedication enhances postoperative analgesia by epidural morphine. Anesth Analg. 1999;89:1487–91. https://doi.org/10.1213/00000539-199912000-00032.
25. Grosu I, Lavand'homme P. Use of dexmedetomidine for pain control. F1000 Med Rep [Internet]. 2010;2. Available from: https://facultyopinions.com/prime/reports/m/2/90/
26. Granfors M, Backman J, Neuvonen M, Neuvonen P. Ciprofloxacin greatly increases concentrations and hypotensive effect of tizanidine by inhibiting its cytochrome P450 1A2? mediated presystemic metabolism. Clin Pharmacol Therap. 2004a;76(6):598–606. https://doi.org/10.1016/j.clpt.2004.08.018.
27. Granfors M, Backman J, Neuvonen M, Ahonen J, Neuvonen P. Fluvoxamine drastically increases concentrations and effects of tizanidine: a potentially hazardous interaction. Clin Pharmacol Therap. 2004b;75(4):331–41. https://doi.org/10.1016/j.clpt.2003.12.005.
28. Guinter JR, Kristeller JL. Prolonged infusions of dexmedetomidine in critically ill patients. Am J Health Syst Pharm. 2010;67(15):1246–53. https://doi.org/10.2146/ajhp090300.
29. Haenecour AS, Seto W, Urbain CM, Stephens D, Laussen PC, Balit CR. Prolonged Dexmedetomidine infusion and drug withdrawal in critically ill children. J Pediatr Pharmacol Therap. 2017;22(6):453–60.
30. Hauber JA, Davis PJ, Bendel LP, et al. Dexmedetomidine as a rapid bolus for treatment and prophylactic prevention of emergence agitation in anesthetized children. Anesth Analg. 2015;121(5):1308–15. https://doi.org/10.1213/ANE.0000000000000931.
31. Ho AMH, Chen S, Karmakar MK. Central apnea after balanced general anaesthesia that included dexmedetomidine. Br J Anaesth. 2005;95(6):773–5.
32. Hsu YW, Cortinez LI, Robertson KM, Keifer JC, Sum-Ping ST, Moretti EW, et al. Dexmedetomidine pharmacodynamics: part I. Anesthesiology. 2004;101(5):1066–76.
33. Ice CJ, Personett HA, Frazee EN, Dierkhising RA, Kashyap R, Oeckler RA. Risk factors for dexmedetomidine-associated hemodynamic instability in noncardiac intensive care unit patients. Anesth Analg. 2016;122(2):462–9. https://doi.org/10.1213/ane.0000000000001125.
34. Jaakola ML, Salonen M, Lehtinen R, Scheinin H. The analgesic action of dexmedetomidine--a novel alpha 2-adrenoceptor agonist--in healthy volunteers. Pain. 1991;46(3):281–5. https://doi.org/10.1016/0304-3959(91)90111-A.
35. Jessen Lundorf L, Korvenius Nedergaard H, Møller AM. Perioperative dexmedetomidine for acute pain after abdominal surgery in adults. Cochrane Anaesthesia Group, editor. Cochrane Database Syst Rev [Internet]. 2016;2016(2). Available from: http://doi.wiley.com/10.1002/14651858.CD010358.pub2
36. Karachalios GN, Charalabopoulos A, Papalimneou V, Kiortsis D, Dimicco P, Kostoula OK, et al. Withdrawal syndrome following cessation of antihypertensive drug therapy: withdrawal syndrome and antihypertensive drug withdrawal. Int J Clin Pract. 2005;59(5):562–70.

37. Kaur M, Singh PM. Current role of dexmedetomidine in clinical anesthesia and intensive care. Anesth Essays Res. 2011;5(2):128–33. https://doi.org/10.4103/0259-1162.94750.
38. Ke HH, Liou JY, Teng WN, Hsu PK, Tsou MY, Chang WK, et al. Opioid-sparing anesthesia with dexmedetomidine provides stable hemodynamic and short hospital stay in non-intubated video-assisted thoracoscopic surgery: a propensity score matching cohort study. BMC Anesthesiol. 2023;23(1):110.
39. Kumar A, Maitra S, Khanna P, Baidya DK. Clonidine for management of chronic pain: a brief review of the current evidences. Saudi J Anaesth. 2014;8(1):92–6. https://doi.org/10.4103/1658-354x.125955.
40. Lee C, Kim YD, Kim JN. Antihyperalgesic effects of dexmedetomidine on high-dose remifentanil-induced hyperalgesia. Korean J Anesthesiol. 2013;64(4):301. https://doi.org/10.4097/kjae.2013.64.4.301.
41. Lee HMD, Ruggoo V, Graudins A. Intrathecal clonidine pump failure causing acute withdrawal syndrome with 'stress-induced' cardiomyopathy. J Med Toxicol. 2016;12(1):134–8.
42. Lee S. Dexmedetomidine: present and future directions. Korean J Anesthesiol. 2019;72(4):323–30.
43. Lin Y, Chen J, Wang Z. Meta-analysis of factors which influence delirium following cardiac surgery. J Card Surg. 2012;27(4):481–92. https://doi.org/10.1111/j.1540-8191.2012.01472.x.
44. Lodenius Å, Maddison KJ, Lawther BK, Scheinin M, Eriksson LI, Eastwood PR, et al. Upper airway collapsibility during dexmedetomidine and propofol sedation in healthy volunteers. Anesthesiology. 2019;131(5):962–73.
45. Malanga GA, Gwynn MW, Smith R, Miller D. Tizanidine is effective in the treatment of myofascial pain syndrome. Pain Physician. 2002;5(4):422–32.
46. Manfredini D, Romagnoli M, Cantini E, Bosco M. Efficacy of tizanidine hydrochloride in the treatment of myofascial face pain. Minerva Med. 2004;95(2):165–71.
47. Manzon L, Nappe TM, DelMaestro C, et al. Clonidine toxicity. [Updated 2023 Jun 26]. In: StatPearls [Internet]. Treasure Island (FL): StatPearls Publishing; 2025.
48. Metz S, Klein C, Morton N. Rebound hypertension after discontinuation of transdermal clonidine therapy. Am J Med. 1987;82(1):17–9. https://doi.org/10.1016/0002-9343(87)90371-8.
49. Miller JL, Allen C, Johnson PN. Neurologic withdrawal symptoms following abrupt discontinuation of a prolonged dexmedetomidine infusion in a child. J Pediatr Pharmacol Therap. 2010;15(1):38–42.
50. Mishima G, Sanuki T, Sato S, Kobayashi M, Kurata S, Ayuse T. Upper-airway collapsibility and compensatory responses under moderate sedation with ketamine, dexmedetomidine, and propofol in healthy volunteers. Physiol Rep [Internet]. 2020;8(10) Available from: https://onlinelibrary.wiley.com/doi/abs/10.14814/phy2.14439
51. Muzyk AJ, Fowler JA, Norwood DK, Chilipko A. Role of α_2-agonists in the treatment of acute alcohol withdrawal. Ann Pharmacother. 2011;45(5):649–57.
52. Neil MJE. Clonidine: clinical pharmacology and therapeutic use in pain management. CCP. 2011;6(4):280–7. https://doi.org/10.2174/157488411798375886.
53. Nguyen M, Tharani S, Rahmani M, Shapiro M. A review of the use of clonidine as a sleep aid in the child and adolescent population. Clin Pediatr (Phila). 2014;53(3):211–6. https://doi.org/10.1177/0009922813502123.
54. Nguyen V, Tiemann D, Park E, Salehi A. Alpha-2 Agonists. Anesthesiol Clin. 2017;35(2):233–45. https://doi.org/10.1016/j.anclin.2017.01.009.
55. Oldfield BJ, Gleeson B, Morford KL, Adams Z, Funaro MC, Becker WC, et al. Long-term use of muscle relaxant medications for chronic pain: a systematic review. JAMA Netw Open. 2024;7(9):e2434835. https://doi.org/10.1001/jamanetworkopen.2024.34835.
56. Owens JA. The practice of pediatric sleep medicine: results of a community survey. Pediatrics. 2001;108(3):E51. https://doi.org/10.1542/peds.108.3.e51.
57. Park J, Forrest J, Kolesar R, Bhola D, Beattie S, Chu C. Oral clonidine reduces postoperative PCA morphine requirements. Can J Anaesth. 1996;43(9):900–6.
58. Pathan S, Kaplan JB, Adamczyk K, Chiu SH, Shah CV. Evaluation of dexmedetomidine withdrawal in critically ill adults. J Crit Care. 2021;62:19–24.
59. Pichot C, Ghignone M, Quintin L. Dexmedetomidine and clonidine: from second- to first-line sedative agents in the critical care setting? J Intensive Care Med. 2012;27(4):219–37. https://doi.org/10.1177/0885066610396815.
60. Pei W, Zou Y, Wang W, Wei L, Zhao Y, Li L. Tizanidine exerts anti-nociceptive effects in spared nerve injury model of neuropathic pain through inhibition of TLR4/NF-κB pathway. Int J Mol Med. 2018;42(6):3209–19. https://doi.org/10.3892/ijmm.2018.3878.
61. Ramasubbu C, Gupta A. Pharmacological treatment of opioid-induced hyperalgesia: a review of the evidence. J Pain Palliat Care Pharmacother. 2011;25(3):219–30. https://doi.org/10.3109/15360288.2011.589490.
62. Riker RR, Shehabi Y, Bokesch PM, Ceraso D, Wisemandle W, Koura F, et al. Dexmedetomidine vs midazolam for sedation of critically ill patients. JAMA. 2009;301(5):489–99.
63. Rostamipoor Z, Nazemi-Rafi M, Mirafzal A, Ilka S, Hosseininasab M. Effect of oral clonidine on pain reduction in patients with opioid use disorder in the emergency department: a randomized clinical trial. Br J Clin Pharmacol. 2024;90(12):3003–9. https://doi.org/10.1111/bcp.15948.
64. Ruffolo RR, Waddell JE, Yaden EL. Postsynaptic alpha adrenergic receptor subtypes differentiated by yohimbine in tissues from the rat. Existence of alpha-2 adrenergic receptors in rat aorta. J Pharmacol Exp Ther. 1981;217(2):235–40.
65. Salah J, Grgurich P, Nault K, Lei Y. Identification of risk factors for hypertension and tachycardia upon dexmedetomidine discontinuation. J Crit Care. 2020 Oct;59:81–5.
66. Saper JR, Lake AE, Cantrell DT, Winner PK, White JR. Chronic daily headache prophylaxis with tizanidine: a double-blind, placebo-controlled, multicenter outcome study. Headache. 2002;42(6):470–82. https://doi.org/10.1046/j.1526-4610.2002.02122.x.
67. Semenchuk MR, Sherman S. Effectiveness of tizanidine in neuropathic pain: an open-label study. J Pain. 2000;1(4):285–92. https://doi.org/10.1054/jpai.2000.9435.
68. Shaw M, Matsa R. Clonidine withdrawal induced sympathetic surge. BMJ Case Rep. 2015; https://doi.org/10.1136/bcr-2015-210325.
69. Smith's Anesthesia for Infants and Children - 10th Edition. Accessed December 10, 2023. https://shop.elsevier.com/books/smiths-anesthesia-for-infants-and-children/davis/978-0-323-69825-2
70. Solanki SL, Goyal VK. Neuraxial dexmedetomidine: wonder drug or simply harmful. Anesth Pain Med [Internet]. 2015;5(2) Available from: https://brieflands.com/articles/aapm-17445.html
71. Srivastava AB, Mariani JJ, Levin FR. New directions in the treatment of opioid withdrawal. Lancet. 2020;395(10241):1938–48.
72. Tabari M, Alipour M, Esalati H. Evaluation of oral tiazinidine effects on [intraoperative] hemodynamic responses during direct laryngoscopy under general anesthesia. Iran Red Crescent Med J. 2013;15(7):541–6. https://doi.org/10.5812/ircmj.11540.
73. Talakoub R, Abbasi S, Maghami E, Zavareh SMHT. The effect of oral tizanidine on postoperative pain relief after elective laparoscopic cholecystectomy. Adv Biomed Res. 2016;5(1):19. https://doi.org/10.4103/2277-9175.175905.
74. Tang C, Xia Z. Dexmedetomidine in perioperative acute pain management: a non-opioid adjuvant analgesic. JPR. 2017;10:1899–904.

75. Terry K, Blum R, Szumita P. Evaluating the transition from dexmedetomidine to clonidine for agitation management in the intensive care unit. SAGE Open Med. 2015;3:2050312115621767. https://doi.org/10.1177/2050312115621767.
76. Themes UFO. Autonomic nervous system: physiology and pharmacology. Anesthesia Key. Published June 16, 2016. Accessed December 10, 2023. https://aneskey.com/autonomic-nervous-system-physiology-and-pharmacology/
77. van Tulder MW, Touray T, Furlan AD, Solway S, Bouter LM. Muscle relaxants for nonspecific low back pain: a systematic review within the framework of the Cochrane collaboration. Spine (Phila Pa 1976). 2003;28(17):1978–92. https://doi.org/10.1097/01.Brs.0000090503.38830.Ad.
78. Venn RM, Hell J, Grounds RM. Respiratory effects of dexmedetomidine in the surgical patient requiring intensive care. Crit Care Lond Engl. 2000;4(5):302–8. https://doi.org/10.1186/cc712.
79. Vongpatanasin W, Kario K, Atlas SA, Victor RG. Central sympatholytic drugs: central sympatholytic drugs in hypertension. J Clin Hypertens. 2011;13(9):658–61.
80. Wagstaff AJ, Bryson HM. Tizanidine: a review of its pharmacology, clinical efficacy and tolerability in the management of spasticity associated with cerebral and spinal disorders. Drugs. 1997;53(3):435–52. https://doi.org/10.2165/00003495-199753030-00007.
81. Weerink MAS, Struys MMRF, Hannivoort LN, Barends CRM, Absalom AR, Colin P. Clinical pharmacokinetics and pharmacodynamics of dexmedetomidine. Clin Pharmacokinet. 2017;56(8):893–913. https://doi.org/10.1007/s40262-017-0507-7.
82. Wrzosek A, Woron J, Dobrogowski, Jakowicka-Wordliczek J, Wordliczek J. Topical clonidine for neuropathic pain. Cochrane Database Syst Rev. 2015, 2015;(8)
83. Wu HH, Wang HT, Jin JJ, Cui GB, Zhou KC, Chen Y, et al. Does dexmedetomidine as a neuraxial adjuvant facilitate better anesthesia and analgesia? a systematic review and meta-analysis. Eldabe S, editor. PLoS ONE. 2014;9(3):e93114.
84. Zhang SJ, Lai G, Griffis CA, Schiltz M, Aroke EN. α2-adrenergic receptor agonist, an attractive but underused ERAS component in improving fast-track recovery and surgical outcomes. AANA J. 2021;89(6):529–37.
85. Zhao Y, He J, Yu N, Jia C, Wang S. Mechanisms of dexmedetomidine in neuropathic pain. Front Neurosci. 2020;14:330.
86. Zhu LL, Wang YH, Zhou Q. Tizanidine: advances in pharmacology & therapeutics and drug formulations. JPR. 2024;17:1257–71. https://doi.org/10.2147/JPR.S461032.

Skeletal Muscle Relaxants

10

Ozgur Karcioglu and Canan Akman

Introduction

Many different diseases and syndromes have the mechanisms to produce pain and spasm. Pain and spasm have a complex dynamic with one another, which has yet to be fully elucidated. Muscular spasm is mostly secondary to a painful lesion in another muscle or joint [1]. Skeletal muscle spasms (SMSs) can have a spinal etiology, such as in the case of lumbar disc herniation (LDH). Spasms can also originate outside the spine, such as a hyperactive pelvic floor.

A. Possible causes of mechanical pain, especially affecting the waist, back, and neck regions, are summarized in Table 10.1.

Pain resulting from conditions associated with SMS can be relieved with nonsteroidal anti-inflammatory drugs (NSAIDs), acetaminophen, and opioid analgesics, while various skeletal muscle relaxants (SMRs), such as cyclobenzaprine, carisoprodol, chlorzoxazone, metaxalone, methocarbamol, orphenadrine, tizanidine, baclofen, thiocolchicoside, and dantrolene, may be administered to directly mediate spasm activity. The use of SMRs has slightly increased in the United States in recent years. Many adult patients are treated with SMRs for long-term and off-label diagnoses, although more research is necessary to highlight the determinants of outcomes associated with these kinds of treatments. Cyclobenzaprine is the dominant agent, accounting for >50% of prescriptions [2].

Table 10.1 Clinical factors causing spasm in the lower lumbar and other spinal regions

Posture disorders
Lack of exercise
Muscle sprain/strain, postexercise pain
Nerve damage
Disc problems
Spondylolisthesis
Spinal stenosis
Arthritis
Fibromyalgia
Hyperactive pelvic floor
Psychological problems, such as stress and anxiety

Lumbar Disc Herniation

These entities including herniated nucleus pulposus and degenerative disc disease are among the most common causes of waist, back, and neck pain. The herniated disc causes pressure and irritation on the nerve root, thus triggering severe and, possibly, chronic pain. Muscle spasm is the body's inherent reflex mechanism to protect that area. This phenomenon is also called the "pain–spasm vicious circle" [3].

In advanced cases, weakness in leg flexion, tingling, and worsening pain are noted. Failure of nonoperative treatments constitutes an indication for surgery. In the multicenter spine

O. Karcioglu (✉)
University of Health Sciences, Department of Emergency Medicine, Istanbul Education and Research Hospital, Istanbul, Turkey
e-mail: Ozgur.Karcioglu@saglik.gov.tr

C. Akman
Canakkale Onsekiz Mart University, Department of Emergency Medicine, Canakkale, Turkey

J. P. Reinert et al. (eds.), *Adjunctive Analgesic Strategies for the Bedside Clinician and Beyond*,
https://doi.org/10.1007/978-3-032-21675-5_10

patient outcomes research trial (SPORT) study, discectomy results in lumbar disc herniation (LDH) cases with root compression have been reported to have more favorable outcomes in regard to pain, functionality, and disability compared to others [4].

Spinal Stenosis

It is the abnormal narrowing of the channels through which the spinal nerves pass. In most cases, this condition develops as a result of degenerative spondylolisthesis. It is accompanied by a degeneration of the facet joints and the intervertebral disc, most commonly encountered in L4 [5].

It progresses more slowly than other causes of low back pain (LBP). Improvement can be achieved with light exercise and changes in routine activity. The patient's pain decreases with sitting and lying and bending forward in flexion and is aggravated with extension and standing. In severe cases, spinal epidural injections cause improvement, while decompressive laminectomy is the most common surgery performed in persistent cases.

Spinal Osteoarthritis

Fluid collection in the intervertebral disc spaces appears due to a deterioration in cartilage structures. Bone protrusions trigger pain by creating pressure on nerve roots. Rest, heat and cold application, and NSAIDs/SMRs may be helpful, while surgery may be reserved for unresponsive cases.

Spinal Fracture

Even "cracks" as thin as a hair can cause spinal collapse and nerve root compression. Sudden onset of severe pain with discomfort mostly constitutes the initial symptom. Bracing or surgery may be required for definitive treatment, along with rest and pain management (NSAIDs/SMRs).

Sprain/Strain

It occurs due to sudden strain, falling, or performing some movements incorrectly or excessively in sports activities. *Sprain* is an injury to the ligaments, while *strain* is used to define torn muscles and tendinous structures. The symptoms mostly respond to proper treatment and rest in a short time. Swimming and physical therapy are helpful in some cases.

Fibromyalgia

Fibromyalgia is a syndrome that causes widespread and severe muscle pain, muscle stiffness, weakness, and focal sensitivity (trigger points) and even prevents sleep. It does not cause actual tissue damage or deformity. The complaints are typically seen in young and middle-aged women who present with anxiety and/or depression and even cognitive problems. The rates of new diagnoses are between 2% and 5% in general outpatient clinics and 10% and 20% in rheumatology clinics [6]. It is theorized that neurochemical changes increase pain sensitization and that the subsequent effects of inhibitory pathways are blunted. As a result of mechanical hyperalgesia, the brain's response to disturbing stimuli becomes sharper. The course typically progresses with flare-ups and extinguishments, while association with irritable bowel syndrome (IBS) and migraine headaches is also common.

A set of criteria for fibromyalgia was published by the American College of Rheumatology (ACR) in 1990 [6].

(a) A history of widespread pain for at least 3 months (common is used to mean tenderness in at least 11 of the 18 designated points, but this criterion is not required in the new guidelines) (Fig. 10.1)
(b) Presence of pain in both the lower and upper halves of the body

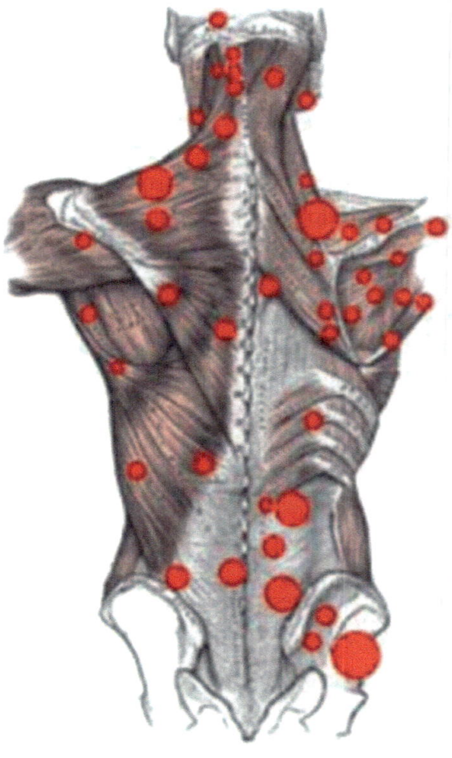

Fig. 10.1 Possible trigger points in a patient with fibromyalgia syndrome

Recently, these criteria have been revised under the name of Widespread Pain Index (WPI) criteria, and new items—fatigue, waking up without adequate sleep, and cognitive symptoms—have been added. NSAIDs, central nervous system (CNS)–active agents, Selective Serotonin Reuptake Inhibitor (SSRI) group antidepressants, muscle relaxants such as cyclobenzaprine, or anticonvulsants can provide successful results. The first US Food and Drug Administration (FDA)—approved agent for the treatment of fibromyalgia was *pregabalin*. However, *amitriptyline* and *cyclobenzaprine* are the most studied agents. These agents have been found to be very effective on sleep patterns, pain, fatigue, and general well-being [7].

Myofascial Pain

Myofascial pain (MP) is a regional muscular pain syndrome characterized by pain transmitted from trigger points within the connective tissue (myofascial structures) around the muscles that separate them from each other. The painful sensation is located exactly at the site of the trigger point, or it can be felt at a distant location, when the muscle is pressed (referred pain) [8].

Cyclobenzaprine, one of the drugs used in the treatment of MP, is a muscle relaxant taken orally to improve sleep quality and reduce pain. It suppresses muscle spasms and can therefore relieve the pain caused by MP without affecting muscle functions.

Leite et al. comprehensively analyzed publications on the subject in their Cochrane review [9]. The authors aimed to assess how effective cyclobenzaprine is at reducing pain and improving sleep in patients with MP. Although they searched extensively through scientific publications, only two trials were available, with a total of 79 participants. The studies tested cyclobenzaprine against a benzodiazepine, clonazepam, and a placebo or local anesthetic, lidocaine. Cyclobenzaprine was better than clonazepam and placebo at reducing jaw pain but had similar effects in improving sleep quality. Participants taking cyclobenzaprine had some improvement of pain intensity compared to those on clonazepam, with a mean difference (MD) of −0.25 (95% CI, −0.41—0.09; *P* value = 0.002), and placebo, with an MD of −0.25 (95% CI, −0.41—0.09; *P* value = 0.002). Because of the discomfort of any form of injection, patients with MP are likely to prefer treatment with cyclobenzaprine tablets. No life-threatening adverse effects were associated with any of the drugs studied. More research is pending before drawing any conclusion on these drugs' usefulness in treating MP.

Botulinum toxin (BTX) type A (onabotulinumtoxinA) is among the agents tried in the treatment of MP. Botulinum toxin injections can have a positive impact on cervicogenic headache resulting from cervical trauma [10]. The agent is a powerful agent inhibiting the innervation of muscles and blocks muscular activity stimulated by the trigger points. This effect may lead to pain relief when it is injected into the affected region.

Soares et al. conducted a Cochrane review in 2014 and pointed out that findings are not sufficiently conclusive to identify the benefits of BTX in the management of myofascial pain syndrome (MPS), based on data from four trials [8].

Hyperactive Pelvic Floor

A hyperactive pelvic floor has been defined as "a condition in which the pelvic floor muscles do not relax or may even contract when relaxation is functionally needed, for example, during micturition or defecation [11]. This condition is based on symptoms such as voiding problems, obstructed defecation or dyspareunia, and on signs like the absence of voluntary pelvic floor muscle relaxation" [12]. There is scarce data on the use of SMRs in the treatment of pelvic floor spasms and related pain, without any concrete recommendations.

A. *The main goals of musculoskeletal pain (MSP) management* are to restore function, prevent recurrent injuries, relieve pain, and regain comfort.

The criteria evaluated for recovery in the studies include:

- Global recovery
- Muscle spasm
- Local pain
- Tenderness with palpation
- Movement ability (range of motion)
- Activity of daily living

Self-care is one of the key points. If the patient rests, applies heat or cold as necessary, has a massage, engages in sufficient activity, and can relieve the pain with the right agents, most of the treatment will have been carried out on its own. In this way, medications or further interventions will not be required in most cases.

There are many treatment options for MSP, especially manifested as LBP. In general, these can be classified as *pharmacological treatments, noninvasive nonpharmacological treatments, injection treatments, and surgical treatments* [13, 14]. In LBP, nonpharmacological treatments are primarily recommended [15, 16].

Most guidelines recommend nonpharmacological treatments first, given that most people with (sub)acute LBP improve over time, regardless of treatment [17]. Nonpharmacological interventions include exercise and similar interventions (e.g., yoga), complementary and alternative therapies (e.g., spinal manipulation, acupuncture, and massage), psychological therapies (e.g., behavioral therapies, relaxation techniques, and Multidisciplinary rehabilitation (MDR)), and physical modalities (e.g., traction, ultrasound, transcutaneous electrical nerve stimulator (TENS), low-level laser therapy, interventional therapy, superficial heat or cold, back braces, and magnets), which can also prove beneficial in selected patients. After that, first NSAIDs and then muscle relaxants are advocated due to well-known analgesic and anti-inflammatory efficacies in these patients. On the other hand, their drawback is the NSAIDs' potential adverse events, particularly gastrointestinal and cardiovascular effects [18].

Pharmacological treatments include NSAIDs, acetaminophen, opioid analgesics, SMRs, antiepileptics, antidepressant agents, and corticosteroids.

Providers caring for patients with LBP face the challenge of selecting medication agents that maximize therapeutic relief while maximizing patient safety, in conjunction with each patient's medical history and medications. Comparative studies of analgesic medicines found little or no evidence favoring one agent over another in treating LBP. In a systematic review and network meta-analysis, Wewege et al. reported that the comparative effectiveness and safety of analgesic medicines for acute nonspecific LBP are uncertain [19]. Low or very low confidence was noted in evidence for reduced pain intensity after treatment with tolperisone (mean difference: −26.1 (95% CI −34.0—18.2)), aceclofenac plus tizanidine (−26.1 (−38.5—13.6)), pregabalin (−24.7 (−34.6—14.7)), and 14 other medicines compared with placebo. Low or very low confidence was noted for no difference between the effects of several of these medicines.

An analysis evaluating the efficacy and tolerability of *SMRs* reported high-level evidence ($n = 496$ in five randomized controlled trials (RCTs)) that this group of drugs provided clinically significant analgesic effects versus placebo (approximately 20 points on a 100-point scale) in patients with LBP [20]. The US guidelines also mentioned certain risks of using SMRs based on data abstracted from RCTs: increased risks related to dizziness, drowsiness, and sedation (RR: 1.50, 95% CI 1.14–1.98). These adverse effects are important to evaluate before administering to certain groups with LBP (e.g., older adults).

Steroids can reduce edema and inflammation of the nerves, which can achieve rapid analgesia within 24 h. Methylprednisolone may be administered orally over 5 days or by injection into the source of pain. Figure 10.2 represents an example of the algorithmic approach employed to manage those patients complaining of LBP.

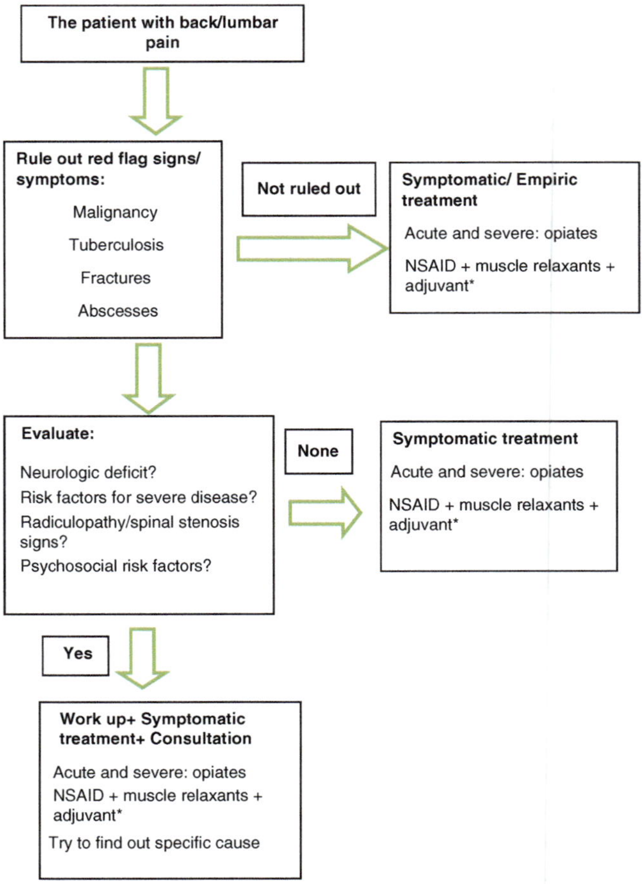

Fig. 10.2 An algorithmic approach scheme for a patient presenting with low back pain. *Adjuvant treatment may include antidepressants or other psychiatric treatments and algology approaches depending on the patient's clinical status

How Should a Patient with Radicular Pain or Neurogenic Claudication (NC) Be Approached?

Nonpharmacological Treatments

Guideline recommendations for the nonpharmacological treatment of radicular pain complicating LBP include staying active and participating in exercise programs [15, 21].

Initial treatment of NC is based on similar principles to radicular pain (algorithm).

In 2010, a Cochrane analysis including two RCTs ($n = 346$) reported little or no effect of such recommendations on pain [22]. However, it may also have other benefits, such as increasing activity, preventing deconditioning, and boosting mood. The US guidelines published low-quality data abstracted from RCTs, suggesting that exercise may have a minor impact on short-term pain improvement relative to conventional care [15].

Exercise may also benefit patients with NC, but evidence is limited: A Cochrane paper could find only one small RCT reporting that a three-week exercise program could benefit patients with limb pain in comparison to no treatment [23].

Mechanical traction is not recommended by either guideline: A Cochrane review reported low-quality findings from two trials (n = 79) that traction proved no more efficacious than placebo traction or no treatment in reducing pain in patients with radicular pain [24].

Pharmacological Treatments

Recent guidelines differ regarding the pharmacological management of radicular pain. Both recommend using opioids either as rescue medication [21] or when nonpharmacological options fail [15].

However, guidelines differ regarding medications for neuropathic pain. While the US guidelines do not advocate antiseizure medications (ASMs) for radicular pain, the UK guidelines have guided clinicians to recommendations regarding the pharmacological treatment of neuropathic pain in nonspecialist conditions, such as the use of some ASMs (e.g., pregabalin and gabapentin) in neuropathic pain [25] (see the gabapentinoid chapter). Gabapentin [26, 27], according to the findings of two small RCTs (n = 143), and pregabalin [28], according to the findings of one high-quality RCT (placebo-controlled; n = 209), are ineffective for cases of radicular acute LBP. There is limited evidence on effective pharmacological options for cases of NC: A 2013 Cochrane review found that there was very low-quality evidence from one trial (N = 152) that methylcobalamin (vitamin B12) plus conservative care improved walking distance in the intermediate- and long-term follow-up compared with conservative treatment alone. From single small trials, there was low-quality evidence for prostaglandins and very low-quality evidence for gabapentin or methylcobalamin that they improved walking distance [23].

Other Treatments

The UK guidelines have approved epidural corticosteroid injection to treat "acute or severe sciatica." On the other hand, a meta-analysis of 14 RCTs (n = 1316) reported that although these interventions led to immediate reductions in pain, these effects were small (approximately 6/100 points) [29]. The UK guidelines do not recommend steroid injections for the treatment of NC due to central spinal stenosis. However, they noted that surgery may be considered for patients with radicular pain. Surgery is indicated only if a lesion consistent with clinical findings is found on diagnostic imaging. A Cochrane review evaluating the efficacy of various surgical procedures versus nonsurgical interventions in adults with symptomatic lumbar spinal stenosis found insufficient evidence to draw conclusions (five RCTs; n = 643; low-quality evidence) [30].

A. *Nonpharmacological Measures Useful in the Treatment of LBP*
   - *TENS application in acute LBP:* It has been reported that there is moderate improvement in acute LBP with approximately 30 minutes of TENS application during emergency transportation to the hospital [31]. Although the data is limited, it is thought to be considered an important option.
   - Spinal manipulation (chiropractic treatment) in acute LBP.
   - Approaches such as exercise, massage, acupuncture, yoga, and cognitive–behavioral treatments are useful in chronic LBP [32].
   - *Cold compresses* are valuable in the first 2 or 3 days. It is recommended to apply an ice pack for 20 minutes. It should be repeated every 2 hours to suppress inflammation.
   - *Warm compresses* can become useful after 3 days. Application for 20 minutes every 2 hours is recommended. A hot bath can function similarly in some patients. It helps relieve both spasm and neural irritation by increasing blood circulation in the area. A Cochrane review analyzing nine studies involving 1100 patients showed that applying a warm blanket had a small positive effect on pain and disability [33].
   - *Elevating the legs* can also be relaxing by reducing the pressure on the nerve roots.
   - *Ultrasonography (USG)/phonophoresis:* Useful results can be obtained in experienced hands in specialized physical therapy clinics.
   - *Spinal cord stimulation:* Stimulation is exerted by placing electrodes in the adjacent epidural space in the spinal region thought to be the source of pain. Electrodes can be placed percutaneously or via a laminectomy. More favorable results were obtained in pain relief compared to conventional treatment [34].
   - *Exercise:* Although almost any type of exercise seems beneficial, the type of exercise that the patient has previously benefited from should take priority. Apart from specific activities such as Pilates, yoga, and tai chi, patients can also try easier and cheaper exercises, such as walking, jogging, swimming, and aerobics. Patients at high risk of chronic LBP should be included in supervised exercise programs.

- *Mobilization exercises* help sustain the range of motion of the joints. It reduces pain through stretching of adhesions, lengthening of shortened muscles, and stimulation of mechanoreceptors, which, in total, relieve muscle spasm. Since the intervertebral disc and synovial facet joints are nourished by movement, cartilage degeneration is prevented by mobilization [35].
- *Spinal manipulation:* Also known as chiropractic manipulation, it is useful in subacute and chronic LBP. It is the manipulation of a joint beyond its accustomed range of motion, without exceeding its anatomical range of motion, which should be supervised and performed by experts. A meta-analysis published in 2018 also confirmed its usefulness [36].

B. *Pharmacological Treatment:* As a general principle, polypharmacy should be avoided as much as possible. The more drugs used, the greater the assumed risks will be. The patient's metabolic status, organ failures, and age must be taken into account.

NSAIDs provide some success in these patients. Ketoprofen, dexketoprofen, ibuprofen, and diclofenac, and are among the most studied. IM administration should be carefully evaluated in terms of the benefit/risk ratio. Depending on the area where IM injection is applied, abscesses, hematomas, and and life-threatening complications, such as Fournier's gangrene, may occur. IV administration is always safer in EDs for most injectable drugs, where adequate precautions are taken against allergy and anaphylaxis.

There are quite a few options for oral use among NSAIDs. Since diclofenac sodium can cause water and salt overload, it may be harmful for middle-aged and older people. In addition, propionic acid derivatives such as flurbiprofen, stand out with their long-lasting efficacy and predictable effectiveness [37].

Corticosteroids are very effective in acute treatment, especially in patients with acute inflammation (e.g., acute exacerbation of OA), but caution should be exercised due to many adverse effects of chronic use, such as Cushing's syndrome, fluid-electrolyte disorders (e.g., hypernatremia and hypokalemia), and disorders of glucose metabolism. Withdrawal after prolonged treatment may result in adrenal insufficiency, which is manifested with hyponatremia, hypoglycemia, hypotension, and weakness. While systemic administration is considerable, intra-articular injections may also be indicated in selected patients with OA.

Opiates constitute the gold standard treatment for severe acute pain. Although IV administration in the ED takes priority, oral therapy will also be appropriate in selected patients. Morphine sulfate, the ancestor of this group, has been downgraded in daily practice due to its adverse effects, such as respiratory depression, hypotension, and histamine release. Semisynthetic derivatives such as fentanyl are at the forefront in practical application due to their safe and predictable effects [38].

Skeletal muscle relaxants (SMRs) consist of CNS depressants, central α2 agonists (tizanidine), and gamma-aminobutyric acid (GABA agonists (baclofen and benzodiazepines). CNS depressants include antihistamines (orphenadrine), chlorzoxazone, metaxalone, methocarbamol, sedatives such as carisoprodol, and tricyclic antidepressant (TCA)-like agents (cyclobenzaprine).

SMR agents can be classified into two genres, including *antispastic* (e.g., for cerebral palsy and multiple sclerosis (MS)) and *antispasmodic* agents (e.g., for primary MSP). Of note, antispastic medications act on the pathways in the spinal cord or skeletal muscle directly to improve hypertonicity and involuntary spasms. Antispasmodics alleviate muscle spasms through receptors in both the brain and the spinal cord.

Antispastic agents such as baclofen and dantrolene should not be used in MSP due to the scarcity of robust data to advocate their application [39, 40]. In these conditions, an antispasmodic agent may be more beneficial (Table 10.2).

Most SMR agents are proven to provide moderate analgesic benefit in acute LBP. Combination therapy is superior to monotherapy, especially when used with NSAIDs or acetaminophen [10, 41]. This effect of SMR is more pronounced in acute pain than in chronic pain. However, SMRs have pharmacological differences from each other; for example, carisoprodol (due to abuse potential) and dantrolene (due to hepatotoxicity) appear to be outdated and are rarely used in clinical practice. Chlorzoxazone is associated with nonfatal, less severe hepatotoxicity [10].

Cashin et al. have recently published a Cochrane review of seven Cochrane reviews (including 103 randomized trials) investigating systemic drug treatment in adult patients with nonspecific LBP until 2021 [42]. The authors found moderate-certainty evidence for a small between-group difference that favored SMRs in comparison with placebo for a higher rate of pain relief (RR: 0.58), improved functionality (RR: 0.55), and increased risk of adverse events (RR: 1.50). The authors concluded that for acute LBP, NSAIDs and SMRs may be associated with small benefits on pain; however, SMRs may cause unwanted effects. On the other hand, acetaminophen had no effect on pain or adverse outcomes. For safety, there was moderate-certainty evidence that SMRs may increase the risk of adverse events, such as CNS depressant activity with cyclobenzaprine; tachycardia, palpitations, urinary retention, and blurred vision with buprenorphine; and sedation and respiratory depression with diazepam. For

Table 10.2 Characteristics of skeletal muscle relaxants. Of note, FDA pregnancy categories of all are recorded as C, except for cyclobenzaprine (B) and diazepam (D) [81, 87, 95]

Agent	Dose	Side effects	Onset of effect	Duration of effect (hr)	Monthly cost	Drug interactions	Additional note
Cyclobenzaprine (antispasmodic + antispastic agent)	5–10 mg PO tid	Drowsiness, urinary retention, dizziness, xerostomia, constipation, and hypotension	1 h	12–24	120–140 (generic) 157 (brand)	AddE with TCAs, barbiturates, and alcohol, seizures with MAOIs and tramadol	The most commonly prescribed SMR; caution should be exercised against psychoactivity
Methocarbamol (antispasmodic agent)	500–1500 mg PO qid, up to 4000–4500 mg/day	Dizziness, blurred vision, and drowsiness	30 min	4–6	15–58 (generic) 176 (brand)	AddE with alcohol and other CNS depressants	Usability of PO, IV, and IM routes is an advantage. It is available as a combination with acetylsalicylic acid (ASA)
Chlorzoxazone (antispasmodic agent)	250–750 mg PO qid	N/V, headache, drowsiness, dizziness, idiosyncratic hepatocellular reaction	1 h	3–4	15–77 (generic) 180 (brand)	AddE with alcohol and other CNS depressants	It has an unclear value in treating muscular spasms and related conditions
Carisoprodol (antispasmodic agent)	250 mg PO qid	Drowsiness, N/V, dizziness, ataxia, withdrawal potential	30 min	4–6	$70–$100 (generic) $600 (brand)	AddE with alcohol and other CNS depressants	It has a quick onset of action after oral ingestion. Take caution with patients with reduced CYP2C19 activity
Metaxalone (antispasmodic agent)	400–800 mg PO qid	Dizziness, headache, drowsiness, leukopenia, nausea, rash, impaired liver function	1 h	4–6	$275	AddE with alcohol and other CNS depressants	Contraindicated in patients with severe renal or hepatic impairment
Diazepam (antispasmodic agent)	2–10 mg PO qid	Sedation, abuse potential, fatigue, hypotension, ataxia, respiratory depression	30 min (PO)	Variable, depending on the route and elimination kinetics	11–23 (generic) 184 (brand)	Effects are potentiated when combined with alcohol, phenothiazines, opioids, barbiturates, MAOIs	IM use should be avoided. Sedation and hypnotic and abuse potential are major drawbacks
Tizanidine (antispasmodic agent)	2–4–8 mg PO qid (max. 36 mg)	Drowsiness, dry mouth, dizziness, hypotension, increased spasm or muscle tone	2 weeks	Variable	330 (generic) 437 (brand)	AddE with alcohol and other CNS depressants; reduced clearance with oral contraceptives	Sedation is the main untoward effect. Coadministration with alcohol can increase the maximum concentration (Cmax) by 15%. Its clearance can be decreased by oral contraceptives
Orphenadrine (antispasmodic agent)	100 mg PO bid	Lightheadedness, anxiety, tachycardia, palpitations, urinary retention, and blurred vision	1 h (PO)	4–6	110–140 (generic) 162 (brand)	Propoxyphene (removed from the US market in 2011) caused confusion, anxiety, tremors, nausea, dry mouth	Contraindicated in patients with underlying neuromuscular junction defects; beware of anaphylaxis in parenteral use
Baclofen (antispastic agent)	5–20 mg PO tid	Drowsiness, slurred speech, hypotension, constipation, urinary retention	3–4 days (PO) 4–6 h (IT) 30 min (IT)	Variable		Antidepressants (short-term memory loss); AddE with imipramine	Be cautious for withdrawal reaction, rebound phenomenon, and withdrawal seizures that can be seen after sudden cessation

AddE Additive effects, *PO* Per oral, *IT* Intrathecal, *CNS* Central nervous system, *MAOIs* Monoaminooxidase inhibitors, *SMRs* Skeletal muscle relaxants, *N/V* Nausea/vomiting acute LBP, the authors reported at least moderate confidence about the effects of paracetamol, NSAIDs, and SMRs on short-term pain and function.

Benzodiazepines are effective agents due to their anxiolytic, peripheral muscle-relaxing effects, and amnestic properties, but they should only be used for a short time in severe cases to break the "pain–spasm vicious cycle" since sedation is not desired in active work life and also since addiction and abuse potentials are major drawbacks. Since they have no pain-relieving effect, they must be combined with analgesics.

Diazepam is one of the most commonly used benzodiazepines in patients with muscle spasms [43]. The agent is characterized by hypnotic, anxiolytic, antiepileptic, and antispasmodic effects. GABA-mediated spinal inhibition is postulated to be the essential action for diazepam in the treatment of muscle spasms. The main drawbacks are sedation and hypnotic and abuse potential, which preclude its use as a first-line SMR. However, the treatments should be tailored for each patient separately. For diazepam, 10–20 mg/day is recommended as an initial dose. The difficulty in predicting the effect mandates that these agents should be titrated individually.

Thiocolchicoside (not available in the Americas and most European countries) has anti-inflammatory and analgesic effects and does not cause sedation, acting on inhibitory neurotransmitters [44]. It has been used in some developing countries in the past decades because it is centrally acting and nonsedating. The side effect profile is similar to colchicine. Almost all of the positive studies were conducted in Russia, India, and Turkey, it has been reported that its use reduces the need for opiates [45]. In the same study, it was noted that patient satisfaction was higher in the group using SMRs. In a systematic review published in 2018, Csiba et al. reported that there is sufficient evidence to recommend thiocolchicoside as monotherapy or combination in patients with LBP [46].

Although concerns about teratogenicity have been rejected by a study from Turkey, more research is needed [47, 48]. Although the agent can be administered via PO and IV routes, there have been reports that topical application has a more positive effect. Other studies have shown that its combined use with the group of *arylpropionic acid derivatives* (profens) has a more positive analgesic effect compared to the use of NSAIDs alone [49]. It is used at a dose of 4–8 mg. There are various toxicity reports after use, ranging from skin findings to convulsions. Early and delayed types of contact hypersensitivity have been reported.

Carisoprodol is a centrally acting skeletal muscle relaxant that indirectly relaxes muscles through interneuronal activity in the descending reticular formation [50]. It is an FDA-approved drug indicated for the relief of discomfort associated with acute MSP. Its use has been limited to a maximum of 3 weeks because of the dependence potential [10]. Its primary metabolite, meprobamate, affects the GABA receptors similarly to benzodiazepines. This action is responsible not only for the agent's beneficial effects but also for its abuse potential [51]. The elimination half-life for carisoprodol is 1.7–2 hours, whereas the half-life for the meprobamate metabolite is around 10 hours. It is used in 250-mg and 350-mg tablets PO, up to three times a day [52].

Important contraindications include acute intermittent porphyria and hypersensitivity reactions to meprobamate, and sulfa allergy can develop due to the conversion of the agent to meprobamate. Patients with reduced CYP2C19 activity are poor metabolizers of carisoprodol, which leads to a significant increase in exposure to carisoprodol and a half-reduced exposure to meprobamate.

Carisoprodol has been sometimes combined with opioids and benzodiazepines [53]. The Drug Enforcement Agency announced carisoprodol as a Schedule IV medication due to its abuse potential, according to the Controlled Substances Act in 2011 [54]. Finally, many countries suspended marketing authorizations for carisoprodol in the past decades following reports that the benefits of the agent no longer outweigh its risks [50].

Cyclobenzaprine is one of the most widely used in the world as an SMR. It is also one of the most researched agents in this group [55]. Its superiority over benzodiazepines has been demonstrated in selected conditions, including muscle spasms, tenderness on palpation, limitation of motion, and limitation of daily living [56]. It is only used orally and has tricyclic antidepressant properties. It works by blocking pain stimulation in the periphery from being sent to the brain. It is postulated to have an effect on noradrenergic and serotonergic systems, spinal 5HT-2 receptors, and somatic motor nerve transmission via gamma and alpha neurons [57, 58].

In a 2001 study, Browning wrote that cyclobenzaprine was found to be significantly more effective than placebo in all five outcomes (local pain, muscle spasm, tenderness to palpation, range of motion, and activities of daily living), with its greatest effect being seen on the fourth day [59]. In a systematic review conducted by Chou in 2007, examining all the evidence to date, cyclobenzaprine was the only agent evaluated as an SMR in the United States in eligible and qualified studies [60]. However, a more recent systematic review reported that SMRs do not improve outcomes more than placebo in patients with acute LBP treated with an NSAID in the ED [61]. Age, sex, or baseline impairment does not impact these results. On the other hand, Childers et al. demonstrated that the agent's use in conjunction with ibuprofen did not provide additional benefits to cyclobenzaprine treatment alone [43].

Cyclobenzaprine is effective in acute neck and waist pain rather than chronic. Its most typical use is in the short-term treatment of fibromyalgia [62]. Although conflicting results have been noted, many studies have found it to be very effective on sleep patterns, pain, fatigue, and general well-being that are associated with fibromyalgia [7]. Although it is accepted that the combination of rest and other painkillers provides higher success, a few studies have also reported that combinations of cyclobenzaprine with acetaminophen or ibuprofen are not superior to a single treatment. It produces a sedative and anticholinergic effect. The recommended dose is 5–20 mg, and after absorption, it undergoes modification in the liver.

The most common toxic effects are lethargy, agitation, and tachycardia. Side effects are more common in the elderly, and confusion and cognitive findings may also occur at treatment doses in these fragile individuals. It is not considered suitable for long treatments durations. It is not recommended for those who have used monoaminooxidase (MAO) inhibitors (MAOIs) in the past 2 weeks, those who have heart block and other cardiac conduction disorders or hyperthyroidism, and those who have recently had a myocardial infarction.

Orphenadrine possesses antihistaminic and anticholinergic effects as a diphenhydramine derivative. The agent is marketed as tablets of 100 mg and in combination with acetylsalicylic acid and caffeine. Orphenadrine is also available in parenteral forms, although there have been reports of severe adverse reactions with parenteral use, including anaphylactoid reactions [10]. Its anticholinergic profile renders orphenadrine use contraindicated in patients with previously known disorders of the neuromuscular junction, such as myasthenia gravis and Lambert–Eaton syndrome [63].

Metaxalone is an SMR agent used to treat discomfort triggered by mechanical muscular pain. The FDA approved it in the 1980s, but there are scarce published data derived from placebo-controlled trials in the management of pain from musculoskeletal spasm [64]. Metaxalone has a favorable side effect profile, although fatal outcomes have also been reported [65, 66]. It necessitates serial liver function testing due to the side effect profile, including hepatotoxicity. As with most SMRs (carisoprodol, chlorzoxazone, cyclobenzaprine, metaxalone, methocarbamol, and orphenadrine), sedation and falls are among the most common side effects [67].

Methocarbamol is an antispasmodic agent used to treat involuntary spasms of striated muscles; therefore, it differs from antispastic drugs such as dantrolene and baclofen, which are primarily used in upper motor neuron disorders. It can be administered via PO, IV, and IM routes. Administration of the injectable form is associated with pain, sloughed skin, and thrombophlebitis [68]. Because the intravenous formulation of methocarbamol contains polyethylene glycol excipient, it is contraindicated in patients with renal impairment due to the risk of metabolic acidosis. The recommended daily dosage is around 4000–4500 mg, divided into three or four doses. While there are no recommended dose adjustments for patients with renal or hepatic impairment, methocarbamol should be used more cautiously in these groups since it undergoes hepatic metabolism and renal elimination. There are few controlled trials comparing methocarbamol with placebo in the management of spasm and resultant pain [69].

Baclofen is effective via the inhibition of monosynaptic and polysynaptic transmission of GABA in the spinal cord. As a GABA-b agonist, the agent triggers hyperpolarization, which decreases the secretion of excitatory neurotransmitters in the CNS and spinal nerves. Baclofen's main indication is spasticity associated with CNS diseases such as MS and some spinal cord lesions. Previous research has demonstrated equal or superior efficacy when compared to diazepam and dantrolene sodium [70]. When compared to benzodiazepines, it causes less hypnotic effect and may alleviate pain by the reduction of substance P release [10].

Baclofen can also be given intrathecally in patients with severe spasticity and for those who do not tolerate oral therapy [39]. Its daily therapeutic dosing range is up to 40–80 mg.

Caution should be exercised in older patients and patients with renal failure. It should be administered at low doses, titrated to effect for patients with stage 3 renal failure (estimated Glomerular Filtration Rate (eGFR) between 30 and 60 mL/min/1.73 m^2) to minimize the risk of neurotoxicity [71]. Since baclofen is linked with an enhanced risk of encephalopathy in patients on dialysis, its use is avoided in this group.

Bulk-flow removal in the cerebrospinal fluid following intrathecal administration of the agent was postulated [72]. After an intrathecal injection of baclofen, the mean elimination half-life is around 90 minutes [73].

Abrupt withdrawal of baclofen treatment is associated with a hypermetabolic state with hyperpyrexia, altered consciousness, muscular rigidity, and rebound spasticity [39]. Severe disease states may progress to rhabdomyolysis and multi-organ failure in vulnerable patients.

Chlorzoxazone acts centrally on muscles to relieve spasms, either through its sedative effects or other unknown mechanisms. Patients may take up to 2 grams daily, in three or four divided doses (Table 10.2). Chlorzoxazone is typically given for 1–4 weeks only and is indicated for therapy of LBP and muscle spasms, although its overall efficacy is considered only fair [74]. van Tulder et al. cited that this agent is viewed as less effective than its counterpart SMRs [41]. Except for possible additive effects when taken with alcohol or other CNS depressants, it is devoid of important drug–drug interactions [10]. In 1986, Powers reported that it can trigger an idiosyncratic hepatocellular reaction [75].

There is conflicting data derived from different studies employing the agent. A study on 393 patients with total knee or hip replacement showed no analgesic effects of postoperative chlorzoxazone administration (250 mg tid for the first

7 days) compared with placebo on acute or chronic postoperative pain in 12 months [76]. On the other hand, Patel et al. reported that fixed-dose combination (FDC) of chlorzoxazone and ibuprofen demonstrated superior efficacy than ibuprofen monotherapy in acute LBP [77].

Its idiosyncratic toxicity profile has been highlighted in medical literature, particularly for hepatotoxicity [78]. In summary, considering the probable lack of effectiveness and high toxicity, this agent's value in the treatment of muscle spasms is vague [79].

Tizanidine inhibits spinal and supraspinal motor neurons and exhibits an agonistic effect at the noradrenergic α2 receptors. Short-acting excitatory effects of tizanidine are linked to its similarity to the antihypertensive agent clonidine, and the cardiovascular properties of tizanidine are mild and transitory in relation to its activity as an SMR [80]. Sedation is known as the main untoward effect [81]. Tizanidine is an FDA-approved drug used in the treatment of increased muscle tone accompanied by spasticity due to CNS diseases, including multiple sclerosis or spinal cord damage. The agent is used in those patients with back pain or muscular spasms. It can be used as a sole agent or in combination with ibuprofen [68–70, 82–84]. The agent results in a greater extent of relief and fewer movement restrictions in comparison to placebo.

In another trial, a hundred and five patients with acute LBP were treated with tizanidine 4 mg PO tid plus ibuprofen 400 mg PO three times a day (tid) or ibuprofen 400 mg PO tid with placebo [83]. The tizanidine–ibuprofen combination was found to be more efficacious than ibuprofen in moderate or severe acute LBP (Table 10.2). The agent's clearance is reduced by up to half in patients with creatinine clearance lower than 25 mL/min. Therefore, it should be used with caution in those with renal failure. Another small-sized study was conducted on myofascial pain syndrome (MPS), which demonstrated that pressure threshold and sleep improved for all study periods ($P < 0.001$) [84]. Tizanidine was rated as good-to-excellent in relieving pain by 89% of subjects and 79% of physicians. No serious adverse events occurred.

Dantrolene is often used for malignant hyperthermia, a life-threatening medical emergency characterized by muscle spasms and rigidity, hyperthermia, tachypnea, tachycardia, acidosis, hyperkalemia, and rhabdomyolysis. It is known as a genetic disorder that induces a hypermetabolic reaction under exposure to a triggering agent, such as volatile inhaled anesthetics or depolarizing neuromuscular blockers [85].

The first-line treatment agent for an MH response is dantrolene. Dantrolene sodium has substantial efficacy in the treatment of MH and should be at hand in procedures under general anesthesia [86]. Further treatment includes managing complications, including hyperkalemia and malignant arrhythmias.

FDA-approved uses for dantrolene include muscle spasticity disorders, as seen with upper motor neuron disorders, including stroke, spinal cord injury, cerebral palsy, and multiple sclerosis [40]. It is the only FDA-approved oral, peripherally acting antispasmodic medication for these disorders. Dantrolene is also used for the treatment of neuroleptic malignant syndrome.

C. Direct Comparisons of SMR

A recent controlled study investigated the effects of fixed-dose combinations (FDCs) of NSAIDs and SMRs in adult patients with LBP [96]. The authors pointed out that dual FDC of etoricoxib (60 mg) and thiocolchicoside (4 mg) and triple FDC of chlorzoxazone (500 mg), diclofenac (50 mg), and acetaminophen (325 mg) were both effective and safe in the treatment of recent-onset LBP. On the other hand, significantly more subjects with very severe pain or functional disability showed improvement after 28 days when treated with dual FDC compared to triple FDC.

D. Chronic MSP

- *Chronic MSP*: It is defined as persistent or recurring pain or discomfort that occurs as part of a disease process that directly affects the musculoskeletal system and/or related soft tissues. Entities included in this approach are those characterized by persistent inflammatory conditions, such as rheumatoid arthritis, and structural changes affecting bones, joints, tendons, or muscles, such as osteoarthrosis.
- *Chronic Neck Pain (CNP):* It is among the main reasons for hospital presentations and physicians' office visits, affecting 10–24% of the population [83]. Although most acute neck pain disappears without significant intervention, some turn into chronic pain.

Management of Chronic MSP

Many pharmacological and nonpharmacological treatments and various noninvasive, surgical, and interventional procedures have been proposed in the management of chronic MSP.

Minor positive effects in chronic lumbar pain (CLP) have been associated with NSAIDs, tramadol (versus placebo) and other opioids, duloxetine, and benzodiazepines. Likewise, NSAIDS, opioids including tramadol, and duloxetine caused minor improvements in function.

In a systematic review published in 2007, Chou et al. reported that there was significant evidence that NSAIDs and SMRs were efficacious and beneficial in acute LBP, and TCAs were valuable in chronic LBP [32]. These agents are mostly useful in short-term treatment.

For chronic LBP, Cashin et al. have recently demonstrated low-certainty findings that NSAIDs and very low–to-high-certainty evidence that opioids can produce a minor impact on painful sensations [42]. As far as safety concerns, the study showed low-certainty evidence or no evidence of difference between NSAIDs and placebo for adverse events and low-certainty evidence that opioids may increase adverse effects.

Reports from major authorities [98] have addressed the biopsychosocial nature of this problem, highlighting the need for evidence-based strategies for the management of chronic pain, including nonpharmacological treatment.

Comorbid Conditions, the Elderly, Spasm, and Pain

Efficient and rational drug selection in the elderly necessitates evaluation of physiological reserves; organ failures; comorbid conditions; socioeconomic status, including self-care; drug interactions; and other factors. NSAIDs and acetaminophen have been found to be useful in arthritis and myofascial pain, gabapentinoids or duloxetine in neuropathic and radicular pain, SMRs for myofascial-based pain, and combination therapies for pain derived from mixed etiologies. Certain SMR agents have drawbacks in the elderly because of the risk of sedation and falls. These include commonly prescribed drugs such as carisoprodol, chlorzoxazone, cyclobenzaprine, metaxalone, methocarbamol, and orphenadrine. On the other hand, tizanidine, baclofen, and dantrolene may be beneficial in the treatment of spasms in those with neck and back pain [67]. Dose reductions may be needed considering organ failures. For example, tizanidine should be avoided in those with hepatic failure, and baclofen dosages must be cut down in those with renal failure.

Conclusions

Skeletal muscle spasms, mostly triggered by tissue injury such as sprains and strains or the irritation of spinal roots, represent various diseases and therapeutic areas. Although nonpharmacological treatments take priority, medications may be needed to improve functional and symptomatic outcomes related to spasms. NSAIDs and muscle relaxants are associated with a variety of potential adverse events that must be taken into account. NSAIDs are beneficial in providing relief in some patients, while SMRs, such as cyclobenzaprine, carisoprodol, chlorzoxazone, metaxalone, methocarbamol, orphenadrine, tizanidine, baclofen, and dantrolene, are more effective in some subgroups. Dose reductions and other measures may be needed to mitigate adverse outcomes in patients with organ failures. Treatments with each agent should be individualized and decided upon its pluses and minuses, after evaluating the patient's specific needs and drawbacks.

References

1. Mense S. Muscle pain: mechanisms and clinical significance. Dtsch Arztebl Int. 2008;105(12):214–9. https://doi.org/10.3238/artzebl.2008.0214.
2. Li Y, Delcher C, Reisfield GM, Wei YJ, Brown JD, Winterstein AG. Utilization patterns of skeletal muscle relaxants among commercially insured adults in the United States from 2006 to 2018. Pain Med. 2021;22(10):2153–61. https://doi.org/10.1093/pm/pnab088.
3. Papadopoulos EC, Khan SN. Piriformis syndrome and low back pain: a new classification and review of the literature. Orthop Clin North Am. 2004;35(1):65–71. https://doi.org/10.1016/S0030-5898(03)00105-6.
4. Weinstein JN, Tosteson TD, Lurie JD, et al. Surgical versus nonoperative treatment for lumbar spinal stenosis four-year results of the spine patient outcomes research trial. Spine (Phila Pa 1976). 2010;35(14):1329–38.
5. Iwasaki M, Akiyama M, Koyanagi I, Niiya Y, Ihara T, Houkin K. Double crush of L5 spinal nerve root due to L4/5 lateral recess stenosis and bony spur formation of lumbosacral transitional vertebra Pseudoarticulation: a case report and review. NMC Case Rep J. 2017;4(4):121–5.
6. Jahan F, Nanji K, Qidwai W, Qasim R. Fibromyalgia syndrome: an overview of pathophysiology, diagnosis and management. Oman Med J. 2012;27(3):192–5.
7. Häuser W, Bernardy K, Uçeyler N, Sommer C. Treatment of fibromyalgia syndrome with gabapentin and pregabalin--a meta-analysis of randomized controlled trials. Pain. 2009;145(1–2):69–81. https://doi.org/10.1016/j.pain.2009.05.014.
8. Soares A, Andriolo RB, Atallah AN, da Silva EM. Botulinum toxin for myofascial pain syndromes in adults. Cochrane Database Syst Rev. 2014;2014(7):CD007533. https://doi.org/10.1002/14651858.CD007533.pub3.
9. Leite FM, Atallah AN, El Dib R, et al. Cyclobenzaprine for the treatment of myofascial pain in adults. Cochrane Database Syst Rev. 2009;2009(3):CD006830. https://doi.org/10.1002/14651858.CD006830.pub3.
10. Jackson KC, Argoff CE, Dubin A. Skeletal muscle relaxants. In: Practical management of pain; 2014. p. 569–574.e1. https://doi.org/10.1016/b978-0-323-08340-9.00041-4.
11. Saga S, Stafne SN, Dons V, Bratlie I, Spetalen S, Hagemann CT. Amsterdam complex pelvic pain symptom scale with subscales: based on a Norwegian translation, psychometric assessment and modification of the Amsterdam hyperactive pelvic floor scale. Acta Obstet Gynecol Scand. 2023;102(10):1409–23. https://doi.org/10.1111/aogs.14665.
12. Messelink B, Benson TB, Berghmans B, et al. Standardization of terminology of pelvic floor muscle function and dysfunction: report from the pelvic floor clinical assessment Group of the International Continence Society. Neurourol Urodynam. 2005;24:374–80.
13. Chou R, Atlas SJ, Stanos SP, et al. Nonsurgical interventional therapies for low back pain: a review of the evidence for an American Pain Society clinical practice guideline. Spine. 2009;34(10):1078–93.
14. Chou R, Baisden J, Carragee EJ, et al. Surgery for low back pain: a review of the evidence for an American pain society clinical practice guideline. Spine (Phila Pa 1976). 2009;34(10):1094–109.
15. Qaseem A, Wilt TJ, McLean RM, Forciea MA, Clinical Guidelines Committee of the American College of Physicians. Noninvasive treatments for acute, subacute, and chronic low

back pain: a clinical practice guideline from the American College of Physicians. Ann Intern Med. 2017;166(7):514–30. https://doi.org/10.7326/M16-2367.
16. Traeger A, Buchbinder R, Harris I, Maher C. Diagnosis an management of low-back pain in primary care. Can Med Assoc J. 2017;189:E1386–95.
17. van der Gaag WH, Roelofs PD, Enthoven WT, van Tulder MW, Koes BW. Non-steroidal anti-inflammatory drugs for acute low back pain. Cochrane Database Syst Rev. 2020;4(4):CD013581. https://doi.org/10.1002/14651858.CD013581.
18. Brune K, Patrignani P. New insights into the use of currently available non-steroidal anti-inflammatory drugs. J Pain Res. 2015;8:105–18. https://doi.org/10.2147/JPR.S75160.
19. Wewege MA, Bagg MK, Jones MD, et al. Comparative effectiveness and safety of analgesic medicines for adults with acute non-specific low back pain: systematic review and network meta-analysis. BMJ. 2023;380:e072962. https://doi.org/10.1136/bmj-2022-072962.
20. Abdel Shaheed C, Maher CG, Williams KA, et al. Efficacy and tolerability of muscle relaxants for low back pain: systematic review and meta-analysis. Eur J Pain. 2017;21:228–37.
21. National Institute for Health and Care Excellence (NICE). Low back pain and sciatica in over 16s: assessment and management. NICE guideline [NG59]. London (UK): NICE; 2016.
22. Dahm KT, Brurberg KG, Jamtvedt G, et al. Advice to rest in bed versus advice to stay active for acute low-back pain and sciatica. Cochrane Database Syst Rev. 2010;(6):CD007612.
23. Ammendolia C, Stuber KJ, Rok E, et al. Nonoperative treatment for lumbar spinal stenosis with neurogenic claudication. Cochrane Database Syst Rev. 2013;(8):CD010712.
24. Wegner I, Widyahening IS, van Tulder MW, et al. Traction for low_ back pain with or without sciatica. Cochrane Database Syst Rev. 2013;8:CD003010.
25. National Institue for Health and Care Excellence (NICE). Neuropathic pain in adults: pharmacological management in nonspeciailist settings. Clinical quideline (CG96). London (UK): NICE; 2010.
26. Yildirim K, Deniz O, Gureser G, et al. Gabapentin monotherapy in patients with chronic radiculopathy: the efficacy and impact on life quality. J Back Musculoskelet Rehabil. 2009;22:17–20.
27. Atkinson JH, Slater MA, Capparelli EV, et al. A randomized controlled trial of gabapentin for chronic low back pain with and without a radiating component. Pain. 2016;157:1499–507.
28. Mathieson S, Maher CG, McLachlan AJ, et al. Trial of pregabalin for acute and chronic sciatica. N Engl J Med. 2017;376:1111–20.
29. Pinto RZ, Maher CG, Ferreira ML, et al. Epidural corticosteroid injections in the management of sciatica: a systematic review and meta-analysis. Ann Intern Med. 2012;157:865–77.
30. Zaina F, Tomkins-Lane C, Carragee E, et al. Surgical versus nonsurgical treatment for lumbar spinal stenosis. Spine. 2016;41:E857–68.
31. Binny J, Joshua Wong NL, Garga S, et al. Transcutaneous electric nerve stimulation (TENS) for acute low back pain: systematic review. Scand J Pain. 2019;19(2):225–33. https://doi.org/10.1515/sjpain-2018-0124.
32. Chou R, Huffman LH, American Pain S, et al. Medications for acute and chronic low back pain: a review of the evidence for an American Pain Society/American College of Physicians clinical practice guideline. Ann Intern Med. 2007;147(7):505–14.
33. French SD, Cameron M, Walker BF, Reggars JW, Esterman AJ. A Cochrane review of superficial heat or cold for low back pain. Spine (Phila Pa 1976). 2006;31(9):998–1006. https://doi.org/10.1097/01.brs.0000214881.10814.64.
34. Kumar A, Felderhof C, Eljamel MS. Spinal cord stimulation for the treatment of refractory unilateral limb pain syndromes. Stereotact Funct Neurosurg. 2003;81(1–4):70–4.
35. Manniche C, Asmussen K, Lauritsen B, et al. Intensive dynamic back exercises with or without hyperextension in chronic back pain after surgery for lumbar disc protrusion. A clinical trial. Spine (Phila Pa 1976). 1993;18(5):560–7.
36. Skelly AC, Chou R, Dettori JR, et al. Noninvasive nonpharmacological treatment for chronic pain: a systematic review update [Internet]. Rockville (MD): Agency for Healthcare Research and Quality (US); 2020. Report No.: 20-EHC009
37. Hanna M, Moon JY. A review of dexketoprofen trometamol in acute pain. Curr Med Res Opin. 2019;35(2):189–202. https://doi.org/10.1080/03007995.2018.1457016. Epub 2018 Apr 24
38. Derry S, Stannard C, Cole P, Wiffen PJ, Knaggs R, Aldington D, Moore RA. Fentanyl for neuropathic pain in adults. Cochrane Database Syst Rev. 2016;10(10):CD011605. https://doi.org/10.1002/14651858.CD011605.pub2.
39. Ghanavatian S, Derian A. Baclofen. [Updated 2024 Aug 11]. In: StatPearls [Internet]. Treasure Island (FL): StatPearls Publishing; 2025. Available from: https://www.ncbi.nlm.nih.gov/books/NBK526037/.
40. Ratto D, Joyner RW. Dantrolene. [Updated 2023 Apr 3]. In: StatPearls [Internet]. Treasure Island (FL): StatPearls Publishing; 2025. Available from: https://www.ncbi.nlm.nih.gov/books/NBK535398/.
41. van Tulder MW, Touray T, Furlan AD, et al. Muscle relaxants for non-specific low back pain. Cochrane Database Syst Rev. 2003;3:CD004252.
42. Cashin AG, Wand BM, O'Connell NE, et al. Pharmacological treatments for low back pain in adults: an overview of Cochrane reviews. Cochrane Database Syst Rev. 2023;4(4):CD013815. https://doi.org/10.1002/14651858.CD013815.pub2.
43. Childers MK, Borenstein D, Brown RL, Gershon S, Hale ME, Petri M, et al. Low-dose cyclobenzaprine versus combination therapy with ibuprofen for acute neck or back pain with muscle spasm: a randomized trial. Curr Med Res Opin. 2005;21(9):1485–93.
44. Priyanka S, Manju J, Girish K. A comparative study of efficacy and tolerability of fixed-dose combination of etoricoxib and thiocolchicoside versus thiocolchicoside alone in patients with painful muscle spasms. Biomed Pharmacol J. 2022;15:353–61. https://doi.org/10.13005/bpj/2374.
45. Bourazani M, Papageorgiou E, Zarkadas G, et al. The role of muscle relaxants—spasmolytic (Thiocochlicoside) in postoperative pain management after mastectomy and breast reconstruction. Asian Pac J Cancer Prev. 2019;20(3):743–9.
46. Csiba L, Zhussupova AS, Likhachev SA, Parfenov VA, Churyukanov MV, Guekht AB. Sistematicheskiĭ obzor po primeneniiu miorelaksantov pri boli v nizhneĭ chasti spiny [A systematic review of using myorelaxants in treatment of low back pain]. Zh Nevrol Psikhiatr Im S S Korsakova. 2018;118(12):100–13. Russian. https://doi.org/10.17116/jnevro2018118121100.
47. Kaplan YC, Keskin-Arslan E, Küçüksolak G, Akyol F, Karadas B, Görgel SN, Kaya-Temiz T. Pregnancy outcomes after maternal use of thiocolchicoside: a case series. Reprod Toxicol. 2018;76:103–8. https://doi.org/10.1016/j.reprotox.2018.01.003. Epub 2018 Jan 31
48. Ozturk Z, Olmez E, Gurpinar T, Vural K. Pregnancy outcomes following the use of thiocolchicoside. Reprod Toxicol. 2016;60:129–32. https://doi.org/10.1016/j.reprotox.2016.02.004. Epub 2016 Feb 12
49. Cigerim L, Kaplan V. Evaluation of the analgesic efficacies of Dexketoprofen Trometamol and Dexketoprofen Trometamol + Thiocolchicoside combinations in the impacted third molar surgery: randomised clinical trial. Med Oral Patol Oral Cir Bucal. 2019;24(1):e114–22.
50. Conermann T, Christian D. Carisoprodol. [Updated 2024 May 2]. In: StatPearls [Internet]. Treasure Island (FL): StatPearls Publishing; 2025. Available from: https://www.ncbi.nlm.nih.gov/books/NBK553077/.
51. Gonzalez LA, Gatch MB, Forster MJ, Dillon GH. Abuse potential of Soma: the GABA(A) receptor as a target. Mol Cell Pharmacol. 2009;1(4):180–6.

52. Berger FM, Kletzkin M, Ludwig BJ, Margolin S. The history, chemistry, and pharmacology of carisoprodol. Ann N Y Acad Sci. 1960;86:90–107.
53. Horsfall JT, Sprague JE. The pharmacology and toxicology of the 'holy trinity'. Basic Clin Pharmacol Toxicol. 2017;120(2):115–9.
54. Sun C, Hollenbach KA, Cantrell FL. Trends in carisoprodol abuse and misuse after regulatory scheduling: a retrospective review of California poison control calls from 2008 to 2015. Clin Toxicol (Phila). 2018;56(7):653–5. https://doi.org/10.1080/15563650.2017.1414950. Epub 2017 Dec 12
55. Braschi E, Garrison S, Allan GM. Cyclobenzaprine for acute back pain. Can Fam Physician. 2015;61(12):1074.
56. Chou R, Peterson K, Helfand M. Comparative efficacy and safety of skeletal muscle relaxants for spasticity and musculoskeletal conditions: a systematic review. J Pain Symptom Manag. 2004;28(2):140–75.
57. Ding X-Q. Drugs affecting nicotinic receptors. In: Dowd FJ, Johnson BS, Mariotti AJ, editors. Pharmacology and therapeutics for dentistry. Amsterdam: Elsevier; 2017. p. 98–109. https://doi.org/10.1016/B978-0-323-39307-2.00007-2.
58. Herrero Babiloni A, Beetz G, Bruneau A, Martel MO, Cistulli PA, Nixdorf DR, Conway JM, Lavigne GJ. Multitargeting the sleep-pain interaction with pharmacological approaches: a narrative review with suggestions on new avenues of investigation. Sleep Med Rev. 2021;59:101459. https://doi.org/10.1016/j.smrv.2021.101459. Epub 2021 Jan 28
59. Browning R, Jackson JL, O'Malley PG. Cyclobenzaprine and back pain: a meta-analysis. Arch Intern Med. 2001;161(13):1613–20.
60. Chou R, Qaseem A, Snow V, et al. Diagnosis and treatment of low back pain: a joint clinical practice guideline from the American College of Physicians and the American Pain Society. Ann Intern Med. 2007;147(7):478–91.
61. Abril L, Zamora C, Cordero M, Williams AR, Friedman BW. The relative efficacy of seven skeletal muscle relaxants. An analysis of data from randomized studies. J Emerg Med. 2022;62(4):455–61. https://doi.org/10.1016/j.jemermed.2021.09.025. Epub 2022 Jan 20
62. Smith B, Peterson K, Fu R, McDonagh M, Thakurta S. Drug class review: drugs for fibromyalgia: final original report [Internet]. Portland (OR): Oregon Health & Science University; 2011.
63. Gareri P, De Fazio P, Cotroneo A, et al. Anticholinergic drug-induced delirium in an elderly Alzheimer's dementia patient. Arch Gerontol Geriatr. 2007;44(suppl 1):199–206.
64. Cherkin DC, Wheeler KJ, Barlow W, et al. Medication use for low back pain in primary care. Spine. 1998;23:607–14.
65. Dent RW, Ervin DK. A study of metaxalone (Skelaxin) vs. placebo in acute musculoskeletal disorders: a cooperative study. Curr Ther Res Clin Exp. 1975;18:433–40.
66. Moore KA, Levine B, Fowler D. A fatality involving metaxalone. Forens Sci Int. 2005;149:49–51.
67. Fu JL, Perloff MD. Pharmacotherapy for spine-related pain in older adults. Drugs Aging. 2022;39(7):523–50. https://doi.org/10.1007/s40266-022-00946-x.
68. Sibrack J, Patel P, Hammer R. Methocarbamol. [Updated 2024 Sep 10]. In: StatPearls [Internet]. Treasure Island (FL): StatPearls Publishing; 2025. Available from: https://www.ncbi.nlm.nih.gov/books/NBK565868/.
69. Tisdale SA, Ervin DK. A controlled study of methocarbamol (Robaxin) in acute painful musculoskeletal conditions. Curr Ther Res Clin Exp. 1975;17:525–30.
70. Waldman HJ. Centrally acting skeletal muscle relaxants and associated drugs. J Pain Symptom Manag. 1994;9(7):434–41. https://doi.org/10.1016/0885-3924(94)90199-6.
71. Vlavonou R, Perreault MM, Barrière O, et al. Pharmacokinetic characterization of baclofen in patients with chronic kidney disease: dose adjustment recommendations. J Clin Pharmacol. 2014;54(5):584–92.
72. Simon MJ, Iliff JJ. Regulation of cerebrospinal fluid (CSF) flow in neurodegenerative, neurovascular and neuroinflammatory disease. Biochim Biophys Acta. 2016;1862(3):442–51.
73. El-Husseini A, Sabucedo A, Lamarche J, Courville C, Peguero A. Baclofen toxicity in patients with advanced nephropathy: proposal for new labeling. Am J Nephrol. 2011;34(6):491–5.
74. LiverTox: Clinical and Research Information on Drug-Induced Liver Injury [Internet]. Bethesda (MD): National Institute of Diabetes and Digestive and Kidney Diseases; 2012. Chlorzoxazone. 2017 Jan 30. PMID: 31643467.
75. Powers BJ, Cattau EL Jr, Zimmerman HJ. Chlorzoxazone hepatotoxic reactions. An analysis of 21 identified or presumed cases. Arch Intern Med. 1986;146(6):1183–6. https://doi.org/10.1001/archinte.146.6.1183.
76. Skrejborg P, Petersen KK, Beck J, Ulrich M, et al. Investigating the effect of perioperative chlorzoxazone on acute postoperative pain after total hip and knee replacement surgery. Clin J Pain. 2020;36(5):352–8. https://doi.org/10.1097/AJP.0000000000000805.
77. Patel HD, Uppin RB, Naidu AR, Rao YR, Khandarkar S, Garg A. Efficacy and safety of combination of NSAIDs and muscle relaxants in the management of acute low back pain. Pain Ther. 2019;8(1):121–32. https://doi.org/10.1007/s40122-019-0112-6.
78. Sun C, Zhang M, Guan C, Li W, Peng Y, Zheng J. In vitro and in vivo metabolic activation and hepatotoxicity of chlorzoxazone mediated by CYP3A. Arch Toxicol. 2024;98(4):1095–110. https://doi.org/10.1007/s00204-023-03674-2. Epub 2024 Feb 18
79. Jackson KC. Low back pain pharmacotherapy. Drugs Today (Barc). 2004;40:765–72.
80. Coward DM. Tizanidine: neuropharmacology and mechanism of action. Neurology. 1994;44(suppl 9):S6–S10.
81. Smith HS, Barton AE. Tizanidine in the management of spasticity and musculoskeletal complaints in the palliative care population. Am J Hospice Palliat Care. 2000;17:50–8.
82. Berry H, Hutchinson DR. A multicentre placebo-controlled study in general practice to evaluate the efficacy and safety of tizanidine in acute low back pain. J Int Med Res. 1988;16:75–82.
83. Berry H, Hutchinson DR. Tizanidine and ibuprofen in acute low back pain: results of a double-blind multicentre study in general practice. J Int Med Res. 1988;16:83–91.
84. Malanga GA, Gwynn MW, Smith R, et al. Tizanidine is effective in the treatment of myofascial pain syndrome. Pain Physician. 2002;5:422–32.
85. Gregory H, Weant KA. Pathophysiology and treatment of malignant hyperthermia. Adv Emerg Nurs J. 2021;43(2):102–10. https://doi.org/10.1097/TME.0000000000000344.
86. Kaur H, Katyal N, Yelam A, Kumar K, Srivastava H, Govindarajan R. Malignant hyperthermia. Mo Med. 2019;116(2):154–9.
87. Carisoprodol (carisoprodol) tablet [package insert]. Philadelphia, PA: Mutual Pharmaceutical Company, Inc.; 2006. http://dailymed.nlm.nih.gov/dailymed/fdaDrugXsl.cfm?id=2774&type=display. Accessed January 14, 2025.
88. Chlorzoxazone (chlorzoxazone) tablet [package insert]. Sellersville, PA: Teva Pharmaceuticals USA; 2003. http://dailymed.nlm.nih.gov/dailymed/fdaDrugXsl.cfm?id=2402&type=display. Accessed January 14, 2025.
89. Cyclobenzaprine hydrochloride (cyclobenzaprine hydrochloride) tablet [package insert]. Corona, CA: Watson Laboratories, Inc.; 2005. http://dailymed.nlm.nih.gov/dailymed/fdaDrugXsl.cfm?id=2794&type=display. Accessed January 14, 2025.
90. Diazepam (diazepam) tablet [package insert]. Miami, FL: IVAX Pharmaceuticals, Inc.; 2004. http://dailymed.nlm.nih.gov/

dailymed/fdaDrugXsl.cfm?id=3430&type=display. Accessed January 14, 2025.
91. Skelaxin (metaxalone) [package insert]. Briston, TN: King Pharmaceuticals; 2007. http://dailymed.nlm.nih.gov/dailymed/drugInfo.cfm?id=4505. Accessed January 14, 2025.
92. Methocarbamol (methocarbamol) tablet [package insert]. Eatontown, NJ: West-ward Pharmaceutical Corp.; 2003. http://dailymed.nlm.nih.gov/dailymed/fdaDrugXsl.cfm?id=2833&type=display. January 14, 2025.
93. Orphenadrine citrate extended-release (orphenadrine citrate) tablet [package insert]. Princeton, NJ: Sandoz, Inc.; 2006. http://dailymed.nlm.nih.gov/dailymed/drugInfo.cfm?id=3665. Accessed January 14, 2025.
94. Tizanidine hydrochloride (tizanidine hydrochloride) tablet [package insert]. Pomona, NY: Barr Laboratories.; 2006. http://dailymed.nlm.nih.gov/dailymed/fdaDrugXsl.cfm?id=1147&type=display. Accessed January 14, 2025.
95. United States Food and Drug Administration. 2007 safety alerts for drugs, biologics, medical devices, and dietary supplements. Zanaflex (tizanidine hydrochloride) tablets and capsules. http://www.fda.gov/medwatch/safety/2007/safety07.htm#Zanaflex. Accessed January 14, 2025.
96. Karmakar A, Arora S, Singal R, et al. The efficacy and safety of a combination of thiocolchicoside and etoricoxib in low back pain (ESCoTEL): a randomized active-controlled trial. Cureus. 2023;15(10):e47621. https://doi.org/10.7759/cureus.47621.
97. Chow RT, Johnson MI, Lopes-Martins RA, Bjordal JM. Efficacy of low-level laser therapy in the management of neck pain: a systematic review and meta-analysis of randomised placebo or active-treatment controlled trials. Lancet. 2009;374(9705):1897–908.
98. Institute of Medicine. Relieving Pain in America: a blueprint for transforming prevention, care, education, and research. Washington, DC: The National Academies Press; 2011.

Anticonvulsants

11

Julie A. Murphy, Loulwa Maktabi, and Coral Matus

Keywords and Definitions

Anticonvulsants:	Also known as antiepileptic drugs, anti-seizure drugs, or anti-seizure medications, they are a diverse group of pharmacological agents used in the treatment of epileptic seizures. Anticonvulsants are also used in the treatment of neuropathic pain.
Neuropathic pain:	It arises from dysfunction or damage to the central or peripheral nervous system and may manifest as abnormal sensations, such as burning, tingling, or shooting pain.
Nociceptive pain:	It is well-localized in response to potentially harmful stimuli and serves as a normal protective mechanism

Abbreviations

CDC	Centers for Disease Control and Prevention
CINP	Chemotherapy-induced neuropathic pain
CLBP	Chronic low back pain
DPN	Diabetic peripheral neuropathy
FDA	Food and Drug Administration
HZV	Herpes zoster virus
NCP	Neuropathic cancer pain
NSAIDs	Nonsteroidal anti-inflammatory drugs
PHN	Postherpetic neuralgia
TGN	Trigeminal neuralgia
VPA	Valproic acid
VAS	Visual analog scale

J. A. Murphy (✉) · L. Maktabi
The University of Toledo College of Pharmacy and Pharmaceutical Sciences, Toledo, OH, USA
e-mail: Julie.murphy@utoledo.edu

C. Matus
The University of Toledo College of Medicine and Life Sciences, Toledo, OH, USA

J. P. Reinert et al. (eds.), *Adjunctive Analgesic Strategies for the Bedside Clinician and Beyond*,
https://doi.org/10.1007/978-3-032-21675-5_11

Background/Introduction

After the publication of the Guideline for Prescribing Opioids for Chronic Pain by the Centers for Disease Control and Prevention (CDC) in 2016, the use of non-opioid pain medications increased by 3% in the first year and 9.7% by the third year after release [1, 2]. By taking advantage of multimodal therapy to improve analgesia, the synergistic action between agents can be utilized to target different mechanisms in the pain perception–modulation system. While gabapentin and pregabalin have been studied extensively and are approved for the treatment of pain in the United States [3], other anticonvulsants have gained interest in the realm of pain management due to their various mechanisms of action in modulating neuronal excitability. Anticonvulsants have been shown to act synergistically with more traditional agents such as nonsteroidal anti-inflammatory drugs (NSAIDs) and opioid analgesics to enhance pain relief. Used in tandem, this can reduce opioid utilization and decrease the risk of opioid-related adverse effects, such as constipation, addiction, tolerance, and respiratory depression.

Pharmacology, Pharmacokinetics, and Pharmacodynamics

The mechanisms of action of anticonvulsants may give some insight regarding the underlying pathophysiology of neuropathic pain and pain due to migraine headache. Safety and adverse effect profiles may limit the use of some medications in this class. Ongoing studies will more clearly define the efficacy of these agents in managing various types of pain.

Figure 11.1 displays the various mechanisms of the anticonvulsants that have been studied for the treatment of pain. Table 11.1 provides a summary of the pharmacology, pharmacokinetics, and pharmacodynamics of those agents.

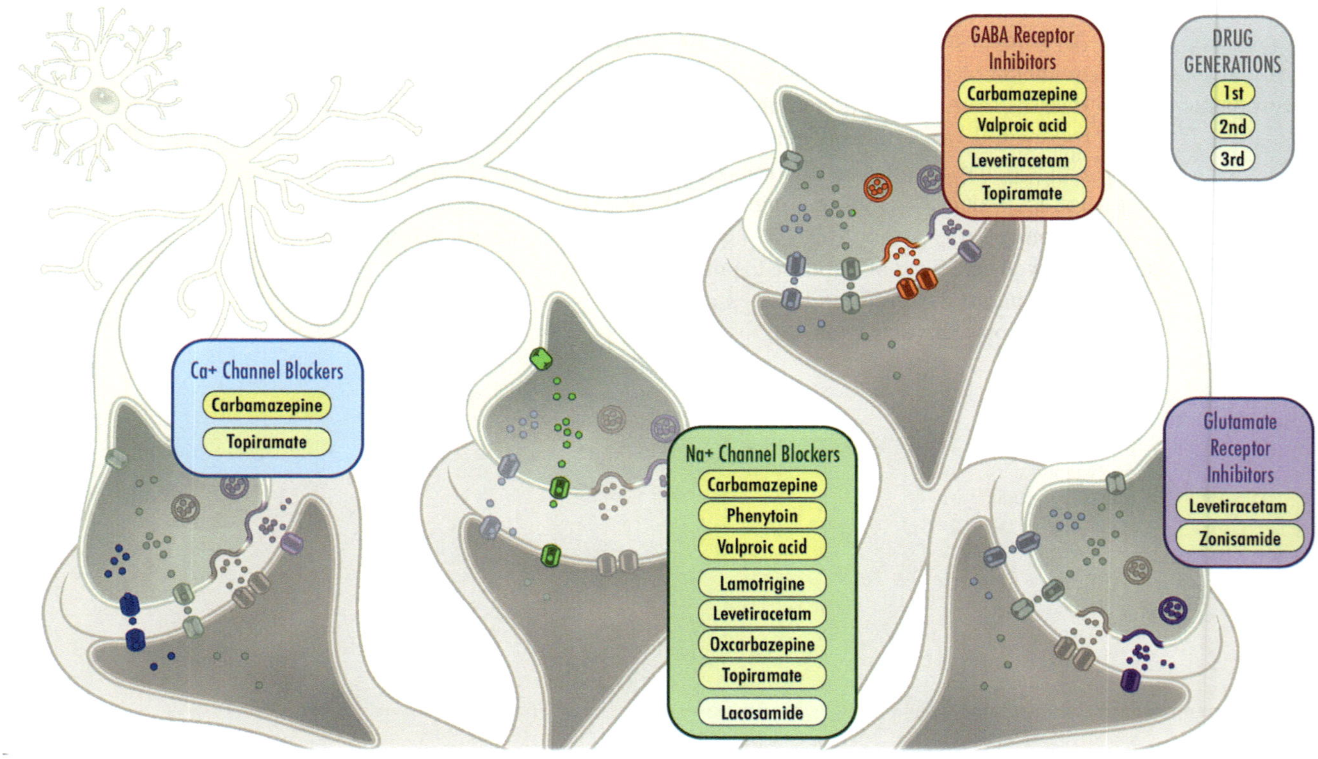

Fig. 11.1 Mechanisms of anticonvulsants used for the treatment of pain

Table 11.1 Summary of the pharmacology, pharmacokinetics, and pharmacodynamics of anticonvulsants

Drug	Pharmacology/ pharmacodynamics	Pharmacokinetics Absorption	Distribution	Metabolism	Excretion
First-generation anticonvulsants					
Carbamazepine [4–7]	Inhibits voltage-sensitive sodium channels, leading to reduction of neuronal signal propagation; potentiates alpha-1, beta-2, and gamma-2 subunits of gamma-aminobutyric acid (GABA) receptors; demonstrates an anti-inflammatory effect, as indicated by decreased plasma extravasation	Absorption from the gastrointestinal tract is slow. Time to peak serum concentrations is unpredictable due to its autoinduction process. Range is 1.5–26 hours	0.59–2 L/kg; 75–90% bound to plasma proteins	Induces liver enzymes to increase metabolism and shorten half-life over time (autoinduction); autoinduction is usually complete 3–5 weeks after the start of a fixed carbamazepine regimen; metabolized by cytochrome P450 3A4 to active epoxide metabolite; epoxide metabolite is metabolized by epoxide hydrolase to the transdiol metabolite	Primarily in the urine (~72%). Elimination half-life is variable due to autoinduction. Initially 25–65 hours but 12–17 hours after multiple doses. The elimination half-life for epoxide metabolite is ~34 hours
Phenytoin [8]	Blocks voltage-dependent sodium channels, leading to a reduction of neuronal signal propagation	Slow and variable, depending on dosage formulation. Peak plasma concentrations occur within 4–12 hours	0.52–0.78 L/kg; ~90% bound to plasma proteins	Follows dose-dependent (Michaelis–Menten) pharmacokinetics. Metabolism is best described in terms of Vmax (metabolic capacity) and Km (a constant equal to the concentration at which the rate of metabolism is half of Vmax)	Primarily in the bile as inactive metabolites. Half-life is dependent upon serum concentration (half-life increases with increasing phenytoin concentrations). Range is 7–29 hours
Valproic acid (VPA) and derivatives [9, 10]	Increases brain gamma-aminobutyric acid (GABA) by inhibiting GABA transaminase; blocks voltage-dependent sodium channels, leading to a reduction of neuronal signal propagation	Absorption rate varies with the formulation administered; this fluctuation is of minor clinical importance. Peak plasma concentrations occur between 2 and 17 hours	Total valproate: 11 L/1.73 m^2; 80–90% bound to plasma proteins	Extensively hepatic via glucuronide conjugation (30–50%) and 40% via mitochondrial beta-oxidation	Urine (30–50% as glucuronide conjugate, <3% unchanged). Elimination half-life ~9–16 hours
Second-generation anticonvulsants					
Lamotrigine [11, 12]	Suggested that it inhibits voltage-sensitive sodium channels and modulates presynaptic neurotransmitter release of glutamate and aspartate	Rapidly and completely absorbed with negligible first-pass metabolism. Peak plasma concentrations occur within 1.4–4.8 hours. Bioavailability is not affected by food.	0.9–1.3 L/kg; ~55% bound to plasma proteins	Hepatic and renal, with >75% metabolized via glucuronidation. Autoinduction may occur	Primarily in the urine (94%; ~90% as glucuronide conjugates and ~10% unchanged). Elimination half-life ~25–33 hours
Levetiracetam [13]	Opposes the activity of negative modulators of GABA- and glycine-gated currents and partially inhibits N-type calcium currents in neuronal cells	Rapidly absorbed with peak plasma concentrations in ~1 hour. Food decreases C_{max} by 20% and delays T_{max} by 1.5 hours	0.5–0.7 L/kg; <10% bound to plasma proteins	Not extensively metabolized. The major pathway is enzymatic hydrolysis of the acetamide group	Primarily unchanged in the urine (~66% of the administered dose). Elimination half-life ~7 hours

(continued)

Table 11.1 (continued)

Drug	Pharmacology/ pharmacodynamics	Pharmacokinetics Absorption	Distribution	Metabolism	Excretion
Oxcarbazepine [14]	Oxcarbazepine and its active metabolite, 10-monohydroxy (MHD), block voltage-sensitive sodium channels, leading to neuronal stabilization; it is a structural derivative of carbamazepine	Completely absorbed. Median T_{max} is 4.5 hours with tablets and 6 hours with suspension. Food has no effect on the rate or extent of absorption	MHD: 49 L; 40% bound to plasma proteins	Rapidly reduced by cytosolic enzymes in the liver to its MHD metabolite. MHD is further metabolized by conjugation with glucuronic acid	Primarily unchanged in the urine (~95% of the dose). Oxcarbazepine elimination half-life is ~2 hours, and the half-life of MHD is 9 hours
Topiramate [15]	Blocks voltage-dependent sodium channels, augments the activity of the neurotransmitter gamma-aminobutyrate at some subtypes of the GABA-A receptor, antagonizes the AMPA/kainate subtype of the glutamate receptor, and inhibits the carbonic anhydrase enzyme, particularly isozymes II and IV	Rapid, with peak concentrations occurring at ~2 hours following a dose. Bioavailability is not affected by food	0.6–0.8 L/kg; 15–41% bound to plasma proteins	Not extensively metabolized. Metabolites are formed via hydroxylation, hydrolysis, and glucuronidation. There is evidence of renal tubular reabsorption of topiramate	Primarily unchanged in the urine (~70% of an administered dose). Elimination half-life is ~21 hours
Zonisamide [16, 17]	Blocks voltage-gated sodium and T-type calcium channels, leading to neuronal stabilization; facilitates serotonergic and dopaminergic neurotransmission	Peak plasma concentrations occur within 2–6 hours. This is delayed (4–6 hours) when taken with food. Food does not impact the bioavailability	1.45 L/kg; ~40% bound to plasma proteins	Undergoes acetylation by N-acetyltransferases to form N-acetyl zonisamide and reduction to form 2-sulfamoylacetyl phenol (SMAP)	Compounds excreted are zonisamide (35%), N-acetyl zonisamide (15%), and the glucuronide of SMAP (50%). Elimination half-life is ~63 hours
		Third-generation anticonvulsants			
Lacosamide [18]	Selectively enhances slow inactivation of voltage-gated sodium channels to help stabilize neuronal membranes; binds to collapsing response mediator protein-2 (CRMP-2), which is involved in neuronal differentiation and control of axonal cell growth	Completely absorbed after oral administration. Bioavailability is not affected by food		Lacosamide is a CYP2C19 substrate	Compounds excreted are unchanged lacosamide (~40%) and inactive O-desmethyl metabolite (~30%). Elimination half-life is ~13 hours

Evidence for Use

Neuropathic Pain

With approximately 20–24% of patients with diabetes in the United States suffering from diabetic peripheral neuropathy (DPN), the management of neuropathic pain has become a common challenge in the clinical setting [19]. Additionally, the incidence of postherpetic neuralgia (PHN) has increased due to increasing cases of herpes zoster virus (HZV) reactivation. Data from the CDC indicates that about one-third of individuals in the United States will develop shingles in their lifetime [20]. Anticonvulsants offer a potential alternative approach to managing neuropathic pain by targeting the underlying aberrant neuronal signals, which are characteristic of neuropathic pain.

Neuropathic pain differs from nociceptive pain not only in its presentation but also in its cause. Neuropathic pain can originate from a peripheral or central source and occurs due to neuronal injury, with subsequent alteration in the function of the nerve [21]. Neuropathic pain provides little to no biological benefit or protection to the organism and can occur in the absence of external stimuli, whereas nociceptive pain is related to the activation of pain receptors that are positioned to provide information to protect the body from potential dangers (such as extreme pressure, chemicals, or heat or cold). The underlying pathogenetic mechanism of neuropathic pain is poorly understood [22].

Phenytoin

Phenytoin was first used in the treatment of trigeminal neuralgia (TGN) in 1942 [23]. The first randomized study in 1977, which evaluated the efficacy of phenytoin in treating DPN, revealed it is no more effective than a placebo [24]. A further crossover study in 1999 evaluated the efficacy of intravenous infusion of phenytoin for acute flare-ups of chronic neuropathic pain and found benefit in 14 of 20 patients, with eight patients reporting "significant" benefit even when consideration was given to side effects [25].

Carbamazepine

Carbamazepine was first approved by the Food and Drug Administration (FDA) for the treatment of trigeminal neuralgia (TGN), with one study demonstrating a response in 70% of patients with TGN compared to 20% response with phenytoin [26]. Additional randomized clinical trials exploring the efficacy of carbamazepine in neuropathic pains of varying quality have been published. In one double-blind, crossover, placebo-controlled trial, 28 of 30 patients with DPN had improved pain relief with carbamazepine compared with placebo, with only two withdrawals for side effects [27]. These studies were no longer than four weeks in length, and in four studies, 65% of participants experienced at least one adverse event with carbamazepine compared with 27% of those receiving a placebo [28]. In studies evaluating the efficacy of carbamazepine in DPN, efficacy was demonstrated at doses between 300 and 2400 mg per day. Dizziness and somnolence were the most frequent but tolerable adverse effects in these studies [22]. In one systematic review of randomized controlled trials, carbamazepine had a number needed to treat (NNT) of 2.6 and a number needed to harm (NNH) of 3.4 [29].

Valproic Acid and Derivatives

In an 8-week, placebo-controlled trial of 48 patients, divalproex sodium showed at least moderate improvement in postherpetic neuralgia (PHN) pain compared to placebo [30]. Another placebo-controlled study evaluating the efficacy of sodium valproate in the management of pain related to DPN enrolled 43 patients. There was significant improvement in pain scores in three quantitative scales for patients treated with sodium valproate, measured after three months of treatment with good medication tolerability [31].

Other Anticonvulsants

In three similar double-blind trials, patients with moderate-to-extreme DPN pain were randomized to receive topiramate or placebo, with the primary outcome of pain reduction measured by a visual analog scale (VAS). None of the three studies reached clinical significance in reducing pain scores, and discontinuation rates due to adverse events were 24% in the topiramate group and 8% in the placebo group [32]. Because of the slow and careful titration required and the associated risk of Stevens–Johnson, lamotrigine is not a first-line medication for neuropathic pain [33]. Lacosamide has not been found to be efficacious in this patient population [34].

Neuropathic Cancer Pain

Neuropathic cancer pain (NCP) is caused by direct damage to the nervous system. A nerve may be compressed by a tumor or strangulated by fibrosis. Cancer treatments, including surgery, chemotherapy, or radiation, may lead to chronic NCP. Once a peripheral nerve is damaged, the pain fibers become abnormally sensitive. When used alone, opioid analgesics are ineffective for the treatment of NCP; the use of adjunctive analgesics is necessary [35].

Levetiracetam

A case series ($N = 7$) described the use of levetiracetam in patients with neoplasms that involved neural structures (brachial plexus or lumbosacral plexus) [36]. Patients had severe pain (8–9 out of 10 on a VAS) despite the use of parenteral opioids. All patients experienced improvement in their level of pain (0–3 out of 10 on the VAS) and a decrease in their overall opioid use within 2 weeks of starting levetiracetam 500–1500 mg twice daily. No adverse events related to levetiracetam were noted, and decreasing opioid use reduced the associated adverse effects. Levetiracetam did not appear to be effective as an adjunctive analgesic in patients with chronic postmastectomy pain syndrome [37].

Oxcarbazepine

A 20-week, randomized, open-label, controlled parallel study ($N = 20$) evaluated the use of oxcarbazepine for chemotherapy-induced neuropathic pain (CINP) in patients who received oxaliplatin for colorectal cancer [38]. The incidence of CINP was lower in patients receiving 1200 mg per day of oxcarbazepine than the control group (31.2% versus 75%; $p = 0.33$). Mild adverse effects of headache and dizziness were reported.

Phenytoin

A randomized, double-blind study compared the efficacy of phenytoin alone (100 mg twice daily) to that of buprenorphine and buprenorphine plus phenytoin ($n = 25$ in each of the three groups) in patients with neuropathic cancer pain (NCP) [39]. For the three groups, more than 50% pain relief was observed for 72%, 84%, and 88% of patients, respectively. Phenytoin may enhance the effects of buprenorphine, enabling the use of lower doses of opioids in patients with NCP.

Two cases of the use of topical phenytoin for the treatment of CINP were described [40]. One patient who experienced CINP in his legs after receiving vincristine for non-Hodgkin's lymphoma did not respond to topical baclofen, amitriptyline, or clonidine. Phenytoin 5% cream was applied three times daily, and he had a reduction in pain within 20 min, which would last at least 5 h. A second patient who suffered from CINP in her feet after receiving bortezomib for immunoglobulin light chain amyloidosis did not respond to oral gabapentin and oxycodone. She experienced a complete reduction in pain using phenytoin 5% cream three times daily and was also able to reduce her gabapentin and oxycodone use. Topical phenytoin is not commercially available in the United States.

Other Anticonvulsants

Lamotrigine was not effective for the relief of pain symptoms in patients with CINP [41]. With nearly one-third of patients experiencing significant weight loss with topiramate, this effect is of concern among patients with cancer who may be struggling with anorexia [42].

Migraine Headache Pain

Most of the data surrounding the use of anticonvulsant medications for migraine headache does not describe their impact on pain. Rather, the data describes a reduction in headache frequency, which ultimately reduces pain.

Valproic Acid and Derivatives

Multiple studies examined the efficacy and safety of valproic acid and its derivatives for the prophylaxis of migraine. In a randomized, double-blind, crossover comparison ($N = 29$), the mean number of headache attacks for patients receiving sodium valproate was 8.8 ± 6 compared to 15.6 ± 8.3 for placebo ($p < 0.001$) [43]. Sodium valproate was well-tolerated, with 7% of patients reporting dyspepsia and nausea. Sodium valproate blood concentrations were between 31.1 and 91.9 ng/mL. No correlation could be determined between concentrations and headache frequency, severity, or duration.

A multicenter, double-blind, randomized, placebo-controlled trial ($N = 107$) with a 4-week baseline phase and 12-week treatment phase was conducted [10]. While patients receiving divalproex sodium had a lower mean 4-week migraine headache frequency than placebo-treated patients (3.5 versus 5.7, $p \leq 0.001$), headache severity at peak intensity (1 = mild, 2 = moderate, 3 = severe, and 4 = excruciating) was not different between the two groups (2.0 versus 2.2). The mean valproate sodium trough concentration during the maintenance period was documented as 66 mg/L (goal 70–120 mg/L).

A similar multicenter, double-blind, placebo-controlled, parallel group study ($N = 176$) was conducted [44]. The mean reduction in 4-week headache frequency was different between placebo and the divalproex sodium groups (−0.5 (placebo), −1.7 (500 mg), −2.0 (1000 mg), and −1.7 (1500 mg)) ($p = 0.05$). Additionally, patients in the 500 mg and 1500 mg treatment groups achieved a greater reduction in migraine attacks impairing usual activities (56% and 55%, respectively) when compared to placebo (26%) ($p = 0.01$). The incidence of nausea, dizziness, and tremor was significantly higher in the 1500 mg group compared to placebo, as was nausea for the 500 mg group. Gastrointestinal events were the primary cause of withdrawal from the study. The valproate sodium trough concentrations were not provided.

In a larger multicenter, double-blind, randomized, placebo-controlled, parallel group study ($N = 237$), the mean reduction in 4-week headache rate was 1.2 for extended-release divalproex sodium versus 0.6 for placebo ($p = 0.006$) [45]. The average dose of extended-release divalproex sodium was 871 mg per day; valproate sodium trough concentrations were not provided. Somnolence, nausea, and asthenia were the primary reasons for divalproex sodium discontinuation and study dropout.

Topiramate

Topiramate was found to be efficacious and safe as an adjunctive treatment for pain associated with migraine headache [46]. In a three-month trial of topiramate ($N = 36$), the average monthly frequency of migraine headaches decreased from 17.04 (SD: 9.36) at baseline to 3.16 (SD: 7.39) ($p < 0.001$) at three months. The mean intensity of headache pain was 9.2 (SD: 1.15) on the VAS of 1–10 (10 being the worst pain possible) at baseline and decreased to 3.2 (SD: 2.19) at the end of three months ($p < 0.001$). In addition, patients rated the severity of their migraine pain as severe-to-incapacitating at the beginning of the trial and mild-to-moderate by the end of the study ($p < 0.001$). This reduction in pain intensity and severity is reflected in the reduction of the average number of analgesics at the beginning of the study (68 doses) compared to the end of the three-month study (30 doses). The most common adverse event reported was a weight loss of 3% of total body weight observed in 8% of patients.

Levetiracetam

A prospective, open-label trial ($N = 16$) evaluated the efficacy of levetiracetam as a preventative treatment for migraine with aura in patients with a high frequency of attacks [47]. Monthly attack frequency decreased from 6.2 ± 1.6 during the run-in period to 0.81 ± 0.8 in the sixth month of the study. Severity of attack (1 = mild, 2 = moderate, and 3 = severe) also decreased from the run-in period (2.56 ± 0.44) to month six (1.32 ± 0.46) of treatment ($p < 0.0001$). Levetiracetam was well-tolerated, with no serious adverse effects or dropouts reported.

Zonisamide

The potential safety and efficacy of zonisamide for patients with refractory migraine headache were explored in an open-label study ($N = 34$) [17]. Headache severity, rated on a 10-point VAS, and frequency were reduced from baseline to three months ($p < 0.01$ and $p < 0.05$, respectively). Zonisamide was well-tolerated, with 11.8% of patients discontinuing therapy due to adverse effects [dysphoria ($n = 2$) and difficulty concentrating ($n = 2$)].

Lamotrigine

The potential efficacy of lamotrigine in the prevention of migraine aura in patients was examined in an open-label study ($N = 47$) [12]. While the monthly frequency of migraine aura reduced from 4.2 (1–15) to 0.7 (0–6), there was no assessment of pain due to migraine headache. Three did not complete the protocol due to the development of a skin rash. A prospective, controlled, open, dose titration study ($N = 59$) investigated whether a reduction in migraine aura frequency would lead to a reduction in migraine attacks [48]. The average monthly frequency of migraine attacks reduced from 2.1 (SD: 1) to 1.2 (SD: 1.1) ($p < 0.001$). The correlation between the reduction of migraine aura and migraine frequency was significant ($p < 0.002$). Due to the slower-than-usual dose titration of lamotrigine, it took almost 5 months for patients to experience a 50% reduction in migraine aura frequency. It is therefore suggested that patients be treated for at least 6 months before lamotrigine is considered ineffective.

Chronic Low Back Pain

While no anticonvulsants are currently FDA-approved for chronic low back pain (CLBP) or other radiculopathies and pain syndromes associated with spinal cord injuries, their impact on such conditions has been explored due to their potential efficacy in managing neuropathic pain, particularly when conventional treatments (i.e., gabapentin, pregabalin, etc.) prove ineffective.

Topiramate

In a 10-week, randomized, placebo-controlled study in patients with CLBP, topiramate was associated with significant changes in pain, mood, and quality of life, according to the McGill Pain Questionnaire, the Oswestry Low Back Pain Disability Questionnaire, and the State-Trait Anger Expression Inventory ($p < 0.001$) [49]. Adverse effects that led to the discontinuation of topiramate included severe somnolence, psychomotor slowing, and problems with vision and memory. In another randomized trial, topiramate reduced average back pain, average overall pain, and worst overall pain scores by 21% ($p = 0.17$), 16% ($p = 0.02$), and 15% ($p = 0.03$), respectively [50]. However, these results were impacted by the high dropout rate attributed to adverse effects such as paresthesias, nausea, anorexia, sedation, and amnesia, concluding that topiramate may be considered as a second-line agent in patients not responding to conventional treatment options. In contrast, case reports and other studies point to the potential role of topiramate in alleviating CLBP due to its effects on weight reduction, making it a favorable adjunctive analgesic in obese patients in comparison to agents such as gabapentin and pregabalin, which may contribute to further weight gain [49, 51].

Lamotrigine

In an open-label trial, lamotrigine led to a reduction in mean spontaneous pain from a baseline of 7.6 ± 1.5 (assessed on a 0–10 Numerical Pain Scale) to 4.5 ± 1.8 in patients with CLBP ($N = 14$) [52]. This effect was observed and reached significance when patients were maintained at 400 mg of lamotrigine for four weeks, after a four-week titration period, which aligns with the suggested lamotrigine dosing in other pain syndromes [53–55]. Mean spontaneous pain reductions, as well as improvement in other measured outcomes such as the Straight Leg Raise (SLR) test and the mechanical range of lumbar motion, were found to correlate with daily lamotrigine doses and mean plasma concentrations, suggesting a dose- and plasma concentration–dependent analgesic effect ($p = 0.001$). In addition, the trial reported a reduction in the utilization of rescue analgesia by the end of the 10-week study period (from 3.5 ± 2.7 pills at baseline to 2.2 ± 1.8 during the last week of study). Adverse effects were reported in four out of 14 patients and included dizziness and diarrhea. This trial points to the potential importance of a prolonged titration period, followed by prolonged maintenance to achieve steady state, in achieving positive analgesic outcomes.

Additionally, in a randomized, placebo-controlled, crossover trial, the efficacy of lamotrigine was investigated in relieving spinal cord injury pain and clinical signs of neuronal hyperexcitability ($N = 22$) [56]. While lamotrigine had no significant effect on the primary outcome of pain intensity in the total sample of patients, including those with complete spinal cord injury, it was found to significantly reduce pain in patients with incomplete lesions ($p = 0.02$), suggesting an effect on neuronal hyperexcitability, one mechanism of neuropathic pain.

Oxcarbazepine

In a small cohort of patients with CLBP that is refractory to gabapentin ($N = 18$), oxcarbazepine exhibited effectiveness in patients reporting symptoms of "burning" pain and allodynia [57]. The main adverse effects observed were dizziness, headache, and nausea. In an open-label trial, oxcarbazepine delivered moderate pain alleviation in 58% of patients overall ($N = 12$) but in 100% of those experiencing allodynia, suggesting a potential benefit of oxcarbazepine in the management of patients particularly burdened by allodynia. The reported adverse effects, such as blurred vision, sedation, dizziness, and hyponatremia, were mild and reversible [58]. Adding to the evidence of targeting specific patient phenotypes, a prospective, randomized, clinical crossover trial compared oxcarbazepine and pregabalin in patients with spinal cord injury of different clinical characteristics ($N = 55$) [59]. Oxcarbazepine showed significant efficacy in patients without evoked pain, notably in patients experiencing electrical, burning, and pricking pain, compared to patients with other types of pain descriptions ($p < 0.05$). Adverse events associated with oxcarbazepine included dizziness, rashes, and elevated liver enzymes. Results of this trial may point to the efficacy of sodium channel blockers in stimulus-independent pain.

Other Anticonvulsants

The effectiveness demonstrated by other anticonvulsants such as carbamazepine, phenytoin, and topiramate in managing neuropathic pain suggests a promising avenue for their utilization in chronic pain due to spinal cord injury [60]. However, further clinical trials are needed to reach a definitive conclusion [61]. Levetiracetam and valproic acid have not been found to be efficacious in this patient population [62–64].

Perioperative Pain Management

While the mainstay of postoperative pain management revolves around the use of opioid analgesics, anticonvulsants may reduce the use of opioids, thereby, minimizing adverse effects, risk of tolerance, and risk of misuse. In addition, anticonvulsants may play a role in postoperative inflammation modulation [65].

Lamotrigine

In a double-blind, randomized, placebo-controlled pilot study conducted in Italy, lamotrigine was employed postoperatively in patients undergoing a transurethral prostatectomy ($N = 20$) [66]. Patients in the lamotrigine group received a dose of 200 mg one hour before spinal anesthesia. Both groups of patients were started on a buprenorphine infusion post-surgery and intramuscular diclofenac as needed. Significant reductions in total analgesic utilization ($p < 0.01$), in addition to serial VAS scores at two ($p = 0.04$), four ($p < 0.01$), and six hours ($p = 0.04$) post-surgery, were observed. No patients in the lamotrigine group required diclofenac in comparison to seven patients in the control group. A mild rash was noted in one participant four hours after the administration of lamotrigine.

Carbamazepine

In another randomized, double-blind, experimental study, carbamazepine was utilized for postoperative pain in patients with an addiction to opioids [67]. This population may especially benefit from adjunctive agents, given their increased risk of opioid tolerance, hyperalgesia, and withdrawal. Patients ($N = 90$) underwent elective surgery for an uncomplicated inguinal hernia, anal fissure, or hemorrhoid. In addition to assessing pain scale scores at baseline and one and 12 h postoperatively, baseline and postoperative serum levels of proinflammatory cytokines interleukin (IL)-6 and IL-10, which may play a role in receptor sensitization and hyperalgesia, were also collected. Patients in the carbamazepine group received a dose of 400 mg two hours prior to surgery. All patients enrolled received morphine as part of general anesthesia. At 12 hours post-surgery, carbamazepine effectively decreased pain and modulated pain behavior in patients with an addiction to opioids ($p < 0.001$). IL-6 (at 12 hours post-surgery; $p < 0.01$) and IL-10 (at one hour post-surgery; $p < 0.001$) levels were also reduced, indicating a possible influence on systemic inflammation and, therefore, pain control.

Applications to Clinical Practice

Considering the diverse array of efficacy data regarding the use of anticonvulsant agents for pain management, it is imperative to assess additional factors when considering the utilization of these adjunctive medications.

Opioid Sparing

While opioids have traditionally been the cornerstone of acute pain management, particularly in perioperative and trauma-related scenarios, a recent transition in care has shifted to opioid-sparing practices, given the proven efficacy of multimodal pain management and the universally acknowledged risks linked to opioid usage [68–71]. In the short term, opioids are notorious for inducing nausea, vomiting, and constipation [71]. Moreover, they pose risks of sedation and respiratory depression, especially when coadministered with other sedative agents [72]. Concerns with the use of opioids in the long term are mainly due to the potential of misuse and abuse, highlighting the necessity for alternative approaches. Although gabapentinoids are frequently cited in the guidelines and literature as the anticonvulsant adjunctive analgesic option in the ICU and trauma setting [73], other anticonvulsants may also play a beneficial role in the management of neuropathic pain associated with trauma and injury.

In one retrospective study evaluating the impact of an inpatient pain pharmacist consult on clinical outcomes, the initiation of adjunctive therapy, such as an anticonvulsant, was a frequently accepted recommendation. Furthermore, significant reductions in morphine milligram equivalents (MMEs) were seen at hospital discharge and after discharge (average MME at admission: 70.5, at discharge: 65.2, and at 90 days after discharge: 50.1) [74]. Embracing multimodal analgesia strategies enables a reduction in opioid requirements and facilitates the judicious use of multiple medications at the lowest and safest possible doses [72]. At the bedside, nurses play an essential role in educating patients about realistic pain management goals and advocating for the implementation of multimodal analgesia approaches. These actions not only foster stronger nurse–patient bonds but also elevate the overall standard of patient care through informed decision-making and collaborative treatment strategies [75].

Comorbidities

Another benefit proposed in the literature of incorporating adjuvants, including anticonvulsants, into pain management strategies is their multifaceted contribution beyond direct pain modulation, particularly in chronic pain scenarios, accompanied by comorbidities [76]. These medications exhibit versatility by addressing various aspects of pain and its associated challenges. For instance, they have demonstrated efficacy in enhancing mood and the overall quality of life, which can be pivotal in managing comorbid conditions that exacerbate pain symptoms, such as psychiatric disorders and obesity [49, 77]. This multifunctional approach not only targets the primary pain experience but also addresses the broader spectrum of factors influencing a patient's well-being, thereby offering a comprehensive and holistic approach to pain management. Furthermore, the use of anticonvulsants for both pain management and psychiatric disorders may be described as rational polypharmacy since pharmacologic and psychiatric interventions are integrated, allowing for improved outcomes and reduced costs, especially in chronic pain [78].

Older Population

Rational polypharmacy is applicable to the older population and those at the end of life, as the use of multiple medications is common and can increase the risk of adverse effects, drug interactions, nonadherence, and increased costs. Rational polypharmacy allows for enhancing pain relief while treating concomitant comorbidities.

Pain management is often poor in the older population, which leads to disability and a decrease in the quality of life [79]. In nursing home residents, reduction in pain intensity is only one of the many targeted outcomes of treatment. Improvement in functional status and prevention of deterioration in psychosocial and cognitive functioning are important outcome measures for pain management, highlighting the importance of multimodal analgesia and the consideration of adjunctive agents [80].

However, the older population is more vulnerable to many of the adverse effects associated with anticonvulsants, such as sedation, dizziness, and falls. For example, carbamazepine has been extensively studied as an effective anticonvulsant for trigeminal neuralgia. Despite this, it may not be considered ideal by many clinicians due to its extensive drug interactions as well as the need for slow titration, given its pharmacokinetics. In addition, side effects such as syndrome of inappropriate antidiuretic hormone (SIADH) and leukopenia could severely impact the older population [80]. Because of this, many clinicians turn to other anticonvulsant agents such as gabapentin. Alternative anticonvulsants such as lamotrigine and topiramate may be trialed if gabapentin is not tolerated or effective [81]. Appropriate pain management should encompass deliberate consideration of adjunctive strategies and, if considered, employing them at the lowest and safest doses possible, given the modest efficacy data in comparison to the increased risk of side effects that may outweigh the proposed benefit of combination therapies [82].

Adverse Drug Reactions

A significant limitation to the utilization of several anticonvulsant agents under discussion stems from the associated adverse effects.

Carbamazepine is associated with a range of adverse effects that warrant careful consideration. Common side effects include nausea, dizziness, drowsiness, ataxia, diplopia, and cognitive effects, such as difficulty concentrating, which may subside with continued use or dosage adjustment [83, 84]. However, more serious adverse effects such as cutaneous drug reactions, including Steven–Johnson syndrome, pose significant risks, especially in patients carrying the HLA-B 1502 allele [28]. Moreover, carbamazepine has been linked to hematological abnormalities, including agranulocytosis, thrombocytopenia, and aplastic anemia, necessitating regular blood monitoring during treatment [76, 84]. Given its metabolism via hepatic CYP3A4 and its potential to cause hepatic dysfunction, carbamazepine may be less preferable to other agents in patients with liver impairment [85]. Finally, carbamazepine can induce hepatic enzyme induction, precipitating drug interactions and altered metabolism of other medications.

Oxcarbazepine presents a favorable alternative to carbamazepine with a reduced risk of cutaneous drug reactions, although prescribers should remain cautious with its use [86]. Studies indicate fewer incidences of rash or hypersensitivity reactions with oxcarbazepine than with carbamazepine or phenytoin, and it also lacks serious idiosyncratic hematologic or hepatic effects, eliminating the need for routine monitoring of hematologic and hepatic profiles [87]. Oxcarbazepine generally exhibits mild and reversible adverse effects, including blurred vision, dizziness, headache, and nausea [87]. However, it may lead to significant hyponatremia, requiring careful monitoring of serum sodium levels, especially with the initiation of therapy [84]. Oxcarbazepine's predictable pharmacokinetics, minimal drug interactions, and lack of autoinduction simplify dose titration and adjustment, facilitating combination therapy if necessary [87].

Topiramate's adverse effect profile encompasses a wide variety of systems that may be affected at different levels of severity, frequently impacting patient tolerability. Common cognitive and nervous system side effects reported with topiramate include paresthesia, vertigo, ataxia, psychomotor slowing, word-finding deficits, amnesia, somnolence, depression, and anxiety [50, 77, 83, 84]. Given its weak carbonic anhydrase inhibitor activity, it is associated with a notable incidence of kidney stones [84]. This activity may also contribute to oligohidrosis, and the resultant hypothermia is particularly concerning for individuals with spinal cord injury who struggle with thermoregulation [88]. Topiramate's unique side effect of weight loss may be beneficial for overweight patients but detrimental for those with conditions like cancer or post-traumatic cachexia. Furthermore, topiramate may induce acute myopathy and fluctuation in intraocular pressures, diminish the efficacy of oral contraceptives, and pose a risk of teratogenicity [88].

Lamotrigine is generally well-tolerated by patients when titrated appropriately. However, a notable adverse effect is the development of a rash, occurring in approximately 5–10% of individuals taking the medication. Certain factors, such as age, concurrent use of valproic acid, and rapid dose escalation, increase the risk of rash development [84]. To mitigate these risks, lamotrigine therapy should commence at a low dose with slow titration [88]. Lamotrigine can also induce ataxia, incoordination, blurred vision, and diplopia [83]. Moreover, lamotrigine carries the risk of decreasing fetal folic acid levels, potentially leading to neural tube malformations [88].

Phenytoin has numerous undesirable adverse effects, such as hypersensitivity, lymphadenopathy, and hepatotoxicity, and the potential for interaction with many other medications, which likely include analgesics [84]. From the standpoint of significant adverse drug reactions, valproic acid is mainly associated with the incidence of hepatotoxicity [76].

Dosing Considerations

Individualized dosing is essential to achieve optimal pain relief while minimizing adverse effects. While many practitioners use dosing guidelines established for treating seizures, titration may be necessary to find the most effective and tolerable dose for each patient. Regular monitoring for both therapeutic efficacy and adverse effects is crucial [76]. Table 11.2 provides a summary of the dosing considerations for the use of anticonvulsants in the treatment of pain.

Table 11.2 Summary of the dosing considerations of anticonvulsants

	Dosing (per manufacturer or used in the literature)	Special considerations
First-generation anticonvulsants		
Carbamazepine		
Neuropathic pain[a]	*TGN*: 200–400 mg/day in two to four divided doses based on chosen formulation, gradually increasing (over several weeks) in increments of 200 mg/day as needed Usual maintenance dose: 600–800 mg/day in two to four divided doses based on chosen formulation; max dosing: 1.2 g/day [4] *Neuropathic pain*: Starting dose of 50–100 mg BID, increasing as needed to a maximum of 1200 mg/day. A dosage of 100–200 mg Q4-6H is usually effective. Higher doses (i.e., 1600 mg) are occasionally required [83] *PHN*: 200–1200 mg daily [4, 28] *DPN*: 300–2400 mg/day, median dose: 600 mg/day [28, 87]	Elderly: 50 mg at bedtime, with 50 mg increments weekly, up to a maximum dosage of 400 mg/day divided into two doses [81] The dosing, titration, and monitoring for PHN are similar to regimens used in TGN and typically lower doses than those needed to achieve anticonvulsant effects [89]
Perioperative pain management	400 mg PO 2 hours prior to surgery [67]	
Phenytoin		
Neuropathic pain	TGN rescue therapy: 250 mg to 1 g as a one-time dose or 15 mg/kg (maximum dose not established) over 30–120 minutes; administer at a rate of ≤50 mg/min [8]	There is no correlation between serum concentrations and the level of pain relief
Cancer pain	100 mg BID [39]	
Valproic acid and derivatives		
Neuropathic pain	*PHN*: 500–1000 mg daily [30] *DPN*: 500 mg daily [31]	There is no correlation between serum concentrations and the level of pain relief
Migraine[a]	250 mg/d, increased by 250 mg Q4 days until a goal dose of 500 mg, 1000 mg, or 1500 mg [9, 44] 250 mg/d, titrated upward at regular increments of 250 mg every other day, with a goal trough plasma concentration of 70–120 mg/L [10] 400 mg BID [43]	

(continued)

Table 11.2 (continued)

	Dosing (per manufacturer or used in the literature)	Special considerations
Second-generation anticonvulsants		
Lamotrigine		
Neuropathic pain	*Neuropathic Pain*: Initial dose is 25–50 mg taken at bedtime, which is increased gradually to 300–500 mg daily in two divided dosages. Suggested regimen: 25 mg/day for 2 weeks; then increase to 25 mg twice daily for 2 weeks; then increase weekly by 25 mg twice daily to a goal of at least 100 mg twice daily [88] *TGN*: 50–400 mg/day [83] *TGN*: Initial: Weeks 1 and 2: 25 mg once daily; increase as needed based on response and tolerability as follows: Weeks 3 and 4: 50 mg/day in one or two divided doses based on the chosen formulation Week 5 and beyond: Increase the daily dose by 50 mg every 1–2 weeks to a maximum of 400 mg/day in one or two divided doses based on the chosen formulation [11]	Initial titration starts from 50 mg/day (recommended for 2 weeks), followed by an increase in dosage to 50 mg BID for the next 2 weeks. Max dosage is 600 mg/day, with a weekly increase of 100 mg. Caution is suggested in patients with renal impairment [83] Consider use in patients who do not respond or with intolerance or contraindications to carbamazepine and/or oxcarbazepine; titration time to effective dose may limit use in patients with severe pain [11] Dose adjustments are required in patients taking medications that alter lamotrigine's metabolism (i.e., valproate, carbamazepine, and phenytoin) [11] Suggested analgesic effect becomes more pronounced with prolonged use at a steady dose [52]
Migraine	*To reduce migraine aura*: 25 mg PO PM to start; then increase by 25 mg per week until reaching a maximum dose of 100 mg [12] *To reduce migraine aura and migraine attacks*: 25 mg daily, during first month; if no improvement, dose was increased by 25 mg monthly, not to exceed 300 mg/day [48]	
Chronic low back pain	*Intractable sciatica*: 400 mg/day; started at 25 mg daily, and dose was doubled weekly till a maximum of 400 mg/day; titrated over 6 weeks Starting week 2, doses were divided into two (morning and evening) [52] *Spinal cord injury*: Gradually increased to 400 mg/day, minimum treatment dose 200 mg/day Weeks 1 and 2: 25 mg/day, weeks 3 and 4: 50 mg/day, week 5: 100 mg/day, week 6: 200 mg/day, week 7: 300 mg/day, weeks 8 and 9: 400 mg/day [56]	
Perioperative pain management	200 mg PO 1 hour prior to spinal anesthesia [66]	
Levetiracetam		
Cancer pain	500 mg–1500 mg twice daily [36]	
Migraine	250 mg per day, increased by 250 mg per week until the final dose of 1000 mg per day (500 mg BID) [47]	

Oxcarbazepine	
Cancer pain	CINP: 1200 mg/day [38]
Chronic low back pain	*Spinal cord injury*: 150 mg PO BID titrated to 300 mg PO BID as tolerated over 1–2 weeks, administered in two dose-escalating phases: up to 900 mg/day in Phase I and up to 1500 mg/day in Phase II [59, 87] *Chronic spinal disorders*: 600–2400 mg [61]
Topiramate	
Neuropathic pain	The usual starting dose is 50 mg taken at bedtime, which is titrated up to 200 mg administered twice daily [84] *DPN*: 100, 200, or 400 mg/day [32] *TGN*: Starting at 25 mg PO BID and increasing by 50 mg per week up to a maximum of 200 mg BID [84]
Migraine[a]	25 mg PO HS, with a weekly increase in dose of 25–50 mg, to a maximum dose of 100 mg per day; some patients may require up to 200 mg/day for optimal response; however, adverse effects may increase [15, 46]
Chronic low back pain	Titrated from 50 mg/day in 50 mg/week increments to a dose of 300 mg/day [49] *Radicular pain*: 50–400 (mean of 200 mg/day) Started at 50 mg QHS and titrated weekly by 50 mg and divided into two doses; maximum of 400 mg a day; titrated over 4 weeks [50] *Spinal disorders*: 25–400 mg, 25 mg BID with a target dose of 100 mg BID (usual maximum dose is 400 mg) [61, 88]
Zonisamide	
Migraine	100 mg daily, increased in 100 mg increments over 3 weeks to 400 mg daily [17]
Third-generation anticonvulsants	
Lacosamide	
Neuropathic pain	50 mg PO twice daily, titrated up to a maximum daily dose of 400mg [34]

[a]FDA-approved indication

Emerging Therapies

Recognizing the prospective role of anticonvulsants in pain management, attributed, among other mechanisms, to their modulation of sodium and calcium ion channels, has led to the pursuit of alternative therapeutic approaches targeting these channels [90]. Novel sodium and calcium channel modulators hold promise for the development of effective pain medications without the adverse effect profile of anticonvulsants [91]. For example, vixotrigine (BIIB074), a novel voltage- and use-dependent sodium channel blocker, was recently studied in a phase II, randomized, placebo-controlled trial assessing its efficacy in patients with neuropathic pain [92]. A significant reduction in average daily pain scores was observed with vixotrigine at a dose of 200 mg twice daily. Additional randomized clinical trials involving larger cohorts of patients are necessary to expand upon the limited body of evidence and establish conclusive insights into the efficacy and therapeutic position of anticonvulsants and other novel therapies in pain management.

Key Themes

- Only a few anticonvulsant agents have received FDA approval for the treatment of pain (carbamazepine is approved for trigeminal neuralgia; valproic acid and topiramate are approved for migraine headache prevention).
- Alternative approaches for pain control, including the use of anticonvulsants, may help mitigate the concerns with the long-term use of opioids.

Conclusions

Anticonvulsants represent a diverse class of medications that, while originally developed for seizure disorders, have demonstrated significant utility in the management of various pain syndromes. Their role in multimodal analgesia strategies is particularly important in the context of opioid-sparing approaches, offering additional benefits in populations with complex comorbidities. While efficacy varies by agent and indication, careful patient selection, individualized dosing, and monitoring for adverse effects are essential to optimizing outcomes. Together, these insights underscore the evolving role of anticonvulsants as important tools in comprehensive pain management.

Acknowledgments The authors would like to thank Tonya Floyd-Bradstock, CMI, MFA, MBA, Certified Medical Illustrator and Biomedical Visualization, VIR & 3D Print Specialist for designing Fig. 11.1.

References

1. Dowell D, Haegerich TM, Chou R. CDC guideline for prescribing opioids for chronic pain - United States, 2016. MMWR Recomm Rep. 2016;65(1):1–49.
2. Goldstick JE, Guy GP, Losby JL, Baldwin GT, Myers MG, Bohnert ASB. Patterns in nonopioid pain medication prescribing after the release of the 2016 guideline for prescribing opioids for chronic pain. JAMA Netw Open. 2022;5(6):e2216475.
3. Moore RA, Wiffen PJ, Derry S, McQuay HJ. Gabapentin for chronic neuropathic pain and fibromyalgia in adults. Cochrane Database Syst Rev. 2011;(3):CD007938.
4. Carbamazepine [package insert]. East Hanover, NJ: Novartis Pharmaceuticals Corporation; 2015.
5. Mehta M, Shah J, Khakhkhar T, Shah R, Hemavathi KG. Anticonvulsant hypersensitivity syndrome associated with carbamazepine administration: case series. J Pharmacol Pharmacother. 2014;5(1):59–62.
6. Al-Quliti KW. Update on neuropathic pain treatment for trigeminal neuralgia. The pharmacological and surgical options. Neurosciences (Riyadh). 2015;20(2):107–14.
7. Bianchi M, Rossoni G, Sacerdote P, Panerai AE, Berti F. Carbamazepine exerts anti-inflammatory effects in the rat. Eur J Pharmacol. 1995;294:71–4.
8. Phenytoin [package insert]. New York, NY: Parke-Davis a division of Pfizer, Inc.; 2018.
9. Valproic acid [package insert]. North Chicago, IL: Abbott Laboratories; 2011.
10. Mathew NT, Saper JR, Silberstein SD, et al. Migraine Prophylaxis with divalproex. Arch Neurol. 1995;52:281–6.
11. Lamotrigine [package insert]. Research Triangle Park, NC: GlaxoSmithKline; 2015.
12. Pascual J, Caminero AB, Mateos V, et al. Preventing disturbing migraine aura with lamotrigine: an open label study. Headache. 2004;44:1024–8.
13. Levetiracetam [package insert]. Smyrna, GA: UCB, Inc.; 2017.
14. Oxcarbazepine [package insert]. East Hanover, NJ: Novartis Pharmaceuticals Corporation; 2017.
15. Topiramate [package insert]. Titusville, NJ: Janssen Pharmaceuticals, Inc.; 2009.
16. Zonisamide [package insert]. St. Michale, Barbados: Concordia Pharmaceuticals, Inc.; 2016.
17. Drake ME, Greathouse NI, Renner JB, Armentbright AD. Open-label zonisamide for refractory migraine. Clin Neuropharmacol. 2004;27(6):278–80.
18. Lacosamide [package insert]. Smyrna, GA: UCB, Inc.; 2008.
19. Schmader KE. Epidemiology and impact on quality of life of postherpetic neuralgia and painful diabetic neuropathy. Clin J Pain. 2002;18:350–4.
20. Centers for Disease Control and Prevention. Shingles Burden and Trends. Accessed March 24, 2024, from https://www.cdc.gov/shingles/surveillance.html.
21. Woolf CJ, Mannion RJ. Neuropathic pain: aetiology, symptoms, mechanisms, and management. Lancet. 1999;353:1959–64.
22. Tremont-Lukats IW, Megeff C, Backonja MM. Anticonvulsants for neuropathic pain syndromes mechanisms of action and place in therapy. Drugs. 2000;60(5):1029–52.
23. Swerdlow M. Anticonvulsant drugs and chronic pain. Clin Neuropharmacol. 1984;7:51–82.
24. Saudek CD, Werns S, Reidenberg MM. Phenytoin in the treatment of diabetic symmetrical polyneuropathy. Clin Pharmacol Ther. 1977;22:196–9.
25. McCleane GJ. Intravenous infusion of phenytoin relieves neuropathic pain: a randomized, double-blinded, placebo-controlled, crossover study. Anesth Analg. 1999;89:985–8.

26. Backonja MM, Serra J. Pharmacologic management part 1: better-studied neuropathic pain diseases. Pain Med. 2004;5(Suppl 1):S28–47.
27. Rull JA, Quibrera H, Gonzalez-Millan H, Lozano CO. Symptomatic treatment of peripheral diabetic neuropathy with carbamazepine (Tegretol): double blind crossover trial. Diabetologia. 1969;5(4):215–8.
28. Wiffen PJ, Derry S, Moore RA, Kalso EA. Carbamazepine for chronic neuropathic pain and fibromyalgia in adults. Cochrane Database Syst Rev. 2014;2014(4):CD005451.
29. McQuay H, Carroll D, Jadad AR, Wiffen P, Moore A. Anticonvulsant drugs for management of pain: a systematic review. BMJ. 1995;311(7012):1047–52.
30. Kochar DK, Garg P, Bumb RA, et al. Divalproex sodium in the management of post-herpetic neuralgia: a randomized double-blind placebo-controlled study. QJM. 2005;98(1):29–34.
31. Kochar DK, Rawat N, Agrawal RP, et al. Sodium valproate for painful diabetic neuropathy: a randomized double-blind placebo-controlled study. QJM. 2004;97(1):33–8.
32. Thienel U, Neto W, Schwabe SK, Vijapurkar U. Topiramate in painful diabetic polyneuropathy: findings from three double-blind placebo-controlled trials. Acta Neurol Scand. 2004;110:221–31.
33. Vadalouca A, Raptis E, Moka E, Zis P, Sykioti P, Siafaka I. Pharmacological treatment of neuropathic cancer pain: a comprehensive review of the current literature. Pain Pract. 2012;12(3):219–51.
34. Carmland ME, Kreutzfeldt MD, Holbech JV, et al. The effect of Lacosamide in peripheral neuropathic pain: a randomized, double-blind, placebo-controlled, phenotype-stratified trial. Eur J Pain. 2024;28:105–19.
35. Yoon SY, Oh J. Neuropathic cancer pain: prevalence, pathophysiology, and management. Korean J Intern Med. 2018;33:1058–69.
36. Dunteman ED. Levetiracetam as an adjunctive analgesic in neoplastic plexopathies: case series and commentary. J Pain Palliat Care Pharmacother. 2005;19(1):35–43.
37. Vilholm OJ, Cold S, Rasmussen L, Sindrup SH. Effect of levetiracetam on the postmastectomy pain syndrome. Eur J Neurol. 2008;15:851–7.
38. Argyriou AA, Chroni E, Polychronopoulos P, et al. Efficacy of oxcarbazepine for prophylaxis against cumulative oxaliplatin-induced neuropathy. Neurology. 2006;67:2253–5.
39. Yajnik S, Singh GP, Singh G, Kumar M. Phenytoin as a coanalgesic in cancer pain. J Pain Symptom Manag. 1992;7(4):209–13.
40. Kopsky DJ, Keppel Hesselink JM. Topical phenytoin for the treatment of neuropathic pain. J Pain Res. 2017;10:469–73.
41. Rao RD, Flynn PJ, Sloan JA, et al. Efficacy of lamotrigine in the management of chemotherapy-induced peripheral neuropathy: a phase 3 randomized, double-blind, placebo-controlled trial, N01C3. Cancer. 2008;112:2802–8.
42. McDonald AA, Portenoy RK. How to use antidepressants and anticonvulsants as adjuvant analgesics in the treatment of neuropathic cancer pain. J Support Oncol. 2006;4:43–52.
43. Hering R, Kuritzky A. Sodium valproate in the prophylactic treatment of migraine: a double-blind study versus placebo. Cephalalgia. 1992;12:81–4.
44. Klapper J, on behalf of the Divalproex Sodium in Migraine Prophylaxis Study Group. Divalproex sodium in migraine prophylaxis: a dose-controlled study. Cephalalgia. 1997;17:103–8.
45. Freitag FG, Collins SD, Carlson HA, etc al. A randomized trial of divalproex sodium extended-release tablets in migraine prophylaxis. Neurology. 2002;58:1652–9.
46. Martinez HR, Londono O, Cantu-Martinez L, Tarin LC, Castillo CD. Topiramate as an adjunctive treatment in migraine prophylaxis. Headache. 2003;43:1080–4.
47. Brighina F, Palermo A, Aloisio A, Francolini M, Giglia G, Fierro B. Levetiracetam in the prophylaxis of migraine with aura: a 6-month open-label study. Clin Neuropharmacol. 2006;29(6):338–42.
48. Lampl C, Katsarava Z, Diener H-C, Limmroth V. Lamotrigine reduces migraine aura and migraine attacks in patients with migraine with aura. J Neurol Neurosurg Psychiatry. 2005;76:1730–2.
49. Muehlbacher M, Nickel MK, Kettler C, et al. Topiramate in treatment of patients with chronic low back pain: a randomized, double-blind, placebo-controlled study. Clin J Pain. 2006;22:526–31.
50. Khoromi S, Patsalides A, Parada S, Salehi V, Meegan JM, Mb M. Topiramate in chronic lumbar radicular pain. J Pain. 2005;6(12):829–36.
51. Gupta A, Kulkarni A, Ramanujam V, Zheng L, Treacy E. Improvement in chronic low back pain in an obese patient with topiramate use. J Pain Palliat Care Pharmacother. 2015;29(2):140–3.
52. Eisenberg E, Damunni G, Hoffer E, Baum Y, Krivoy N. Lamotrigine for intractable sciatica: correlation between dose, plasma concentration and analgesia. Eur J Pain. 2003;7(6):485–91.
53. Eisenberg E, Lurie Y, Braker C, Daoud D, Ishay A. Lamotrigine reduces painful diabetic neuropathy: a randomized, controlled study. Neurology. 2001;57(3):505–9.
54. McCleane GJ. Lamotrigine in the management of neuropathic pain: a review of the literature. Clin J Pain. 2000;16(4):321–6.
55. Simpson DM, Olney R, McArthur JC, Khan A, Godbold J, Ebel-Frommer K. A placebo-controlled trail of lamotrigine for painful HIV-associated neuropathy. Neurology. 2000;54(11):2115–9.
56. Finnerup NB, Sindrup SH, Bach FW, Johannesen IL, Jensen TS. Lamotrigine in spinal cord injury pain: a randomized controlled trial. Pain. 2002;96(3):375–83.
57. Ward S, Royal M, Jenson M, Bhakta B, Gunyea I, Movva V. An open-label trial of oxcarbazepine in patients with radiculopathy refractory to gabapentin. J Pain. 2002;3(2):42.
58. Jenkins K, Kaplan SE, Leahy LF, et al. Oxcarbazepine in central neuropathic pain with allodynia following spinal cord injury. J Pain. 2002;3:10.
59. Min K, Oh Y, Lee S-H, Ryu JS. Symptom-based treatment of neuropathic pain in spinal cord injured patients: a randomized, crossover clinical trial. Am J Phys Med Rehabil. 2016;95(5):330–8.
60. Dinoff B, Richards S, Ness TJ. Clinical notes use of topiramate for spinal cord injury-related pain. J Spinal Cord Med. 2003;26:401–3.
61. Polatin PB, Dersh J. Psychotropic medication in chronic spinal disorders. Spine J. 2004;4(4):436–50.
62. Finnerup NB, Grydehøj J, Bing J, et al. Levetiracetam in spinal cord injury pain: a randomized controlled trial. Spinal Cord. 2009;47:861–7.
63. Guy S, Mehta S, Leff L, Teasell R, Loh E. Anticonvulsant medication use for the management of pain following spinal cord injury: systematic review and effectiveness analysis. Spinal Cord. 2014;52:89–96.
64. Drewes AM, Andreasen A, Poulsen LH. Valproate for treatment of chronic central pain after spinal cord injury. A double-blind crossover study. Paraplegia. 1994;32:565–9.
65. Gilron I. Review article: the role of anticonvulsant drugs in postoperative pain management: a bench-to-bedside perspective. Can J Anaesth. 2006;53(6):562–71.
66. Bonicalzi V, Canavero S, Cerutti F, Piazza M, Clemente M, Chio A. Lamotrigine reduces total postoperative analgesic requirement: a randomized double-blind, placebo-controlled pilot study. Surgery. 1997;122(3):567–70.
67. Salimi A, Sabetkasaei M, Raisi H, et al. Carbamazepine effects on pain management and serum IL-6, IL-10 evaluation in addicted patients undergoing surgery. Eur J Pharmacol. 2017;812:184–8.
68. American Society of Anesthesiologists Task Force on Acute Pain Management. Practice guidelines for acute pain management in the perioperative setting: an updated report by the American Society

of Anesthesiologists Task Force on Acute Pain Management. Anesthesiology. 2012;116(2):248–73.
69. Cho C, Song K, Min B, et al. Multimodal approach to postoperative pain control in patients undergoing rotator cuff repair. Knee Surg Sports Traumatol Arthrosc. 2011;19(10):1744–8.
70. Beaudoin FL, Straube S, Lopez J, Mello MJ, Baird J. Prescription opioid misuse among ED patients discharged with opioids. Am J Emerg Med. 2014;32(6):580–5.
71. Keene DD, Rea WE, Aldington D. Acute pain management in trauma. Trauma. 2011;13(3):167–79.
72. Jarzyna D, Jungquist CR, Pasero C, et al. American Society for Pain Management Nursing guidelines on monitoring for opioid-induced sedation and respiratory depression. Pain Manag Nurs. 2011;12(3):118–45.
73. Barr J, Fraser GL, Puntillo K, et al. Clinical practice guidelines for the management of pain, agitation, and delirium in adult patients in the intensive care unit. Crit Care Med. 2013;41(1):263–306.
74. Joe CD, Pham TC, Sevak RJ, Moon YSK. Impact of inpatient pain pharmacist e-consults on post-discharge morphine equivalent daily doses. Presented at: PAINWeek 2020 Live Virtual Conference; September 11–13; virtual.
75. Sullivan D, Lyons M, Montgomery R, Quinlan-Colwell A. Exploring opioid-sparing multimodal analgesia options in trauma: a nursing perspective. J Trauma Nurs. 2016;23(6):361–75.
76. Rummans TA. Nonopioid agents for treatment of acute and sub-acute pain. Mayo Clin Proc. 1994;69:481–90.
77. Chang V, Gonzalez P, Akuthota V. Evidence-informed management of chronic low back pain with adjunctive analgesics. Spine J. 2008;8(1):21–7.
78. Bras M, Dordevic V, Gregurek R, Bulajic M. Neurobiological and clinical relationship between psychiatric disorders and chronic pain. Psychiatr Danub. 2010;22(2):221–6.
79. Dalacorte RR, Rigo JC, Dalacorte A. Pain management in the elderly at the end of life. North Am J Med Sci. 2011;3(8):348–54.
80. Weiner D, Hanlon J. Pain in nursing home residents: management strategies. Drugs Aging. 2001;18(1):13–29.
81. Nikolaus T, Zeyfang A. Pharmacological treatments for persistent non-malignant pain in older persons. Drugs Aging. 2004;21(1):19–41.
82. Chaparro LE, Wiffen PJ, Moore RA, Gilron I. Combination pharmacotherapy for the treatment of neuropathic pain in adults. Cochrane Database Syst Rev. 2012;(7):CD008943.
83. Colombo B, Annovazzi POL, Comi G. Neuropathic cranial pain. Neurol Sci. 2003;24(Suppl 2):S132–7.
84. Vu TH. Current pharmacologic approaches to treating neuropathic pain. Curr Pain Headache Rep. 2004;8(1):15–8.
85. Dwyer JP, Jayasekera C, Nicoll A. Analgesia for the cirrhotic patient: a literature review and recommendations. J Gastroenterol Hepatol. 2014;29(7):1356–60.
86. Reinert JP, Cook E. Oxcarbazepine-induced cutaneous reaction in a female of Mexican ancestry. J Pharm Technol. 2019;35(4):179–83.
87. Carrazana E, Mikoshiba I. Rationale and evidence for the use of oxcarbazepine in neuropathic pain. J Pain Symptom Manag. 2003;25(5 Suppl):S31–5.
88. Kupfer M, Formal CS. Non-opioid pharmacologic treatment of chronic spinal cord injury-related pain. J Spinal Cord Med. 2022;45(2):163–72.
89. Bennetto L, Patel NK, Fuller G. Trigeminal neuralgia and its management. BMJ. 2007;334(7586):201–5.
90. Kaye AD, Cornett EM, Hart B, et al. Novel pharmacological nonopioid therapies in chronic pain. Curr Pain Headache Rep. 2018;22(4):31.
91. Bialer M. Why are antiepileptic drugs used for nonepileptic conditions? Epilepsia. 2012;53(Suppl 7):26–33.
92. Faber CG, Attal N, Lauria G, et al. Efficacy and safety of vixotrigine in idiopathic or diabetes-associated painful small fibre neuropathy (CONVEY): a phase 2 placebo-controlled enriched-enrolment randomised withdrawal study. EClinicalMedicine. 2023;59:101971.

12 Ketamine

Abagail Barazi

Abbreviations

ADE	Adverse drug event
CYP450	Cytochrome P450
FDA	Food and Drug Administration
GABA	γ-aminobutyric acid
ICP	Intracranial pressure
IM	Intramuscular
IN	Intranasal
IV	Intravenous
IVP	Intravenous push
MME	Morphine milligram equivalents
NMDA	N-methyl-D-aspartate
NR2B	N-methyl-D-aspartate receptor subtype 2B
NRS	Numeric rating scale
OUD	Opiate-use disorder
PCA	Patient-controlled analgesia
PCP	Phencyclidine
PO	Oral
RCT	Randomized controlled trial
VAS	Visual analog scale

Introduction

Ketamine is an N-methyl-D-aspartate (NMDA) receptor antagonist that was first approved for use as an anesthetic in 1970 but has been found to be useful for many other indications since, including analgesia. In 1962, Parke Davis and Calvin Stevens developed ketamine as a structural analog with one-tenth of the potency of phencyclidine (PCP). It was first used in human trials in 1962 [1]. Since it is derived from PCP, ketamine can still trigger dissociative effects, although not as intensely as PCP [2]. In a 1966 study, ketamine was found to be a useful analgesic with a distinct altered consciousness and a limited duration of action. Compared to PCP, they found that ketamine did not cause severe emergence delirium or major side effects [1]. The Food and Drug Administration (FDA)–approved indication for ketamine is the induction and maintenance of anesthesia, although there are countless off-label uses [3].

Ketamine is commonly used for its sedative properties in the operating room and emergency department (ED) during procedures. However, when used for analgesia, ketamine is administered in low doses to avoid dissociative effects that can occur with higher doses. Its use has been found to be favorable in many clinical scenarios as it has little effect on hemodynamic stability and respiratory drive [4]. Multiple guidelines recommend ketamine as an appropriate adjunct analgesic agent in the perioperative setting, in critically ill patients, and in the sickle cell patient population, specifically when used in subanesthetic doses [5–7]. Many prospective, randomized controlled trials (RCTs) have also been performed, demonstrating the efficacy and safety of ketamine as an adjunct analgesic in various clinical scenarios. The remainder of this chapter will review the pharmacology of ketamine in pain, the evidence supporting its use, and safety considerations.

A. Barazi (✉)
Bon Secours Mercy Health St. Vincent Medical Center, Toledo, OH, USA
e-mail: akirwen@mercy.com

J. P. Reinert et al. (eds.), *Adjunctive Analgesic Strategies for the Bedside Clinician and Beyond*,
https://doi.org/10.1007/978-3-032-21675-5_12

Pharmacology, Pharmacokinetics, and Pharmacodynamics

Pain is processed through many receptors and routes in the body. Figure 12.1 provides a visual of this pathophysiology. NMDA receptors are located throughout the central nervous system, especially in areas responsible for the perception of pain [8]. Glutamate is released in response to a painful event, which then binds to NMDA receptors. This triggers a cascade, which may lead to opioid tolerance and opioid-induced hyperalgesia [4]. The activation of NMDA receptors can lead to central sensitization, which makes neurons more responsive to all inputs [9]. There are four subtypes of the NMDA receptor, labeled A through D. Type N-methyl-D-aspartate receptor subtype 2B (NR2B) is found in the limbic system, which is responsible for emotions and memory. The transmission of pain messages to the thalamus, spinal cord, and extrasynaptic locations is also facilitated by the NR2B receptor [8]. With prolonged opioid use, some patients develop opioid-induced hyperalgesia. When hyperalgesia occurs, the patient becomes hypersensitive to all stimuli, including stimuli that may not normally produce pain. Hyperalgesia is distinguishably different from opioid tolerance because it cannot be resolved by increasing the medication dose [10]. Phosphorylation of the NMDA receptor is essential for activation but also contributes to hyperalgesia and morphine interactions with the NMDA receptor. Ketamine's NMDA antagonism works against the hyperalgesia that can occur with prolonged opioid use, making it a useful resource for patients experiencing this phenomenon [8].

Ketamine's mechanism of action is depicted in Fig. 12.2. The primary receptor responsible for ketamine's mechanism of action is the NMDA receptor, where it is a noncompetitive antagonist. However, ketamine has been found to act on many other receptors as well, such as γ-aminobutyric acid (GABA), acetylcholine, dopamine, serotonin, and opioid receptors. The effects on the NMDA and opioid receptors are believed to be responsible for its analgesic effects [2]. Nociceptor stimulation signals the release of glutamate, which binds to postsynaptic NMDA

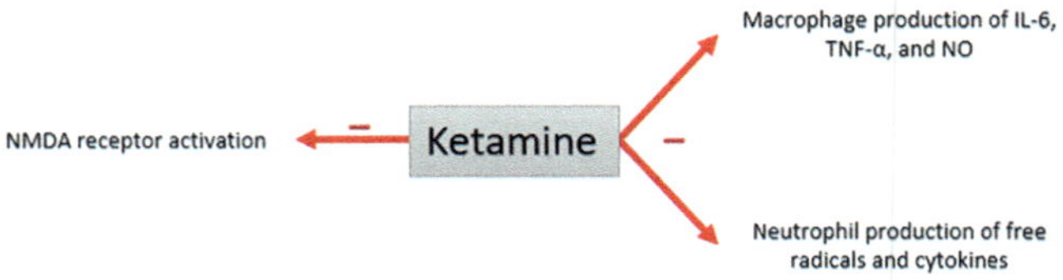

Fig. 12.2 Ketamine's mechanism of action [2, 9, 11]

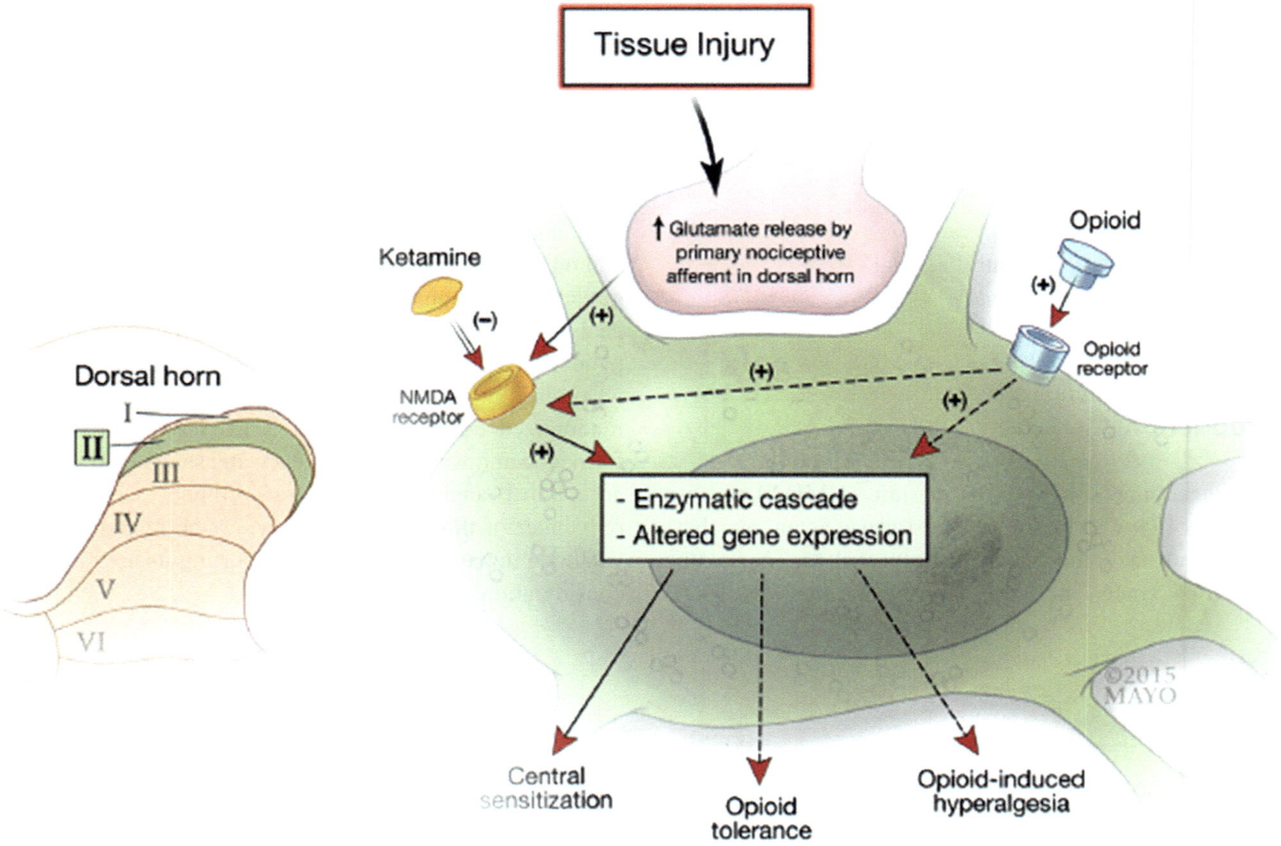

Fig. 12.1 Pain pathophysiology [3]

receptors, causing neuronal excitation and propagated pain signaling. Ketamine non-competitively antagonizes postsynaptic NMDA receptors through binding to the PCP binding site located within the NMDA receptor's Ca^{2+} ion channel pore. This decreases the channel's opening time and frequency, subsequently inhibiting glutamate's excitatory effects [9]. NMDA inhibition also reduces the activity of nitric oxide (NO) synthase, which is implicated in the downregulation and blunted response of opioid receptors that are associated with the pathophysiology of opioid-induced hyperalgesia [11]. Ketamine is believed to decrease the hypersensitization that occurs during opioid-induced hyperalgesia because of its effects on the NMDA receptor [2]. Ketamine modulates the production of inflammatory mediators in the central nervous system associated with pain through inhibiting the production of interleukin-6 (IL-6), tumor necrosis factor-α (TNF-α), and NO by macrophages, as well as the production of free radicals and cytokines by neutrophils [10]. Ketamine is formulated as a racemic mixture of S- and R-enantiomers [4]. However, it has been found that the S-enantiomer has a higher affinity for the PCP site of the NMDA receptor, with approximately three times the analgesic potency of R-ketamine [2]. The S-enantiomer, esketamine, is available as a nasal solution and has been approved for treatment-resistant depression but is not commonly used for analgesia. [12]

There are many routes of administration available for ketamine, including intravenous (IV), intramuscular (IM), oral (PO), and intranasal (IN), although the most common route is IV. When administered orally, racemic ketamine has a bioavailability of about 17–24%, whereas the S-enantiomer has an oral bioavailability of about 8–11% [13]. Fortunately, other routes have a higher bioavailability, with the IM route producing 90–93% bioavailability. Additionally, the IN route has around 45% bioavailability [14]. Distribution occurs rapidly, with a relatively large volume of distribution of approximately 3 L/kg. When given intravenously, ketamine has a rapid onset of action of 10–30 seconds and a duration of action of about 5–15 minutes. However, when given IM, the onset of action increases to 3–5 minutes, with a duration of action of about 15–30 minutes [15]. Metabolism occurs primarily in the liver though cytochrome P450 (CYP450) enzymes CYP2B6 and CYP3A4 via N-dealkylation to active and inactive metabolites. The active metabolite norketamine possesses approximately one-third the effects of ketamine. In addition to being metabolized by CYP enzymes, it is a major substrate of CYP2B6 and CYP3A4, which influences drug–drug interactions [11]. The alpha half-life of the drug is approximately 10–15 minutes [3]. Elimination occurs primarily via the kidneys, with the parent drug and metabolites excreted via the urine [2].

Evidence for Use

The 2018 consensus guidelines on the use of intravenous ketamine infusions for acute pain management from the American Society of Regional Anesthesia and Pain Medicine, the American Academy of Pain Medicine, and the American Society of Anesthesiologists provide multiple evidence-based recommendations on ketamine use. They state that subanesthetic ketamine infusion should be considered for patients undergoing painful surgery (grade B recommendation, moderate level of certainty). These guidelines also recommend that ketamine boluses should not exceed 0.35 mg/kg and infusions for acute pain generally should not exceed1 mg/kg/hour in settings without intensive monitoring (grade C recommendation, moderate level of certainty). Ketamine, at these subanesthetic doses, can be used as an adjunct to opioids for perioperative analgesia (grade B recommendation, moderate level of certainty) [6]. The use of ketamine is also included in the 2018 clinical practice guidelines for the prevention and management of pain, agitation/sedation, delirium, immobility, and sleep disruption in adult patients in the intensive care unit (ICU). These guidelines suggest using low-dose ketamine (0.5 mg/kg IV push × 1, followed by 1–2 mcg/kg/minute infusion) as an adjunct to opioid therapy when seeking to reduce opioid consumption in postsurgical adults admitted to the ICU (conditional recommendation, very low quality of evidence) [5]. The American Society of Hematology's 2020 guidelines for sickle cell disease management of acute and chronic pain also provide recommendations on ketamine use. These guidelines state that they suggest subanesthetic ketamine infusion as an adjunctive treatment of pain that is refractory or not effectively treated with opioids alone for adults and children presenting with sickle cell disease who are hospitalized (conditional recommendation based on very low certainty in the evidence about effects). The recommended dose starts at 0.1–0.3 mg/kg/hour, with a maximum of 1 mg/kg/hour [7].

Many randomized controlled trials have been conducted to evaluate the use of ketamine for the management of acute pain. These trials have included various populations, doses, and administration methods to determine the most effective treatment option(s). Low-dose ketamine is commonly described as a dose of <1 mg/kg, but an optimal dose for pain management has not been widely accepted. Some studies have evaluated various weight-based doses of ketamine that have helped guide clinicians on sub-dissociative dosing for analgesia.

Table 12.1 Ketamine versus placebo

Study	Design/population	Study groups	Results	Conclusion
16	Double-blind RCT Acute pain ≥6/10 in the ED n = 116	*Intervention* Ketamine 0.1 mg/kg IVP over 1 min + IV opioids *Comparator* Placebo + IV opioids	Average total opioid dose 2.86 MME lower in the ketamine group ($p = 0.0241$); final average pain scores 0.65 points lower in the ketamine group ($p = 0.0083$)	Ketamine reduces pain scores and overall MME requirements, although a higher ketamine dose may be needed
17	Double-blind RCT Nephrolithiasis and acute pain ≥6/10 in the ED $n = 106$	*Intervention* Ketamine 0.15 mg/kg IV + morphine 0.1 mg/kg IV (MK) *Comparator* Morphine 0.1 mg/kg IV + placebo (MP)	Lower pain scores at 10 ($p = 0.0019$) and30 min ($p = 0.003$) in the MK group; higher incidence of repeated morphine doses at 10 ($p = 0.005$) and 30 min ($p = 0.02$) in the MP group; the MP group experienced more side effects (oxygen saturation < 90%, nystagmus, nausea/vomiting, and hypotension)	Adjunct ketamine provides more pain relief than morphine monotherapy while reducing MME and adverse effects
18	Double-blind RCT Acute pain ≥5/10 in the ED $n = 60$	*Intervention* 1. Ketamine 0.15 mg/kg IV 2. Ketamine 0.3 mg/kg IV *Comparator* Morphine 0.1 mg/kg IV + placebo	Larger difference in pain intensity reduction from baseline in both ketamine doses versus placebo ($p = 0.02$); pain reduction was more sustained with ketamine 0.3 mg/kg; no difference in outcomes when comparing ketamine doses	Adjunct ketamine provides more pain relief than morphine monotherapy; 0.3 mg/kg may be the optimal ketamine dose
19	Double-blind RCT Acute on chronic pain ≥70/100 on VAS in the ED $n = 106$	*Intervention* 1. Ketamine 0.25 mg/kg IV over 20 min 2. Ketamine 0.5 mg/kg IV over 20 min *Comparator* Placebo	Pain reduction in both ketamine groups superior to placebo ($p = 0.001$); placebo required more rescue medications ($p = 0.03$); no difference in pain control at 24–48 hr. after treatment initiation; more ADEs associated with ketamine	Ketamine is superior to placebo in the treatment of acute on chronic pain but increases the risk of ADEs
20	Double-blind RCT Age ≥ 65 with three or more rib fractures from blunt force trauma $n = 59$	*Intervention* Ketamine 2 mcg/kg/min × 48 hr. + IV opioids *Comparator* Placebo + IV opioids	Majority of patients required ICU admission (86.4%) No difference in pain at 12–24 hr. ($p = 0.61$) or 24–48 hr. ($p = 0.17$); median opioid requirements reduced by 17 MME in the first 24 hr. with ketamine in the ISS ≥15 subgroup ($p = 0.04$)	Adjunct ketamine reduces opioid requirements in severe trauma patients but does not improve pain control

ADE Adverse drug event, *CI* Confidence interval, *ED* Emergency department, *IV* Intravenous, *RCT* Randomized control trial

Ketamine Monotherapy or as an Adjunct to Opioids

To establish the efficacy of ketamine as an analgesic, it has been compared to placebo as monotherapy or as an adjunct to opioid analgesics. These articles are summarized in Table 12.1. A randomized, double-blind, placebo-controlled trial was performed by Bowers and colleagues evaluating low-dose ketamine for pain [16]. Patients in the emergency department with a pain score of at least six out of ten who were being treated with IV opioids were randomized to ketamine 0.1 mg/kg IV push over one minute or an equivalent volume of normal saline. Although there was a significant difference in pain scores compared to placebo, there was only a difference of 0.65 points on a numeric rating scale (NRS) of 0–10. Patients in the ketamine group also required significantly lower doses of rescue opioids for pain management. The results of this trial still support the use of IV ketamine for analgesia but suggest that it may be more effective at doses higher than 0.1 mg/kg.

Ketamine has also been evaluated for use in the treatment of renal colic at a slightly higher dose. Abbasi and colleagues conducted a randomized, double-blind trial in adult patients with nephrolithiasis in the emergency department with a pain score of at least six out of ten [17]. Ketamine 0.15 mg/kg IV plus morphine 0.1 mg/kg IV was compared to placebo plus morphine 0.1 mg/kg IV. Significantly lower pain scores were reported in the ketamine group at 10 and 30 minutes after administration. Additionally, the placebo group required significantly more repeated doses of morphine at 10 and 30 minutes. In this trial, the addition of low-dose ketamine to morphine significantly decreased pain scores and opioid requirements.

To further evaluate the most appropriate dose of ketamine for pain, Beaudoin and colleagues conducted a randomized, double-blind, placebo-controlled trial in patients with acute pain in the emergency department [18]. Patients were included if they had a documented pain score of at least five out of ten on an NRS. Ketamine was administered IV at a dose of either 0.15 mg/kg, 0.3 mg/kg, or placebo as an adjunct to 0.1 mg/kg of IV morphine. Sixty patients were included in the study, and they found significantly better pain intensity differences in both ketamine groups. However, the group that received the 0.3-mg/kg dose of ketamine showed sustained pain relief at 2 hours after administration, whereas the 0.15-mg/kg dose of ketamine only showed more pain relief than placebo up to 30 minutes. The results of this trial support a dose of 0.3 mg/kg of ketamine as an adjunct to morphine for the treatment of moderate-to-severe pain.

Another trial compared a ketamine IV infusion of 0.25 mg/kg or 0.5 mg/kg to placebo in 106 patients with acute on chronic pain is an appropriate phrase this represents patients who have chronic pain that are experiencing a new episode of acute pain in addition to their already existing chronic pain-with a visual analog scale (VAS) score of at least 70 mm in the emergency department [19]. Both ketamine groups experienced superior pain reduction compared to placebo and required fewer rescue medications. Patients who received ketamine were more likely to experience adverse effects, including dizziness and nausea. Three patients in the 0.5-mg/kg group discontinued the study drug due to adverse effects and were not included in the analysis. Ketamine appears to be safe and effective for the treatment of acute on chronic pain, with the lower 0.25 mg/kg potentially being safer than 0.5 mg/kg.

Most trials evaluated ketamine as a single-dose IV push or IV infusion, but ketamine may also be administered as a continuous infusion to decrease opioid requirements [20]. Elderly patients with at least three rib fractures after blunt force trauma were randomized to either ketamine IV infusion 2 mcg/kg/min for 48 hours or placebo. There were 59 patients included; both groups were also given IV opioids, and the majority of these patients were admitted to the ICU. Numeric pain scores and opioid requirements were not different between groups at any time point. However, once patients were separated into two groups based on injury severity score (ISS), more severely injured patients (ISS ≥15) required lower doses of opioids. Based on these studies, ketamine may be used as an adjunct to opioids for moderate-to-severe acute pain in the emergency department and intensive care unit. The most effective and most commonly used dose appears to be approximately 0.3 mg/kg IV.

Ketamine Versus Morphine

There have also been studies conducted comparing ketamine to an active treatment such as morphine. These articles are summarized in Table 12.2. Jennings and colleagues evaluated the use of ketamine in the out-of-hospital setting for trauma analgesia [21]. Patients were included if they reported a pain score of at least five after receiving 5 mg of IV morphine. They included 135 patients who were then randomized to either ketamine 10–20 mg IV and then 10 mg every 3 minutes until pain-free or morphine 5 mg IV every 5 minutes until pain-free. Patients received a median total ketamine dose of 35 mg and a median total morphine dose of 15 mg. The ketamine group had significantly better reductions in pain scores on arrival to the emergency department (−5.6 for ketamine versus −3.2 for morphine), but the ketamine group had a higher rate of adverse effects. The most notable differences in adverse effects were disorientation, emergence phenomena, and increased systolic blood pressure (>180 mmHg). This study showed that ketamine significantly improved uncontrolled pain better than morphine alone in trauma patients in the out-of-hospital setting.

Table 12.2 Ketamine versus morphine

Study	Design	Study groups	Results	Conclusion
21	Open-label RCT Acute traumatic pain with a score > 5/10 after 5 mg morphine before hospital arrival *n* = 135	*Intervention* Ketamine 10–20 mg IV +10 mg every 3 min *Comparator* Morphine 5 mg IV every 5 min	Ketamine reduced mean pain scores by 2.4 points more than morphine (95% CI - 3.2—1.6); 26% had an increased risk of ADEs with ketamine (95% CI - 40.70—10.59)	Ketamine + morphine provides more pain reduction than morphine alone; adjunct ketamine may increase ADE risks
22	Double-blind RCT Acute pain ≥5/10 in the ED *n* = 45	*Intervention* Ketamine 0.3 mg/kg IV (max 25 mg) over 5 min every 20 min up to three doses *Comparator* Morphine 0.1 mg/kg IV (max 8 mg) over 5 min every 20 min up to three doses	No difference in overall pain reduction; the ketamine group achieved maximum pain reduction at 5 min, morphine achieved maximum at 100 min	Ketamine does not produce greater pain reduction than morphine; peak pain reduction occurs more rapidly with ketamine

ADE adverse drug event, *CI* confidence interval, *ED* emergency department, *IV* intravenous, *RCT* randomized control trial

Another prospective, randomized trial was performed by Miller and colleagues that compared ketamine to morphine in the emergency department [22]. Patients were included if they had pain of the back, flank, abdomen, or extremity that the treating clinician felt warranted IV opioids. Ketamine 0.3 mg/kg (max 25 mg) IV over 5 minutes was compared to morphine 0.1 mg/kg (max 8 mg) IV over 5 minutes. Both agents could be repeated every 20 minutes for a maximum of three doses. Similar numbers of patients in each group required repeat doses of their agents. Although ketamine did not show superior pain reduction compared to morphine, it was comparable to morphine and produced sustained pain control for two hours. Nearly all high-quality studies currently published in the literature compare ketamine to morphine or as an adjunct to opioid analgesics, so there is limited data on ketamine versus other opioid or non-opioid analgesics.

Perioperative Pain

Consensus guidelines were created by multiple organizations regarding the use of IV ketamine infusions for acute pain management [6]. They recommend the use of IV ketamine in perioperative patients with moderate-to-severe postoperative pain, opioid-tolerant patients, and as an adjunct to opioids for patients with sickle cell disease or obstructive sleep apnea. The optimal doses include a bolus of up to 0.35 mg/kg and/or an infusion rate of up to 1 mg/kg/hour, acknowledging that many patients may only need 0.1–0.5 mg/kg/hour. Relative contraindications for use include patients with poorly controlled cardiovascular disease, pregnancy, psychosis, hepatic disease, elevated intracranial pressure, and elevated intraocular pressure. Similarly, the Critical Care Medicine guidelines suggest low-dose ketamine (0.5-mg/kg IV push, followed by 1–2-mcg/kg/min infusion) as an adjunct to opioid therapy in postoperative intensive care unit patients [5]. When administered as a continuous infusion, ketamine is dosed in units of either mcg/kg/min or mg/kg/hour, which may lead to confusion among providers. For perspective, 1 mcg/kg/min is equivalent to 0.06 mg/kg/hour, whereas 1 mg/kg/hour is equivalent to 16.67 mcg/kg/min. Both guidelines recommend starting the infusion with low doses and increasing as needed or as tolerated.

Clinical trials have produced conflicting evidence on the benefits of ketamine in the perioperative setting, although most have shown positive results. These articles are summarized in Table 12.3. When compared to lidocaine in a randomized, double-blind, placebo-controlled trial of adults with opiate-use disorder (OUD), ketamine was found to provide inferior analgesia and opioid-sparing effects. Ketamine was administered as a 0.35 mg/kg IV bolus, followed by 0.2 mg/kg/hr. IV infusion, and lidocaine was administered as 1.5 mg/kg IV, followed by 2 mg/kg/hr. IV infusion. Additionally, ketamine led to higher rates of drowsiness [23]. Despite these

Table 12.3 Perioperative pain

Study	Design	Study groups	Results	Conclusion
23	Double-blind, double-dummy, parallel-group RCT Age 20–40 with OUD undergoing orthopedic surgery $n = 180$	*Intervention* 1. Ketamine 0.35 mg/kg IV bolus +0.2 mg/kg/hr 2. Lidocaine 1.5 mg/kg IV bolus +2 mg/kg/hr *Comparator* Placebo	Reduced pain scores and MME requirements in the lidocaine group versus the ketamine and placebo groups ($p < 0.001$); higher incidence of drowsiness with ketamine	Lidocaine provides better analgesia and is more opioid-sparing than ketamine and placebo in patients with OUD undergoing orthopedic surgery
24	Double-blind, parallel-group RCT Mechanically ventilated patients undergoing major abdominal surgery $n = 93$	*Intervention* 1. Ketamine 0.5 mg/kg IV +2 mcg/kg/min × 24 hr. +1 mcg/kg/min × 24 hr 2. Morphine PCA—2 mg bolus +1 mg every 7 min without limitation *Comparator* Morphine PCA—2 mg bolus +1 mg every 7 min without limitation	VAS similar throughout the first 48 hr.; total MME administration 22 ± 8 mg lower in the ketamine group ($p < 0.05$); similar incidence of ADEs between groups	Adjunct ketamine reduces opioid consumption by up to 25–30% in mechanically ventilated patients undergoing major abdominal surgery without increasing the incidence of ADEs
25	Meta-analysis of 70 randomized, double-blind, placebo-controlled trials Perioperative IV ketamine use $n = 4701$	*Intervention* IV ketamine + opioids *Comparator* Placebo + opioids	Ketamine decreased MME requirements ($p < 0.001$); greater effect in upper abdominal and thoracic surgeries, less effect in head and neck surgeries; largest reduction in MME seen in patients with baseline pain scores of 7/10 ($p < 0.001$); no reduction in MME seen in patients with baseline of 4/10 ($p = 0.268$)	Adjunct ketamine reduces postoperative opioid consumption with more efficacy in patients with severe pain; ketamine may be more efficacious for specific types of surgery

ADE adverse drug event; *IV* intravenous; *MME* morphine milligram equivalents; *OUD* opiate-use disorder; *PCA* patient-controlled analgesia; *RCT* randomized control trial; *VAS* visual analogue scale results, other trials and meta-analyses have shown that ketamine can be beneficial in surgical patient populations.

Surgical intensive care unit patients have been found to benefit from ketamine for analgesia after major abdominal surgery while mechanically ventilated. Ketamine, given as a 0.5-mg/kg IV bolus, followed by a 2-mcg/kg/min IV infusion for 24 hours, and then 1 mcg/kg/min for an additional 24 hours, reduced opioid consumption by approximately 25%–30% when compared to morphine patient-controlled analgesia. Despite reduced morphine requirements, visual analog scale pain scores were similar throughout the 48 hours of analgesia [24]. A large meta-analysis of randomized, double-blind, controlled trials found similar results with the use of perioperative ketamine. There were 70 studies with a total of 4701 patients included in the analysis. Ketamine significantly decreased opioid consumption, with the largest reduction seen in upper abdominal and thoracic surgery. Patients with higher pain scores of at least seven out of ten had the highest reduction in opioid consumption, while those with pain scores of four or lower had no reduction in consumption. It did not appear that the dose or method of administration (bolus versus infusion) produced any impact on efficacy [25]. In the perioperative setting, it appears that ketamine has the most benefit in critically ill patients with severe pain as an adjunct analgesic to reduce opioid consumption. More data is needed, but there may be no benefit with ketamine in the orthopedic surgery population and/or patients with a history of opiate-use disorder.

Special Populations

In addition to the surgical population, ketamine has been found to be beneficial for use in patients with sickle cell disease. The 2020 American Society of Hematology guidelines on the management of acute and chronic pain in sickle cell disease suggest that a subanesthetic ketamine infusion may be used as an adjunctive treatment of pain in hospitalized patients with sickle cell disease [7]. Most available studies on ketamine for sickle cell crisis have been conducted in the pediatric population, but there was a study published in 2022 in adult patients [26]. This was a blinded randomized trial in adult patients with acute sickle vaso-occlusive crisis in the emergency department. A total of 278 patients were randomized to either ketamine 0.3 mg/kg IV (138 patients) or morphine 0.1 mg/kg IV (140 patients)—both prepared in 100 mL of normal saline. There was not a significant difference in numeric pain scores between groups in Intention to treat and per protocol are how the study groups were analyzed and evaluated. This just explains different statistic methods utilized. Would not make any changes here ($p = 0.780$). However, cumulative morphine doses were significantly lower in the ketamine group (0.07 mg/kg in the ketamine group versus 0.13 mg/kg in the morphine group, $p < 0.001$), so it was concluded that ketamine may be used as an adjunct analgesic for sickle cell crisis in adult patients.

In pediatric patients, the highest-quality evidence for ketamine use in sickle cell disease comes from a study published in 2018 [27]. This was a prospective, randomized, double-blind trial in children aged 7–18 years with severe acutely painful sickle cell crisis. A total of 240 children (120 in each group) were enrolled and received either ketamine 1 mg/kg IV or morphine 0.1 mg/kg IV. There was no significant difference between groups in the primary outcome of percentage change in numeric pain score ($p = 0.18$). However, ketamine did provide maximum pain relief significantly faster than morphine (19.8 minutes with ketamine versus 34.1 minutes with morphine, $p < 0.001$). Another smaller retrospective study of 22 patients aged three years or older admitted to the hospital for vaso-occlusive sickle cell crisis was published in 2024 [28]. Ketamine infusions ranging from 0.02 to 0.21 mg/kg/hour led to significantly lower pain scores ($p < 0.05$) and reduced opioid requirements. Further studies are required in both sickle cell crisis and pediatric patients to determine the utility of ketamine as an analgesic agent, although currently available data shows promising results with its use as an adjunct to opioid analgesics.

Alternative Routes of Administration

While the IV route is the most common route of administration, IN administration may be favorable in some clinical scenarios. Patients may benefit from IN administration in the setting of difficult IV access, prehospital scenarios, or the pediatric population. An observational study of ketamine 0.5–0.75 mg/kg IN was conducted in emergency department patients who were six years or older, with a visual analog scale (VAS) score of 50 mm or greater [29]. Of the forty patients included, 35 patients (88%) achieved the primary outcome of a reduction in VAS of 13 mm or more within 30 minutes. Adverse effects were mild and transient, including dizziness, feelings of unreality, and nausea.

Intranasal ketamine has also been found to be effective in the out-of-hospital setting in a randomized, placebo-controlled trial [30]. A fixed dose of ketamine based on the patient's weight (approximately 0.5–1 mg/kg) was given to adult patients with an NRS of at least five in addition to usual care, which included nitrous oxide based on paramedic protocols. Significantly more patients in the ketamine group experienced a clinically significant reduction in their pain scores at 30 minutes, defined as a reduction of at least two points. Despite higher rates of mild adverse effects, patient satisfaction scores were higher in the ketamine group.

Finally, IN ketamine was compared to active comparators in a single-center, randomized trial [31]. Adult patients with VAS scores of at least 80 were randomized to either 1 mg/kg of IN ketamine, 0.1 mg/kg of IV morphine, or 0.15 mg/kg of IM morphine. Intranasal ketamine showed a

Table 12.4 Dosing considerations

	Dose	Additional considerations
Intravenous	0.25–0.5 mg/kg IV piggyback	Administer over 15 minutes
Intranasal	0.5–1 mg/kg IN	Use a high concentration formulation, such as 50 mg/mL or 100 mg/mL, to decrease volume
Intramuscular	Not studied well enough to provide a dose recommendation at this time Consider IV doses, given the high IM bioavailability	Use a high concentration formulation, such as 50 mg/mL or 100 mg/mL, to decrease volume

similar time to onset of pain relief of approximately 14 minutes, whereas IV morphine was effective in approximately 9 minutes and IM morphine in 26 minutes. Higher rates of adverse effects were seen with IN ketamine, including dizziness, confusion, and difficulty concentrating. The results of these trials prove that a dose of 0.75–1 mg/kg of IN ketamine may be a favorable alternative to opioids in settings where IV access is difficult or not possible.

Dosing Considerations

There are many uses for ketamine, and its various effects are dose-dependent. In addition to its many uses, there are many routes and methods of administration, which can lead to confusion and potential for error. Most importantly, when being used for analgesia, ketamine should be administered at a dose of <1 mg/kg IV to avoid dissociative and anesthetic effects. Table 12.4 includes dose recommendations and additional considerations for the various routes of administration. With a wide variety of concentrations available, dual-verification methods should be considered to ensure that the correct dose and volume are being administered. Finally, when administering as a continuous infusion, the units should be carefully reviewed (mcg/kg/min versus mg/kg/hour) to confirm the appropriate units.

Safety

Although ketamine generally has a favorable safety profile, there are still concerning side effects to monitor patients for. Ketamine has the potential to cause transient increases in blood pressure and heart rate, and vital signs should be monitored during use. Important monitoring parameters include blood pressure, heart rate, pulse oximetry, and mental status. Fortunately, patients seem to have a preserved respiratory drive, unlike in other analgesics such as opioids, which is an advantage of ketamine over other analgesics. Ketamine does not have a therapeutic range, so there is no need to monitor blood levels for efficacy or toxicity. It was initially believed that ketamine causes an increase in intracranial pressure (ICP); however, many studies have since proven this is likely not the case. A review of the literature that included small, prospective, randomized trials in ventilated patients showed that continuous infusion of ketamine does not lead to an increase in ICP. In fact, this review found that bolus doses of ketamine may actually lower ICP. Ketamine may be considered for use in patients with traumatic brain injury or other populations with elevated ICP [32].

Some patients may experience an emergence reaction while recovering from anesthetic doses, which can manifest as excitement, delirium, irrational behavior, and other symptoms [8]. Some side effects can be prevented or reduced depending on how the medication is administered. Slower administration times have been associated with a decreased risk of hallucinations and feelings of unreality. For instance, Motov and colleagues conducted a prospective, randomized, double-blind, double-dummy trial in patients with abdominal, flank, back, traumatic chest, or musculoskeletal pain [33]. Ketamine 0.3 mg/kg was administered as either an IV push over 5 minutes or an IV infusion over 15 minutes. Adverse effects were relatively similar between groups, but the IV push group experienced higher rates of feeling of unreality and higher rates of sedation. There were no reported differences in rates of agitation. This trial supports a slower administration of IV ketamine to reduce the risk of side effects. Additionally, Clattenburg and colleagues evaluated IV push versus IV infusion ketamine in a prospective, randomized, double-blind, double-dummy trial [34]. Ketamine 0.3 mg/kg was administered as either an IV push over 1 minute or an IV infusion over 15 minutes. There were 59 patients included in the trial who had a pain score of at least five out of ten. When administered as an IV push, ketamine led to higher rates of unreality and hallucinations than the IV infusion group. Pain scores were similar between groups at 60 minutes. Based on the results of this trial, an IV infusion of ketamine produces similar pain control and fewer side effects than an IV push.

Drug–drug interactions are an additional aspect to consider. Ketamine is a major substrate of both CYP2B6 and CYP3A4, which may influence drug interactions [7]. However, nearly all drug–drug interactions of concern with ketamine are due to its effects on mental status. Use of concomitant medications that cause sedation and central nervous system depression should be considered carefully, with potentially increased monitoring. Special populations require additional attention to determine the appropriate use of medications. The use of ketamine in the pediatric population was discussed earlier and is considered safe and effective for analgesia in pediatric patients with sickle cell disease. Another special population to consider is pregnant patients [25–27]. Ketamine use in pregnancy, including obstetrics, is not recommended because safe use has not been well-established [3].

Conclusions

Ketamine has plenty of evidence supporting its use as an adjunct agent for analgesia in various settings, such as the emergency department, intensive care unit, perioperative setting, and sickle cell vaso-occlusive crisis. Importantly, it may not be effective when used as a first-line analgesic, and most of the available data supports its use in addition to an opioid or after the patient has failed opioid therapy. When used as an adjunct analgesic agent, ketamine has also been shown to produce opioid-sparing effects. It appears that the most effective dose for the treatment of pain is approximately 0.3 mg/kg, which should be given as an IV infusion over 15 minutes, as opposed to IV push, to avoid negative psychoactive effects. In the perioperative setting, the same bolus dose is appropriate, which may then be followed by a dose of 1–2 mcg/kg/min (0.06–1.2 mg/kg/hr), titrated to effect. Although the intramuscular route appears to be a promising route of administration with high bioavailability, it has not been widely studied for pain management. An intranasal dose of 0.75–1 mg/kg may be considered in settings where IV access is not preferred.

Ketamine has been proven to be relatively safe, with preserved respiratory drive unlike other commonly used analgesics. Important monitoring parameters during and after ketamine administration include blood pressure, heart rate, pulse oximetry, and mental status. Patients should also be monitored for emergence reactions, although they are less common with slowly administered sub-dissociative doses used for analgesia, as opposed to anesthetic doses.

Acknowledgments We would like to acknowledge Cole Jerousek, PharmD candidate for compiling literature into tables and creating a mechanism of action figure.

References

1. Li L, Vlisides PE. Ketamine: 50 years of modulating the mind. Front Hum Neurosci. 2016;10(612)
2. Zanos P, Moaddel R, Morris PJ, et al. Ketamine and ketamine metabolite pharmacology: insights into therapeutic mechanisms. Pharmacol Rev. 2018;70(3):621–60.
3. Ketalar (ketamine) [Package insert]. Chestnut Ridge: Par Pharmaceutical, Inc; Updated 3/2022.
4. Gorlin AW, Rosenfeld DM, Ramakrisna H. Intravenous sub-anesthetic ketamine for perioperative analgesia. J Anaesthesiol Clin Pharmacol. 2016;32(2):160–7.
5. Devlin JW, Skrobik Y, Gelinas C, et al. Clinical practice guidelines for the prevention and management of pain, agitation/sedation, delirium, immobility, and sleep disruption in adult patients in the ICU. Crit Care Med. 2018;46(9):e825–73.
6. Schwenk ES, Viscusi ER, Buvanendran A, et al. Consensus guidelines on the use of intravenous ketamine infusions for acute pain management from the American society of regional anesthesia and pain medicine, the American academy of pain medicine, and the American society of anesthesiologists. Reg Anesth Pain Med. 2018;43:456–66.
7. Brandow AM, Carroll CP, Creary S, et al. American Society of Hematology 2020 guidelines for sickle cell disease: management of acute and chronic pain. Am Soc Hematol. 2020;4(12):2656–701.
8. Mion G, Villevielle T. Ketamine pharmacology: an update (pharmacodynamics and molecular aspects, recent findings). CNS Neurosci Ther. 2013;19(6):370–80.
9. Bennett GJ. Update on the neurophysiology of pain transmission and modulation: focus on the NMDA-receptor. J Pain Symptom Manag. 2000;19:S2–6.
10. Mercadante S, Arcuri E, Santoni A. Opioid-induced tolerance and hyperalgesia. CNS Drugs. 2019;33:943–55.
11. Nowacka A, Borcyk M. Ketamine applications beyond anesthesia. Eur J Pharmacol. 2019;860:172547.
12. Spravato (esketamine) [package insert]. Titusville: Janssen Pharmaceuticals, Inc. Updated 10/2023.
13. Fanta S, Kinnunen M, Backman JT, et al. Population pharmacokinetics of S-ketamine and norketamine in healthy volunteers after intravenous and oral dosing. Eur J Clin Pharmacol. 2015;71:441–7.
14. Yanagihara Y, Ohtani M, Kariya S, et al. Plasma concentration profiles of ketamine and norketamine after administration of various ketamine preparations to healthy Japanese volunteers. Biopharm Drug Dispos. 2003;24:37–43.
15. Rosenbaum SB, Gupta V, Patel P, et al. In: StatPearls [Internet]. Treasure Island: StatPearls Publishing; 2024. Available from: https://www.ncbi.nlm.nih.gov/books/NBK470357/.
16. Bowers KJ, McAllister KB, Ray M, et al. Ketamine as an adjunct to opioids for acute pain in the emergency department: a randomized controlled trial. Acad Emerg Med. 2017;24(6):676–85.
17. Abbasi S, Bidi N, Mahshidfar B, et al. Can low-dose of ketamine reduce the need for morphine in renal colic? A double-blind randomized clinical trial. Am J Emerg Med. 2018;36:376–9.
18. Beaudoin FL, Lin C, Guan W, et al. Low-dose ketamine improves pain relief in patients receiving intravenous opioids for acute pain in the emergency department: results of a randomized, double-blind, clinical trial. Acad Emerg Med. 2014;21(11):1193–202.
19. Lumanauw DD, Youn S, Horeczko T, et al. Subdissociative ketamine is effective for treating acute exacerbations of chronic pain. Acad Emerg Med. 2019;26(9):1044–51.
20. Kugler NW, Carver TW, Juul J, et al. Ketamine infusion for pain control in elderly patients with multiple rib fractures: results of a randomized controlled trial. J Trauma Acute Care Surg. 2019;87(5):1181–8.
21. Jennings PA, Cameon P, Bernard S, et al. Morphine and ketamine is superior to morphine for out-of-hospital trauma analgesia: a randomized controlled trial. Ann Emerg Med. 2012;59:497–503.
22. Miller JP, Schauer SG, Ganem VJ, et al. Low-dose ketamine vs morphine for acute pain in the ED: a randomized controlled trial. Am J Emerg Med. 2015;33:402–8.
23. Sahmeddini MA, Khosravi MB, Farbood A. Comparison of perioperative systemic lidocaine or systemic ketamine in acute pain management of patients with opioid use disorder after orthopedic surgery. J Addict Med. 2019;13:220–6.
24. Guillou N, Tanguy M, Seguin P, et al. The effects of small-dose ketamine on morphine consumption in surgical intensive care unit patients after major abdominal surgery. Anesth Analg. 2003;97:843–7.
25. Laskowski K, Stirling A, McKay WP, et al. A systematic review of intravenous ketamine for postoperative analgesia. Can J Anesth. 2011;58:911–23.

26. Alshahrani MS, AlSulaibikh AH, ElTahan MR, et al. Ketamine administration for acute painful sickle cell crisis: a randomized controlled trial. Acad Emerg Med. 2022;29:150–8.
27. Lubega FA, DeSilva MS, Munube D, et al. Low dose ketamine versus morphine for acute severe vaso occlusive pain in children: a randomized controlled trial. Scand J Pain. 2018;18(1):19–27.
28. Onyebuchi CO, Chumpitazi CE, Placencia JK, et al. Ketamine for pain in sickle cell disease reduces opioid usage. J Pain Symptom Manag. 2024;67(3):e169–75.
29. Andolfatto G, Willman E, Joo D, et al. Intranasal ketamine for analgesia in the emergency department: a prospective observational series. Acad Emerg Med. 2013;20:1050–4.
30. Andolfatto G, Innes K, Dick W, et al. Prehospital analgesia with intranasal ketamine (PAIN-K): a randomized, double-blind trial in adults. Ann Emerg Med. 2019;74:241–50.
31. Shimonovich S, Gigi R, Shapira A, et al. Intranasal ketamine for acute traumatic pain in the emergency department: a prospective, randomized clinical trial of efficacy and safety. BMC Emerg Med. 2016;16(43):1–9.
32. Zeiler FA, Teitelbaum J, West M, et al. The ketamine effect on ICP in traumatic brain injury. Neurocrit Care. 2014;21:163–73.
33. Motov S, Mai M, Pushkar I, et al. A prospective, randomized, double-dummy trial comparing IV push low dose ketamine to short infusion of low dose ketamine for treatment of pain in the ED. Am J Emerg Med. 2017;35:1095–100.
34. Clattenburg EJ, Hailozian C, Haro D, et al. Slow infusion of low-dose ketamine reduces bothersome side effects compared to intravenous push: a double-blind, double-dummy, randomized controlled trial. Acad Emerg Med. 2018;25(9):1048–52.

Antipsychotics

13

Austin Smith and Justin P. Reinert

Abbreviations

5-HT	Serotonin
ACh	Acetylcholine
BPS	Bladder pain syndrome
CGli	Clinical Globcal Impression
CNS	Central nervous system
CPK	Creatinine phosphokinase
CVD	Cardiovascular disease
D	Dopamine
EPS	Extrapyramidal symptoms
FGA	First-generation antipsychotic
FGI	Fibromyalgia Impact Questionnaire
FGID	Functional gastrointestinal disorder
FM	Fibromyalgia
mAChRs	Muscarinic acetylcholine receptors
MORs	μ-opioid receptors
NMDA	N-methyl-D-aspartate
NMS	Neuroleptic malignant syndrome
PAG	Periaqueductal gray
PSQI	Pittsburgh Sleep Quality Index
SGA	Second-generation antipsychotic
SSRI	Selective serotonin reuptake inhibitor
TD	Tardive dyskinesia
XR	Extended-release

A. Smith (✉)
Robert J. Dole VA Medical Center, Wichita, KS, USA
e-mail: AustinM.Smith@va.gov

J. P. Reinert
The University of Toledo, College of Pharmacy and Pharmaceutical Sciences, Toledo, OH, USA

Background/Introduction

The perception of pain is a complex process impacted by various factors. It is a physical and emotional experience, involving peripheral and central desensitization. Beginning at nociceptors, or nerve endings that interpret pain, pain travels an ascending pathway from the periphery to the dorsal horn of the spinal cord. Pain can lead to extreme debilitation, impacting functioning and quality of life. Pain can also directly influence mood, emotions, and psychiatric symptoms. Furthermore, underlying psychiatric conditions can exacerbate and influence the experience of pain [1]. Not surprisingly, chronic pain is a predictor of comorbid psychiatric diagnoses, and psychiatric diagnoses are a strong predictive factor of persisting chronic pain [2].

Treatment of pain remains suboptimal. In a cohort study examining the rates of acute and chronic pain among over 10,000 adults in the United States from 2019 to 2020, 38.9% of patients reported experiencing non-chronic pain and 20.8% reported experiencing chronic pain [3]. Certain types of pain conditions, such as fibromyalgia, can be particularly difficult to treat and have limited treatment options [4].

Consideration of alternative treatments and augmentation strategies is important to expand options for pain treatment. Due to risks of chronic opioid use for pain, adjunctive medication options that may lower both pain and opioid requirements may be preferred [5].

Antipsychotic medications can be considered for use as an adjunctive option for the treatment of pain. While limited literature exists and their use is somewhat controversial, there is evidence suggesting benefit in certain types of pain, including fibromyalgia, cancer pain, neuropathic pain, and headaches [6]. While having a likely lower risk than chronic opioid use, antipsychotic medications carry certain risks to patients, which may impact utility in practice.

J. P. Reinert et al. (eds.), *Adjunctive Analgesic Strategies for the Bedside Clinician and Beyond*,
https://doi.org/10.1007/978-3-032-21675-5_13

Pharmacology, Pharmacokinetics, and Pharmacodynamics

Antipsychotics are complex due to their expansive receptor-binding profiles [6]. While some studies exist evaluating the use of first-generation antipsychotics (FGAs), or typical antipsychotic medications, there is greater available literature evaluating the use of second-generation antipsychotic (SGA) medications, or atypical antipsychotic medications, which will be focused on in this chapter. FGAs have less selectivity at dopamine receptors than SGAs, allowing for antagonism of dopamine at various unintended sites. Dopamine blockade downstream can lead to undesirable side effects. SGAs have lower binding affinity at the dopamine D_2 receptors and greater binding at 5-HT_{2a} serotonin receptors, corresponding with fewer side effects than FGAs [2, 6]. While the receptor-binding profile of antipsychotics is extensive, the focus of this chapter will be on receptor systems that are theorized to impact pain. Due to variation in receptor binding and potency, the mechanism of pain relief may vary between specific antipsychotics [6].

Dopamine (D)

Dopamine action has an established role in the experience of pain. It is thought to contribute to the experience of "priming," which is a state in which neuroplastic changes prolong hyperalgesia. Dopamine antagonism may reverse this priming [7]. There is evidence that migraine with aura is associated with increased frequency of D_2 allele genes, and people experiencing migraine are more likely to experience dopaminergic symptoms (nausea, vomiting, sedation, dizziness, and sweating) after dopamine agonist administration [7]. Supporting this theory, certain dopamine antagonist medications can be used for the treatment of migraines. Antidopaminergic properties of SGAs, such as olanzapine, may explain evidence suggesting the efficacy of use in the treatment of migraines and other pain conditions [8]. While D_2 receptors are most commonly implicated with antipsychotic medications, all of the dopamine receptor subtypes may have a clinical role in analgesia.

Dopamine receptors, classified into D_1-like (D_1 and D_5) and D_2-like (D_2, D_3, and D_4) families, play nuanced and region-specific roles in pain perception and modulation [9]. These G protein–coupled receptors are distributed throughout key nociceptive and modulatory regions of the central nervous system (CNS), including the striatum, nucleus accumbens, periaqueductal gray (PAG), thalamus, spinal cord, and prefrontal cortex. The involvement of dopamine in pain is biphasic, contributing both to the facilitation and inhibition of nociception, depending on the receptor subtype, site of action, and disease state [9].

D_1-like receptors (D_1 and D_5) are typically excitatory, coupling to G proteins and stimulating adenylate cyclase activity, leading to increased intracellular cyclic adenosine monophosphate (cAMP). Preclinical studies indicate that D_1 receptor activation in the spinal cord and basal ganglia can facilitate nociceptive transmission, particularly under acute pain conditions [10, 11]. However, in supraspinal areas, such as the prefrontal cortex and the limbic system, D_1 receptor activation may contribute to pain inhibition by enhancing cognitive and emotional coping mechanisms [11]. The role of D_5 receptors in pain remains less well-characterized, but their co-localization with D_1 receptors suggests a possible synergistic role in modulating both motor and affective components of pain [10].

D_2-like receptors (D_2, D_3, and D_4) are generally inhibitory, reducing cAMP production and modulating ion channel activity. D_2 receptors are the most well-studied in this group and have a prominent role in descending inhibitory pain pathways. Activation of D_2 receptors in the PAG and spinal cord can lead to antinociceptive effects by inhibiting excitatory neurotransmitter release and enhancing inhibitory tone [12].

D_3 receptors, predominantly located in the limbic system, appear to regulate the emotional and motivational–affective dimensions of pain. D_3 receptor agonism has shown analgesic effects in neuropathic and inflammatory pain models, potentially by modulating mesolimbic reward circuits that influence pain salience and affective distress [13]. D_4 receptors, while less well-understood, are implicated in modulating cortical and thalamic excitability and may contribute to the sensory–discriminative aspects of pain. Some experimental models suggest that D_4 receptor modulation could influence response to chronic stress–induced hyperalgesia [14].

Collectively, the dopamine system exerts layered control over multiple dimensions of pain: sensory, affective, cognitive, and motivational. Pharmacologic manipulation of dopamine receptors, either through agonism or antagonism, may yield therapeutic benefits depending on the pain phenotype. Importantly, the analgesic effect of dopamine receptor modulation appears context-dependent, and an agent's net impact on pain can vary based on its receptor selectivity, central versus peripheral action, and interaction with other neurotransmitter systems, such as serotonin, norepinephrine (NE), and opioids.

Serotonin (5-HT)

One of the most important functions of SGAs is binding at serotonin receptors, including 5-HT_{2A}, 5-HT_{1A}, and 5-HT_{2C}. As discussed within the antidepressant chapter, the serotoninergic system helps maintain homeostasis [15].

Nociceptors and neurons in the central nervous system (CNS) that receive input show neuroplasticity in response to injury. In this case, serotonergic effects may potentiate pain [16]. It is reasonable to conclude that medications that impact the serotonergic system may offer benefit in the treatment of pain.

Activation of the 5-HT_{1A} receptor, which is primarily inhibitory and widely expressed in the dorsal raphe nucleus and limbic regions, has been associated with antinociceptive effects in both preclinical and clinical models. This receptor modulates descending serotonergic pathways, promoting inhibitory neurotransmission in the spinal cord and reducing the transmission of nociceptive signals [17]. Partial agonism at 5-HT_{1A}, seen with some second-generation antipsychotics such as aripiprazole, may contribute to analgesic effects and enhanced tolerability.

In contrast, 5-HT_{2A} receptors are primarily excitatory and are implicated in the facilitation of pain, particularly in chronic and inflammatory states [18]. These receptors are expressed in high densities in the cortex, limbic system, and dorsal horn of the spinal cord, where they potentiate glutamatergic transmission and enhance central sensitization. Antagonism of 5-HT_{2A} receptors, common among SGAs such as risperidone, olanzapine, and quetiapine, has been shown to attenuate hyperalgesia and allodynia in animal models, suggesting a beneficial role in chronic pain states [15]. Antagonism by SGAs at 5-HT_{2A} receptors also stimulates downstream dopamine release, leading to lower side effect incidence with SGAs when compared to FGAs and greater tolerability in practice [19]. Similarly, 5-HT_{2C} receptors, which are predominantly inhibitory, also modulate pain signaling, though their role appears to be context- and region-dependent. In some cases, 5-HT_{2C} receptor activation has been linked to antinociception, likely through the modulation of gamma-aminobutyric acid (GABA)ergic interneurons and descending monoaminergic pathways. However, overstimulation may produce anxiety and exacerbate pain perception under certain conditions. Therefore, antagonism at 5-HT_{2C}, also seen with SGAs, may contribute to anxiolysis and indirect pain relief, particularly in patients with comorbid mood disorders [6]. Together, the modulation of these serotonergic receptors by antipsychotic medications reflects a promising, though underutilized, avenue for adjuvant analgesia in complex pain syndromes.

α-Adrenoreceptors (α_1 and α_2)

There is some evidence within animal models that the antinociceptive effect of antipsychotic medications is mediated by agonistic activity at a_1-adrenorecetpors [20, 21]. An understanding of the role of alpha-receptors in the context of pain is important in recognizing the utility of antipsychotics that mediate these receptors.

α-adrenergic receptors, specifically α_1 and α_2 subtypes, play significant but divergent roles in pain modulation, with growing clinical and preclinical evidence supporting their relevance in analgesia [20, 21]. These G protein–coupled receptors mediate the effects of norepinephrine in the peripheral and central nervous systems and are differentially expressed in key pain pathways, including the spinal dorsal horn, brain stem, and locus coeruleus. Their activation can either facilitate or inhibit nociception, depending on the receptor subtype and location [20, 21].

α_1-adrenergic receptors are postsynaptic and typically excitatory, coupling to Gq proteins and stimulating phospholipase C, leading to increased intracellular calcium. Although α_1 receptor activation is traditionally associated with vasoconstriction and sympathomimetic effects, there is some evidence suggesting that it may contribute to analgesic effects via non-opioid pathways, particularly in the context of atypical antipsychotics. For example, olanzapine, which exhibits modest α_1 antagonism, demonstrated antinociceptive effects in rodent models independent of the endogenous opioid system [22]. The mechanism may involve downstream inhibition of excitatory neurotransmission in the spinal cord or modulation of stress-related arousal circuits that influence pain perception. While direct clinical trials are limited, the sedative and anxiolytic properties of α_1 antagonism, common to agents like quetiapine and risperidone, may provide indirect benefit in chronic pain conditions, where anxiety and hypervigilance contribute to pain amplification [23].

Histaminergic Receptors (H1 and H2)

Histaminergic pathways, particularly via H1 and H2 receptors, are also implicated in pain transmission and modulation. Histamine (HA) exerts a pro-nociceptive effect peripherally but may have both excitatory and inhibitory roles in the CNS, depending on the receptor subtype and site of action. Activation of H1 receptors is generally associated with increased nociception, while H2 receptor activation has been shown in animal models to exert an analgesic effect, possibly through the modulation of cAMP and downstream signaling in the spinal cord and thalamus [24]. While H1 receptor antagonists are known to contribute to sedation and weight gain, they may also play a role in pain perception. Sedation itself may indirectly modulate pain by improving sleep and reducing the subjective experience of pain, particularly in chronic conditions [25].

Moreover, H1 antagonism may decrease neuronal excitability, thereby reducing central sensitization.

Acetylcholine (M1)

Acetylcholine (ACh) plays a nuanced role in nociceptive signaling, with both pro- and antinociceptive effects depending on the receptor subtype and anatomic location [26]. Muscarinic acetylcholine receptors (mAChRs), particularly the M1 subtype, are widely distributed in the central nervous system and contribute to cognitive processing, arousal, and the modulation of pain [26]. Medications such as clozapine and olanzapine possess high affinity for muscarinic receptors and act predominantly as M1 antagonists [27]. While anticholinergic effects are often associated with undesirable outcomes such as cognitive impairment and dry mouth, preclinical and translational research suggests that central muscarinic antagonism may also contribute to analgesia by dampening cortical arousal and reducing the emotional–affective component of pain perception [28]. Muscarinic blockade in the anterior cingulate cortex and spinal cord resulted in decreased nociceptive behavior, implicating ACh in central sensitization and chronic pain states [26]. SGAs with antimuscarinic properties may offer a unique analgesic mechanism through the attenuation of central cholinergic tone, especially in chronic or neuropathic pain contexts where affective processing is heightened. While the analgesic contribution of ACh antagonism by SGAs requires further clinical validation, existing evidence supports its relevance as part of the multimodal receptor activity that may underlie the pain relief observed with certain SGAs [26–28].

Glutamate (N-Methyl-D-Aspartate)

Glutamate is the principal excitatory neurotransmitter in the central nervous system and plays a pivotal role in pain processing, particularly in central sensitization, hyperalgesia, and the development of chronic pain states [29]. The N-methyl-D-aspartate (NMDA) receptor, a subtype of glutamate receptor, is especially important in the amplification and persistence of nociceptive signals. While second-generation antipsychotics (SGAs) do not directly antagonize glutamate receptors, emerging evidence suggests that they may modulate glutamatergic transmission indirectly, contributing to antinociceptive effects [30]. For instance, clozapine and olanzapine have been shown to downregulate cortical glutamate levels and may influence NMDA receptor function via their modulatory effects on dopaminergic and serotonergic pathways, both of which tightly regulate glutamate release and reuptake [31]. Additionally, SGAs may reduce glutamate excitotoxicity and central sensitization by enhancing GABAergic tone and reducing neuroinflammation, processes that are increasingly recognized in chronic pain syndromes [30, 31]. Preclinical models support this mechanism; for example, clozapine was found to inhibit pain behavior in animal models of neuropathy through mechanisms partially dependent on glutamatergic modulation [32]. Thus, although indirect, the impact of SGAs on glutamate signaling represents a potential mechanism for analgesia, particularly in conditions involving dysfunctional excitatory neurotransmission, such as fibromyalgia, neuropathic pain, and migraine [33, 34]. Further clinical studies are warranted to delineate which SGAs offer the most robust glutamate-mediated analgesic benefit [34].

Endogenous Opioids

Neurotransmitter interactions with endogenous opioids and opioid receptors represent a compelling and biologically plausible mechanism through which SGAs may exert antinociceptive effects [35]. Several lines of evidence suggest that SGAs modulate pain not only through classical dopaminergic and serotonergic pathways but also by influencing the opioidergic system, a key component of the body's intrinsic pain control network [35].

As elucidated by Schreiber et al., antinociceptive effects observed with SGAs such as olanzapine may, in part, be mediated through indirect interactions with μ-opioid receptors (MORs) [22]. In rodent models, olanzapine demonstrated significant analgesic activity in the formalin pain test, an established model of inflammatory pain, even when administered in the absence of exogenous opioids. Interestingly, this effect was attenuated but not abolished by naloxone, an opioid receptor antagonist, suggesting that SGAs may enhance or modulate the function of endogenous opioids rather than acting as direct opioid receptor agonists. This implies a synergistic or facilitatory role of SGAs in endogenous opioid signaling pathways [22].

Further support comes from clinical and neurochemical studies demonstrating that dopaminergic neurotransmission is functionally interconnected with opioid receptor activity, especially in pain-related brain regions such as the periaqueductal gray (PAG), nucleus accumbens, and anterior cingulate cortex [36]. Disturbances in dopamine pathways, such as those observed in fibromyalgia and other chronic pain conditions, may lead to reduced activation of opioid-mediated descending pain inhibition. This is consistent with findings that dopaminergic activity enhances the release of endogenous opioids, contributing to analgesia via indirect activation of MORs [37]. Therefore, D_2 receptor antagonism by SGAs may help restore balance in dopaminergic–opioidergic circuits, thereby normalizing pain processing in certain patient populations.

While more research is warranted to fully elucidate these mechanisms, the available preclinical and clinical data sug-

Table 13.1 SGA receptor activity [7–37]

Neurotransmitter	Receptor subtype(s)	SGA activity	Clinical/pharmacologic effects	Examples of SGA-targeting receptors
Dopamine (DA)	D_2	Antagonist (low-to-moderate affinity)	Antipsychotic effect; less extrapyramidal symptoms; modulates pain via opioid–dopaminergic pathways	Risperidone, olanzapine, quetiapine, clozapine, paliperidone
	D_2/D_3	Partial agonist	Stabilizes dopamine tone; may reduce hyperalgesia	Aripiprazole, brexpiprazole, cariprazine
	D_3	Antagonist/partial agonist	Modulation of emotional pain, reward, and cognition	Cariprazine (high D_3 affinity)
	D_1/D_4	Antagonist (less studied)	Potential cognitive and mood modulation	Clozapine (moderate D_4 affinity)
Serotonin (5-HT)	5-HT_2A	Antagonist	Enhances dopamine release; contributes to analgesia and reduced side effects	Risperidone, olanzapine, quetiapine, clozapine, ziprasidone
	5-HT_1A	Partial agonist	Anxiolysis; mood enhancement; facilitates descending pain inhibition	Aripiprazole, ziprasidone, lurasidone
	5-HT_2C	Antagonist	Improves sleep and mood; modulates dopaminergic tone	Clozapine, olanzapine, quetiapine
Norepinephrine (NE)	α_1	Antagonist	Sedation; hypotension; indirectly reduces pain via CNS depressant effects	Quetiapine, clozapine, olanzapine, risperidone
	α_2	Indirect modulation	Facilitates descending analgesic pathways	Quetiapine (modest α_2 antagonism), clozapine
Histamine (HA)	H_1	Antagonist	Sedation; weight gain; thalamic deactivation may contribute to analgesia	Clozapine, olanzapine, quetiapine
Acetylcholine (ACh)	M_1 (muscarinic)	Antagonist	Cognitive dulling; sedation; contributes to sedative synergy	Clozapine, olanzapine
Glutamate (Glu)	NMDA (indirect)	Indirect modulation	Glutamate–dopamine interaction may influence central sensitization and chronic pain	Clozapine (possible indirect effect), experimental SGAs
Endogenous opioids	μ-opioid (indirect)	Indirect enhancement via DA/5-HT	May upregulate endogenous opioid activity; synergistic analgesia with dopaminergic effect	Olanzapine, quetiapine (preclinical data: Schreiber 1999)

gest that the opioid-modulating effects of SGAs represent a promising avenue for adjunctive pain management, particularly in patients with overlapping psychiatric and chronic pain disorders. A summary of pharmacologic targets and the SGAs that mediate them can be found in Table 13.1.

Evidence for Use

The most studied antipsychotics for pain include olanzapine, quetiapine, and ziprasidone. While smaller SGA studies indicate potential analgesic effect, there are few double-blind, placebo-controlled studies with greater than 50 patients. One condition with the largest number of existing studies is fibromyalgia. It should also be noted that many of the existing studies utilize SGAs in combination with other multimodal pain treatments, including opioids [38, 39].

Olanzapine

Olanzapine appears to have the largest positive data available of SGAs for various pain diagnoses, with studies evaluating cancer pain, headache, migraine prophylaxis, back pain, fibromyalgia, and neck pain. One small study (eight patients) indicated potential benefit from olanzapine when used to treat cancer-related pain. Patients experienced a reduction in pain scores and opioid requirements. All patients included in this study were experiencing severe pain, not controlled with opioid medication treatment. The study concluded that olanzapine may be particularly beneficial in patients with pain, in addition to severe anxiety and/or mild cognitive impairment [40]. Furthermore, one case report showed that olanzapine may reduce the craving behavior of opioids in pain secondary to advanced cancer [41]. Limited research on this topic is available, and further research is warranted. A larger study evaluating olanzapine use in pain evaluated 51 patients treated with olanzapine for fibromyalgia. Many patients had comorbid psychiatric diagnoses. While 48.2% of patients reported "excellent" improvement in pain levels, 52% of patients discontinued due to weight gain, somnolence or sedation, or lack of benefit [42]. It has been suggested that olanzapine may have greater efficacy in chronic pain syndromes that feature central sensitization and/or psychiatric comorbidity [43].

Quetiapine

Quetiapine also has evidence supporting its use as an adjunctive in fibromyalgia treatment. In a larger, double-blind, randomized, placebo-controlled study of 120 patients not experiencing psychosis, quetiapine extended-release (XR) showed significant decreases in pain, improvement in depression scores, and improvement in quality of life [44]. Another open-label study of quetiapine in a fibromyalgia population of 35 patients noted that while patients did not experience significant improvement in pain scores, they did report improvement in fatigue, stiffness, sleep, anxiety, and depression [45]. While the existing literature does not show substantial differences in pain scores with quetiapine use, quetiapine may offer secondary benefits for psychiatric comorbidities, which can ultimately impact the experience of pain.

Ziprasidone

A case series of 32 primarily female patients prescribed ziprasidone showed a non-statistically significant improvement on the Fibromyalgia Impact Questionnaire (FGI) and Pittsburgh Sleep Quality Index (PSQI). Patients prescribed ziprasidone did report lower rates of stiffness, sadness, and anxiety. The study concluded that ziprasidone could be considered in patients with fibromyalgia who are experiencing significant anxiety or depression [46].

Other SGAs, including aripiprazole and risperidone, also have existing case studies and series indicating potential benefit in conditions such as chronic pain, headache, and medication overuse headache [47–49].

Safety

As previously mentioned, FGA use is limited in practice due to nonselective binding at dopamine receptors. Antipsychotic-induced extrapyramidal symptoms (EPS), otherwise known as drug-induced movement disorders, are possible with both FGA and SGA use. EPS can cause short-lasting or chronic impairment. Symptoms range from akathisia to Parkinsonism, dystonia, and tardive dyskinesia (TD). They can range from mild to severe, with the potential to significantly impact functioning, social interactions, and medication adherence. Symptoms are most likely to occur when first initiating an antipsychotic medication or after a dose increase [50]. This risk is significantly greater with the use of FGAs, but patients initiated on SGAs should still be monitored for EPS.

While SGAs offer a lower risk of EPS than FGAs due to lower specificity for dopamine antagonism and broader mechanism of action, there are other side effects which may impact use. As noted in several studies examining SGA use in pain, metabolic side effects frequently limit the long-term use of these medications. SGAs have been associated with weight gain and increased waist circumference, hyperglycemia, cholesterol elevations, and elevated blood pressure. Metabolic syndrome, which occurs when three of the previously mentioned criteria are present, puts patients at a greater risk of cardiovascular disease (CVD) [51].

Sedation is another common side effect of SGAs due to their action at histamine receptors, among other receptor interactions. Sedation can impact the adherence and utility of SGAs for some patients [51]. SGAs also carry risk for elderly patients with dementia due to increased risk of cerebrovascular events and death when compared to placebo [51].

Neuroleptic malignancy syndrome (NMS) is also associated with antipsychotic use. NMS is a life-threatening condition, more common with FGA use but possible with SGA use as well. It includes initial signs of hyperthermia, rigidity, elevated creatinine phosphokinase (CPK), changes in mental status, and autonomic dysregulation. The risk of development is greater with high doses, polypharmacy, older age, previous history of NMS, and specific family and personal historical comorbidities [51]. Rarely, the symptomatology of serotonin syndrome and NMS may overlap. Judicious monitoring is warranted [52].

SGA use may increase the risk of developing serotonin syndrome, specifically when used in combination with other serotonergic medications. This risk is much less common with SGA use compared to highly serotonergic medication classes, such as selective serotonin reuptake inhibitors (SSRIs). Partial agonism at 5-HT_{1A} occurs with certain SGAs and theoretically contributes to serotonin syndrome. Combining multiple serotonergic medications or drugs, leading to increased exposure of one or more medications, may cause excessive serotonin exposure, leading to toxicity. Most cases of serotonin syndrome observed with SGA use are found in cases with concomitant drug use (for example, in combination with SSRIs). Side effects are often mild but can progress and become life-threatening, particularly if the offending agents are not discontinued. Prescribers should monitor for signs of serotonin syndrome, including autonomic hyperactivity and neuromuscular abnormalities [53–55].

Limited evidence exists evaluating the specific risks of SGA use in combination with opioid use. Many patients in studies evaluating SGA use for pain conditions were on concomitant opioid treatment, without reported increase in opioid overdose or CNS-related side effects. One population-based, cohort study advised caution when utilizing sedating antipsychotics in combination with prescribed opioids due to an increased rate of overdose compared with nonsedating antipsychotics. Authors suggested choosing nonsedating antipsychotic treatment when able, if utilizing in combination with opioid treatment [56].

Table 13.2 Dosing considerations

Drug	Indication	Minimum dose	Average dose	Maximum dose
Aripiprazole [49, 57, 58]	Chronic pain, mixed	2 mg	–	15 mg
	Chronic pain, mixed	2 mg	–	6 mg
	Migraine	5 mg	–	20 mg
	Medication overuse headache	6 mg	–	12 mg
Olanzapine [8, 33, 40–42, 59, 60]	FM	>5 mg	5–10 mg	>20 mg
	Headache	10 mg	10 mg	10 mg
	Cancer pain	2.5 mg	–	7.5 mg
	FM	5 mg	–	10 mg
	FM	2.5 mg	10 mg	20 mg
	Headache	2.5 mg	10 mg	25 mg
	Cancer pain	10 mg	10 mg	10 mg
	Headache/migraine cluster	2.5 mg	5–10 mg	35 mg
Quetiapine [44, 45, 61–64]	For weaning sedation	25 mg	100 mg	200 mg
	Bladder pain syndrome	50 mg (XR)	–	150 mg (XR)
	FGID	25 mg	50 mg	100 mg
	FM	25 mg	–	100 mg
	Migraine	25 mg	75 mg	75 mg
	Migraine prophylaxis	25 mg	–	400 mg
	FM	50 mg (XR)	224 mg (XR)	300 mg (XR)
Risperidone [47]	Chronic pain	0.25 mg	–	1.5 mg
Ziprasidone [46, 65]	Chronic migraine	20 mg	–	60 mg
	FM	20 mg	40 mg	80 mg

Applications to Clinical Practice

The treatment of pain, anxiety, and depression can often overlap in clinical practice. SGAs have less evidence than other medication classes that exist for the treatment of pain conditions, and all use of SGAs for the treatment of pain is considered off-label.

While SGAs do not consistently show statistically significant pain relief in the existing literature, there are certain conditions in which they are more likely to provide benefit. Comorbid psychiatric disorders are higher in patients with fibromyalgia compared to other pain conditions. Patients with higher rates of depression, anxiety, and insomnia at baseline may be more likely to experience a favorable response from SGAs. Noted improvement in anxiety, sleep, and/or stress tolerability may contribute to noted reductions in pain and improvement in functioning.

Dosing of antipsychotics was variable in clinical trials but often fell within a low-dose-to-moderate-dose range. Clinical trials evaluating olanzapine included doses between 2.5 mg and 20 mg daily [33]. Quetiapine was often initiated at 50 mg and titrated up to 300 mg daily as tolerated [44]. The range of ziprasidone utilized was between 20 and 80 mg per day, one trial indicating a median dose of 40 mg [46]. Benefits from medication use were often noted after use for four weeks or longer. When used for treatment of psychotic disorders, antipsychotics can take 6–8 weeks or longer to reach their full benefit. Therefore, medications should be utilized for an extended period, if tolerated, to evaluate the full benefit for pain. Table 13.2 provides specific dosing strategies that have been used in randomized controlled trials and case reports/series.

Certain populations may be poor candidates for antipsychotic use, including those with a history of cardiovascular disease, elderly patients and those with dementia, or those with a history of EPS or NMS with past antipsychotic use. Robust clinical trial data remain limited, and this should be considered when evaluating potential antipsychotic use. Despite more favorable side effect profiles of SGAs compared to FGAs, side effects of SGAs can still limit treatment. Risks and benefits of SGA use should be carefully weighed with patients and families prior to initiation in practice.

Key Themes

- Evidence supporting the use of antipsychotics for pain management is limited to small trials and case series.
- Some evidence does point toward the potential benefit of SGAs when used as an augmentation strategy for specific pain conditions, including fibromyalgia, cancer pain, and chronic headaches.
- Side effects often limit the use of SGAs in practice and should be considered prior to treatment.

Conclusions

Antipsychotic medications have potential utility in difficult-to-treat pain conditions. Certain conditions with higher rates of psychiatric comorbidity may be more likely to respond to antipsychotic use. SGAs are preferred over FGAs due to their side effect profile but still carry the risk of metabolic syndrome, EPS, and NMS, among other side effects. Further research is necessary to fully understand the mechanism of antipsychotics in pain treatment and the overall impact of SGAs on pain conditions.

References

1. National Institute of Neurological Disorders and Stroke. Pain. National Institute of Neurological Disorders and Stroke. Published 2023. https://www.ninds.nih.gov/health-information/disorders/pain.
2. Khouzam HR. Psychopharmacology of chronic pain: a focus on antidepressants and atypical antipsychotics. Postgrad Med. 2016;128(3):323–30.
3. Nahin RL, Feinberg T, Kapos FP, Terman GW. Estimated rates of incident and persistent chronic pain among us adults, 2019-2020. JAMA Netw Open. 2023;6(5):e2313563.
4. Calandre EP, Rico-Villademoros F. The role of antipsychotics in the management of fibromyalgia. CNS Drugs. 2012;26(2):135–53.
5. CDC. Assess Risks and Potential Harms of Opioid Use. Overdose Prevention. Published June 24, 2024. https://www.cdc.gov/overdose-prevention/hcp/clinical-care/assess-risks-of-opioid-use.html
6. De La Cruz A, Vo K. Antipsychotics for Pain Management. US Pharmacist Published March 19, 2020. https://www.uspharmacist.com/article/antipsychotics-for-pain-management
7. Kim JYV, Tillu DV, Quinn TL, et al. Spinal dopaminergic projections control the transition to pathological pain plasticity via a d1/d5-mediated mechanism. J Neurosci. 2015;35(16):6307.
8. Silberstein SD, Peres MFP, Hopkins MM, Shechter AL, Young WB, Rozen TD. Olanzapine in the treatment of refractory migraine and chronic daily headache. Headache. 2002;42(6):515–8.
9. Mishra A, Singh S, Shukla S. Physiological and functional basis of dopamine receptors and their role in neurogenesis: possible implication for parkinson's disease. J Exp Neurosci. 2018;12:1179069518779829.
10. Megat S, Shiers S, Moy JK, et al. A critical role for dopamine d5 receptors in pain chronicity in male mice. J Neurosci. 2018;38(2):379–97.
11. Zhao F, Cheng Z, Piao J, Cui R, Li B. Dopamine receptors: is it possible to become a therapeutic target for depression? Front Pharmacol. 2022;13:947785.
12. Wood MD, Scott C, Clarke K, et al. Aripiprazole and its human metabolite are partial agonists at the human dopamine D2 receptor, but the rodent metabolite displays antagonist properties. Eur J Pharmacol. 2006;546(1–3):88–94.
13. Sokoloff P, Le Foll B. The dopamine D3 receptor, a quarter century later. Herman J, ed. Eur J Neurosci. 2017;45(1):2–19.
14. Ho AM-C, Tang NL-S, Cheung BK-L, Stadlin A. Dopamine receptor d4 gene −521c/t polymorphism is associated with opioid dependence through cold-pain responses. Ann N Y Acad Sci. 2008;1139(1):20–6.
15. Liu QQ, Yao XX, Gao SH, et al. Role of 5-HT receptors in neuropathic pain: potential therapeutic implications. Pharmacol Res. 2020;159:104949.
16. Kandasamy R, Price TJ. The pharmacology of nociceptor priming. Handb Exp Pharmacol. 2015;227:15.
17. Millan M, Marin P, Bockaert J, Mannourylacour C. Signaling at G-protein-coupled serotonin receptors: recent advances and future research directions. Trends Pharmacol Sci. 2008;29(9):454–64.
18. Courteix C, Dupuis A, Martin PY, Sion B. 5-ht2a receptors and pain. In: Guiard BP, Di Giovanni G, editors. 5-HT2A Receptors in the Central Nervous System. Springer International Publishing; 2018. p. 339–52.
19. Stahl SM. Stahl's Essential Psychopharmacology: Neuroscientific Basis and Practical Application. 4th ed. Cambridge University Press; 2013.
20. Campbell JN, Meyer RA, Raja SN. Is nociceptor activation by alpha-1 adrenoreceptors the culprit in sympathetically maintained pain? APS J. 1992;1(1):3–11.
21. Carroll I, Mackey S, Gaeta R. The role of adrenergic receptors and pain: The good, the bad, and the unknown. Sem Anesth Perioper Med Pain. 2007;26(1):17–21.
22. Schreiber S, Getslev V, Backer MM, Weizman R, Pick CG. The atypical neuroleptics clozapine and olanzapine differ regarding their antinociceptive mechanisms and potency. Pharmacol Biochem Behav. 1999;64(1):75–80.
23. Proudman RGW, Pupo AS, Baker JG. The affinity and selectivity of α-adrenoceptor antagonists, antidepressants, and antipsychotics for the human α1A, α1B, and α1D-adrenoceptors. Pharmacol Res Perspect. 2020;8(4):e00602.
24. Sanna MD, Ghelardini C, Thurmond RL, Masini E, Galeotti N. Behavioural phenotype of histamine H4 receptor knockout mice: Focus on central neuronal functions. Neuropharmacology. 2017;114:48–57.
25. Kumar K, Kirksey MA, Duong S, Wu CL. A review of opioid-sparing modalities in perioperative pain management: methods to decrease opioid use postoperatively. Anesth Analg. 2017;125(5):1749–60.
26. Naser PV, Kuner R. Molecular, cellular and circuit basis of cholinergic modulation of pain. Neuroscience. 2018;387:135–48.
27. Weiner DM, Meltzer HY, Veinbergs I, et al. The role of M1 muscarinic receptor agonism of N-desmethylclozapine in the unique clinical effects of clozapine. Psychopharmacology. 2004;177(1–2):207–16.
28. Vecera SP, O'Reilly RC. Figure-ground organization and object recognition processes: an interactive account. J Exp Psychol Hum Percept Perform. 1998;24(2):441–62.
29. Wozniak KM, Rojas C, Wu Y, Slusher BS. The role of glutamate signaling in pain processes and its regulation by GCP II inhibition. Curr Med Chem. 2012;19(9):1323–34.
30. Schmitt A, Zink M, Müller B, et al. Effects of long-term antipsychotic treatment on NMDA receptor binding and gene expression of subunits. Neurochem Res. 2003;28(2):235–41.
31. Goff DC, Hennen J, Lyoo IK, et al. Modulation of brain and serum glutamatergic concentrations following a switch from conventional neuroleptics to olanzapine. Biol Psychiatry. 2002;51(6):493–7.
32. Fukuyama K, Kato R, Murata M, Shiroyama T, Okada M. Clozapine normalizes a glutamatergic transmission abnormality induced by an impaired NMDA receptor in the thalamocortical pathway via the activation of a group iii metabotropic glutamate receptor. Biomolecules. 2019;9(6):234.
33. Rico-Villademoros F, Hidalgo J, Dominguez I, García-Leiva JM, Calandre EP. Atypical antipsychotics in the treatment of fibromyalgia: a case series with olanzapine. Prog Neuro-Psychopharmacol Biol Psychiatry. 2005;29(1):161–4.
34. Walitt B, Klose P, Üçeyler N, Phillips T, Häuser W. Antipsychotics for fibromyalgia in adults. Cochrane Database Syst Rev. 2016;2016(6):CD011804.

35. Urban-Kowalczyk M, Kotlicka-Antczak M, Strzelecki D, Rudecka E, Śmigielski J. Plasma β-endorphin concentration and antipsychotic treatment outcome in schizophrenia: 1-year follow-up. Med Sci Monit. 2020;26:e924307.
36. Reeves KC, Shah N, Muñoz B, Atwood BK. Opioid receptor-mediated regulation of neurotransmission in the brain. Front Mol Neurosci. 2022;15:919773.
37. Schmauss C, Emrich HM. Dopamine and the action of opiates: A reevaluation of the dopamine hypothesis of schizophrenia with special consideration of the role of endogenous opioids in the pathogenesis of schizophrenia. Biol Psychiatry. 1985;20(11):1211–31.
38. Fishbain DA, Cutler RB, Lewis J, Cole B, Rosomoff RS, Rosomoff HL. Do the second-generation "atypical neuroleptics" have analgesic properties? A structured evidence-based review. Pain Med. 2004;5(4):359–65.
39. Coronado B, Dunn J, Veronin MA, Reinert JP. Efficacy and safety considerations with second-generation antipsychotics as adjunctive analgesics: a review of literature. J Pharm Technol. 2021;37(4):202.
40. Khojainova N, Santiago-Palma J, Kornick C, Breitbart W, Gonzales GR. Olanzapine in the management of cancer pain. J Pain Symptom Manag. 2002;23(4):346–50.
41. Go SI, Song HN, Lee SJ, Bruera E, Kang JH. Craving behavior from opioid addiction controlled with olanzapine in an advanced cancer patient: a case report. J Palliat Med. 2018;21(9):1367–70.
42. Freedenfeld RN, Murray M, Fuchs PN, Kiser RS. Decreased pain and improved quality of life in fibromyalgia patients treated with olanzapine, an atypical neuroleptic. Pain Pract. 2006;6(2):112–8.
43. Jimenez XF, Sundararajan T, Covington EC. A systematic review of atypical antipsychotics in chronic pain management: olanzapine demonstrates potential in central sensitization, fibromyalgia, and headache/migraine. Clin J Pain. 2018;34(6):585–91.
44. McIntyre A, Paisley D, Kouassi E, Gendron A. Quetiapine fumarate extended-release for the treatment of major depression with comorbid fibromyalgia syndrome: a double-blind, randomized, placebo-controlled study. Arthritis Rheumatol. 2014;66(2):451–61.
45. Hidalgo J, Rico-Villademoros F, Calandre EP. An open-label study of quetiapine in the treatment of fibromyalgia. Prog Neuro-Psychopharmacol Biol Psychiatry. 2007;31(1):71–7.
46. Calandre EP, Hidalgo J, Rico-Villademoros F. Use of ziprasidone in patients with fibromyalgia: a case series. Rheumatol Int. 2007;27(5):473–6.
47. Fe-Bornstein M, Watt SD, Gitlin MC. Improvement in the level of psychosocial functioning in chronic pain patients with the use of risperidone: table 1. Pain Med. 2002;3(2):128–31.
48. Yamada K, Makihara Y, Imamura Y. Effectiveness of aripiprazole for medication overuse headache: A case report. Psychiatry Clin Neurosci. 2011;65(3):296–8.
49. Fei L, Abrardi L, Mediati RD. Unexpected effect of aripiprazole on nociceptive pain. Ther Adv Psychopharmacol. 2012;2(5):211–2.
50. Ali T, Sisay M, Tariku M, Mekuria AN, Desalew A. Antipsychotic-induced extrapyramidal side effects: A systematic review and meta-analysis of observational studies. PLoS One. 2021;16(9):e0257129.
51. Solmi M, Murru A, Pacchiarotti I, et al. Safety, tolerability, and risks associated with first- and second-generation antipsychotics: a state-of-the-art clinical review. Ther Clin Risk Manag. 2017;13:757.
52. Maktabi L, Shipman D, Reinert JP. Serotonin syndrome and neuroleptic malignant syndrome: a case report of intersecting symptomatology. Mental Health Clin. 2024;14(1):23–7.
53. Mikkelsen N, Damkier P, Pedersen SA. Serotonin syndrome-A focused review. Basic Clin Pharmacol Toxicol. 2023;133(2):124–9.
54. Charles H. Brown. Drug-induced Serotonin Syndrome. U.S. Pharmacist. Published November 17, 2010. https://www.uspharmacist.com/article/drug-induced-serotonin-syndrome
55. Racz R, Soldatos TG, Jackson D, Burkhart K. Association between serotonin syndrome and second-generation antipsychotics via pharmacological target-adverse event analysis. Clin Transl Sci. 2018;11(3):322–9.
56. Szmulewicz AG, Bateman BT, Levin R, Huybrechts KF. Risk of overdose associated with co-prescription of antipsychotics and opioids: a population-based cohort study. Schizophr Bull. 2022;48(2):405–13.
57. Kasahara S, Kunii Y, Mashiko H, Otani K, Konno SI, Niwa SI. Four cases of chronic pain that improved dramatically following low-dose aripiprazole administration. Prim Care Companion CNS Disord. 2011;13(2):PCC.10l01078.
58. LaPorta LD. Relief from migraine headache with aripiprazole treatment. Headache. 2007;47(6):922–6.
59. Hill CH, Miner JR, Martel ML. Olanzapine versus droperidol for the treatment of primary headache in the emergency department. Acad Emerg Med. 2008;15(9):806–11.
60. Rozen TD. Olanzapine as an abortive agent for cluster headache. Headache. 2001;41(8):813–6.
61. Assadoon MS, Kovacevic MP, Dube KM, Szumita PM, Lupi KE, DeGrado JR. Evaluation of atypical antipsychotics for the facilitation of weaning sedation in mechanically ventilated critically ill patients. J Intensive Care Med. 2024;39(1):52–8.
62. Grover M, Dorn SD, Weinland SR, Dalton CB, Gaynes BN, Drossman DA. Atypical antipsychotic quetiapine in the management of severe refractory functional gastrointestinal disorders. Dig Dis Sci. 2009;54(6):1284–91.
63. Krymchantowski AV, Jevoux C, Moreira PF. An open pilot study assessing the benefits of quetiapine for the prevention of migraine refractory to the combination of atenolol, nortriptyline, and flunarizine: table 1. Pain Med. 2010;11(1):48–52.
64. 11th European headache federation congress jointly with 31st congress of the Italian society for the study of headaches: Rome, Italy. 01–03 December 2017. J Headache Pain. 2017;18(S1):111, s10194-017-0817-z.
65. Cahill C, Hardiman O, Murphy K. Treatment of refractory chronic daily headache with the atypical antipsychotic ziprasidone — a case series. Cephalalgia. 2005;25(10):822–6.

14 Calcium Channel Blockers

Justin P. Reinert

Definitions

Term	Definition
Calcium Ions (Ca^{2+})	Essential ions involved in neuronal excitability, neurotransmitter release, and intracellular signaling
Voltage-Gated Calcium Channels (VGCCs)	Protein channels in nerve cells that open in response to voltage changes, allowing calcium influx critical for neurotransmitter release
N-type Calcium Channels	VGCC subtype located at presynaptic terminals, facilitating release of neurotransmitters like glutamate and substance P involved in pain signaling
T-type Calcium Channels	Low-voltage activated VGCCs involved in neuronal firing, excitability, and thalamocortical rhythms, linked to pain transmission
L-type Calcium Channels	High-voltage activated VGCCs expressed in muscle, cardiac, and some neurons, with limited role in pain modulation
Ziconotide	A synthetic ω-conotoxin that selectively blocks N-type VGCCs, used intrathecally for severe chronic neuropathic pain
Ethosuximide	An antiepileptic drug that selectively inhibits T-type calcium channels, with investigational use in neuropathic pain
Opioid-Sparing Effect	Reduction in opioid requirements achieved by an adjunct therapy, lowering risk of opioid-related side effects
Intrathecal Administration	Delivery of medication directly into the spinal canal, allowing targeted effect on the central nervous system
Neuropsychiatric Adverse Effects	Side effects affecting mood, cognition, or behavior, including dizziness, hallucinations, and mood changes
Polypharmacy	The concurrent use of multiple medications, increasing risk of drug interactions
Calcium Channel Blockers (CCBs)	A class of drugs that inhibit VGCCs, primarily used for cardiovascular diseases but investigated for analgesia
Hyperalgesia	Increased sensitivity to painful stimuli
Allodynia	Pain due to stimuli that normally do not provoke pain

Background and Introduction

Calcium ions (Ca^{2+}) play an essential role in neuronal excitability, neurotransmitter release, and intracellular signaling within both the peripheral and central nervous systems [1]. Given their integral function, disruptions in calcium ion homeostasis have been implicated in various pain states, particularly neuropathic and inflammatory pain [1]. This mechanistic understanding has prompted interest in calcium channel blockers (CCBs), a drug class traditionally used in cardiovascular medicine, as potential adjunctive agents in pain management [2]. The rationale for their use lies in their ability to modulate pain pathways by inhibiting voltage-gated calcium channels (VGCCs), which are critical to the propagation and amplification of nociceptive signals [2–4] (Tables 14.1 and 14.2).

Building upon this mechanistic rationale, several subtypes of VGCCs, most notably the N-type and T-type calcium channels, have been identified as key contributors to pain transmission and sensitization [1–4]. N-type calcium channels, primarily located at presynaptic terminals of nociceptive neurons, facilitate the release of neurotransmitters such as glutamate and substance P, both of which are involved in the development and maintenance of chronic pain [5, 6]. T-type channels are implicated in neuronal firing and excitability, particularly in dorsal horn neurons and peripheral sensory fibers [7–9]. Preclinical studies have demonstrated that selective blockade of these channels can attenuate hyper-

J. P. Reinert (✉)
The University of Toledo College of Pharmacy and Pharmaceutical Sciences, Toledo, OH, USA
e-mail: justin.reinert@utoledo.edu

J. P. Reinert et al. (eds.), *Adjunctive Analgesic Strategies for the Bedside Clinician and Beyond*,
https://doi.org/10.1007/978-3-032-21675-5_14

Table 14.1 Calcium channels

Calcium channel type	Mechanism in pain transmission	Medications
N-type (Cav2.2)	Located on presynaptic terminals of peripheral and spinal neurons; mediates release of pro-nociceptive neurotransmitters (e.g., glutamate, substance P, CGRP); inhibition reduces pain signaling	Ziconotide
T-type (Cav3.1–3.3)	Low-voltage activated; contributes to thalamocortical oscillations, neuronal excitability, and visceral/inflammatory pain; implicated in chronic and diabetic neuropathic pain	Ethosuximide
P/Q-type (Cav2.1)	Found in CNS synapses; regulates neurotransmitter release; mutations linked to familial hemiplegic migraine; experimental role in chronic pain (e.g., CRPS, migraine)	No selective clinical agents currently available
R-type (Cav2.3)	Expressed in the spinal cord, dorsal horn, and sensory ganglia; involved in synaptic transmission and possibly chronic pain sensitization	No approved agents currently available
L-type (Cav1.1–1.4)	Involved in muscle contraction and cardiovascular function; minor/modest role in nociception; not primarily involved in pain signaling pathways	Amlodipine, Nifedipine, Verapamil

Table 14.2 Summary of efficacy and safety data

Type of Calcium Channel Blocker (CCB)	Mechanism of action	Pain types potentially managed
Ziconotide (N-type selective, intrathecal)	Blocks N-type VGCC at presynaptic terminals, inhibiting release of pro-nociceptive neurotransmitters (glutamate, substance P, CGRP)	Severe chronic neuropathic pain, cancer-related pain, complex regional pain syndrome, failed back surgery syndrome
Nifedipine (Dihydropyridine, systemic)	Blocks L-type VGCC, affecting neuronal excitability and muscle contraction	Postoperative pain (gynecological, orthopedic), adjunct to opioids; limited efficacy due to cardiovascular side effects
Nimodipine (Dihydropyridine, systemic)	Blocks L-type VGCC with some opioid-sparing effects via calcium channel blockade	Cancer-associated chronic pain, perioperative pain (cardiac surgery); variable results depending on setting
Ethosuximide (T-type, systemic)	Selective inhibition of T-type VGCC involved in neuronal excitability and thalamocortical rhythms	Experimental use in neuropathic and inflammatory pain; limited clinical efficacy and tolerability
Non-dihydropyridine (verapamil, diltiazem)	Blocks L-type and other VGCC subtypes with limited analgesic effect	Mixed results; generally no consistent benefit in pain management; may increase opioid requirements in some cases

algesia and allodynia in animal models of neuropathic and inflammatory pain [10–12]. These findings underscore the therapeutic potential of targeting VGCCs to disrupt maladaptive nociceptive signaling and improve pain control in select patient populations.

Pharmacology, Pharmacokinetics, Pharmacodynamics

VGCCs are subdivided into several types based on their biophysical properties and pharmacologic sensitivities, including L-type, N-type, P/Q-type, R-type, and T-type channels [5]. Each subtype contributes uniquely to nociceptive transmission and central sensitization. L-type calcium channels, which are high-voltage activated, are widely expressed in muscle and cardiac tissues but are also present in dorsal horn neurons [6, 7]. Their contribution to pain processing is modest, with systemic agents like amlodipine and nifedipine demonstrating only limited analgesic effects in some neuropathic pain models [2, 8]. The clinical data supporting their use in chronic pain are sparse and inconclusive, and dose escalation is frequently constrained by cardiovascular side effects such as hypotension and bradycardia [2, 7, 8].

In contrast, N-type calcium channels have a well-established role in pain modulation [5]. These channels are predominantly located at presynaptic terminals in the spinal cord and peripheral nerves, where they facilitate the release of key pro-nociceptive neurotransmitters, including glutamate, substance P, and calcitonin gene-related peptide (CGRP) [9–12]. Inhibition of these channels significantly reduces pain transmission. Ziconotide, a synthetic ω-conotoxin that selectively blocks N-type calcium channels, is approved for intrathecal administration in cases of severe chronic pain, particularly in patients refractory to opioids [9–12]. Clinical trials have demonstrated its efficacy in conditions such as cancer-related and neuropathic pain; however, its narrow therapeutic window and potential for serious neuropsychiatric adverse effects, such as confusion, hallucinations, and suicidal ideation, necessitate careful dose titration and monitoring [9–12].

T-type calcium channels are low-voltage-activated and play an important role in thalamocortical rhythm regulation and neuronal excitability [13, 14]. These channels are increasingly recognized for their role in visceral and inflammatory pain. While clinical agents targeting T-type channels are not yet widely available, compounds such as ethosuximide and newer experimental agents have demonstrated analgesic effects in animal models of diabetic neuropathy and inflammatory pain [15]. Human trials are limited but ongoing, and further research is required to translate these findings into clinical practice. The potential for central nervous system depression and off-target effects remains a concern with systemic T-type channel inhibition [13–15].

P/Q-type and R-type calcium channels are less well understood in the context of pain but are known to influence neurotransmitter release in the central nervous system [16, 17]. Preclinical studies suggest that these channels may contribute to the development of chronic pain syndromes such as migraine and complex regional pain syndrome, but the lack of selective pharmacologic agents has limited their clinical application. The future development of subtype-specific antagonists may provide new opportunities for therapeutic intervention [16, 17].

Evidence for Use

Ziconotide

Ziconotide is a synthetic peptide analog of ω-conotoxin MVIIA, a marine snail venom-derived compound that selectively inhibits N-type voltage-gated calcium channels [18]. This selective inhibition blocks calcium influx at presynaptic nerve terminals in the dorsal horn of the spinal cord, thereby suppressing the release of pro-nociceptive neurotransmitters such as glutamate, substance P, and CGRP [18–20]. Ziconotide's mechanism is fundamentally distinct from that of opioids, making it a valuable tool in cases of opioid-refractory pain. Importantly, it is non-opioid, nonaddictive, and does not induce tolerance, a significant advantage in chronic pain populations [18–20].

The 2006 study by Rauck et al. evaluated the efficacy of intrathecal ziconotide in 220 patients with severe chronic pain, predominantly of neuropathic origin [21]. The study demonstrated a statistically significant reduction in pain scores via evaluation with the visual analog scale of pain intensity (VASPI) compared to placebo ($p < 0.001$), with 32.2% of patients in the treatment arm achieving ≥30% pain reduction versus 17.6% in the placebo group [21]. These findings were corroborated in earlier trials, including a 2004 study by Staats et al., which also reported significant pain relief in cancer and AIDS patients receiving ziconotide [22]. Collectively, these studies established ziconotide as an effective agent for managing chronic, treatment-resistant pain [21, 22].

Beyond its efficacy in cancer-related pain, ziconotide has shown utility in nonmalignant pain conditions. A 2016 pooled analysis by McDowell et al. reviewed data from three controlled trials and confirmed that ziconotide provided meaningful analgesia in both cancer-related and non-cancer pain, including complex regional pain syndrome and failed back surgery syndrome [23]. Importantly, responders often had durable pain control over extended periods, with some patients maintaining benefit beyond six months [23]. These results have led to the inclusion of ziconotide in pain management guidelines, such as those from the Polyanalgesic Consensus Conference (PACC), which recommend it as a first-line intrathecal agent in select patients, particularly those with neuropathic pain who are not candidates for intrathecal opioids [24].

Ethosuximide

Ethosuximide, a succinimide-class antiepileptic drug, has traditionally been used for the treatment of absence seizures due to its selective inhibition of T-type calcium channels, particularly in thalamocortical neurons [25]. In recent years, this mechanism of action has drawn interest in pain research [25, 26].

Preclinical studies have provided compelling evidence for the analgesic effects of ethosuximide in models of neuropathic pain. A study by Bourinet et al. demonstrated that mice with genetic knockouts of Cav3.2, a major T-type channel isoform, exhibited reduced mechanical and thermal hypersensitivity after nerve injury [27]. Ethosuximide replicated this phenotype pharmacologically, reducing allodynia and hyperalgesia in chronic constriction injury (CCI) and spinal nerve ligation (SNL) models [28]..

The EDONOT trial, a randomized, double-blind, placebo-controlled study, was the first to evaluate the efficacy and safety of ethosuximide in patients with nondiabetic peripheral neuropathic pain [29, 30]. Conducted across multiple centers in France, the trial enrolled 220 adults experiencing chronic neuropathic pain, with a Numeric Rating Scale (NRS) score of ≥4 and a Douleur Neuropathique 4 (DN4) score of ≥4, persisting for at least three months. Participants were randomly assigned to receive either ethosuximide or a placebo for a duration of six weeks, following a one-week run-in period. The primary endpoint was the change in pain intensity, assessed using the NRS, while secondary endpoints included quality of life measures and safety evaluations. Safety concerns led to the early termination of the study and are discussed later in this chapter [29, 30].

Antihypertensive Agents

A double-blind, randomized controlled trial by Carta et al. evaluated the analgesic adjunct effect of sustained-release nifedipine in patients undergoing abdominal hysterectomy or orthopedic surgery [31]. Patients received nifedipine or a placebo before and shortly after surgery, along with morphine as needed for pain. The nifedipine group experienced statistically significant improvements in analgesia across multiple pain scales compared to placebo. However, this benefit was accompanied by an increased risk of systolic hypotension within 60–90 minutes post-procedure, indicating a need for careful hemodynamic monitoring [31]. Pereira et al. further confirmed the potentiation of morphine analgesia by nifedipine in a double-blind, placebo-controlled study of women undergoing gynecological surgery [32]. Patients receiving combined intrathecal morphine and sublingual nifedipine experienced a markedly prolonged time to first pain complaint (428 minutes), compared to morphine alone (105 minutes) or nifedipine alone (15 minutes). Despite these positive analgesic effects, significant hypotension was again observed in nifedipine-treated patients, necessitating fluid resuscitation in some cases [32].

Similarly, nimodipine has demonstrated promising opioid-sparing effects in cancer patients with chronic pain. In a prospective observational study, Santillán et al. reported a significant reduction in baseline morphine requirements in 16 of 23 patients receiving nimodipine alongside oral morphine, with morphine doses nearly halving on average [33]. This finding was corroborated by a subsequent randomized controlled trial by the same authors in which nimodipine prevented further morphine dose escalation in a majority of patients with cancer-associated pain, with no changes observed in morphine metabolism, supporting a direct analgesic mechanism attributable to calcium channel blockade [34]. In perioperative cardiac surgery patients, Boldt et al. demonstrated that nimodipine coadministration with fentanyl reduced opioid requirements by approximately 70%, a profound opioid-sparing effect not seen with nifedipine or placebo [35]. This trial reported no significant cardiovascular adverse events, highlighting nimodipine's favorable safety profile in this context [35].

Evidence Against Use

Contrary to these positive findings, other studies have not confirmed the analgesic benefits of CCBs. Nitahara et al. studied IV diltiazem infusion combined with epidural fentanyl in gynecological surgery patients and found no difference in opioid consumption or pain scores compared to placebo, with a higher incidence of nausea in the diltiazem group [36]. Similarly, Casey et al. observed that nimodipine administration before and after total knee arthroplasty unexpectedly increased morphine requirements compared to placebo, without any improvement in subjective pain scores [37]. This suggests potential negative interactions between nimodipine and opioid analgesics in certain surgical settings.

Roca et al. conducted a crossover trial in cancer patients comparing morphine with nimodipine versus morphine with placebo over eight days but found no significant difference in pain intensity or analgesic efficacy between the regimens [38].

Vaupel et al. evaluated intravenous verapamil's effect on morphine analgesia in opioid-tolerant polydrug users, finding that verapamil increased pain thresholds but did not affect pain endurance or response, indicating a limited role for verapamil in enhancing opioid analgesia [39].

Finally, Hasegawa et al. performed a randomized, double-blind crossover study testing oral diltiazem, verapamil, and nimodipine administered after morphine [40]. None of the CCBs potentiated morphine analgesia during cold pressor testing, suggesting that these agents do not universally enhance opioid-induced pain relief [40].

Safety

Safety remains a principal limitation in the clinical application of CCBs for pain management. Systemic administration of these agents is often associated with cardiovascular side effects, particularly hypotension and bradycardia, which can be dose-limiting [2, 41]. Neuropsychiatric adverse effects are especially concerning with intrathecal agents like ziconotide, necessitating close monitoring [42]. Additionally, CCBs are metabolized via the cytochrome P450 3A4 pathway, which presents a risk for drug-drug interactions in populations frequently burdened by polypharmacy [41].

Despite its efficacy, ziconotide's clinical adoption has been cautious due to its narrow therapeutic window and potential for serious central nervous system (CNS) adverse effects. These include dizziness, confusion, hallucinations, mood changes, and, in rare cases, suicidal ideation. The risk of neuropsychiatric side effects is strongly dose-dependent. To mitigate this, contemporary protocols emphasize slow titration, often starting at doses as low as 0.5 mcg/day, with increments of no more than 0.5–1.0 mcg/week. This approach reduces the likelihood of adverse effects while allowing therapeutic benefit to emerge gradually [41–43].

The results of the EDONOT trial indicated that ethosuximide did not significantly reduce the severity of neuropathic pain compared to the placebo [29, 30]. Furthermore, the study reported a higher incidence of adverse events in the ethosuximide group, including gastrointestinal disturbances and central nervous system symptoms such as drowsiness and dizziness. These findings suggest that, at the doses tested, ethosuximide may not be an effective or well-tolerated treatment for nondiabetic peripheral neuropathic pain [29, 30].

Applications to Clinical Practice

Calcium channel blockers represent a promising yet complex adjunct in clinical pain management due to their ability to modulate voltage-gated calcium channels (VGCCs), which are integral to nociceptive signaling. The blockade of N-type calcium channels, in particular, has been clinically validated by the intrathecal use of ziconotide, a selective N-type VGCC inhibitor, for severe refractory neuropathic and cancer-related pain. Its non-opioid mechanism offers a valuable alternative in patients intolerant or unresponsive to opioids, though its narrow therapeutic window and neuropsychiatric side effects necessitate cautious dosing and vigilant monitoring. This underscores the importance of individualized therapy and slow titration protocols to balance efficacy and safety.

Other CCBs, such as the dihydropyridines nifedipine and nimodipine and the non-dihydropyridines verapamil and diltiazem, have demonstrated variable analgesic effects largely limited by cardiovascular adverse events like hypotension and bradycardia, which restrict dose escalation. Nimodipine shows particular promise in opioid-sparing during cancer pain and perioperative settings, with a comparatively favorable safety profile. However, inconsistent clinical trial outcomes suggest that CCB analgesic efficacy may depend heavily on pain etiology, patient population, and concomitant opioid use, highlighting the need for further targeted research.

Key Themes

- VGCCs, especially N-type and T-type subtypes, have a role in pain transmission and represent therapeutic targets for pain modulation.
- Intrathecal ziconotide, a selective N-type calcium channel blocker, is effective for severe, refractory neuropathic and cancer-related pain but requires careful dose titration due to a narrow therapeutic window and risk of neuropsychiatric side effects.
- Dihydropyridine CCBs like nimodipine and nifedipine show opioid-sparing effects in certain pain conditions, but their analgesic benefits are inconsistent and limited by cardiovascular adverse effects such as hypotension and bradycardia.
- T-type calcium channel blockers such as ethosuximide demonstrated preclinical analgesic potential but lack robust clinical efficacy and are associated with central nervous system adverse events.
- Safety concerns, including cardiovascular effects and drug interactions via CYP3A4 metabolism, remain significant barriers to the broader clinical use of systemic CCBs for pain management.

Conclusions

Calcium channel blockers offer valuable potential in pain treatment by targeting critical mechanisms involved in pain transmission. Intrathecal ziconotide has shown clear benefits for patients with difficult-to-treat neuropathic and cancer-related pain, though its use requires cautious dosing due to significant neuropsychiatric side effects. Systemic CCBs like nifedipine and nimodipine may reduce opioid needs in some cases but show variable effectiveness and carry risks such as hypotension and bradycardia. Research into T-type calcium channel inhibitors is ongoing, with promising preclinical results but limited clinical data so far. Ultimately, the successful integration of CCBs into clinical practice depends on individualized therapy, careful titration, and close monitoring to balance efficacy with safety concerns.

References

1. Zhang Y, Shannonhouse J, Son H, Park JT, Kim YS. Regulatory action of calcium and calcium channels in pain pathways. Int J Biol Sci. 2025;21(8):3726–39.
2. Reinert JP, Tiemann AR, Barlow ML, Veronin MA. Evaluating the efficacy and safety of calcium channel blockers as adjunctive analgesics to opioid therapy: a literature review. Pharm Pract Res. 2022;52(1):7–18.
3. Snutch TP, Peloquin J, Mathews E, McRory J. Molecular properties of voltage-gated calcium channels. In: Zamponi G, editor. Voltage-gated calcium. New York: Landes Bioscience; 2005. p. 61–94.
4. Westenbroek RE, Hell JW, Warner C, Dubel SJ, Snutch TP, Catterall WA. Biochemical properties and subcellular distribution of an N-type calcium channel α1 subunit. Neuron. 1992;9:1099–115.
5. Snutch TP. Targeting chronic and neuropathic pain: The N-type calcium channel comes of age. Neurotherapeutics. 2005;2(4):662–70.
6. Antunes FTT, Campos MM, Carvalho V de PR, et al. Current drug development overview: targeting voltage-gated calcium channels for the treatment of pain. IJMS. 2023;24(11):9223.
7. Manzar A, Sic A, Banh C, Knezevic NN. Therapeutic potential of calcium channel blockers in neuropsychiatric, endocrine and pain disorders. Cells. 2025;14(14):1114.
8. Lipman AG. Analgesic drugs for neuropathic and sympathetically maintained pain. Clin Geriatr Med. 1996;12(3):501–15.
9. Webster LR. The relationship between the mechanisms of action and safety profiles of intrathecal morphine and ziconotide: a review of the literature: intrathecal mechanisms of action and safety. Pain Med. 2015;16(7):1265–77.
10. Matis G, De Negri P, Dupoiron D, Likar R, Zuidema X, Rasche D. Intrathecal pain management with ziconotide: Time for consensus? Brain Behav. 2021;11(S1):e02055.
11. Nair AS, Poornachand A, Kodisharapu PK. Ziconotide: indications, adverse effects, and limitations in managing refractory chronic pain. Indian J Palliat Care. 2018;24(1):118–9.
12. Rubiu E, Restelli F, Nazzi V, et al. A benefit/risk assessment of intrathecal ziconotide in chronic pain: a narrative review. JCM. 2024;13(6):1644.
13. Lee S. Pharmacological inhibition of voltage-gated ca(2+) channels for chronic pain relief. Curr Neuropharmacol. 2013;11(6):606–20.
14. Todorovic SM, Jevtovic-Todorovic V. T-type voltage-gated calcium channels as targets for the development of novel pain therapies. Br J Pharmacol. 2011;163(3):484–95.

15. Barton ME, Eberle EL, Shannon HE. The antihyperalgesic effects of the T-type calcium channel blockers ethosuximide, trimethadione, and mibefradil. Eur J Pharmacol. 2005;521(1-3):79–85.
16. Nimmrich V, Gross G. P/Q-type calcium channel modulators. Br J Pharmacol. 2012;167(4):741–59.
17. de Amorim Ferreira M, Ferreira J. Role of cav2. 3(R-type) calcium channel in pain and analgesia: a scoping review. CN. 2024;22(11):1909–22.
18. Lin J, Chen S, Butt UD, Yan M, Wu B. A comprehensive review on ziconotide. Heliyon. 2024;10(10):e31105.
19. Ohashi N, Uta D, Ohashi M, Hoshino R, Baba H. Omega-conotoxin MVIIA reduces neuropathic pain after spinal cord injury by inhibiting N-type voltage-dependent calcium channels on spinal dorsal horn. Front Neurosci. 2024;18:1366829.
20. Williams JA, Day M, Heavner JE. Ziconotide: an update and review. Exp Opin Pharmacother. 2008;9(9):1575–83.
21. Rauck RL, Wallace MS, Leong MS, et al. A randomized, double-blind, placebo-controlled study of intrathecal ziconotide in adults with severe chronic pain. J Pain Symp Manage. 2006;31(5):393–406.
22. Staats PS, Yearwood T, Charapata SG, et al. Intrathecal ziconotide in the treatment of refractory pain in patients with cancer or aids: a randomized controlled trial. JAMA. 2004;291(1):63.
23. McDowell GC, Pope JE. Intrathecal ziconotide: dosing and administration strategies in patients with refractory chronic pain. Neuromodulation. 2016;19(5):522–32.
24. Deer TR, Hayek SM, Grider JS, et al. The polyanalgesic consensus conference (Pacc)®: intrathecal drug delivery guidance on safety and therapy optimization when treating chronic noncancer pain. Neuromodulation. 2024;27(7):1107–39.
25. Gören MZ, Onat F. Ethosuximide: from bench to bedside. CNS Drug Rev. 2007;13(2):224–39.
26. Rogawski MA. New evidence supporting a role for t-type ca(2+) channels in absence epilepsy and in the action of ethosuximide. Epilepsy Curr. 2002;2(2):57.
27. Bourinet E, Alloui A, Monteil A, et al. Silencing of the Cav3.2 T-type calcium channel gene in sensory neurons demonstrates its major role in nociception. EMBO J. 2005;24(2):315–24.
28. Hamidi GA, Ramezani MH, Arani MN, Talaei SA, Mesdaghinia A, Banafshe HR. Ethosuximide reduces allodynia and hyperalgesia and potentiates morphine effects in the chronic constriction injury model of neuropathic pain. Eur J Pharmacol. 2012;674(2-3):260–4.
29. Kerckhove N, Mallet C, Pereira B, et al. Assessment of the effectiveness and safety of Ethosuximide in the Treatment of non-Diabetic Peripheral Neuropathic Pain: EDONOT—protocol of a randomised, parallel, controlled, double-blinded and multicentre clinical trial. BMJ Open. 2016;6(12):e013530.
30. Kerckhove N, Pereira B, Soriot-Thomas S, et al. Efficacy and safety of a T-type calcium channel blocker in patients with neuropathic pain: A proof-of-concept, randomized, double-blind and controlled trial. Eur J Pain. 2018;22(7):1321–30.
31. Carta F, Argenton S, Cervi D, et al. Potentiation of morphine analgesia by nifedipine in postoperative pain. Minerva Anestesiol. 1988;54(4):127–30.
32. Pereira IT, Prado WA, Dos Reis MP. Enhancement of the epidural morphine-induced analgesia by systemic nifedipine. Pain. 1993;53(3):341–5.
33. Santillán R, Maestre JM, Hurlé MA, Flórez J. Enhancement of opiate analgesia by nimodipine in cancer patients chronically treated with morphine: a preliminary report. Pain. 1994;58(1):129–32.
34. Santillán R, Hurlé MA, Armijo JA, de los Mozos R, Flórez J. Nimodipine-enhanced opiate analgesia in cancer patients requiring morphine dose escalation: a double-blind, placebo-controlled study. Pain. 1998;76(1):17–26.
35. Boldt J, von Bormann B, Kling D, Russ W, Ratthey K, Hempelmann G. Low-dose fentanyl analgesia modified by calcium channel blockers in cardiac surgery. Eur J Anaesthesiol. 1987;4(6):387–94.
36. Nitahara K, Matsunaga M, Katori K, Yotsui H, Higuchi H, Higa K. Effect of continuous low-dose intravenous diltiazem on epidural fentanyl analgesia after lower abdominal surgery. Br J Anaesth. 2003;90(4):507–9.
37. Casey G, Nortcliffe SA, Sharpe P, Buggy DJ. Perioperative nimodipine and postoperative analgesia. Anesth Analg. 2006;102(2):504–8.
38. Roca G, Aguilar LJ, Gomar C, Mazo V, Costa J, Vidal F. Nimodipine fails to enhance the analgesic effect of slow release morphine in the early phases of cancer pain treatment. Pain. 1996;68(2):239–43.
39. Vaupel DB, Lange WR, London ED. Effects of verapamil on morphine-induced euphoria, analgesia and respiratory depression in humans. J Pharmacol Exp Ther. 1993;267(3):1386–94.
40. Hasegawa AE, Zacny JP. The influence of three l-type calcium channel blockers on morphine effects in healthy volunteers. Anesth Analg. 1997;85(3):633–8.
41. Sica DA. Calcium channel blocker class heterogeneity: select aspects of pharmacokinetics and pharmacodynamics. J Clin Hypertens (Greenwich). 2005;7(4 Suppl 1):21–6.
42. Burdge G, Leach H, Walsh K. Ziconotide-induced psychosis: A case report and literature review. Ment Health Clin. 2018;8(5):242–6.
43. Howard Smith H. Safety and efficacy of intrathecal ziconotide in the management of severe chronic pain. TCRM. Published online July 2009:521.

Magnesium

15

Thomas J. Papadimos, Scott M. Pappada, and Justin P. Reinert

Abbreviations

AUC	Area Under the Curve
BOX-11	A pain assessment tool used in CRPS studies
CNS	Central Nervous System
CRPS	Complex Regional Pain Syndrome
CRPS-1	Complex Regional Pain Syndrome Type 1
CS	Central Sensitization
GABA	Gamma-Aminobutyric Acid
HADS	Hospital Anxiety and Depression Scale
IL-6	Interleukin 6
IL-β1	Interleukin Beta 1
IT	Intrathecal
IV	Intravenous
Mg	Magnesium
$MgSO_4$	Magnesium Sulfate
NFkB	Nuclear Factor Kappa B
NMDA	N-Methyl-D-Aspartate
NSAIDs	Nonsteroidal Anti-Inflammatory Drugs
PHN	Postherpetic Neuralgia
RCT	Randomized Controlled Trial
TKA	Total Knee Arthroplasty
TNF-α	Tumor Necrosis Factor Alpha
VAS	Visual Analog Scale

T. J. Papadimos (✉)
Departments of Surgery and Anesthesiology, University of Toledo College of Medicine and Life Sciences, Toledo, OH, USA
e-mail: Thomas.Papadimos@UToledo.edu

S. M. Pappada
Department of Anesthesiology, University of Toledo College of Medicine and Life Sciences, Toledo, OH, USA
e-mail: Scott.Pappada@UToledo.edu

J. P. Reinert
Department of Pharmacy Practice, The University of Toledo College of Pharmacy and Pharmaceutical Sciences, Toledo, OH, USA
e-mail: Justin.Reinert@UToledo.edu

Introduction

Management of pain perioperatively involves a plethora of interventions including opioids and non-opioids in combination or alone, as well as neuraxial and regional techniques. In all instances, while pain must be addressed, the risk of over-prescription of opioids and their consumption and related adverse events must be taken into consideration. Multimodal analgesic techniques have a new emphasis in view of the opioid epidemic that has engulfed the USA. Magnesium infusions should be considered as a part of such an approach.

The cost of the opioid epidemic in the US has taken its toll on patients, their families, and communities. This epidemic is costing the US more than $78 billion dollars a year [1, 2]. While the same crisis is not manifest in Europe up to now, the synthetic opioid crisis may be reaching its doorstep in the near future [3]. This crisis, in addition to the recent shortage of medications for surgical theaters, has required anesthesiologists to search for non-opiate solutions for their institutions and practices [4].

Conventional analgesic strategies, including opioids and nonsteroidal anti-inflammatory drugs (NSAIDs), are commonly used but may be associated with significant side effects, such as sedation, respiratory depression, gastrointestinal complications, and an increased risk of dependency [5–8]. As a result, there is growing interest in adjunctive therapies that can enhance analgesic efficacy while minimizing adverse effects [9, 10]. Magnesium infusions and injections have been studied extensively and used in multiple postoperative settings [10–27], as well as in chronic, neuropathic, and migraine pain [28–32], and chemotherapy-induced peripheral neuropathy, trigeminal neuralgia, and complex regional pain syndrome [28–34].

It has also been used as an antiarrhythmic in atrial fibrillation and ventricular tachycardia [35], eclampsia and pre-eclampsia for its anticonvulsant and vasodilatory properties, [36], as well as severe asthma [37].

However, its application in pain control through its potential ability to limit the use of perioperative opioids in surgery,

J. P. Reinert et al. (eds.), *Adjunctive Analgesic Strategies for the Bedside Clinician and Beyond*,
https://doi.org/10.1007/978-3-032-21675-5_15

especially trauma, needs serious consideration. For instance, there are over seven million orthopedic injuries in the US each year, usually caused by motor vehicle crashes, sports injuries, and occupational accidents, resulting in 3.6 million hospital visits, 800,000 inpatient stays, and 600,000 emergency surgeries annually [38]. Intravenous (IV) magnesium can be incorporated into multimodal analgesic regimens to enhance pain control and reduce reliance on opioids. Pain management following surgery and trauma is a critical aspect of patient care, as inadequate control of postoperative pain can impair recovery, increase the risk of complications, prolong hospital length of stay, and cost institutions thousands of dollars in excess care and expenses [39–47].

Magnesium and Pain

Magnesium sulfate, administered via IV infusion, has emerged as a promising adjuvant in the management of postoperative pain. Magnesium has demonstrated effectiveness in reducing postoperative pain intensity, potentially decreasing the need for opioids, improving patient comfort, and reducing opioid side effects (e.g., nausea, constipation). IV magnesium may also reduce opioid consumption by providing an analgesic effect and thereby reducing opioid-related complications through an *opioid sparing effect* [48–50]. Such infusions may also *reduce the inflammatory response* [51–54], which may delay recovery and contribute to further pain. Additionally, magnesium acts as a *muscle relaxant* [24, 55, 56] and may assist orthopedic surgeons by providing significant muscle relaxation, allowing more effective intraoperative manipulation and reduction of spasms. Patients with chronic pain from various conditions may benefit from magnesium's *neuromodulatory effect* [50, 57].

More specifically, magnesium plays a vital role in modulating pain through its actions as a noncompetitive antagonist of the N-methyl-D-aspartate (NMDA) receptor [58]. By blocking NMDA receptors in a voltage-dependent manner, magnesium inhibits central sensitization (CS), which leads to pain hypersensitivity and reduces the transmission of pain signals.

The concept of CS, and magnesium's role in its mitigation, is important [59]. Previously, there were two major pain models. The first was the "pain pathway model," in which peripheral pathways were activated by pain stimuli, and the duration and intensity of pain were determined by the strength and timing of these inputs [59]. The second was the "gate control theory" of pain, which proposed that pain transmission pathways could be opened or closed by a gating mechanism [59]. However, it is now evident that there are also specific paths where facilitation and inhibition provide controls. Both concepts were partially correct. CS is an augmentation of circuit function in neurons and pain tracts caused by an augmentation in membrane excitability and the effectiveness of synapses, along with reduced inhibition. When the functional properties of the neurons change, normal innocuous stimuli can be painful. This occurs secondary to inflammation and injury; it is a manifestation of the exceptional plasticity of the somatosensory system. CS recruits previously subthreshold synaptic inputs to pain neurons, thereby causing such inputs to be augmented and amplified. This will generate pain hypersensitivity. In effect, these changes in the subthreshold neurons cause the patient's pain to be disassociated with the normal acute pain response. In other words, CS creates a hypersensitive pain state by changing the sensory response of normal inputs because the normal acute pain response is no longer coupled to the "presence, intensity, or duration of noxious peripheral stimuli [59]." Magnesium's role in the interference of CS may be of understated importance.

Magnesium also inhibits voltage-gated calcium channels, thereby decreasing neurotransmitter release (e.g., glutamate) and dampening nociceptive signaling [60]. This competition with calcium at the neuromuscular junction facilitates muscle relaxation and alleviates muscle tension or spasm. Furthermore, magnesium downregulates pro-inflammatory cytokines such as Tumor Necrosis Factor [TNF-α], Interleukin-6 [IL-6], and Interleukin beta 1 [IL-β1], potentially minimizing postoperative pain and swelling [52, 54, 61–64]. These cytokines are involved in the pathology of pain. There is evidence that IL-β1 causes hyperalgesia after intraperitoneal, intracerebroventricular, and intraplantar administration. IL-β1 increases production of substance P and prostaglandin PGE_2 in neural and glial cells [62, 64].

Addressing the positive attributes of adding magnesium infusions to patients in the perioperative period that arguably decrease opioid administration and pain should be accompanied by a perspective of what a lack of magnesium can cause. Magnesium is the fourth most abundant cation in the body, so the connection of hypomagnesemia to inflammation is not surprising. It is important for cell proliferation, cell homeostasis, and cell death and is associated with metabolism [65]. Hypomagnesemia impairs the immune system, especially adaptive immune cells, and promotes an inflammatory response through activation of the innate immune system [65]. Hypomagnesemia occurs because of dietary imbalances, chronic disease, and various medications [52]. Magnesium deficiency has an impact on leukocytes and microvascular endothelial cells, which are actors in acute inflammation, through activation of NFkB pathway in these cells, resulting in the substantial release of inflammatory mediators (nitric oxide and prostacyclin) [66]. These mediators lead to vasodilation, edema, and hyperemia (signs of inflammation). Also, by activating NFkB, hypomagnesemia will cause adhesion molecules to proliferate and allow adherence of leukocytes, which leads to cytokine and chemokine release that attracts white blood cells that will then migrate to the site of injury [66, 67]. IL-6 is important in the neuronal response to nerve injury. It also activates microglia and astrocytes and regulates neuronal peptide expression [62]. TNF-α is found in the neurons and glia and is important in neuropathic and inflammatory hyperalgesia. Magnesium sulfate was also found to suppress inflammation after coronary artery bypass grafting by decreasing IL-6 and TNF-α [61].

While it is evident that magnesium plays a major role in regulating the immune response to pain, hypomagnesemia must be acknowledged because it can create a nonspecific immune response when the immune system is challenged, which is associated with low-grade chronic inflammation, calcium deregulation, and redox imbalance, which are all associated with dysregulated magnesium transporters that contribute to the inflammatory response [52].

Magnesium infusions can be given before anesthetic induction, after anesthetic induction, or postoperatively to mitigate intraoperative and postoperative pain [68]. Furthermore, by minimizing CS, magnesium infusions may reduce the risk of developing chronic pain after surgery [22, 25, 47]. While magnesium infusions have been used for over a decade, there are limitations and other considerations that must be examined. While magnesium infusions are generally safe [45], they require monitoring for side effects such as hypotension, bradycardia, and respiratory depression, especially in those patients with organ dysfunction [69]. For instance, patients with renal dysfunction or preexisting electrolyte disorders need careful consideration due to the risk of hypermagnesemia; magnesium levels exceeding 4–5 mmol/L [9.7–12.2 mg/dl] are considered toxic. The prevalence of hypermagnesemia clinically is 3.0% in the general population, and in hospitals it is 5.7–9.3%. Additionally, optimal dosing protocols are not standardized, with multiple variations in preoperative, intraoperative, and postoperative regimens; and, furthermore, some studies report that the presumed efficacy of the antinociceptive effect of magnesium is not readily evident [68–73].

Efficacy

Magnesium Sulfate in Acute Pain and the Perioperative Period

Besides its role as an antiarrhythmic medication [35], its use in preeclampsia and eclampsia, and its use in asthmatic exacerbations [37], its role as an analgesic and antispasmodic medication is evolving [26]. In the perioperative setting, IV magnesium infusions are administered as a bolus dose followed by continuous infusion (30–50 mg/kg; 6–20 mg/kg/h) [50]. While the use of magnesium infusions has increased over time, some examples of the evidence for its use follows.

In 2007, a systematic review by Lysakowski et al. conducted the first attempt meta-analysis on the use of magnesium for postoperative pain, but it yielded inconclusive results as to magnesium's effectiveness [27]. Six years later, Albrecht et al. published the first comprehensive systematic review and meta-analysis assessing the analgesic effects of perioperative IV magnesium administration, which demonstrated promising results [74]. They concluded that magnesium reduced opioid consumption for postoperative pain and, to a lesser extent, also decreased pain scores. However, they could not determine whether bolus, bolus and infusion, or just infusion was the best approach.

The methodological approaches in determining the opioid sparing effect and analgesic effects of magnesium infusions have been difficult because of the heterogeneity of research efforts as documented by Puch et al. in their review of 42 studies [68]. They complained that only 55% of the studies demonstrated a definite decrease in pain scores and morphine consumption. The remainder (45%) showed no clear effect. Puch et al. stressed the need for a uniform methodological approach.

Several interesting systematic reviews and meta-analyses on the value of magnesium as a pain adjuvant in orthopedic surgery have been published. These studies highlight the need for more randomized controlled trials (RCTs) while underscoring magnesium's potential benefits and comparing optimal dosing strategies, including timing and route of administration (intravenous vs. intrathecal).

Gormley et al. reviewed the reduction of opioids dispensed after orthopedic surgery [81]. The authors impetus to limit opioid use was the severe, ongoing opioid epidemic in North America [1, 2]. They reviewed 141 studies of 20,963 patients; 113 were RTCs. While all the studies they reviewed had used multiple interventions to reduce opioid use after orthopedic surgery, only 4/141 (2.8%) addressed magnesium sulfate use. After review of their data, the authors came to the same conclusion as others: there is a need for a rigorous and consistent application of methodology to RCTs in orthopedic pain control to enable a thoughtful and helpful evidence-based approach to pharmacologic and non-pharmacologic interventions in clinical practice. This is especially true as it applies to magnesium sulfate infusions.

Peng et al. screened 2350 articles and found 11 RTCs ($N = 535$ patients) in their review that also addressed perioperative IV administration of magnesium sulfate in orthopedic surgery [44]. Their review in support of magnesium yielded mixed results. They reported that six of the trials demonstrated a reduction in pain intensity, while five studies did not. Nonetheless, a reduction of nausea, vomiting, and shivering with the use of magnesium sulfate was evident. The authors concluded that there is a need for further research.

Sbitan et al. performed a narrative review to compare the intrathecal (IT) and IV administration of magnesium sulfate as a pain adjuvant in orthopedic procedures [41]. They identified nine RCTs that addressed IT and IV administration of magnesium sulfate, but only three trials directly compared the IT vs. IV approach. Their conclusion in this regard, for both approaches, was that there is evidence for the efficacy of magnesium. However, the choice of the mode of administration remained a critical question, and they too called for further studies.

There are two reviews on spinal surgery that are noteworthy. The first, Campos et al., published a recent systematic review on the safety and efficacy of magnesium in spinal surgery [24]. They reported that the neuroprotective and anti-inflammatory effects of magnesium, compared to steroids, caused a decrease in pain. In doing so, magnesium also significantly decreased opioid consumption. Hemodynamically, when compared to steroids, magnesium demonstrated a lower mean arterial pressure (which may be a surgical advantage). Furthermore, magnesium also lowered the consumption of muscle relaxants and enhanced the effect of vecuronium. This analysis also confirmed that magnesium can be used in combination with other medications or strategies to elicit synergistic effects. Finally, the authors concluded that there is no agreement in the scientific community on whether to use a bolus, bolus plus infusion, or infusion only. Loading doses, maintenance dosing, and protocols varied. Most loading doses were initiated IV just prior to anesthetic induction and ranged from 30 to 50 mg/kg in saline and were infused over 10–30 min; maintenance infusions were administered continuously throughout the surgery at a rate of 10–20 mg/kg/h with few side effects.

Yue et al. performed a systematic review and meta-analysis of 14 trials (781 patients) that reported the use of IV magnesium infusions during spinal surgery [82]. They determined that magnesium infusions reduced morphine consumption at 24 h compared to controls, which matched findings in previous reviews of various surgical procedured [27, 74, 83–86]. However, they concluded that although the morphine consumption was less, the evidence of pain relief was of low quality. Their work demonstrated that postsurgical analgesic use of magnesium infusions shorter than 24 h did not demonstrate effective pain relief. Furthermore, their review also documented a decreased rate of nausea and vomiting and a delay in anesthetic awakening. Again, the authors argued for more RCTs.

The second, a systematic review and meta-analysis by Azimi et al., explored RCTs and magnesium use in total knee arthroplasties (TKA) [40]. They evaluated eight RCTs regarding pain management and analgesic use in 536 patients. They found that in the first 24 h postoperatively, there was a significant decrease in opioid consumption but low to moderate evidence that administration of magnesium intraoperatively for postoperative pain control in TKAs was effective. The authors likewise noted significant heterogeneity across studies in terms of methods, dosing regimens, and routes of administration.

Elhouty et al. were concerned that toxic goiter resection would lead to inadequate pain control on manipulation of the thyroid gland, through a neurohumoral response, that would lead to hemodynamic instability [87]. They compared IV magnesium sulphate infusions vs. lidocaine infusions and vs. a control group. They found that the magnesium and the lidocaine groups significantly prolonged the requests for initial analgesia in the postanesthesia care unit, but the beneficial effects were more prominent in the magnesium group.

In patients undergoing bilateral inguinal hernia repair under spinal anesthesia, Farouk et al. studied the effects of IV magnesium sulfate vs. dexmedetomidine vs. a control group [15]. Infusion of either magnesium or dexmedetomidine improved the quality of the spinal anesthetic and increased the duration of postoperative analgesia and decreased the consumption of morphine over the ensuing 24 h. Magnesium infusions resulted in better hemodynamic stability, while dexmedetomidine provided slightly longer pain control.

Akbudak et al. studied the preemptive use of magnesium sulfate on postoperative pain in women undergoing mastectomy [16]. The experimental group was given 50 mg/kg of magnesium sulfate in 250 ml of isotonic fluid 30 min before induction of anesthesia, and the control group was given the same isotonic fluid, but without magnesium sulfate. The magnesium group had lower pain scores without affecting hemodynamic measurements during induction or maintenance of general anesthesia.

There is clearly a positive effect in the use of magnesium sulfate infusions. It can be documented in individual studies and in systematic reviews and meta-analyses. However, the effects of surgery type, patient demographics, physiologic status, and dosing require further investigation.

Magnesium in Chronic Pain

Complex Regional Pain Syndrome

Complex Regional Pain Syndrome (CRPS) is a severe, chronic neuropathic pain condition that typically develops after trauma, surgery, or fractures and is characterized by disproportionate regional pain alongside sensory abnormalities such as allodynia and hyperalgesia, motor dysfunction, and autonomic disturbances [88–90]. It is divided into type 1 (without confirmed nerve injury) and type 2 (with nerve injury), diagnosed using criteria such as the Budapest Criteria [91–93]. One proposed mechanism, central nervous system sensitization, is driven largely by NMDA receptor-mediated neuroplasticity, which enhances pain transmission and perception [89, 91, 93–95]. Considering its mechanism of action, magnesium sulfate presents as a promising treatment option for CRPS, especially given the limited efficacy and complexity of current therapies.

A pilot study conducted by Collins et al. investigated the effects of IV magnesium sulfate on pain and functional outcomes in patients with Complex Regional Pain Syndrome type 1 (CRPS 1). Ten patients were enrolled, with eight receiving magnesium sulfate and two receiving a placebo. Exclusion criteria addressed comorbid conditions and potential treatment interferences. The magnesium group received 70 mg/kg of magnesium sulfate IV over 4 h daily for 5 days, while placebo patients received saline. All participants continued standardized physical therapy and were permitted to use non-opioid analgesics. Pain assessments, sensory testing, functional evaluations, and quality of life measures were conducted at baseline and up to 12 weeks posttreatment. Significant reductions in median daily pain scores were observed at all time points following magnesium treatment, with four patients meeting the predefined criterion of ≥50% pain reduction by week 12. The findings suggested that magnesium infusions may offer analgesic benefit and led to a subsequent randomized controlled trial by the same team of investigators [96].

That randomized, double-blind, placebo-controlled trial evaluated the effects of IV magnesium sulfate in 56 patients with CRPS-1, using the same protocol as the Collins et al. study, with participants receiving either 70 mg/kg of magnesium sulfate IV or a placebo over 4 h for five consecutive days. Pain, impairment, function, participation, and quality of life were assessed at baseline and at 1, 3, 6, and 12 weeks posttreatment. While both groups experienced a modest improvement in pain scores after the first week, no significant differences were observed between the magnesium and placebo groups in pain or impairment outcomes overall. Also, the magnesium sulfate group showed short-term within-group improvements as well as enhanced job participation at 12 weeks. Notably, patients with lower anxiety and depression scores (HADS ≤10) experienced greater functional improvement with magnesium [97].

Based on the paucity of current evidence, IV magnesium sulfate shows some potential for short-term pain relief and functional improvement in patients with CRPS type 1, though no significant differences between magnesium and placebo in overall pain and impairment outcomes were identified in a randomized trial. Routine use of IV magnesium sulfate for CRPS-1 cannot be broadly recommended at this time, but it may warrant further investigation in select patient subgroups or as part of a multimodal treatment approach [96, 97] (Table 15.1).

Neuropathic Pain

A randomized, double-blind study by Kim et al. investigated the effectiveness and safety of IV ketamine and magnesium sulfate infusions in treating severe, intractable postherpetic neuralgia (PHN) in 30 patients who had failed multiple conventional pharmacological and interventional therapies, including nerve blocks and systemic medications such as anticonvulsants and antidepressants. These patients reported persistent, spontaneous neuropathic pain with high intensity, classified as a visual analog scale (VAS) score > 7, lasting at least 6 months, despite ongoing treatments. Participants were randomly assigned to receive either ketamine 1 mg/kg per hour or magnesium sulfate 30 mg/kg infusions, each administered IV over 1 hour, under sedation with midazolam to ensure unconsciousness during the pro-

Table 15.1 Dosing considerations for magnesium as an analgesic

Pain syndrome/setting	Magnesium dose/regimen	Route of administration	Notes/outcome
Perioperative pain (general)	30–50 mg/kg bolus, then 6–20 mg/kg/h	Intravenous (IV)	Administered as a bolus before/after induction, followed by continuous infusion during surgery
Complex regional pain syndrome (CRPS type 1)	70 mg/kg over 4 h daily ×5 days	IV	Pilot and RCT studies; some improvement in pain and function in subgroups
Postherpetic neuralgia (PHN)	30 mg/kg over 1 h ×3 sessions	IV	Compared to ketamine; effective with a 39.6% average pain reduction
Spinal surgery (various procedures)	Loading dose: 30–50 mg/kg over 10–30 min; Maintenance: 10–20 mg/kg/h	IV	Reduced opioid consumption; variation in protocols across studies
Mastectomy (preemptive use)	50 mg/kg in 250 mL isotonic fluid 30 min preinduction	IV	Lower pain scores without affecting hemodynamics
Orthopedic surgery (general)	Variable; some used bolus + infusion	IV and intrathecal (IT)	Efficacy varies; further studies needed for standardization
Neuropathic pain (refractory)	3 grams over 30 min, adjunct to ketamine	IV	No added benefit over ketamine alone in crossover study
Trigeminal neuralgia	Not specified	IV	Preliminary evidence suggests benefit

cedure. Each patient underwent three infusion sessions, given every other day. Both treatment groups showed statistically significant reductions in pain compared to baseline: ketamine patients' mean VAS scores decreased from 8.0 to 4.33, while magnesium patients' scores fell from 7.7 to 3.1. Although ketamine achieved a higher average percentage reduction in pain (51%) compared to magnesium (39.6%), the difference was not statistically significant. Using a predefined criterion of response (≥50% reduction in VAS), 10 of 15 ketamine-treated patients and 7 of 15 magnesium-treated patients were classified as responders, indicating that magnesium provided substantial analgesic benefit in a majority of cases. This finding is significant in that it compares two NMDA-receptor antagonists for an analgesic effect and demonstrates nonsignificant differences in their analgesic effects [98].

A second randomized, placebo-controlled, crossover, double-blind clinical study was completed by Pickering and colleagues to determine the impact of ketamine vs. ketamine with concomitant magnesium sulfate in the management of refractory neuropathic pain. The majority of included patients were seeking relief from postsurgical neuropathies, followed by radiculopathies and post-traumatic neuropathies. Patients received three treatments in random order by IV infusion every 35 days: placebo with 0.9% saline, ketamine at 0.5 mg/kg over 2 h, and the same ketamine regimen in addition to 3 grams of magnesium sulfate over 30 min. The primary objective was to evaluate the analgesic effect of IV ketamine compared to placebo, with the primary endpoint being the area under the curve (AUC) of average daily pain intensity over 35 days post-infusion. From the 20 enrolled patients, no statistically significant difference in average daily pain intensity AUC was observed over the 35-day evaluation window between either intervention or placebo. Both ketamine regimens demonstrated a modest but statistically significant reduction in pain at 7 days post-infusion compared to placebo; however, the addition of magnesium sulfate did not provide an additional analgesic benefit. Mild to moderate adverse events such as fatigue, nausea, and dizziness occurred more frequently with ketamine and ketamine/magnesium than with placebo [99].

These studies highlight the potential role of magnesium as an adjunctive analgesic in managing severe neuropathic pain, particularly when conventional treatments have failed. These trials suggest that magnesium sulfate may have standalone analgesic properties for neuropathic pain, though it does not appear to significantly potentiate ketamine's effects when used concomitantly. Further research is warranted to refine dosing regimens, identify patient subgroups most likely to benefit, and better understand the duration and mechanisms of analgesia.

A summary of magnesium doses, comparators, and outcomes can be found in Table 15.1.

Safety Considerations

Tolerability

As is evident from the clinical data presented within this chapter, magnesium sulfate is well tolerated and considered to have a favorable safety profile, with the majority of demonstrated adverse effects being associated with minor, noncritical occurrences. Significant adverse effects, including respiratory arrest or depression, have only been sparsely documented in the literature, while dizziness and nausea were relatively common. From an IV administration standpoint, it is reasonable to consider magnesium sulfate injections or infusions to have the potential to cause itching, swelling, and erythema; however, these localized reactions should not prevent clinicians from using magnesium sulfate. Oral preparations may be more associated with gastrointestinal adverse effects, including nausea and constipation [100].

Practice Implications

While magnesium sulfate is widely considered to be an electrolyte, supplement, or elemental ion, it must be recognized that in the setting of therapeutic intervention, magnesium sulfate is a drug. As such, the consideration of drug-drug and drug-disease state interactions must be investigated to ensure the safety of administration, as well as to ensure that the desired efficacy can be readily attained.

Magnesium sulfate, especially when provided IV, has notable central nervous system (CNS) depressant properties that can potentiate the sedative and respiratory depressant effects of opioids and benzodiazepines. This interaction is primarily pharmacodynamic in nature and is mediated through magnesium's ability to antagonize NMDA receptors, block calcium channels, and enhance GABAergic neurotransmission [101, 102]. This combination may result in amplified sedative effects and an increased risk of respiratory depression.

Clinical evidence supports these interactions. In a randomized controlled trial by Koinig et al., patients undergoing gynecologic surgery who received IV magnesium sulfate 50 mg/kg boluses followed by 15 mg/kg/h infusions required significantly less propofol and fentanyl for adequate anesthesia and analgesia, indicating that magnesium potentiated the effects of both agents [101]. Similarly, Telci et al. found that perioperative magnesium sulfate reduced postoperative opioid consumption and pain scores but was associated with increased sedation [102]. While specific studies on magnesium with benzodiazepines are limited, pharmacologic data and clinical observations suggest that magnesium's GABA-enhancing effects can intensify benzodiazepine-induced sedation. This potentiation is particularly concerning in vulnerable populations such as the elderly, patients with respiratory disease, or those receiving high doses of opioids or benzodiazepines [101]. While needing to be fully investigated in a clinical capacity, it may be reasonable to consider decreasing concomitant opioid and benzodiazepine doses while patients are receiving magnesium as an adjunctive analgesic to prevent oversedation or respiratory depression.

With specific regard to interactions with other adjunctive analgesics, magnesium salts have been implicated in decreasing the gastrointestinal absorption of gabapentin, potentially reducing its bioavailability and therapeutic effect. This interaction occurs due to the formation of chelate complexes in the gastrointestinal tract. Gabapentin's absorption is mediated by the L-amino acid transport system in the small intestine, and concurrent administration of magnesium, as found in antacids or magnesium-containing supplements, can significantly reduce peak plasma concentrations and the AUC of gabapentin [103]. In a study by Yagi et al., coadministration of an aluminum-magnesium hydroxide antacid reduced the bioavailability of gabapentin by approximately 20%. To mitigate this interaction, it is recommended that oral magnesium-containing products and gabapentin be administered at least 2 h apart. This interaction has not been documented with IV preparations of magnesium sulfate [104].

From a drug-disease perspective, magnesium sulfate must be used cautiously in renal impairment, as impaired excretion can lead to hypermagnesemia, manifesting as hypotension, bradycardia, respiratory depression, and, in severe cases, cardiac arrest [105]. Patients with myasthenia gravis are also at heightened risk, as magnesium can worsen neuromuscular transmission and precipitate severe muscle weakness or respiratory failure [106]. In obstetric patients, magnesium is often used for seizure prophylaxis in preeclampsia; however, coexisting conditions such as hypocalcemia can be exacerbated, particularly with prolonged therapy, since magnesium inhibits parathyroid hormone secretion and calcium release [107].

A Call for Future Research

Future research can span broad focus areas. An initial area of research could involve studies aimed at the optimization of dosing protocols. There have been numerous studies that report significant variability in loading doses, maintenance infusions, and timing of doses during preoperative, perioperative, or postoperative periods [41, 108]. The significant variability among these studies complicates standardization and the identification of an optimal dosing protocol leading to the best patient outcomes. Future studies evaluating whether a fixed-dose or weight-based dosing approach yields more favorable outcomes among different surgical patient populations would be welcome [109].

Another important area of examination is the execution of comparative efficacy studies, which investigate the potential for magnesium to serve as an adjuvant to other non-opioid analgesics like ketamine, lidocaine, or NSAIDs currently used in multimodal pain management strategies [110, 111]. Specific focuses of research may be encouraged by prior efforts, for example, to evaluate the differential effects of IV versus IT magnesium sulfate administration to determine the most effective administration routes for specific surgical procedures [41, 112].

Additionally, it is important to evaluate the effectiveness of magnesium in the management of surgical patients with chronic pain. To this end, it would be fruitful to investigate magnesium's role in managing chronic pain conditions such as complex regional pain syndrome, neuropathic pain, and fibromyalgia. Current studies have demonstrated mixed results, which necessitate the execution of larger, higher-quality clinical trials with patient follow-up over extended periods of time [28, 108, 113]. It would be beneficial if some aspects of inquiry would target magnesium's ability to reduce central sensitization mechanisms in chronic pain states, considering its N-methyl-D-aspartate (NMDA) receptor antagonism and calcium channel blocking properties [50, 57].

Studies of magnesium's safety, broader benefits, and potential side effects should be undertaken to evaluate its impact on the comorbid conditions of surgical patient populations such as those with chronic kidney disease, acute kidney injury, cardiovascular disease, and gastrointestinal disorders [114–118]. Further examination of the long-term implications or side effects of repeated magnesium use in chronic conditions to establish safety guardrails for prolonged treatment regimens would also be helpful. Investigative trials should be directed at the execution of comprehensive clinical trials focusing on long-term safety and efficacy across diverse patient groups, which are essential to evaluate and optimize its therapeutic use.

Conclusion

There is considerable evidence that IV magnesium infusions are effective in orthopedic surgery, consistently demonstrating a reduction of postoperative opioid consumption and an improvement in pain scores when used in the first 24 h. However, the results should be interpreted cautiously because of various clinical shortcomings and the variable methodological approaches that have been applied to the available research. Further clinical studies need to be performed using uniform methodological approaches (RCTs, surgery type, route of administration, dosing, etc.), and if possible, correlated with immunological (cytokine) findings. Multicenter trials examining the use of magnesium sulfate infusions for pain control and reduced requests for analgesic medications in the perioperative period are worth pursuing. We encourage our colleagues in the surgery, anesthesiology, and critical care communities to actively engage in clinical investigations to answer these questions.

References

1. Shipton EA, Shipton EE, Shipton AJ. A review of the opioid epidemic: what do we do about it? Pain Ther. 2018;7:23–36.
2. Chen LH, Hedegaard H, author Warner M. Drug-poisoning deaths involving opioid analgesics: United States, 1999–2011. US Department of Health and Human Services, Centers for Disease Control and …; 2014.
3. Griffiths PN, Seyler T, De Morais JM, Mounteney JE, Sedefov RS. Opioid problems are changing in Europe with worrying signals that synthetic opioids may play a more significant role in the future. Wiley Online Library; 2023.
4. Mitra S, Carlyle D, Kodumudi G, Kodumudi V, Vadivelu N. New advances in acute postoperative pain management. Curr Pain Headache Rep. 2018;22(5):35.
5. Daoust R, Paquet J, Cournoyer A, Piette É, Morris J, Lessard J, et al. Side effects from opioids used for acute pain after emergency department discharge. Am J Emerg Med. 2020;38(4):695–701.
6. Gharibo C, Drewes AM, Breve F, Rekatsina M, Tamayo MAN, Varrassi G, et al. Iatrogenic side effects of pain therapies. Cureus. 2023;15(9):e44583.
7. Benyamin R, Trescot AM, Datta S, Buenaventura RM, Adlaka R, Sehgal N, et al. Opioid complications and side effects. Pain Physician. 2008;11(2S):S105.
8. Paul AK, Smith CM, Rahmatullah M, Nissapatorn V, Wilairatana P, Spetea M, et al. Opioid analgesia and opioid-induced adverse effects: a review. Pharmaceuticals. 2021;14(11):1091.
9. Gupta K, Vohra V, Sood J. The role of magnesium as an adjuvant during general anaesthesia. Anaesthesia. 2006;61(11):1058–63.
10. Tsaousi G, Nikopoulou A, Pezikoglou I, Birba V, Grosomanidis V. Implementation of magnesium sulphate as an adjunct to multimodal analgesic approach for perioperative pain control in lumbar laminectomy surgery: a randomized placebo-controlled clinical trial. Clin Neurol Neurosurg. 2020;197:106091.
11. Ferasatkish R, Dabbagh A, Alavi M, Mollasadeghi G, Hydarpur E, Moghadam AA, et al. Effect of magnesium sulfate on extubation time and acute pain in coronary artery bypass surgery. Acta Anaesthesiol Scand. 2008;52(10):1348–52.
12. Salkaya A, Oba S, Altınay M, Türk HŞ, Kılınç L, Yılmaz A. The effects of perioperative low-dose magnesium sulfate infusion on postoperative pain in lumbar surgery. Signa Vitae. 2024;20(1):50.
13. Jerkovic D, Tadin A, Gavic L, Vladislavic NZ, Grgic N, Macan D. Effect of orally administered magnesium on postoperative pain level and trismus after surgical removal of the lower third molars: a randomized, double-blind, placebo-controlled trial. Clin Oral Investig. 2020;24(12):4649–59.
14. El Mourad MB, Arafa SK. Effect of intravenous versus intraperitoneal magnesium sulfate on hemodynamic parameters and postoperative analgesia during laparoscopic sleeve gastrectomy–a prospective randomized study. J Anaesthesiol Clin Pharmacol. 2019;35(2):242–7.
15. Farouk I, Hassan MM, Fetouh AM, Elgayed AEA, Eldin MH, Abdelhamid BM. Analgesic and hemodynamic effects of intravenous infusion of magnesium sulphate versus dexmedetomidine in patients undergoing bilateral inguinal hernial surgeries under spinal anesthesia: a randomized controlled study. Braz J Anesthesiol. 2021;71(5):489–97.
16. Akbudak IH, Yilmaz S, Ilhan S, Tanriverdi SY, Erdem E. The effect of preemptive magnesium sulfate on postoperative pain in patients undergoing mastectomy: a clinical trial. Eur Rev Med Pharmacol Sci. 2023;27(17):7907–13.
17. Sousa AM, Rosado GM, Neto Jde S, Guimaraes GM, Ashmawi HA. Magnesium sulfate improves postoperative analgesia in laparoscopic gynecologic surgeries: a double-blind randomized controlled trial. J Clin Anesth. 2016;34:379–84.
18. Jokar A, Cyrus A, Babaei M, Taheri M, Almasi-Hashiani A, Behzadinia E, et al. The effect of magnesium sulfate on renal colic pain relief; a randomized clinical trial. Emerg (Tehran). 2017;5(1):e25.
19. Kamel EZ, Abd-Elshafy SK, Sayed JA, Mostafa MM, Seddik MI. Pain alleviation in patients undergoing cardiac surgery; presternal local anesthetic and magnesium infiltration versus conventional intravenous analgesia: a randomized double-blind study. Korean J Pain. 2018;31(2):93–101.
20. Celenlioglu AE, Sir E, Ors-Yildirim N, Yildirim AK, Ince ME, Doganci S. Effect of perioperative intravenous magnesium sulfate on postoperative pain after iliac venous stenting. J Vasc Surg Venous Lymphat Disord. 2023;11(3):517–24.
21. Oh TK, Oh AY, Ryu JH, Koo BW, Lee YJ, Do SH. Retrospective analysis of the association between intraoperative magnesium sulfate infusion and postoperative acute kidney injury after major laparoscopic abdominal surgery. Sci Rep. 2019;9(1):2833.
22. Ghezel-Ahmadi V, Ghezel-Ahmadi D, Schirren J, Tsapopiorgas C, Beck G, Bölükbas S. Perioperative systemic magnesium sulphate to minimize acute and chronic post-thoracotomy pain: a prospective observational study. J Thorac Dis. 2019;11(2):418.
23. Lee C, Song YK, Jeong HM, Park SN. The effects of magnesium sulfate infiltration on perioperative opioid consumption and opioid-induced hyperalgesia in patients undergoing robot-assisted laparoscopic prostatectomy with remifentanil-based anesthesia. Korean J Anesthesiol. 2011;61(3):244–50.
24. Campos J, Bas JL, Campos C, Mariscal G, Bas T, Bas P. Efficacy and safety of intravenous magnesium sulfate in spinal surgery: a systematic review and meta-analysis. J Clin Med. 2024;13(11):3122.
25. Kido K, Katagiri N, Kawana H, Sugino S, Konno D, Suzuki J, et al. Effects of magnesium sulfate administration in attenuating chronic postsurgical pain in rats. Biochem Biophys Res Commun. 2021;534:395–400.
26. Kim RK, Kim JW, Angelotti T, Esquivel M, Tsui BC, Hwang JH. Magnesium and esophageal pain after Peroral endoscopic Myotomy of the esophagus: a randomized, double-blind, placebo-controlled trial. Anesth Analg. 2022; https://doi.org/10.1213/ANE.0000000000006990.
27. Lysakowski C, Dumont L, Czarnetzki C, Tramèr MR. Magnesium as an adjuvant to postoperative analgesia: a systematic review of randomized trials. Anesth Analg. 2007;104(6):1532–9.
28. Fischer SG, Collins S, Boogaard S, Loer SA, Zuurmond WW, Perez RS. Intravenous magnesium for chronic complex regional pain syndrome type 1 (CRPS-1). Pain Med. 2013;14(9):1388–99.

29. Pachman DR, Barton DL, Watson JC, Loprinzi CL. Chemotherapy-induced peripheral neuropathy: prevention and treatment. Clin Pharmacol Ther. 2011;90(3):377–87.
30. Piccolo J, Kolesar JM. Prevention and treatment of chemotherapy-induced peripheral neuropathy. Am J Health Syst Pharm. 2014;71(1):19–25.
31. Brill S, Sedgwick PM, Hamann W, Di Vadi PP. Efficacy of intravenous magnesium in neuropathic pain. Br J Anaesth. 2002;89(5):711–4.
32. Chiu HY, Yeh TH, Huang YC, Chen PY. Effects of intravenous and Oral magnesium on reducing migraine: a meta-analysis of randomized controlled trials. Pain Physician. 2016;19(1):E97–112.
33. Urits I, Jung JW, Amgalan A, Fortier L, Anya A, Wesp B, et al. Utilization of magnesium for the treatment of chronic pain. Anesth Pain Med. 2021;11(1):e112348.
34. Xu M, Chen P, Zhu X, Wang CZ. Efficacy of intravenous lidocaine and magnesium in intractable trigeminal neuralgia: a preliminary report. J Neurol Sci. 2016;371:149–51.
35. Onalan O, Crystal E, Daoulah A, Lau C, Crystal A, Lashevsky I. Meta-analysis of magnesium therapy for the acute management of rapid atrial fibrillation. Am J Cardiol. 2007;99(12):1726–32.
36. Witlin AG, Sibai BM. Magnesium sulfate therapy in preeclampsia and eclampsia. Obstet Gynecol. 1998;92(5):883–9.
37. Cheuk D, Chau T, Lee S. A meta-analysis on intravenous magnesium sulphate for treating acute asthma. Arch Dis Child. 2005;90(1):74–7.
38. Jarman MP, Weaver MJ, Haider AH, Salim A, Harris MB. The national burden of orthopedic injury: cross-sectional estimates for trauma system planning and optimization. J Surg Res. 2020;249:197–204.
39. Heidari B, Salimi R, Saremi H, Arab Ghahestani M. Assessment of magnesium sulfate infusion in combination with ketorolac for the pain Management in Intertrochanteric Fractures; a randomized clinical trial. Arch Bone Jt Surg. 2023;11(6):414–20.
40. Azimi A, Tabatabaei FS, Azimi A, Mazloom H, Foruzanfar MM, Mahdavi NS. Intra-operative adjunctive magnesium sulfate in pain management of total knee arthroplasty; a systematic review and meta-analysis. Arch Acad Emerg Med. 2023;11(1):e58.
41. Sbitan L, Nabhan AI, Alafandi BZ, Alzraikat O, Alzraikat N. Magnesium sulfate for postoperative pain in orthopedic surgery: a narrative review. Medicine (Baltimore). 2024;103(24):e38522.
42. Zhao C, Wang L, Chen L, Wang Q, Kang P. Effects of magnesium sulfate on periarticular infiltration analgesia in total knee arthroplasty: a prospective, double-blind, randomized controlled trial. J Orthop Surg Res. 2023;18(1):301.
43. Frassanito L, Messina A, Vergari A, Colombo D, Chierichini A, Della Corte F, et al. Intravenous infusion of magnesium sulfate and postoperative analgesia in total knee arthroplasty. Minerva Anestesiol. 2015;81(11):1184–91.
44. Peng YN, Sung FC, Huang ML, Lin CL, Kao CH. The use of intravenous magnesium sulfate on postoperative analgesia in orthopedic surgery: a systematic review of randomized controlled trials. Medicine (Baltimore). 2018;97(50):e13583.
45. Rodriguez-Rubio L, Nava E, Del Pozo JSG, Jordan J. Influence of the perioperative administration of magnesium sulfate on the total dose of anesthetics during general anesthesia. A systematic review and meta-analysis. J Clin Anesth. 2017;39:129–38.
46. Soeding P, Morris A, Soeding A, Hoy G. Effect of intravenous magnesium on post-operative pain following Latarjet shoulder reconstruction. Shoulder Elbow. 2024;16(1):46–52.
47. Oh TK, Chung SH, Park J, Shin H, Chang CB, Kim TK, et al. Effects of perioperative magnesium sulfate administration on postoperative chronic knee pain in patients undergoing Total knee arthroplasty: a retrospective evaluation. J Clin Med. 2019;8(12):2231.
48. Arumugam S, Lau CS, Chamberlain RS. Perioperative adjunct magnesium decreases postoperative opioid requirements—a meta-analysis. Int J Clin Med. 2016;7(5):297–308.
49. Steinlechner B, Birkenberg B, Dworschak M, Grubhofer G, Schiferer A, Rajek A. The opioid-sparing effect of magnesium after cardiac surgery: P-95. Eur J Anaesthesiol I EJA. 2005;22:37.
50. Shin HJ, Na HS, Do SH. Magnesium and pain. Nutrients. 2020;12(8):2184.
51. Nielsen FH. Magnesium deficiency and increased inflammation: current perspectives. J Inflamm Res. 2018;11:25–34.
52. Maier JA, Castiglioni S, Locatelli L, Zocchi M, Mazur A, editors. Magnesium and inflammation: advances and perspectives. In Seminars in cell & developmental biology; 2021: Elsevier.
53. Veronese N, Pizzol D, Smith L, Dominguez LJ, Barbagallo M. Effect of magnesium supplementation on inflammatory parameters: a meta-analysis of randomized controlled trials. Nutrients. 2022;14(3):679.
54. Sugimoto J, Romani AM, Valentin-Torres AM, Luciano AA, Ramirez Kitchen CM, Funderburg N, et al. Magnesium decreases inflammatory cytokine production: a novel innate immunomodulatory mechanism. J Immunol. 2012;188(12):6338–46.
55. Gutiérrez-Román CI, Carrillo-Torres O, Pérez-Meléndez ES. Uses of magnesium sulfate in anesthesiology. Revista Médica del Hospital General de México. 2022;85(1):25–33.
56. Ersal M, Altan HA. The effects of intravenous magnesium sulfate infusion on perioperative hemodynamics, postoperative recovery, and analgesia in arthroscopic knee surgery during spinal anesthesia. J Bursa Fac Med. 2023;1(2):57–64.
57. Morel V, Pickering ME, Goubayon J, Djobo M, Macian N, Pickering G. Magnesium for pain treatment in 2021? State of the art. Nutrients. 2021;13(5):1397.
58. Aditya R, Indriasari I, Limawan MA. Comparison of the effect of magnesium sulfate 50 mg/kg with 30 mg/kg on opioid requirement and blood magnesium level after abdominal hysterectomy. Anaesth Pain Intensive Care. 2024;28(3):517–23.
59. Latremoliere A, Woolf CJ. Central sensitization: a generator of pain hypersensitivity by central neural plasticity. J Pain. 2009;10(9):895–926.
60. Franzoni S, Rossi SMP, Cassinadri A, Sangaletti R, Benazzo F. Perioperative pain management in total knee arthroplasty: a narrative review of current multimodal analgesia protocols. Appl Sci. 2023;13(6):3798.
61. Aryana P, Rajaei S, Bagheri A, Karimi F, Dabbagh A. Acute effect of intravenous administration of magnesium sulfate on serum levels of interleukin-6 and tumor necrosis factor-α in patients undergoing elective coronary bypass graft with cardiopulmonary bypass. Anesthesiol Pain Med. 2014;4(3):e16316.
62. Zhang J-M, An J. Cytokines, inflammation, and pain. Int Anesthesiol Clin. 2007;45(2):27–37.
63. Singh M, Kim A, Young A, Nguyen D, Monroe CL, Ding T, et al. The mechanism and inflammatory markers involved in the potential use of N-acetylcysteine in chronic pain management. Life (Basel). 2024;14(11):1361.
64. Lim EF, Hoghooghi V, Hagen KM, Kapoor K, Frederick A, Finlay TM, et al. Presence and activation of pro-inflammatory macrophages are associated with CRYAB expression in vitro and after peripheral nerve injury. J Neuroinflammation. 2021;18(1):82.
65. de Baaij JH, Hoenderop JG, Bindels RJ. Magnesium in man: implications for health and disease. Physiol Rev. 2015;95(1):1–46.
66. Castiglioni S, Cazzaniga A, Maier JA. Potential interplay between NFkappaB and PPARgamma in human dermal microvascular endothelial cells cultured in low magnesium. Magnes Res. 2014;27(2):86–93.
67. Bernardini D, Nasulewic A, Mazur A, Maier JA. Magnesium and microvascular endothelial cells: a role in inflammation and angiogenesis. Front Biosci. 2005;10:1177–82.

68. Puch Oernskov M, Gaspar Santos S, Sohail Asghar M, Wildgaard K. Is intravenous magnesium sulphate a suitable adjuvant in postoperative pain management?–A critical and systematic review of methodology in randomized controlled trials. Scand J Pain. 2023;23(2):251–67.
69. Geroge RCJM, Wilson SHH. "Oh Mg!" magnesium: a powerful tool in the perioperative setting: ASRA Pain Medicine News; 2018. Available from: https://www.asra.com/news-publications/asra-newsletter/newsletter-item/asra-news/2018/07/23/-oh-mg!-magnesium-a-powerful-tool-in-the-perioperative-setting.
70. Wilder-Smith CH, Knopfli R, Wilder-Smith OH. Perioperative magnesium infusion and postoperative pain. Acta Anaesthesiol Scand. 1997;41(8):1023–7.
71. Ko SH, Lim HR, Kim DC, Han YJ, Choe H, Song HS. Magnesium sulfate does not reduce postoperative analgesic requirements. Anesthesiology. 2001;95(3):640–6.
72. O'Flaherty JE, Lin CX. Does ketamine or magnesium affect posttonsillectomy pain in children? Paediatr Anaesth. 2003;13(5):413–21.
73. Choi GJ, Kim YI, Koo YH, Oh HC, Kang H. Perioperative magnesium for postoperative analgesia: an umbrella review of systematic reviews and updated meta-analysis of randomized controlled trials. J Pers Med. 2021;11(12):1273.
74. Albrecht E, Kirkham KR, Liu SS, Brull R. Peri-operative intravenous administration of magnesium sulphate and postoperative pain: a meta-analysis. Anaesthesia. 2013;68(1):79–90.
75. James MF, Cronje L. Pheochromocytoma crisis: the use of magnesium sulfate. Anesth Analg. 2004;99(3):680–6.
76. Masamune T, Ishiyama T, Kawamura A, Suzuki M, Oguchi T, Kashimoto S, et al. Use of magnesium sulfate during resection of pheochromocytoma. Masui. 2002;51(5):516–7.
77. Pitt-Miller P, Primus E. Use of magnesium sulphate as adjunctive therapy for resection of phaeochromocytoma. West Indian Med J. 2000;49(1):73–5.
78. Kara H, Sahin N, Ulusan V, Aydogdu T. Magnesium infusion reduces perioperative pain. Eur J Anaesthesiol. 2002;19(1):52–6.
79. Tauzin-Fin P, Sesay M, Delort-Laval S, Krol-Houdek MC, Maurette P. Intravenous magnesium sulphate decreases postoperative tramadol requirement after radical prostatectomy. Eur J Anaesthesiol. 2006;23(12):1055–9.
80. Bakhsh M, Abbas S, Hussain RM, Ali Khan S, Naqvi SM. Role of magnesium in preventing post-operative atrial fibrillation after coronary artery bypass surgery. J Ayub Med Coll Abbottabad. 2009;21(2):27–9.
81. Gormley J, Gouveia K, Sakha S, Stewart V, Emmanuel U, Shehata M, et al. Reduction of opioid use after orthopedic surgery: a scoping review. Can J Surg. 2022;65(5):E695.
82. Yue L, Lin Z-M, Mu G-Z, Sun H-L. Impact of intraoperative intravenous magnesium on spine surgery: A systematic review and meta-analysis of randomized controlled trials. EClinicalMedicine. 2022;43:101246.
83. Chen C, Tao R. The impact of magnesium sulfate on pain control after laparoscopic cholecystectomy: a meta-analysis of randomized controlled studies. Surg Laparosc Endosc Percutan Tech. 2018;28(6):349–53.
84. Ng KT, Yap JLL, Izham IN, Teoh WY, Kwok PE, Koh WJ. The effect of intravenous magnesium on postoperative morphine consumption in noncardiac surgery: a systematic review and meta-analysis with trial sequential analysis. Eur J Anaesthesiol. 2020;37(3):212–23.
85. De Oliveira GS Jr, Castro-Alves LJ, Khan JH, McCarthy RJ. Perioperative systemic magnesium to minimize postoperative pain: a meta-analysis of randomized controlled trials. Anesthesiology. 2013;119(1):178–90.
86. Guo BL, Lin Y, Hu W, Zhen CX, Bao-Cheng Z, Wu HH, et al. Effects of systemic magnesium on post-operative analgesia: is the current evidence strong enough? Pain Physician. 2015;18(5):405–18.
87. Elhouty MG, Elbahrawy K, Sakr A. Analgesic and hemodynamic effects of intravenous magnesium sulfate infusion versus lidocaine infusion in patients undergoing thyroid surgery for toxic goiter resection: a randomized controlled study. Res Opin Anesth Intensive Care. 2024;11(1):9–15.
88. Goebel A. Complex regional pain syndrome in adults. Rheumatology. 2011;50(10):1739–50.
89. Smart KM, Wand BM, O'Connell NE. Physiotherapy for pain and disability in adults with complex regional pain syndrome (CRPS) types I and II. Cochrane Database Syst Rev. 2016;2(2):CD010853.
90. de Rooij AM, Perez RS, Huygen FJ, van Eijs F, van Kleef M, Bauer MC, van Hilten JJ, Marinus J. Spontaneous onset of complex regional pain syndrome. Eur J Pain. 2010;14(5):510–3.
91. Iolascon G, de Sire A, Moretti A, Gimigliano F. Complex regional pain syndrome (CRPS) type I: historical perspective and critical issues. Clin Cases Miner Bone Metab. 2015;12(Suppl 1):4–10.
92. Shim H, Rose J, Halle S, Shekane P. Complex regional pain syndrome: a narrative review for the practising clinician. Br J Anaesth. 2019;123(2):e424–33.
93. Harden NR, Bruehl S, Perez RSGM, Birklein F, Marinus J, Maihofner C, Lubenow T, Buvanendran A, Mackey S, Graciosa J, Mogilevski M, Ramsden C, Chont M, Vatine JJ. Validation of proposed diagnostic criteria (the "Budapest criteria") for complex regional pain syndrome. Pain. 2010;150(2):268–74.
94. Bruehl S. An update on the pathophysiology of complex regional pain syndrome. Anesthesiology. 2010;113(3):713–25.
95. Bruehl S. Complex regional pain syndrome. BMJ. 2015;351:h2730.
96. Collins S, Zuurmond WWA, De Lange JJ, Van Hilten BJ, Perez RSGM. Intravenous magnesium for complex regional pain syndrome type 1 (CRPS 1) patients: a pilot study. Pain Med. 2009;10(5):930–40.
97. Fischer SGL, Collins S, Boogaard S, Loer SA, Zuurmond WWA, Perez RSGM. Intravenous magnesium for chronic complex regional pain syndrome type 1(CRPS-1). Pain Med. 2013;14(9):1388–99.
98. Kim YH, Lee PB, Oh TK. Is magnesium sulfate effective for pain in chronic postherpetic neuralgia patients comparing with ketamine infusion therapy? J Clin Anesth. 2015;27(4):296–300.
99. Pickering G, Pereira B, Morel V, et al. Ketamine and magnesium for refractory neuropathic pain: a randomized, double-blind, crossover trial. Anesthesiology. 2020;133(1):154–64.
100. Zygmunt M, Heilmann L, Berg C, et al. Local and systemic tolerability of magnesium sulphate for tocolysis. Eur J Obstet Gynecol Reprod Biol. 2003;107(2):168–75.
101. Koinig H, Wallner T, Marhofer P, Andel H, Hörauf K, Mayer N. Magnesium sulfate reduces intra- and postoperative analgesic requirements. Anesth Analg. 1998;87(1):206–10.
102. Telci L, Esen F, Akcora D, Erden T, Canbolat AT, Akpir K. Evaluation of effects of magnesium sulphate in reducing intraoperative anaesthetic requirements. Br J Anaesth. 2002;89(4):594–8.
103. Gidal BE, DeCerce J, Bockbrader HN, et al. Gabapentin bioavailability: effect of dose and frequency of administration in adult patients with epilepsy. Epilepsy Res. 1998;31(2):91–9.
104. Yagi T, Naito T, Mino Y, Umemura K, Kawakami J. Impact of concomitant antacid administration on gabapentin plasma exposure and oral bioavailability in healthy adult subjects. Drug Metab Pharmacokinet. 2012;27(2):248–54.
105. Tangvoraphonkchai K, Davenport A. Magnesium and cardiovascular disease. Adv Chronic Kidney Dis. 2018;25(3):251–60.

106. Singh P, Idowu O, Malik I, Nates JL. Acute respiratory failure induced by magnesium replacement in a 62-year-old woman with myasthenia gravis. Tex Heart Inst J. 2015;42(5):495–7.
107. Sawhney H, Aggarwal N, Biswas R, Vasishta K, Gopalan S. Maternal mortality associated with eclampsia and severe pre-eclampsia of pregnancy. J Obstet Gynaecol. 2000;26(5):351–6.
108. Onyeaka H, Adeola J, Xu R, Pappy AL, Smucker M, Ufondu W, et al. Intravenous magnesium for the management of chronic pain: an updated review of the literature. Psychopharmacol Bull. 2024;54(4):81–105.
109. Peng Y-N, Sung F-C, Huang M-L, Lin C-L, Kao C-H. The use of intravenous magnesium sulfate on postoperative analgesia in orthopedic surgery: a systematic review of randomized controlled trials. Medicine. 2018;97(50):e13583.
110. Toumia M, Sassi S, Dhaoui R, Kouraichi C, Bel Haj Ali K, Sekma A, et al. Magnesium sulfate versus lidocaine as an adjunct for renal colic in the emergency department: a randomized, double-blind controlled trial. Ann Emerg Med. 2024;84(6):670–7.
111. Shetty A, Delanerolle G, Cavalini H, Deng C, Yang X, Boyd A, et al. A systematic review and network meta-analysis of pharmaceutical interventions used to manage chronic pain. Sci Rep. 2024;14(1):1621.
112. Sbitan L, Nabhan AI, Alafandi BZ, Alzraikat O, Alzraikat N. Magnesium sulfate for postoperative pain in orthopedic surgery: a narrative review. Medicine. 2024;103(24):e38522.
113. Soleimanpour H, Imani F, Dolati S, Soleimanpour M, Shahsavarinia K. Management of pain using magnesium sulphate: a narrative review. Postgrad Med. 2022;134(3):260–6.
114. Navarro-González JF, Mora-Fernández C, García-Pérez J, editors. Reviews: clinical implications of disordered magnesium homeostasis in chronic renal failure and dialysis. In Seminars in dialysis; 2009. Wiley Online Library.
115. Al Shukri Z, Al-Maqbali JS, Al Alawi AM, Al Riyami N, Al Riyami S, Al Alawi H, et al. Incidence of dysmagnesemia among medically hospitalized patients and associated clinical characteristics: a prospective cohort study. Int J Endocrinol. 2023;2023(1):6650620.
116. Chan M-J, Chen J-J, Lee C-C, Fan P-C, Su Y-J, Cheng Y-L, et al. Clinical impact of hypermagnesemia in acute kidney injury patients undergoing continuous kidney replacement therapy: a propensity score analysis utilizing real-world data. J Crit Care. 2025;85:154947.
117. Cheungpasitporn W, Thongprayoon C, Qian Q, editors. Dysmagnesemia in hospitalized patients: prevalence and prognostic importance. Mayo Clin Proc; 2015: Elsevier.
118. Asai Y, Yanagawa T, Yamamoto T, Sato Y. Exploratory study of pharmacists' monitoring methods based on left ventricular function for hypermagnesemia by magnesium oxide in heart failure. J Clin Pharmacol. 2023;63(1):48–56.

Lidocaine

16

Wenxin Zhuo

Introduction

Lidocaine, also known as lignocaine, is a class Ib Vaughan-Williams antiarrhythmic agent and one of the most widely used local anesthetics. It was first synthesized by Nils Löfgren and Bengt Lundqvist in 1943 and 1946 to meet the demands of anesthetic agents with a rapid local anesthetic onset and low toxicity in surgical procedures [18]. Prior to the discovery of lidocaine, several older local anesthetic agents, such as procaine, were developed to replace the undesirable toxicity and addictive properties brought by cocaine [9]. However, procaine presented several challenges: it was difficult to preserve, required bedside reconstitution before administration, and had a shorter duration of action necessitates frequent redosing [18]. Therefore, lidocaine quickly gained popularity as a local anesthetic agent due to its improved efficacy and safer toxicity profile. In this chapter, the author will emphasize the use of lidocaine in pain management and regional anesthesia, rather than its antiarrhythmic applications in cardiac dysrhythmia management.

Pharmacology, Pharmacokinetics, Pharmacodynamics

Unlike older local anesthetic agents such as procaine or benzocaine, which contain an ester linkage, lidocaine is synthesized from xylidine and contains both hydrophilic and hydrophobic side-chain moieties connected by an amide linkage [4]. The hydrophilic amine portion allows diffusion to the neuronal membrane, while the hydrophobic aromatic portion enables penetration of the neuronal membrane [4].

The mechanism of action of lidocaine works by reversibly blocking axonal sodium channels and reducing the inward current of sodium ions in the nerve fiber to deter the impulse of action potential [8]. Three local anesthetic inhibitory mechanisms are voltage-dependent block, cumulative frequency-dependent block, and slow sodium inactivation [24]. In the resting state, the equilibrium of the membrane potential is established by balancing the amount of potassium and sodium ions across the membrane [8]. During an action potential, the opening of the voltage-gated sodium channel allows the inward flow of sodium ions, causing depolarization of the cell membrane [8], which conducts information signals to the peripheral nervous system or the central nervous system. Lidocaine exerts its anesthetic effect by blocking the sodium channel to disrupt the inward flow of sodium ions into the cell membrane, preventing the conduction of nerve impulses [8, 23]. Tertiary amine local anesthetics, such as lidocaine, produce phasic inhibition, also known as "use-dependent blockade," by selectively binding to the voltage-gated sodium channel, resulting in the increased sodium channel depolarization frequency [8]. The positively charged form provided by the tertiary amine structure has a higher affinity and binds to the sodium channel when opened [8, 24]. Therefore, the degree of blockade is greatly enhanced with repetitive stimulation, due to tighter binding between lidocaine and the opened sodium channel [8, 24]. Additionally, the sodium channel undergoes a structural conformation change during an action potential that allows more sodium ions to pass through [8]. However, local anesthetic molecules can fit into an amphipathic pocket or between the membrane and the pore-forming regions of the channel [8]. The binding of lidocaine to the channel locks the sodium channel to slow down the structural rearrangement [8] to block further neuronal firing.

Lidocaine's distribution to the site of action and ability to inhibit axonal sodium channels depend on its hydrophobicity [8, 24], the pH [25], and the rate of dissociation from the receptor. As previously mentioned, lidocaine consists of a hydrophilic and a hydrophobic portion connected by an amide linkage. Hille [23] proposed and tested a

W. Zhuo (✉)
UToledo Health, Toledo, OH, USA
e-mail: Wenxin.zhuo@utoledo.edu

J. P. Reinert et al. (eds.), *Adjunctive Analgesic Strategies for the Bedside Clinician and Beyond*,
https://doi.org/10.1007/978-3-032-21675-5_16

hypothesis that amide-type local anesthetics could provide inhibitory effects through both hydrophilic and hydrophobic pathways. The hydrophilic pathway only functions when the sodium voltage-gated channel is open, whereas the hydrophobic pathways are always available to lipid-soluble molecules [24]. The hydrophobic aromatic portion of the local anesthetic enables membrane penetration and binds to the site of action on the cytosolic side of the sodium channel [24]. Once lidocaine crosses the cytosolic membrane, the lower pH inside the cell will recharge the lidocaine and bind to the sodium channel [8]. This mechanism may also explain why amide-type local anesthetics could provide a longer duration of action compared to ester-type local anesthetics due to the plasma esterase rapid degradation of the ester linkage, leading to the loss of amphipathic structure [24]. Local anesthetics must be hydrophilic enough to diffuse to axonal neurons and sufficiently hydrophobic to penetrate the neuronal membrane. To diffuse through the membrane, the molecule must be neutral and unionized. However, lidocaine (pKa 7.9) and many other local anesthetics are weak bases [23, 25], with pKa values above the human physiologic pH of 7.4. At a high pH, such as 8, the rate of action for lidocaine could be as fast as within one second after administration in animal models [25]. Conversely, the rate and depth of blockade decrease when the pH becomes more acidic [25]. Thus, certain disease states, such as metabolic acidosis, could attenuate the lidocaine local anesthetic effects and may require a larger dose.

To maximize the local anesthetic effects, vasoconstrictors, commonly epinephrine, are often added to local anesthetics to delay systemic absorption and prolong the duration of action by decreasing the local blood circulation through vasoconstriction [37]. The addition of anesthetic effects varied from different injection sites and the concentration of epinephrine [37]. Systemic absorption was reduced by approximately 50% in patients who received subcutaneous lidocaine 2% with epinephrine, compared to intercostal and epidural injections [37]. As far as the impact of different epinephrine concentrations on safety and efficacy, Scott et al. found no significant efficacy superiority in 1:80,000 to 1:200,000 [37]. In a recent double-blind randomized controlled trial comparing lidocaine 2% with epinephrine 1:80,000 versus 1:200,000 for inferior alveolar nerve block, the 1:80,000 concentration also did not demonstrate superior efficacy [1]. Evidence supporting the use of lidocaine with epinephrine concentrations above 1:200,000 is limited. The current commercially available lidocaine products only come with 1:100,000 and 1:200,000. In terms of the impact of the mean duration of action with epinephrine, the mean duration of analgesic effect was 128 minutes in plain lidocaine 1%, but the duration of analgesia was significantly prolonged to 231 minutes in lidocaine 1% with epinephrine (1:200,000) in a small clinical study by Swerdlow and Jones [38].

Lidocaine exhibits a two-compartment pharmacokinetic model, and 90% metabolizes through the liver [6]. The half-life was about 90 minutes after a lidocaine continuous infusion discontinued [6]. This was similar to the mean half-life of 108 minutes in Rowland's study in subjects after receiving two intravenous lidocaine boluses [35]. The volume of distribution at steady state is 0.6–4.5 L/kg [5, 35]. The oral absorption of lidocaine ranges between 0.19 and 0.38 due to the extensive hepatic first-pass effect [5]. This raised concern about the candidacy of oral lidocaine administration that goes through the extensive hepatic first-pass effect and requires a more frequent dosing schedule or a larger dose to compensate for the low systemic concentration [35]. Additionally, lidocaine is deethylated by the cytochrome P-450 1A2 and 3A4 to 3-hydroxylation of lidocaine and monoethylglycinexylidide (MEGX) [40] and subsequently 2,6-xylidine [3]. In Higuchi's in vitro study, 2,6-xylidine could be further metabolized by CYP 2E1 to 4-hydroxyxylidine and enter the pathway to form methemoglobin, which could cause methemoglobinemia [22]. Therefore, lidocaine oral administration is not routinely used due to the concern of accumulation of toxic metabolites that could bring more harm than benefit [35].

Evidence for Use

Lidocaine is one of the most versatile local anesthetic and analgesic agents and has been widely used in local infiltration, peripheral nerve block, and epidural injections. In recent years, there has been some growing interest in intravenous lidocaine infusions in postoperative pain management [42] and refractory neuropathic pain [39]. Many randomized controlled trials have been performed with perioperative intravenous lidocaine in the past two decades (see Table 16.1 for a summary of continuous IV lidocaine randomized controlled trials). However, the designs and methodologies of these trials vary significantly, leading to substantial heterogeneity and difficulty in systematic analysis [17]. Weibel et al. performed the first systematic review in 2015 [30] and updated it in 2018 [42], including a total of 68 trials with 4525 randomized participants in the continuous intravenous perioperative lidocaine infusion for postoperative pain and the recovery setting. Weibel et al. reported that IV lidocaine reduced postoperative pain scores at 0–4 hours with a standardized mean difference (SMD) of −0.50 (95% confidence interval −0.72 to −0.28) in 29 studies involving 1656 participants [42]. The reduction equates to 0.37 cm to 2.48 cm on a 0 cm to 10 cm Visual Analogue Scale (VAS) pain score, assuming the change of 1 cm on the VAS is clinically meaningful [42].

Table 16.1 Summary of continuous intravenous lidocaine randomized controlled trials

Study	Surgery type	Intervention	Comparison	Outcomes
Ahn et al. [2]	Laparoscopic colectomy	*n* = 25 1.5 mg/kg IV lidocaine bolus followed by 2 mg/kg/hr. continuous infusion + fentanyl PCA	*n* = 25 Saline bolus injection followed by infusion + fentanyl PCA	Lidocaine group patients had significantly lower VAS scores and fentanyl consumption compared to the placebo group at 24 hours after surgery No patient had postoperative complications related to lidocaine infusion
Kang and Kim [28]	Inguinal herniorrhaphy	*n* = 32 1.5 mg/kg IV lidocaine bolus followed by 2 mg/kg/hr. continuous infusion + fentanyl PCA	*n* = 32 Saline bolus injection followed by infusion + fentanyl PCA	Patients in the lidocaine group had significantly lower VAS and fentanyl consumption 12 hours after surgery compared to the control group
Farag et al. [15]	Spine surgery	*n* = 57 Lidocaine 2 mg/kg/hr. (max 200 mg/hr) continuous infusion + morphine PCA	*n* = 58 Saline infusion + morphine PCA	Lidocaine mean verbal response scale pain scores decreased from 5.3 to 4.4 (95% CI, $P < 0.01$), and morphine equivalent dosage reduced from 74 to 55 mg ($p = 0.011$) in 48 hours after extensive spine surgery
Grigoras et al. [19]	Breast surgery	*n* = 17 1.5 mg/kg IV lidocaine bolus followed by 1.5 mg/kg/hr. continuous infusion until 60 minutes post-surgery	*n* = 19 Equal volume of saline	Two patients in the lidocaine group had greater pain intensity (VAS) and significantly less hyperalgesia at 3 months compared to nine patients in the control group
Dewinter et al. [11]	Laparoscopic sterilization	*n* = 40 1.5 mg/kg IV lidocaine bolus followed by 1.5 mg/kg/hr. continuous infusion until 30 minutes post-surgery	*n* = 40 Equal volume of saline	No difference in numeric rating scale (NRS) and perioperative opioid consumption between groups Lidocaine group had a significantly lower time to meet hospital discharge criteria (median 177 minutes vs. 221 minutes, p = 0.02)
Koppert et al. [29]	Major abdominal surgery	*n* = 20 1.5 mg/kg IV lidocaine bolus followed by 1.5 mg/kg/hr. continuous infusion until 60 minutes post-surgery	*n* = 20 Equal volume of saline	No patient's lidocaine plasma concentration exceeds the toxic level (>5 mcg/mL) Patients who received lidocaine infusion have less pain during observed movement and needed less morphine during the first 72 hours post-surgery (103.1 ± 72.0 mg versus 159.0 ± 73.3 mg, $P < 0.05$)
Herroeder et al. [20]	Colorectal surgery	*n* = 31 1.5 mg/kg IV lidocaine bolus followed by 2 mg/min continuous infusion until 4 hours post-surgery	*n* = 29 Equal volume of saline	Patients who received lidocaine infusions had a significantly shorter return of bowel function (66.6 ± 26.4 versus 82.1 ± 33.8 hours for control patients after surgery, $P < 0.05$) and hospital length of stay by 1 day (7 days versus 8 days, respectively, $P = 0.004$) No difference observed in terms of daily pain scales
Bryson et al. [7]	Abdominal hysterectomy	*n* = 44 1.5 mg/kg IV lidocaine bolus followed by 3 mg/kg/hr. continuous infusion until 4 hours post-surgery	*n* = 46 Equal volume of saline	No difference observed in hospital length of stay, opioid consumption, pain scores, and recovery in both groups
El-Tahan et al. [14]	Cesarean section	*n* = 45 1.5 mg/kg IV lidocaine bolus 30 minutes before induction followed by 1.5 mg/kg/hr. continuous infusion until 60 minutes post-surgery	*n* = 45 Equal volume of saline	Lidocaine-treated patients had smaller increases in heart rate and mean arterial blood pressure ($P < 0.02$) Lidocaine is safe and effective in cesarean delivery stress reduction for both neonates and maternal patients
Insler et al. [26]	Coronary Artery Bypass Surgery	*n* = 36 1.5 mg/kg IV lidocaine bolus 30 minutes before induction, followed by 30 mcg/kg/min (1.8 mg/kg/hr) continuous infusion up to 48 hours in the ICU unless earlier ICU discharge	*n* = 34 Equal volume of placebo substitute	No significant difference observed in VAS, opioid consumption, time to extubation, ICU length of stay, and hospital length of stay between study groups
Wang et al. [41]	Coronary Artery Bypass Surgery	*n* = 43 1.5 mg/kg IV lidocaine bolus followed by 4 mg/min continuous infusion until the end of surgery	*n* = 45 Equal volume of placebo substitute	Lidocaine-treated patients had a significant reduction in postoperative cognitive dysfunction compared with that in the placebo group. (18.6% versus 40.0%, $P = 0.028$)

(continued)

Table 16.1 (continued)

Study	Surgery type	Intervention	Comparison	Outcomes
Weinberg et al. [43]	Open radical prostatectomy	*n* = 38 1.5 mg/kg IV lidocaine bolus followed by 1.5 mg/kg/hr. continuous intraopperative infusion and then transition to subcutaneous infusion at 1.5 mg/kg/hr. post-surgery for 24 hours	*n* = 38 Equal volume of saline	No difference in pain at rest at 24 hours in both groups. Lidocaine-treated patients decreased 13.9 (2.2–25.7, 95% CI, *P* = 0.021) mg of morphine
Martin et al. [32]	Total hip arthroplasty	*n* = 28 1.5 mg/kg IV lidocaine bolus followed by 1.5 mg/kg/hr. continuous infusion until 1 hour post-surgery	*n* = 30 Equal volume of saline	No significant difference in postoperative morphine consumption in 24–48 hours, pain scores, duration of hospital stay, and hyperalgesia in both groups
Kaba et al. [27]	Laparoscopic colectomy	*n* = 20 1.5 mg/kg IV lidocaine bolus followed by 2 mg/kg/hr. continuous infusion intraoperatively and 1.33 mg/kg/hr. continuous infusion until 24 hours post-surgery	*n* = 20 Equal volume of saline	Lidocaine-treated patients had quicker bowel function recovery (28 versus 51 hours, *P* = 0.001), shorter hospital length of stay (2 versus 3 days, *P* = 0.005), and decreased pain and fatigue scores when compared to the placebo group
Lee et al. [31]	Off-pump coronary artery surgery	*n* = 49 1.5 mg/kg IV lidocaine bolus followed by 2 mg/kg/hr. continuous infusion intraoperatively	*n* = 50 Equal volume of saline	Patients who received lidocaine continuous infusion reduced myocardial injury, demonstrated by lower creatinine kinase-myocardial band (CK-MB) (*P* = 0.005) and troponin concentration (*P* = 0.027)
Sakata et al. [36]	Bariatric surgery	*n* = 29 1.5 mg/kg IV lidocaine bolus followed by 2 mg/kg/hr. continuous infusion intraoperatively	*n* = 29 Equal volume of saline	Lidocaine-treated patients had less intraoperative sevoflurane requirements and decreased morphine consumption over 24 hours
Herzog et al. [21]	Robotic colorectal surgery	*n* = 29 1.5 mg/kg IV lidocaine bolus followed by 1.5 mg/kg/hr. continuous infusion until 2 hours post-surgery	*n* = 29 Equal volume of saline	No difference between both groups in postoperative morphine consumption at 24 and 72 hours

PCA patient-controlled analgesia; *VAS* Visual Analog Scale; *NRS* numeric rating scale; *ICU* intensive care unit

There were no significant benefits of using IV lidocaine at both 24 hours (SMD −0.14) and 48 hours (SMD −0.11), equating to 0.10 to 0.48 cm and 0.08 to 0.42 cm on the VAS, respectively [42]. Although the SMD of pain scores did not show significant differences, lidocaine reduced the risk of ileus in four studies (risk ratio 0.37; 95% CI: 0.15 to 0.87), improved the time to first defecation or bowel movements by a mean difference of −7.92 hours (95% CI: −12.71 to −3.13) in 12 studies, reduced the risk of postoperative nausea within 72 hours (risk ratio 0.78; 95% CI: −0.67 to 0.91) in 35 studies, and decreased overall opioid consumption by a mean difference of −4.52 mg morphine equivalents (95% CI: −6.25 to −2.79) in 40 studies [42].

Even though the reviews show some numerically significant benefits of IV lidocaine, the authors ultimately concluded that the effect of IV lidocaine on early postoperative pain reduction, gastrointestinal recovery, postoperative nausea, and opioid consumption has beneficial impacts due to very low-quality evidence [42].

Outside of perioperative pain management, lidocaine has been studied in neuropathic pain management as well. Ten randomized control trials were included in the systematic review by Tremont-Lukats et al. of patients with neuropathic pain [39]. Lidocaine (most commonly administered as 5 mg/kg IV over 30 to 60 minutes) reduced the VAS pain scores, with a weighted mean difference of 1.0 cm (95% CI: −1.7 to −0.04) compared to the placebo group [39]. Although the study result was statistically significant, it is difficult to draw a conclusion about the clinically meaningful impacts of IV lidocaine in patients with neuropathic pain [39]. The short serum half-life of lidocaine limits its use for chronic neuropathic pain, as the analgesic effect diminishes within a few hours after the stop of the infusion. Due to the risk of severe adverse events, the Association of Anaesthetists recommends that patients receiving IV lidocaine should have a monitored bed space in a high-dependency unit [17]. Therefore, the benefits and risks of utilizing intravenous lidocaine in patients with neuropathic pain should be carefully assessed and balanced by the clinician prior to initiation.

In terms of the safety and adverse events reported in the systematic review of continuous IV lidocaine in postoperative pain management, 27 out of 50 studies reported adverse events such as drowsiness, lightheadedness, perioral numbness, tinnitus, and bradycardia [42]. Similarly, the most common IV lidocaine adverse effects reported in the Tremont-Lukats et al. study [39] were drowsiness, fatigue, nausea, and dizziness. Although the incidence of lidocaine adverse events is relatively low, lidocaine still carries the risk of local anesthetic systemic toxicity (LAST), like other local anesthetic agents. The incidence of LAST is currently estimated to be 0.03%, or 27 cases in 10,000 peripheral nerve blocks [13]. The two major body organs prone to lidocaine systemic toxicity are the heart and brain [12]. The increased local anesthetic plasma concentrations can induce central nervous system (CNS) toxicity by disrupting the balance between excitatory and inhibitory neurotransmission [12]. Early clinical symptoms of CNS toxicity include lightheadedness, dizziness, blurry vision, and tinnitus [12]. As blood plasma concentration increases, CNS toxicity could manifest as muscle twitching and tremors [12]. Toxic plasma concentration of lidocaine is typically above 5 mcg/mL [12, 17]. When the plasma lidocaine concentration is above 8 mcg/mL [10], CNS toxicity could include convulsive seizures or even comas due to the inhibition of both inhibitory and excitatory neurotransmission [12]. Further increase of plasma lidocaine concentrations may result in cardiac toxicity, including tachycardia, ventricular arrhythmia, myocardial conduction delays, and profound contractile dysfunction [34].

If LAST is suspected, the American Society of Regional Anesthesia and Pain Medicine recommends administering 100 mL of 20% lipid emulsion bolus over 2–3 minutes, followed by a continuous infusion of 0.25 mL/kg/min (based on ideal body weight) until cardiac stability is maintained for at least 10 minutes [33]. Lipid emulsion provides scavenging effects by shuttling the drug away from organs susceptible to lidocaine toxicity [16]. Non-scavenging benefits by activating prosurvival kinases to protect tissue from ischemic damage [16].

Applications to Clinical Practice

The current commercially available lidocaine products in the United States include topical lidocaine, oral lidocaine solution, and intravenous lidocaine. Topical lidocaine has been formulated into cream, gel, jelly, patch, and spray, allowing flexibility to meet patient needs. It provides localized pain relief, reduces systemic exposure, and is easy to apply. These advantages make it a preferred choice for many patients experiencing pain or discomfort. Additionally, most topical lidocaine products are available over the counter, making them easily accessible to patients. See Tables 16.2 and 16.3 for a summary of common topical lidocaine and local anesthetic lidocaine dosing and their indications.

In early parental lidocaine pharmacokinetic studies, an infusion rate of 40 mcg/kg/min (equivalent to 2.4 mg/kg/hr) was required to attain a plateau plasma concentration of 4 mcg/mL [35]. In 62 studies of IV lidocaine, the most common dosing was a bolus dose ranging from 1 mg/kg to 3 mg/kg (most commonly 1.5 mg/kg) of body weight or a fixed dose of 100 mg lidocaine, followed by 1 mg/kg/hr. to 5 mg/kg/hr. continuous infusion [42].

Conclusions

The consensus recommendation for IV lidocaine continuous infusion from the Association of Anaesthetists advises a bolus loading dose of no more than 1.5 mg/kg over 10 minutes, followed by an infusion of no more than 1.5 mg/kg/hour for less than 24 hours [17]. Intravenous lidocaine dosing should be based on the patient's ideal body weight and should not be administered to patients less than 40 kg [17]. This regimen is intended to avoid toxic plasma concentration, as discussed above.

Table 16.2 Lidocaine topical product dosing and indications

Delivery mechanisms	Strength	Max dose	Indication and usage
Cream	4%, 5%	Three to four applications in 24 hours	Apply to intact skin for minor cuts, burns, and insect bites
Gel	3%, 4%, 5%	Product-specific	Topical pain, postsurgical pain, and pain associated with various types of closed or open wounds
Jelly	2%	30 mL (600 mg) in any 12-hour period	Topical treatment of painful urethritis Male urethra: 5–30 mL (100–600 mg) Female urethra: 3–5 mL (60–100 mg) Anesthetic lubricant for endotracheal intubation
Patch	4%, 5% (Rx only)	Max of three patches for up to 12 hours within 24 hours	Pain associated with postherpetic neuralgia. Commonly used for back pain.
Ointment	5%	20 g of ointment/day (max 5 g in a single application)	Intubation or topical pain (e.g., skin irritation, sunburn)
Topical solution	4%	Three applications in 24 hours	Topical pain
Spray	4%	Four applications in 24 hours	Topical pain, commonly used for joint, ankle, or wrist sprains
Oral solution	2% viscous	Max 4.5 mg/kg or 300 mg/dose; max eight doses within 24 hours	Anesthesia of the mouth or pharynx

Table 16.3 Lidocaine infiltration, nerve blocks, caudal, and epidural dosing[a]

Procedure	Conc. (%)	Vol. (mL)	Total Dose (mg)
Infiltration			
Percutaneous	0.5 or 1	1–60	5–300
IV regional	0.5	10–60	50–300
Peripheral nerve blocks			
Brachial	1.5	15–20	225–300
Dental	2	1–5	20–100
Intercostal	1	3	30
Paravertebral	1	3–5	30–50
Pudendal (each side)	1	10	100
Sympathetic nerve blocks			
Cervical (stellate ganglion)	1	5	50
Lumbar	1	5–10	50–100
Central neural blocks			
Epidural			
Thoracic	1	20–30	200–300
Lumbar analgesia	1	25–30	250–300
Lumbar anesthesia 1.5%	1.5	15–20	225–300
Lumbar anesthesia 2%	2	10–15	200–300
Caudal obsterical analgesia	1	20–30	200–300
Caudal surgical analgesia	1.5	15–20	225–300

[a]Adapted from the lidocaine manufacturer's package insert

Key Themes

- Local anesthetics must be sufficiently hydrophilic to diffuse to neurons and sufficiently lipophilic to diffuse across the neuronal membrane (cytosolic side) to the site of action.
- The mechanism of action is the binding of ionized (cationic nitrogen) local anesthetic to the sodium channel.
- Diffusion away from the injection site can be slowed by the vasoconstrictor, commonly epinephrine.
- The choice and dose of local anesthetic depend on the treatment duration and condition.
- The benefits of parental lidocaine (both bolus and continuous infusion) remain unclear. Clinicians should carefully balance the benefits and risks prior to initiating IV lidocaine.
- Diffusion to organs that have cells with sodium channels can produce LAST, which is a medical emergency and could be managed by infusing 20% lipid emulsion.

References

1. Aggarwal V, Singla M, Miglani S, Kohli S. Comparison of the anaesthetic efficacy of epinephrine concentrations (1: 80 000 and 1: 200 000) in 2% lidocaine for inferior alveolar nerve block in patients with symptomatic irreversible pulpitis: a randomized, double-blind clinical trial. Int Endod J. 2014;47(4):373–9. https://doi.org/10.1111/iej.12157. https://www.ncbi.nlm.nih.gov/pubmed/23895176
2. Ahn E, Kang H, Choi GJ, Park YH, Yang SY, Kim BG, Choi SW. Intravenous lidocaine for effective pain relief after a laparoscopic colectomy: a prospective, randomized, double-blind, placebo-controlled study. Int Surg. 2015;100(3):394–401. https://doi.org/10.9738/INTSURG-D-14-00225.1.
3. Alexson SE, Diczfalusy M, Halldin M, Swedmark S. Involvement of liver carboxylesterases in the in vitro metabolism of lidocaine. Drug Metab Dispos. 2002;30(6):643–7. https://doi.org/10.1124/dmd.30.6.643. https://www.ncbi.nlm.nih.gov/pubmed/12019189
4. Becker DE, Reed KL. Local anesthetics: review of pharmacological considerations. Anesth Prog. 201259(2):90–101; quiz 102–3. https://doi.org/10.2344/0003-3006-59.2.90. https://www.ncbi.nlm.nih.gov/pubmed/22822998
5. Bennett PN, Aarons LJ, Bending MR, Steiner JA, Rowland M. Pharmacokinetics of lidocaine and its deethylated metabolite: dose and time dependency studies in man. J Pharmacokinet Biopharm. 1982;10(3):265–81. https://doi.org/10.1007/BF01059261. https://www.ncbi.nlm.nih.gov/pubmed/7175699
6. Boyes RN, Scott DB, Jebson PJ, Godman MJ, Julian DG. Pharmacokinetics of lidocaine in man. Clin Pharmacol Ther. 1971;12(1):105–16. https://doi.org/10.1002/cpt1971121105. https://www.ncbi.nlm.nih.gov/pubmed/5099888
7. Bryson GL, Charapov I, Krolczyk G, Taljaard M, Reid D. Intravenous lidocaine does not reduce length of hospital stay following abdominal hysterectomy. Can J Anaesth. 2010;57(8):759–66. https://doi.org/10.1007/s12630-010-9332-2.
8. Butterworth JF, Strichartz GR. Molecular mechanisms of local anesthesia: a review. Anesthesiology. 1990;72(4):711–34. https://doi.org/10.1097/00000542-199004000-00022. https://www.ncbi.nlm.nih.gov/pubmed/2157353
9. Calatayud J, González A. History of the development and evolution of local anesthesia since the coca leaf. Anesthesiology. 2003;98(6):1503–8. https://doi.org/10.1097/00000542-200306000-00031. https://www.ncbi.nlm.nih.gov/pubmed/12766665
10. Davison R, Parker M, Atkinson AJ. Excessive serum lidocaine levels during maintenance infusions: mechanisms and prevention. Am Heart J. 1982;104(2 Pt 1):203–8. https://doi.org/10.1016/0002-8703(82)90193-4. https://www.ncbi.nlm.nih.gov/pubmed/7102503
11. Dewinter GB, Teunkens A, Vermeulen K, Al Tmimi L, Van de Velde M, Rex S. Systemic lidocaine fails to improve postoperative pain, but reduces time to discharge readiness in patients undergoing laparoscopic sterilization in day-case surgery: a double-blind, randomized, placebo-controlled trial. Reg Anesth Pain Med. 2016;41(3):362–7. https://doi.org/10.1097/AAP.0000000000000398.
12. Dillane D, Finucane BT. Local anesthetic systemic toxicity. Can J Anaesth. 2010;57(4):368–80. https://doi.org/10.1007/s12630-010-9275-7. https://www.ncbi.nlm.nih.gov/pubmed/20151342
13. El-Boghdadly K, Pawa A, Chin KJ. Local anesthetic systemic toxicity: current perspectives. Local Reg Anesth. 2018;11:35–44. https://doi.org/10.2147/LRA.S154512. https://www.ncbi.nlm.nih.gov/pubmed/30122981
14. El-Tahan MR, Warda OM, Diab DG, Ramzy EA, Matter MK. A randomized study of the effects of perioperative i.v. lidocaine on hemodynamic and hormonal responses for cesarean section. J Anesth. 2009;23(2):215–21. https://doi.org/10.1007/s00540-009-0738-3.
15. Farag E, Ghobrial M, Sessler DI, Dalton JE, Liu J, Lee JH, Zaky S, Benzel E, Bingaman W, Kurz A. Effect of perioperative intravenous lidocaine administration on pain, opioid consumption, and quality of life after complex spine surgery. Anesthesiology. 2013;119(4):932–40. https://doi.org/10.1097/ALN.0b013e318297d4a5.
16. Fettiplace MR, Weinberg G. The mechanisms underlying lipid resuscitation therapy. Reg Anesth Pain Med. 2018;43(2):138–49. https://doi.org/10.1097/AAP.0000000000000719. https://www.ncbi.nlm.nih.gov/pubmed/29356774

17. Foo I, Macfarlane AJR, Srivastava D, Bhaskar A, Barker H, Knaggs R, Eipe N, Smith AF. The use of intravenous lidocaine for postoperative pain and recovery: international consensus statement on efficacy and safety. Anaesthesia. 2021;76(2):238–50. https://doi.org/10.1111/anae.15270. https://www.ncbi.nlm.nih.gov/pubmed/33141959
18. Gordh T. Lidocaine: the origin of a modern local anesthetic. 1949. Anesthesiology. 2010;113(6):1433–7. https://doi.org/10.1097/ALN.0b013e3181fcef48. https://www.ncbi.nlm.nih.gov/pubmed/21068652
19. Grigoras A, Lee P, Sattar F, Shorten G. Perioperative intravenous lidocaine decreases the incidence of persistent pain after breast surgery. Clin J Pain. 2012;28(7):567–72. https://doi.org/10.1097/AJP.0b013e31823b9cc8.
20. Herroeder S, Pecher S, Schönherr ME, Kaulitz G, Hahnenkamp K, Friess H, Böttiger BW, Bauer H, Dijkgraaf MG, Durieux ME, Hollmann MW. Systemic lidocaine shortens length of hospital stay after colorectal surgery: a double-blinded, randomized, placebo-controlled trial. Ann Surg. 2007;246(2):192–200. https://doi.org/10.1097/SLA.0b013e31805dac11.
21. Herzog J, Schou M, Jensen KM, Lauridsen JT, Jensen AG. A randomised controlled trial of lidocaine infusion on post-operative opioid consumption in patients undergoing robotic colorectal surgery. Dan Med J. 2020;67(1):A06190342.
22. Higuchi R, Fukami T, Nakajima M, Yokoi T. Prilocaine- and lidocaine-induced methemoglobinemia is caused by human carboxylesterase-, CYP2E1-, and CYP3A4-mediated metabolic activation. Drug Metab Dispos. 2013;41(6):1220–30. https://doi.org/10.1124/dmd.113.051714. https://www.ncbi.nlm.nih.gov/pubmed/23530020
23. Hille B. Common mode of action of three agents that decrease the transient change in sodium permeability in nerves. Nature. 1966;210(5042):1220–2. https://doi.org/10.1038/2101220a0. https://www.ncbi.nlm.nih.gov/pubmed/5967794
24. Hille B. Local anesthetics: hydrophilic and hydrophobic pathways for the drug-receptor reaction. J Gen Physiol. 1977a;69(4):497–515. https://doi.org/10.1085/jgp.69.4.497. https://www.ncbi.nlm.nih.gov/pubmed/300786
25. Hille B. The pH-dependent rate of action of local anesthetics on the node of Ranvier. J Gen Physiol. 1977b;69(4):475–96. https://doi.org/10.1085/jgp.69.4.475. https://www.ncbi.nlm.nih.gov/pubmed/16078
26. Insler SR, O'Connor M, Samonte AF, Bazaral MG. Lidocaine and the inhibition of postoperative pain in coronary artery bypass patients. J Cardiothorac Vasc Anesth. 1995;9(5):541–6. https://doi.org/10.1016/s1053-0770(05)80138-7.
27. Kaba A, Laurent SR, Detroz BJ, Sessler DI, Durieux ME, Lamy ML, Joris JL. Intravenous lidocaine infusion facilitates acute rehabilitation after laparoscopic colectomy. Anesthesiology. 2007;106(1):11–6. https://doi.org/10.1097/00000542-200701000-00007.
28. Kang H, Kim BG. Intravenous lidocaine for effective pain relief after inguinal herniorrhaphy: a prospective, randomized, double-blind, placebo-controlled study. J Int Med Res. 2011;39(2):435–45. https://doi.org/10.1177/147323001103900211.
29. Koppert W, Weigand M, Neumann F, Sittl R, Schuettler J, Schmelz M, Hering W. Perioperative intravenous lidocaine has preventive effects on postoperative pain and morphine consumption after major abdominal surgery. Anesth Analg. 2004;98(4):1050–5. https://doi.org/10.1213/01.ANE.0000104582.71710.EE.
30. Kranke P, Jokinen J, Pace NL, Schnabel A, Hollmann MW, Hahnenkamp K, Eberhart LH, Poepping DM, Weibel S. Continuous intravenous perioperative lidocaine infusion for postoperative pain and recovery. Cochrane Database Syst Rev. 2015;7:CD009642. https://doi.org/10.1002/14651858.CD009642.pub2. https://www.ncbi.nlm.nih.gov/pubmed/26184397
31. Lee EH, Lee HM, Chung CH, Chin JH, Choi DK, Chung HJ, Sim JY, Choi IC. Impact of intravenous lidocaine on myocardial injury after off-pump coronary artery surgery. Br J Anaesth. 2011;106(4):487–93. https://doi.org/10.1093/bja/aeq416.
32. Martin F, Cherif K, Gentili ME, Enel D, Abe E, Alvarez JC, Mazoit JX, Chauvin M, Bouhassira D, Fletcher D. Lack of impact of intravenous lidocaine on analgesia, functional recovery, and nociceptive pain threshold after total hip arthroplasty. Anesthesiology. 2008;109(1):118–23. https://doi.org/10.1097/ALN.0b013e31817b5a9b.
33. Neal JM, Barrington MJ, Fettiplace MR, Gitman M, Memtsoudis SG, Mörwald EE, Rubin DS, Weinberg G. The third American Society of Regional Anesthesia and Pain Medicine practice advisory on local anesthetic systemic toxicity: executive summary 2017. Reg Anesth Pain Med. 2018;43(2):113–23. https://doi.org/10.1097/AAP.0000000000000720. https://www.ncbi.nlm.nih.gov/pubmed/29356773
34. Reiz S, Nath S. Cardiotoxicity of local anaesthetic agents. Br J Anaesth. 1986;58(7):736–46. https://doi.org/10.1093/bja/58.7.736. https://www.ncbi.nlm.nih.gov/pubmed/2425836
35. Rowland M, Thomson PD, Guichard A, Melmon KL. Disposition kinetics of lidocaine in normal subjects. Ann N Y Acad Sci. 1971;179:383–98. https://doi.org/10.1111/j.1749-6632.1971.tb46915.x. https://www.ncbi.nlm.nih.gov/pubmed/5285383
36. Sakata RK, de Lima RC, Valadão JA, Leal PC, Moura EC, Cruz VP, de Oliveira CM. Randomized, double-blind study of the effect of intraoperative intravenous lidocaine on the opioid consumption and criteria for hospital discharge after bariatric surgery. Obes Surg. 2020;30(4):1189–93. https://doi.org/10.1007/s11695-019-04340-2.
37. Scott DB, Jebson PJ, Braid DP, Ortengren B, Frisch P. Factors affecting plasma levels of lignocaine and prilocaine. Br J Anaesth. 1972;44(10):1040–9. https://doi.org/10.1093/bja/44.10.1040. https://www.ncbi.nlm.nih.gov/pubmed/4639822
38. Swerdlow M, Jones R. The duration of action of bupivacaine, prilocaine and lignocaine. Br J Anaesth. 1970;42(4):335–9. https://doi.org/10.1093/bja/42.4.335.
39. Tremont-Lukats IW, Challapalli V, McNicol ED, Lau J, Carr DB. Systemic administration of local anesthetics to relieve neuropathic pain: a systematic review and meta-analysis. Anesth Analg. 2005;101(6):1738–49. https://doi.org/10.1213/01.ANE.0000186348.86792.38. https://www.ncbi.nlm.nih.gov/pubmed/16301253
40. Wang JS, Backman JT, Taavitsainen P, Neuvonen PJ, Kivistö KT. Involvement of CYP1A2 and CYP3A4 in lidocaine N-deethylation and 3-hydroxylation in humans. Drug Metab Dispos. 2000;28(8):959–65. https://www.ncbi.nlm.nih.gov/pubmed/10901707
41. Wang D, Wu X, Li J, Xiao F, Liu X, Meng M. The effect of lidocaine on early postoperative cognitive dysfunction after coronary artery bypass surgery. Anesth Analg. 2002;95(5) https://doi.org/10.1097/00000539-200211000-00002.
42. Weibel S, Jelting Y, Pace NL, Helf A, Eberhart LH, Hahnenkamp K, Hollmann MW, Poepping DM, Schnabel A, Kranke P. Continuous intravenous perioperative lidocaine infusion for postoperative pain and recovery in adults. Cochrane Database Syst Rev. 2018;6(6):CD009642. https://doi.org/10.1002/14651858.CD009642.pub3. https://www.ncbi.nlm.nih.gov/pubmed/29864216
43. Weinberg L, Rachbuch C, Ting S, Howard W, Yeomans M, Gordon I, McNicol L, James K, Story D, Christophi C. A randomised controlled trial of peri-operative lidocaine infusions for open radical prostatectomy. Anaesthesia. 2016;71(4):405–10. https://doi.org/10.1111/anae.13368.

17 Cannabidiol

Austin De La Cruz, Olajumoke Olateju, Dipali Rinker, Mina Shrestha, and Douglas Thornton

Definitions/Abbreviations

2018 Farm Bill	Agriculture Improvement Act of 2018
ASHP	American Society of Health-System Pharmacists
CBD	Cannabidiol
CSA	Controlled Substances Act
DEA	Drug Enforcement Administration
FDA	Food and Drug Administration
USDA	United States Department of Agriculture

Introduction

Cannabidiol, commonly abbreviated as CBD, is a naturally occurring product that can be derived from multiple sources, including the cannabis plant. Use of CBD products has skyrocketed in the United States, with sales topping $4 billion in 2022 [1]. The cannabis policy landscape in the US has undergone significant changes in the recent years, marked by a divergence between federal and state laws on cannabis use. Despite cannabis, including all its components and derivatives such as THC and CBD, being generally illegal under US federal law due to concerns about misuse and health effects, states have increasingly adopted more liberal policies toward cannabis.

A. De La Cruz · O. Olateju · D. Rinker · M. Shrestha
D. Thornton (✉)
University of Houston College of Pharmacy, Houston, TX, USA
e-mail: aidelacruz@uh.edu; oolateju@cougarnet.uh.edu; dvrinker@central.uh.edu; mshrest9@central.uh.edu; jdthornt@central.uh.edu

History of Regulatory Landscape

The regulation of cannabis use traces its origins to the early 1900s, when smoked cannabis, commonly referred to informally as marihuana or marijuana, was linked to certain marginalized ethnic and racial minorities [2]. This association led to many states prohibiting cannabis use, culminating in the enactment of the Marihuana Tax Act of 1937 [3]. This legislation imposed taxes and administrative burdens on cannabis production and sales, covering both medical and nonmedical uses. Following the Marihuana Tax Act, global recognition of the therapeutic effects of cannabis increased, but concerns about its potential for abuse persisted. Negative attitudes toward cannabis, notably in the US, prompted the enactment of the *Single Convention on Narcotic Drugs* in 1961 [4, 5]. This international agreement placed cannabis and cannabis resin in the most restrictive category, prohibiting their manufacture, distribution, and sale [5]. The US, being a party to the Single Convention, repealed the Marijuana Tax Act to comply with its provisions. In 1970, the *Controlled Substances Act* (CSA)[6] was enacted, partly to fulfill US obligations under the Single Convention. It designated marijuana, defined as cannabis compounds, derivatives, and synthetic versions, and THC as hallucinogens, categorizing them as Schedule I substances with no accepted medical use and a high potential for abuse [6, 7]. Federal law stipulates that the production, sale, possession, and distribution of cannabis can incur fines and prison time.

Modern Regulation

Over time, the federal government eased enforcement of cannabis-related crimes through initiatives such as the Cole Memorandum of 2013 and the Rohrabacher-Farr Amendment of 2014 [7]. In 2018, the Agriculture Improvement Act, commonly known as the "2018 Farm Bill, " differentiated hemp from cannabis, legalized hemp cultivation and removed

J. P. Reinert et al. (eds.), *Adjunctive Analgesic Strategies for the Bedside Clinician and Beyond*,
https://doi.org/10.1007/978-3-032-21675-5_17

hemp and certain cannabinoids extracted from hemp from the US Controlled Substances Act, effectively legalizing hemp [8]. Hemp, as defined in the bill, includes any cannabis plant or derivative containing not more than 0.3% THC. Consequently, CBD and CBD products derived from hemp are no longer federally illegal, while those from other cannabis varieties remain prohibited [7]. In the same year, the DEA designated FDA-approved cannabis-derived CBD products with not more than 0.1% THC as Schedule V substances. Under the Farm Bill authority, the FDA approved Epidiolex® (cannabidiol), the first CBD product, for treating childhood seizures [9]. Currently, the FDA has approved only Epidiolex® and three cannabis-related drugs (Marinol® [dronabinol], Syndros® [dronabinol], and Cesamet® [nabilone]) for use with a prescription from a licensed healthcare provider. The dronabinol products are approved to treat anorexia associated with weight loss in AIDS patients, while nabilone is indicated for nausea and vomiting associated with cancer chemotherapy in patients who have not responded adequately to conventional antiemetic treatments.

State cannabis policies exhibit inconsistency across jurisdictions and often clash with federal regulations [7, 10]. In accordance with the 2018 Farm Bill and the Agricultural Marketing Act, states possess the authority to enact state-specific regulations governing hemp production for commercial purposes. However, any state-promulgated regulations on hemp production, including those implemented before federal legalization under the 2018 Farm Bill, must undergo review and preapproval by the USDA [7]. States are not obligated to implement their hemp regulations, and in the absence of a state-specific plan, the USDA is empowered by the 2018 Farm Bill to regulate hemp production in those states. There are four primary categories of state cannabis policies: (1) prohibition of all supply, (2) decriminalization, (3) legalization for medical purposes, and (4) legalization for recreational purposes [7]. The liberalization of policies has largely replaced the *prohibition* of cannabis cultivation, distribution, and possession due to concerns about addiction and crime. Idaho and Kansas, however, stand as two states that maintain a complete cannabis ban and impose criminal penalties, even for minimal possession. Some states allow the use of cannabis products with low THC but high CBD content while upholding prohibitions and criminal penalties for other cannabis activities. *Decriminalization* entails the removal of criminal penalties associated with cannabis possession for personal use and nonprofit exchange. *Legalization for medical purposes* permits patients with "qualifying conditions, " as certified by a medical professional, to purchase cannabis from state-operated dispensaries. California pioneered medical cannabis legislation in 1996, and the adoption of such programs has steadily increased in various jurisdictions [6]. The global phenomenon of *recreational legalization* was initiated in Colorado and Washington. It generally grants adults aged 21 and older permission to cultivate four to six cannabis plants while restricting possession and purchase to one to two ounces. Most states with recreational laws impose a minimum 19% retail excise tax on sales and prohibit cannabis use while operating a motor vehicle, with four states implementing specific per se THC limits for driving. In recent years, a growing number of states have taken steps to decriminalize cannabis possession and legalize its medical and recreational uses [7, 10]. As of November 2020, 16 states had decriminalized cannabis possession and casual exchange, 36 states had legalized cannabis for medical use, and 15 states had legalized cannabis for recreational purposes [7].

The Supremacy Clause of the US Constitution establishes that federal law takes precedence over state laws that are inconsistent or in conflict with federal law in specific ways [6, 7]. However, a provision in the federal Controlled Substances Act (CSA) specifies that state drug laws are only preempted in cases of an "affirmative conflict" with the CSA. State law serves as the primary enforcement authority for drug-related offenses [6]. Individuals and entities engaging in cannabis-related activities would technically violate the federal CSA, but the federal government generally refrains from prosecuting individuals possessing or sharing small amounts of cannabis. Instead, enforcement priorities focus on larger commercial cannabis entities or drug trafficking organizations, particularly those involved in interstate transport or foreign importation. The disparity between federal and state laws on cannabis use has facilitated the commercialization of cannabis without sufficient efforts to ensure product safety [6]. With limited evidence on the effects of cannabis liberalization on population health, it becomes crucial for policymakers to adopt a public health-informed approach to legalized cannabis supply. This approach should address inconsistencies between federal and state laws, provide regulatory oversight to enhance the safety of the cannabis supply, and address inequities stemming from the war on drugs and disparities in access to newly legalized supply chains [7].

Healthcare organizations, including the Institute of Medicine (IOM) and the American Society of Health-System Pharmacists (ASHP), express opposition to the use of medical marijuana [11]. Despite this stance, both organizations actively promote increased research into medical marijuana [11]. In 2011, the ASHP issued a statement emphasizing the need for expanded research on the clinical applications and safety of medical marijuana [11, 12]. The organization called for the standardization of potency and formulations in medical marijuana research. Moreover, both organizations advocate for ongoing education for pharmacists, addressing therapeutic and legal aspects related to the use of medical marijuana. Notably, the ASHP opposes the preparation and distribution of medical marijuana by licensed pharmacists, except when it is conducted for research purposes. This nuanced approach reflects a commitment to advancing scientific understanding while maintaining cautious and well-informed perspectives within the healthcare community. Given the legal variations related to cannabis use, pharmacists must comprehend the intricate legal framework associated with cannabis regulations to safeguard themselves and enhance their ability to serve patients effectively [13].

Pharmacology, Pharmacokinetics, Pharmacodynamics

Pharmacology

Cannabidiol (CBD), a phytocannabinoid, modulates the activity of several cellular effectors like cannabinoid receptors type 1 (CB1) and type 2 (CB2), serotonergic ($5HT_{1A}$) receptors, GPR55, the μ- and δ-opioid receptors, the transient receptor potential cation channel subfamily v member 1 (TRPV1), peroxisome proliferator-activated receptors (PPAR2, PPARγ), and fatty acid amide hydroxylase (FAAH) enzyme [14].

CBD produces analgesic effects by interacting with two G protein-coupled receptors, namely the cannabinoid receptor type 1 (CB1) and type 2 (CB2), within the endocannabinoid system that regulates many physiological functions, including pain and mood [15–18]. These receptors are responsible for regulating the perception of pain, dopamine and glutamatergic regulation, immune function, and energy metabolism [16, 17]. CB1 receptors are responsible for pain perception at the midbrain and spinal cord regions [16, 19]. CB2 receptors are mainly expressed in peripheral immune cells and the gastrointestinal system and regulate the release of inflammatory cytokines like interleukin (IL)-1β, IL-6, and tumor necrosis factor (TNF)-α [18]. By weakly binding to the orthosteric agonist binding site of the CB1 and CB2 receptors, CBD exerts an allosteric modulating effect on these receptors. The negative allosteric effect of CBD on CB1 receptors acts as an antagonist of cannabinoid antagonists to produce an analgesic effect. The interaction of CBD with CB2 receptors exhibits an anti-inflammatory effect in suppressing mast cell degranulation and neutrophil propagation around pain centers [16, 19, 20]. Moreover, CBD suppresses the FAAH enzyme, thereby increasing the availability of anandamide, which is responsible for activating the CB1 receptors [21]. Additionally, CBD interacts with TRPV1 to control pain signals.

CBD also modulates various non-endocannabinoid signaling systems. CBD also interacts with other receptors like PPAR2 and PPARγ receptors, monoamine transporters (norepinephrine, dopamine, and serotonin 1A receptors), fatty acid amide hydrolase, monoacylglycerol lipase, transport fatty acid-binding proteins, adenosine equilibrative nucleoside transporters, and glycine receptors α1 and α3 [22, 23].

CBD interacts with several other receptors to exhibit different physiological effects, including anxiolytic, anticonvulsant, neuroprotective, and antioxidant effects [15]. CBD exerts antianxiety effects through activation of adenosine receptors, anticancer effects by blocking GPR55 signals and weakening bone reabsorption and cancer cell proliferation, and helps in reducing breast cancer proliferation and metastasis by blocking Id-1 gene expression [21]. Additionally, CBD interacts with several other receptors. CBD binds to serotonergic $5HT_{1A}$ receptors, inhibits adenosine uptake, and can activate TRPV1 receptors at micromolar concentrations [17, 21, 24, 25].

Pharmacokinetics

CBD can be administered via oral, inhalation, intravenous, or transdermal routes. The pharmacokinetics of CBD vary depending on its route of administration. Oral administration of CBD can cause an intense rise in hepatic metabolism, and mucosal administration can increase plasma concentrations [15].

CBD has low bioavailability, can achieve a quick maximal concentration, and has a relatively long half-life. The bioavailability after oral consumption is approximately 6%, whereas it ranges between 11% and 45% (mean 31%) after inhalation [22, 26, 27]. It is a highly lipophilic drug, with 10% of absorption occurring on the surface of erythrocytes. It has rapid tissue distribution with high accumulation in the brain, adipose tissues, and other organs [17, 22]. CBD has a high distribution volume of approximately 32 L/kg [17]. Due to its low water solubility and absorption, the pharmacokinetics of CBD are more variable when given in capsules and less variable when delivered as oil products, sprays, or lozenges [17, 22, 27].

The peak concentration of CBD depends on its dose. CBD is mostly administered via the oral route at a 20 to 6000 mg dose [28]. The maximum concentration (C_{max}) after oral administration of 1500 mg CBD (Epidiolex®) was reported to be 292 ng/ml, and 6000 mg CBD was 782 ng/ml [29]. The C_{max} of a single dose of 800 mg oral CBD among regular users ranged between 1.6 and 271.9 ng/ml [28]. Following oral administration of CBD, the mean time to reach maximum (T_{max}) concentration can range from 1 to 6.13 hours, with maximum concentration reaching around 3–5 hours after single oral administration, 4.07–5.11 hours among polydrug users, and 3 hours among regular users. The T_{max} is 2.17 hours after sublingual administration, which is shorter than that of oral administration [17].

CBD has a long half-life ranging between 18 and 32 hours, with a half-life of 2 to 5 days after repeated oral consumption

[17, 22, 27]. The half-life of the CBD (Epidiolex®) after acute dosing was 14.39–16.61 hours [28]. The half-life of CBD after oromucosal spray is about 1.4 to 10.9 hours, 31 hours when smoked, and 2 to 5 days after chronic oral consumption [26].

CBD metabolizes in the liver and intestines. CBD undergoes CYP3A- and CYP2C-dependent phase I metabolism to form three main metabolites—predominantly 7-hydroxy-CBD, 7-carboxy-CBD, and 6-hydroxy-CBD. CBD metabolites are then excreted either intact or by further metabolizing to glucuronide conjugates in feces and urine [17, 22, 27]. CBD and other metabolites achieve maximum concentration around 0–4 hours with the level peaking around 2.5 hours post-administration [17, 26]. The clearance of CBD is 57.6–93.6 L/h [17]. CBD exposure increases by fourfold with food intake, especially after a high-fat meal, with the half-life changing to 24.4 hours [28].

Pharmacodynamics

CBD is relatively safe and well-tolerated up to oral doses of 1600 mg. Adverse effects of cannabidiol can range from mild to lethal depending on the route of administration. The most common side effects of CBD include diarrhea, sedation, diminished appetite, and elevated liver enzymes when repeatedly consumed at high doses [27]. Some rare side effects include thrombocytopenia, respiratory infections, and changes in liver enzymes [30]. Some studies reported limited effects of CBD on physiological outcomes like heart rate and blood pressure, but a couple of studies showed a modest decline in arterial pressure and systolic blood pressure following acute administration that returned to baseline after a week of use [28].

CBD inhibits hepatic cytochrome P450 enzymes, including CYP2C19 and CYP2A4, which are involved in the metabolism of many drugs. Thus, CBD interacts with many prescriptions as well as over-the-counter drugs. CBD, when concomitantly used with clobazam and norclobazam, increased serum concentration of clobazam by 500% and norclobazam by 60%. CBD, when concomitantly used with the anticonvulsant valproate, can cause an increase in liver enzymes. CBD, when used in children with epilepsy, was associated with higher rates of pneumonia, and when used at higher doses (≥20 mg/kg), it was associated with abnormal liver function [28]. Due to the low affinity of CBD with CB1 receptors, CBD does not have any intoxicating effects [27] and has limited abuse potential [28]. However, more studies are required to identify long-term adverse effects and drug-drug interactions of CBD.

One of the concerns associated with CBD is the availability of unregulated CBD in different formulations, including oral capsules or tinctures, sublingual oils, topical creams, e-liquids, or crystallized formulations, and dietary supplement forms. However, it is not known whether these formulations contained CBD. Moreover, there is concern about the possibility of hazardous chemicals being present in these unregulated CBD formulations. There have been reports that 21% of CBD formulations contained THC, which can have intoxicating and other side effects [28].

Evidence for Use

There has been a significant increase in demand and consumption of CBD in recent years. Data suggest that past-12-month use of CBD was as high as 26% in the United States. CBD has been used in the form of drops, topicals, edibles/foods, vape oils, capsules, and dried flower. Although many individuals reported using CBD for depression and anxiety, the majority reported using CBD to manage chronic pain [31].

The market for CBD has grown exponentially. It is estimated that by 2030, CBD will be a 60-billion-dollar industry, with a projected annual growth of 20% [32]. CBD is commonly believed by the public to be "healthy, " in large part due to advertising. Two surveys of CBD advertising in the US and Canada found that most advertising claims focused on perpetuating the idea that CBD was "natural" and effective in pain management [33, 34]. Clearly, the use of CBD is on the rise, based on the belief that it is a safe way to manage pain and mental health conditions. What is less clear is whether CBD is truly as safe and effective as advertised.

Prior to 2020, most studies on CBD focused on nabiximols (which is a combined product of THC/CBD in a 1:1 ratio), sometimes comparing THC/CBD to CBD alone [35–37]. The results are mixed, with some studies finding that nabiximols are slightly more effective than CBD in reducing pain, and others finding no significant difference. Due to the popularity of CBD, there have been several trials examining the efficacy and safety of CBD alone on pain levels and quality of life, among other outcomes. There have also been several studies on the safety of CBD alone. A review of 16 randomized controlled trials (RCTs) examined the overall impact of CBD on several outcomes. Ten studies were parallel group RCTs (randomized, double-blind, placebo-controlled trials) and six were crossover studies (randomized, double-blind, placebo-controlled trials within patients). The outcomes of these studies are summarized below:

Efficacy of CBD

Parallel Studies

A study by Alaia et al. (2022) [38] conducted a multicenter trial to examine the ability of CBD to reduce pain among those who have undergone arthroscopic rotator cuff repair.

One hundred and one patients were randomized to either receive oral, buccally absorbed CBD at 25 mg or 50 mg per day three times a day for 14 days postoperatively, while the control group received an identical placebo. Pain was assessed using the Visual Analog Scale (VAS), as well as opioid consumption and satisfaction with pain control. Additionally, liver function and nausea were tested to assess safety. Results indicated that while there were significantly lower pain scores and greater satisfaction with pain control between the two groups on day 1, this difference disappeared by day 2. The quantity of opioids consumed was low in both groups to begin with. By days 7 and 14, there were no statistically significant differences in VAS scores, opioid consumption, or pain satisfaction between the two groups. Additionally, there were no significant differences in liver function tests. The authors concluded that CBD might show promise in the reduction of pain in the immediate postoperative period for patients with orthopedic conditions, with an acceptable safety profile (VAS scores $p = 0.04$) [38].

Atieh and colleagues [39] conducted a study to examine the use of CBD versus placebo along with the interaction effects of two gene variants on patients with functional dyspepsia (indigestion). Forty-eight patients with functional dyspepsia and non-delayed gastric emptying were randomized to either 20 mg per kg per day of oral CBD or placebo. Self-reported symptoms of dyspepsia, including abdominal pain, nausea, and bloating, as well as postprandial (i.e., after a meal) distress and quality of life, were measured over the course of four weeks. At the end of four weeks, all patients underwent measures of physiological functions, including gastric emptying, gastric volumes, and a nutrient satiation test. Results indicated that there were no significant differences in either physiological functions or patient response outcomes between the two groups [39].

Bebee and colleagues [40] evaluated the efficacy and safety of a single dose of CBD for patients presenting to the emergency department in Melbourne, New Zealand, with acute lower back pain. One hundred patients were randomized to receive either a single dose of 400 mg of oral CBD or a placebo, in addition to standard analgesic medication. Outcomes assessed included pain, length of stay in the emergency department, need for additional analgesics (e.g., opioid use), and adverse events. Results indicated that there were no significant differences in mean pain scores two hours after administration, length of hospital stay, use of opioids, or reporting of adverse events between the two groups [40].

Haffar and colleagues [41] examined the use of multiple analgesics postoperatively among patients receiving total knee arthroplasty. Eighty patients were assigned to receive either applied topical CBD (120 mg), essential oil, CBD plus essential oil, or placebo three times daily around the treated knee for two weeks. Primary outcomes included scores on the visual analog pain scale (VAS), a numeric rating scale of sleep scores, and opioid use. Data were collected within 42 days post-surgery. Results indicated that there were no differences in VAS or sleep scores, nor were there any differences in opioid use among the four groups [41].

Hansen et al. (2023) [42] investigated the use of cannabis-based medicine on neuropathic pain in spasticity in Danish patients with multiple sclerosis and spinal cord injury. One hundred and thirty-four patients were randomized to receive either oral THC, CBD, a combination of THC and CBD, or a placebo. The duration of treatment was six weeks, followed by a one-week washout. The primary outcomes of interest were patient-reported neuropathic pain and/or spasticity, and secondary outcomes included global perceptions of change and quality of life. The authors concluded that there were no differences in primary or secondary outcomes between the four groups [42].

Hardy et al. (2023) [43] evaluated the use of CBD to reduce symptoms associated with advanced cancer among patients receiving palliative care. In a multicenter trial, 142 Australian patients were randomized to receive either 100 mL oral CBD oil, 0.5 mL once daily to 2 mL three times per day, or a matched placebo. Patients were followed over two weeks, and the primary outcome was self-report of symptoms on day 14, defined by a score on the Edmonton Symptom Assessment Scale (ESAS) ≥ 6 on day 14. Secondary outcomes were overall ESAS scores, opioid use, perceptions of effective dosage, overall perceptions of improvement, depression, anxiety, quality of life, and adverse events. The authors concluded that there was no difference in the proportion of patients with an ESAS score ≥ 6 between the two groups ($p = 0.24$). ESAS symptoms decreased over time for both groups. Additionally, there were no differences in levels of depression, anxiety, or quality of life between the two groups. There were also no differences in reported adverse events between the two groups, with only a slightly larger proportion of patients in the CBD group reporting dyspnea (i.e., difficulty breathing) than the placebo group [43].

Narang and colleagues [44] tested the efficacy of CBD among patients undergoing ureteroscopy with stent placement for urinary stone disease. Ninety patients across five sites in the US and Canada who had undergone ureteroscopy with stent placement were randomized to receive 20 mg of oral CBD oil daily for three days postoperatively or a placebo. Additionally, all patients were prescribed rescue medications, including narcotics. Primary outcomes were levels of pain, use of other medications, and ureteral stent symptoms. Secondary outcomes were the impact on physical activity, sleep, urination, and activities of daily living. Results indicated that there were no differences between the two groups in pain levels, opioid use, physical activity, sleep, urination, and activities of daily living [44].

Vela and colleagues [45] tested the efficacy of CBD as an adjunctive treatment for pain management. One hundred and thirty-six Danish patients with hand osteoarthritis or psoriatic arthritis who reported experiencing moderate pain intensity were randomized to receive adjunctive oral CBD between 20 and 30 mg or placebo daily for 12 weeks. The primary outcomes of interest were pain intensity within the last 24 hours, sleep quality, depression, anxiety, pain catastrophizing, and disability. Additionally, the researchers looked at differences in the proportion of patients reporting adverse and serious adverse events between the two groups. The results indicated that there was no significant difference in pain intensity between the two groups ($p = 0.96$). Additionally, there were no significant differences found on sleep quality, depression, anxiety, or pain catastrophizing scores. Moreover, there was no difference in the percentage of adverse events and serious adverse events experienced between the two groups [45].

Xu and colleagues [46] examined the impact of CBD on reducing pain symptoms associated with symptomatic peripheral neuropathy (damage to nerves causing weakness and pain in extremities). Twenty-nine patients were randomized to receive 250 mg of topical CBD or a placebo. Patients were followed for four weeks, after which time patients in the placebo condition then transitioned to the treatment group. Primary outcomes were self-reports of neuropathic pain. The results indicated a significant reduction in intense pain, sharp pain, and cold/itchy sensations in the CBD group. Additionally, there were no adverse events reported in this study [46].

Zubcevic et al. [47] also conducted a study to examine the effect of CBD and the combination of CBD/THC on peripheral neuropathic pain. One hundred and 15 Danish participants with painful polyneuropathy, postherpetic neuralgia, and peripheral nerve injury due to either trauma or surgery who had failed at least one previous evidence-based pharmacological treatment were included in the study. Patients were randomized to either receive oral CBD (5 to 50 mg), THC (2.5 to 25 mg), CBD/THC (5 mg/2.5 mg–50 mg/25 mg), or placebo over eight weeks. The primary outcome was average weekly pain. The results indicated that none of the treatments reduced pain compared to the placebo [47].

Crossover Studies

Crossover studies are a type of research design where patients who are initially randomized to the treatment group or groups are then "switched over" to the placebo, while those who were initially randomized to the placebo condition are simultaneously "switched over" to the treatment condition or conditions. Patients essentially serve as their own controls and comparisons, which is why these studies are often also called "within-study" designs. The advantage of a crossover study is that both between-patient and within-patient effects can be determined.

Arout et al. [48] examined the analgesic impact of CBD on healthy, noncannabis-using patients. In this preclinical study, 17 patients were randomized to receive an oral single dose of 200 mg, 400 mg, or 800 mg CBD or no CBD. Outcomes included pain threshold and pain tolerance, self-perceptions of pain, and perceptions of mood and cardiovascular outcomes. The results suggested that all doses of CBD *increased* pain relative to the placebo ($p < 0.01$). The authors did indicate that CBD had a dose-dependent, albeit modest, effect on mood. Measures of safety indicated that oral CBD was safe and well-tolerated, producing only small decreases in blood pressure ($p < 0.01$) [48].

In another preclinical study, DeVita and colleagues [49] also examined the impact of CBD on human pain reactivity. The purpose of this study was to test the interaction effects of CBD and expectancies for receiving CBD on human pain reactivity. Using a 2 × 2 design, 15 healthy adults were randomly assigned to four different conditions: sublingual single-dose CBD plus being told they were receiving CBD, a placebo plus being told they were receiving CBD, CBD plus being told that what they were given was a placebo, and a placebo plus being told what they were given was a placebo. Primary outcomes were pain threshold, tolerance, pain intensity, and unpleasantness. The results indicated that there was a main effect of expectancies on pain outcomes, such that the impact of pain was significantly larger when patients were told that they were receiving CBD. Pain and unpleasantness were reduced in the condition where patients were receiving CBD and were told that they were receiving CBD, relative to the control group [49].

A study by Schneider et al. [50] examined the therapeutic potential of CBD for reducing acute pain, hyperalgesia (a condition where patients experience higher-than-normal levels of pain), and allodynia (neuropathic pain that makes people extremely sensitive to touch). Twenty healthy volunteers in Switzerland were randomized to receive either a single dose of 800 mg of orally administered CBD or a placebo. Primary outcomes included pain, hyperalgesia, and allodynia. Self-reported pain did not differ between the CBD and placebo groups ($p = 0.928$), nor did levels of hyperalgesia ($p = 0.597$) or allodynia ($p = 0.884$). [50] Dieterle and colleagues [51] also examined the impact of oral CBD on opioid-induced hyperalgesia in healthy volunteers. Twenty-four Swiss participants were randomized to receive either a 1600 mg single-dose oral CBD or placebo. Primary outcomes included hyperalgesia and pain that was induced by electrical stimulation. Patients were given an infusion of opioids over 30 minutes, starting approximately an hour and a half after receiving either the oral CBD or placebo. The results indicated that although CBD was well-tolerated, it had no significant effect on hyperalgesia, allodynia, or pain when compared to placebo [51].

Heineman and colleagues [52] sought to evaluate the potential of CBD for the treatment of pain associated with thumb joint arthritis in a two-phase study. During Phase 1, ten healthy patients were monitored for one week after receiving 6.2 mg of topical CBD. No adverse events were identified, so the researchers proceeded to Phase 2, where 18 participants with thumb joint arthritis were randomized to either two weeks of twice-daily treatment of 6.2 mg topical CBD or shea butter alone. Following a two-week washout period, patients were switched to the other treatment arm. Primary outcomes included scores on the Visual Analog Scale for pain (VAS) as well as scores on the disabilities of the arm, shoulder and hand scale. Additionally, physical parameters were identified, such as range of motion, grip, and pinch strength. Results indicated that patients in the CBD arm reported significant improvements in pain and reductions in disabilities of the arms, shoulders, and hands. Additionally, there were significant improvements in range of motion, grip, and pinch strength [52].

Finally, a study by van Orten-Luiten et al. [53] sought to examine the impact of CBD in reducing abdominal pain and increasing perceived well-being among female patients with irritable bowel syndrome, one of the most common gastrointestinal disorders and one associated with lowered quality of life. In this study, 32 female Irritable Bowel Syndrome (IBS) patients from the Netherlands were randomized to receive a chewing gum formulation containing either 50 mg of CBD or a placebo. Patients were instructed to chew gum as and when it was needed to reduce their pain symptoms. Pain intensity was measured on the Visual Analog Scale (VAS), and quality of life was measured on the IBS-36 questionnaire. Results indicated that there was no statistically significant difference in pain scores or quality of life between the CBD and placebo group [53].

Safety of CBD

In addition to the studies outlined above, there are several clinical studies that have examined the safety of CBD. Specifically, several studies have examined Epidiolex® (cannabidiol), a purified CBD medicine formulated for oral administration. A systematic review in 2019 [54] was conducted to examine the risk for adverse events (AEs), severe adverse events (SAEs), or toxicity because of CBD. The results of the review identified 29 studies that evaluated the safety of CBD. Of those 29, 13 were clinical human trials. Nine were focused on neurological outcomes, and four were focused on psychiatric outcomes. Among the studies that focused on the safety of CBD on neurological outcomes, the percentage of adverse events varied between 16% and 93%. A moderate number of adverse events were identified, defined as sufficiently discomforting to the point of limiting or interfering with daily activities and possibly requiring interventional treatment, with the most common adverse events being lightheadedness, dizziness, headache, drowsiness, weight gain, lethargy, changes in appetite, diarrhea, vomiting, and rash. Six studies identified severe adverse events, including epileptic seizures and elevated aminotransferase concentration levels, a sign of potential hepatotoxicity.

Summary of Risks and Benefits of CBD for Pain Management

In summary, it does not appear that CBD is more effective than a placebo in reducing pain or symptoms associated with pain across a variety of diseases and symptom conditions. This is consistent across study design type, countries, variable dosing frequencies and dosages, and variable administrations. The studies by Xu et al. [46] and Heineman et al. [52] are the only exceptions. It is unclear what stands out about these studies, as all the studies identified had very small sample sizes, rendering a definitive outcome difficult to report.

The risks associated with CBD are mixed. Although most clinical trials did not identify any significant differences in the proportion of patients reporting adverse events between placebo and CBD conditions, there are several studies that have identified moderate to severe adverse events, with a considerable percentage of patients reporting experiencing at least moderate adverse events. Combined with the evidence to suggest that CBD is not associated with reductions in pain or associated symptoms, clinicians may want to consider the risks and benefits of administering CBD to patients who report pain.

Applications to Clinical Practice

Place in Pain Management

In June 2018, the US Food and Drug Administration approved the first CBD medication, Epidiolex® (cannabidiol), for the treatment of two rare and severe seizure disorders, Lennox-Gastaut Syndrome and Dravet Syndrome, in patients two years of age and older [55]. This drug approval marked a turning point for the use of CBD as a viable therapeutic preparation, offering hope to many children who suffer from the rare genetic condition that may result in hundreds of seizures per day. These positive trials for this product further ignited the possibility of using CBD as a remedy for multiple other ailments and syndromes. Since then, CBD has been studied for various disease states, including, but not limited to, chronic pain, spasticity, social anxiety disorder, substance use disorders, Parkinson's disease, nausea and vomiting in chemotherapy, weight gain in HIV infection, sleep disorders, and Tourette syndrome [56, 57]. Unfortunately, the evidence of CBD's effectiveness for indications other than drug-resistant pediatric epilepsy conditions remains scarce and inadequate [57]. Many states with medical cannabis laws in place may encourage the use of CBD and/or cannabis in place of a prescription opioid or non-opioid pain medication for chronic noncancer pain. A study sought to answer this question using data from 12 states that implemented the medical cannabis laws, as well as 17 comparison states. In the first 3 years of implementation of the medical cannabis law, there was no significant change in the receipt of opioid or nonopioid pain treatment among patients with chronic noncancer pain [58].

Since the peak of the opioid epidemic, most clinical practice guidelines have deemphasized prescription opioids as a first-line treatment option for chronic noncancer pain management, yet none have referenced or recommended CBD as a viable treatment option [58]. The 2022 Veterans Affairs/Department of Defense Clinical Practice Guideline for the Use of Opioids in the Management of Chronic Pain does not list CBD or cannabis as a potential non-opioid treatment option for chronic pain [59]. The 2020 American College of Physicians and American Academy of Family Physicians guidelines fail to mention CBD as a treatment option for pharmacological and non-pharmacological management [60]. Additionally, the 2022 Centers for Disease Control Clinical Practice Guideline for Prescribing Opioids for Pain does not recommend CBD and states that the evidence of cannabis for painful conditions is limited and inconsistent across studies, citing that some studies have reported adverse events such as dizziness, nausea, and sedation [61].

One of the many unknown aspects of CBD use in the over-the-counter setting includes proper dosing. With an entirely unregulated product, it becomes difficult to standardize dosing practices given the variability associated with differing manufacturing practices, dosage forms, CBD potency, use of excipients, and low bioavailability. Unlike the prescription product, there is not enough information regarding labeling accuracy, lot-to-lot variability, and long-term safety of cannabidiol products, which can further complicate dosing. Twenty global experts across nine countries used a multistage Delphi process to develop consensus-based recommendations on how to dose and administer medical cannabis safely and effectively [62]. The protocols were developed with a focus on the safety of what the prescribers observed in their respective practices to be effective. The Delphi process led to a consensus that a patient may be treated with CBD for the treatment of neuropathic pain, inflammatory pain, nociplastic pain, and mixed pain, with clinicians titrating, adapting, and managing individualized treatment goals for each patient. Table 17.1 includes dosing information. One of the primary reasons for the recommendation of CBD-predominant varieties is due to their safety, tolerability, lack of euphoria induction, and low risk of adverse effects [62]. It is recommended that clinicians follow the patient every 2–4 weeks, and, once the patient is stable, appointments may occur every 3 weeks or longer depending on tolerability and safety [62].

Table 17.1 Example CBD dosing regimen

	Routine protocol	Conservative protocol
Starting CBD type	CBD-predominant	
Starting CBD dose	5 mg twice daily	5 mg once or twice daily
CBD titration	Increase to 10 mg/day (total daily dose) every 2 to 3 days	Increase to 5–10 mg/day (total daily dose) every 2 to 3 days

Consider discontinuing therapy if the patient experiences any intolerable, moderate, or severe side effects, or if the maximum agreed-upon dose is reached and no longer offers any benefit to the patient, or if the patient has misuse or diversion associated with cannabis or cannabidiol products [62]. Cannabidiol doses up to 300 mg per day have been used safely for up to 6 months, and doses of 1200 to 1500 mg/day up to 4 weeks [56]. In larger studies of Epidiolex® (cannabidiol) treatment, CBD was associated with the following adverse effects in 36% of patients: somnolence, decreased appetite, and diarrhea. Additionally, a considerable number of patients had elevated liver function tests as well, resulting in a recommendation to obtain serum transaminases (ALT and AST) and total bilirubin levels in all patients prior to starting Epidiolex® (cannabidiol) oral therapy, as well as 1 month and 3 months after the start of treatment [56, 63].The FDA label contains additional warnings and precautions, contraindications, drug interactions, dosing, and adverse reactions that may be useful for reference to CBD inquiries in clinical practice [63]. Safety considerations, such as the possibility of resulting drug interactions without the supervision of a healthcare provider, remain perilous in the hands of the potentially inexperienced consumer.

As mentioned previously, CBD is known to interfere with cytochrome P450 drug metabolism pathways, which can result in diminished, additive, or synergistic properties that can be harmful to the patient [64]. CBD is extensively metabolized by CYP450 enzymes in the liver, including CYP3A4 and CYP2C19 isoforms. Many CYP3A4 inhibitor medications exist in the market today (e.g., ketoconazole, ritonavir, and clarithromycin) and may lead to significantly increased levels of CBD if consumed together. Furthermore,

CBD inhibits CYP2C19, CYP2D6, and CYP2C9. As a result, CBD may increase the serum concentrations of some commonly prescribed medications, including cyclosporine, sildenafil, antihistamines, haloperidol, antidepressants, and some statins (e.g., atorvastatin and simvastatin) [64]. Even though prescription CBD is used as an adjunct in epilepsy, its prescribing should still be carefully considered, given the multiple interactions that CBD has with other antiepileptic drugs, including clobazam, stiripentol, and valproate [64]. A few studies support the use of CBD for various pain syndromes, although it is important to note that CBD may have interacting effects when coadministered with common opioids (e.g., morphine, codeine) used in pain syndromes [64]. UDP-glucuronosyltransferase (UGT) 2B7 and 2B4 are major enzymes that lead to the metabolism of codeine and morphine and may result in subsequent interactions when used with CBD [65]. CBD may potentially inhibit UGT2B7 activity, which may require dose adjustments if adjunct use is indicated [64].

There is a consensus that individuals with psychotic disorders, unstable cardiovascular disorders, pregnant patients, and those planning to become pregnant and/or breastfeeding should avoid medical cannabis products. The prevalence of cannabis use among pregnant women has almost doubled in the past two decades, with approximately 10% of pregnancies being associated with maternal cannabis exposure in the US and Canada. This change in beliefs about cannabis may be due to expanding legalization, decriminalization, and medicalization, in addition to the decrease in the perceived risk of harm [66]. Although cannabidiol has evidence to support its use in certain indications, it should be noted that this does not generalize to the larger population, especially when considering the special populations outlined above.

If a patient and/or physician chooses to utilize CBD and hemp oils, it is vital that providers direct them to the highest quality product [56]. Table 17.2 includes a Checklist for Finding a High Quality Cannabidiol and Hemp Oil Product that can help determine a reputable company.

Given the lack of consensus among clinical trials and major guidelines regarding the efficacy and safety of CBD, patients should be upfront with their healthcare providers about their use and ask their pharmacists to check for the possibility of drug interactions, which may be present with a multitude of their maintenance medications.

Table 17.2 Checklist for Finding a High Quality Cannabidiol and Hemp Oil Product

1. Does it meet the following quality standards?
(a) Current Good Manufacturing Practices (CGMP) certification from the US Food and Drug Administration
2. Does the company have an independent adverse event reporting program?
3. Is the product certified organic or ecofarmed?
4. Have their products been laboratory tested by batch to confirm tetrahydrocannabinol levels <0.3% and no pesticides or heavy metals?

Key Themes

- Cannabidiol, commonly known as CBD, is a naturally occurring product that has exploded in popularity after passing the 2018 Farm Bill, which removed hemp from the federal Controlled Substances Act.
- There are no FDA-approved CBD-containing products that are indicated for pain.
- Nonprescription products containing CBD are heavily marketed but poorly regulated, with many products being mislabeled, impure, or contaminated [67].
- The vast majority of clinical trials that have evaluated CBD have found there is no evidence for use in treating pain [68].
- Clinicians need to be prepared to have a discussion with their patients who are looking to CBD to treat their pain, as the risks outweigh the benefits.

Conclusions

After a long history of cannabis products being prohibited, the use of cannabidiol (CBD) has quickly grown in popularity since the legalization of hemp in 2018. CBD is an extensively used product for pain management that is not supported by evidence. Lacking efficacy in this disease state, the risks associated with CBD use far outweigh the benefits. Healthcare providers need to be well-informed about the risks and benefits of these products, as their use is projected to continue growing in the near future.

References

1. Prohibition Partners. Dollar sales of cannabidiol (CBD) products in the United States from 2022 to 2026 (in million U.S. dollars) [Graph]. Statista Inc. Statista Web site. https://www.statista.com/statistics/1067467/cbd-product-dollar-sales-us/. Published 2022. Accessed 4 Dec 2023.
2. Bonnie RJ, Whitebread CH. Marihuana conviction - a history of Marihuana prohibition in the United States. U.S. Department of Justice Office of Justice Programs. https://www.ojp.gov/ncjrs/virtual-library/abstracts/marihuana-conviction-history-marihuana-prohibition-united-states. Published 1974. Accessed 23 Jan 2023.
3. Musto DF. The Marihuana Tax Act of 1937. Arch Gen Psychiatry. 1972;26(2):101–8.
4. Lande A. The single convention on narcotic drugs, 1961. Int Organ. 1962;16(4):776–97.
5. Pertwee RG. Pharmacological actions of cannabinoids. Handb Exp Pharmacol. 2005;168:1–51.
6. Mead A. Legal and regulatory issues governing cannabis and cannabis-derived products in the United States. Front Plant Sci. 2019;10:697.

7. Haffajee RL, Mauri A. Cannabis liberalization in the US: the policy landscape. Health Affairs Health Policy Brief. 2021;
8. Wiley JL Camille K, Thomas BF. Cannabidiol: science, marketing, and legal perspectives. In: Research Triangle Park: RTI Press; 2020. https://www.ncbi.nlm.nih.gov/books/NBK565434/
9. U.S. Food and Drug Administration. FDA Regulation of Cannabis and Cannabis-Derived Products, including Cannabidiol (CBD). https://www.fda.gov/news-events/public-health-focus/fda-regulation-cannabis-and-cannabis-derived-products-including-cannabidiol-cbd. Published 2023. Updated September 28, 2023. Accessed 23 Jan 2024.
10. Smart R, Pacula RL. Early evidence of the impact of cannabis legalization on cannabis use, cannabis use disorder, and the use of other substances: findings from state policy evaluations. Am J Drug Alcohol Abuse. 2019;45(6):644–63.
11. Moeller KE, Woods B. Pharmacy students' knowledge and attitudes regarding medical marijuana. Am J Pharm Educ. 2015;79(6):85.
12. Traynor K. Medical cannabis sparks treatment conversations. ASHP News Center. https://news.ashp.org/news/ashp-news/2019/03/14/medical-cannabis-sparks-treatment-conversations. Published 2019. Accessed 23 Jan 2024.
13. Seamon MJ, Fass JA, Maniscalco-Feichtl M, Abu-Shraie NA. Medical marijuana and the developing role of the pharmacist. Am J Health Syst Pharm. 2007;64(10):1037–44.
14. Laprairie RB, Bagher AM, Kelly ME, Denovan-Wright EM. Cannabidiol is a negative allosteric modulator of the cannabinoid CB1 receptor. Br J Pharmacol. 2015;172(20):4790–805.
15. Bartončíková M, Lapčíková B, Lapčík L, Valenta T. Hemp-derived CBD used in food and food supplements. Molecules. 2023;28(24).
16. National Center for Biotechnology Information. PubChem compound summary for: CID 644019, Cannabidiol. https://pubchem.ncbi.nlm.nih.gov/compound/Cannabidiol. Published 2024. Accessed 9 Jan 2024.
17. Dixon T, Cadenhead KS. Cannabidiol versus placebo as adjunctive treatment in early psychosis: study protocol for randomized controlled trial. Trials. 2023;24(1):775.
18. Erridge S, Leung O, Holvey C, et al. An observational study of clinical outcome measures in patients treated with cannabis-based medicinal products on the UK medical cannabis registry. Neuropsychopharmacol Rep. 2023;43(4):616–32.
19. Peng J, Fan M, An C, Ni F, Huang W, Luo J. A narrative review of molecular mechanism and therapeutic effect of cannabidiol (CBD). Basic Clin Pharmacol Toxicol. 2022;130(4):439–56.
20. Guo Y, Wei R, Deng J, Guo W. Research progress in the management of vascular disease with cannabidiol: a review. J Cardiothorac Surg. 2024;19(1):6.
21. Lee MA. CBD: how it works. O'Shaughnessy's [Internet] 2011.
22. Chayasirisobhon S. Mechanisms of action and pharmacokinetics of cannabis. Perm J. 2020;25:1–3.
23. Faraj M, Dautrich T, Lundahl L, Marusak H. Effects of two cannabidiol oil products on self-reported stress relief: a quasi-experimental study. Med Cannabis Cannabinoids. 2023;6(1):138–47.
24. Cannabidiol. https://www.mercy.net/content/dam/mercy/en/pdf/springfield-tdo/cannabidiol.pdf. Accessed 8 Jan 2024.
25. World Health Organization. Cannabidiol (CBD): Critical review report. https://www.who.int/docs/default-source/controlled-substances/whocbdreportmay2018-2.pdf?sfvrsn=f78db177_2. Published 2018. Accessed 11 Jan 2024.
26. Meissner H CM. Cannabidiol (CBD). In: StatPearls [Internet]. Treasure Island: StatPearls Publishing; 2023.
27. Sideris A, Doan LV. An overview of cannabidiol. Anesth Analg. 2024;138(1):54–68.
28. Britch SC, Babalonis S, Walsh SL. Cannabidiol: pharmacology and therapeutic targets. Psychopharmacology. 2021;238(1):9–28.
29. Taylor L, Gidal B, Blakey G, Tayo B, Morrison G. A phase I, randomized, double-blind, placebo-controlled, single ascending dose, multiple dose, and food effect trial of the safety, tolerability and pharmacokinetics of highly purified cannabidiol in healthy subjects. CNS Drugs. 2018;32(11):1053–67.
30. Cannabidiol. 2019;44(3):13–14. Published March 15, 2019.
31. Goodman S, Wadsworth E, Schauer G, Hammond D. Use and perceptions of cannabidiol products in Canada and in the United States. Cannabis Cannabinoid Res. 2022;7(3):355–64.
32. Cannabinoids market to triple to $60 billion by 2030, CBD segment leads U.S. Sales Global Cannabis Times; 2022. https://globalcannabistimes.com/cannabinoids-market-to-triple-to-60-billion-by-2030-cbd-segment-leads-u-s-sales/. Accessed 21 Mar 2023.
33. Amann L, Kruse E, Lazard AJ, Reboussin BA, Wagoner KG, Romero-Sandoval EA. CBD retailers in NC promote CBD online to treat pain violating FDA rules about medical claims and offer low-CBD/high-price products J Pain Res. 2022;15(null):3847–58.
34. Zenone MA, Snyder J, Crooks V. Selling cannabidiol products in Canada: a framing analysis of advertising claims by online retailers. BMC Public Health. 2021;21(1):1285.
35. Serpell M, Ratcliffe S, Hovorka J, et al. A double-blind, randomized, placebo-controlled, parallel group study of THC/CBD spray in peripheral neuropathic pain treatment. Eur J Pain. 2014;18(7):999–1012.
36. Überall MA. A review of scientific evidence for THC:CBD oromucosal spray (Nabiximols) in the management of chronic pain. J Pain Res. 2020;13:399–410.
37. Boyaji S, Merkow J, Elman RNM, Kaye AD, Yong RJ, Urman RD. The role of cannabidiol (CBD) in chronic pain management: An assessment of current evidence. Curr Pain Headache Rep. 2020;24(2):4.
38. Alaia MJ, Hurley ET, Vasavada K, et al. Buccally absorbed cannabidiol shows significantly superior pain control and improved satisfaction immediately after arthroscopic rotator cuff repair: a placebo-controlled, double-blinded, randomized trial. Am J Sports Med. 2022;50(11):3056–63.
39. Atieh J, Maselli D, Breen-Lyles M, et al. Cannabidiol for functional dyspepsia with normal gastric emptying: a randomized controlled trial. Am J Gastroenterol. 2022;117(8):1296–304.
40. Bebee B, Taylor DM, Bourke E, et al. The CANBACK trial: a randomised, controlled clinical trial of oral cannabidiol for people presenting to the emergency department with acute low back pain. Med J Aust. 2021;214(8):370–5.
41. Haffar A, Khan IA, Abdelaal MS, Banerjee S, Sharkey PF, Lonner JH. Topical Cannabidiol (CBD) after Total knee arthroplasty does not decrease pain or opioid use: a prospective randomized double-blinded placebo-controlled trial. J Arthroplast. 2022;37(9):1763–70.
42. Hansen JS, Gustavsen S, Roshanisefat H, et al. Cannabis-based medicine for neuropathic pain and spasticity-a multicenter, randomized, double-blinded, placebo-controlled trial. Pharmaceuticals (Basel). 2023;16(8).
43. Hardy J, Greer R, Huggett G, Kearney A, Gurgenci T, Good P. Phase IIb randomized, placebo-controlled, dose-escalating, double-blind study of cannabidiol oil for the relief of symptoms in advanced cancer (MedCan1-CBD). J Clin Oncol. 2023;41(7):1444–52.
44. Narang G, Moore J, Wymer K, et al. Effect of cannabidiol oil on post-ureteroscopy pain for urinary calculi: a randomized, double-blind, placebo-controlled trial. J Urol. 2023;209(4):726–33.
45. Vela J, Dreyer L, Petersen KK, Arendt-Nielsen L, Duch KS, Kristensen S. Cannabidiol treatment in hand osteoarthritis and psoriatic arthritis: a randomized, double-blind, placebo-controlled trial. Pain. 2022;163(6):1206–14.
46. Xu DH, Cullen BD, Tang M, Fang Y. The effectiveness of topical cannabidiol oil in symptomatic relief of peripheral neuropathy of the lower extremities. Curr Pharm Biotechnol. 2020;21(5):390–402.

47. Zubcevic K, Petersen M, Bach FW, et al. Oral capsules of Tetra-hydro-cannabinol (THC), Cannabidiol (CBD) and their combination in peripheral neuropathic pain treatment. Eur J Pain. 2023;27(4):492–506.
48. Arout CA, Haney M, Herrmann ES, Bedi G, Cooper ZD. A placebo-controlled investigation of the analgesic effects, abuse liability, safety and tolerability of a range of oral cannabidiol doses in healthy humans. Br J Clin Pharmacol. 2022;88(1):347–55.
49. De Vita MJ, Maisto SA, Gilmour CE, McGuire L, Tarvin E, Moskal D. The effects of cannabidiol and analgesic expectancies on experimental pain reactivity in healthy adults: a balanced placebo design trial. Exp Clin Psychopharmacol. 2022;30(5):536–46.
50. Schneider T, Zurbriggen L, Dieterle M, et al. Pain response to cannabidiol in induced acute nociceptive pain, allodynia, and hyperalgesia by using a model mimicking acute pain in healthy adults in a randomized trial (CANAB I). Pain. 2022;163(1):e62–71.
51. Dieterle M, Zurbriggen L, Mauermann E, et al. Pain response to cannabidiol in opioid-induced hyperalgesia, acute nociceptive pain, and allodynia using a model mimicking acute pain in healthy adults in a randomized trial (CANAB II). Pain. 2022;163(10):1919–28.
52. Heineman JT, Forster GL, Stephens KL, Cottler PS, Timko MP, DeGeorge BR Jr. A randomized controlled trial of topical cannabidiol for the treatment of thumb basal joint arthritis. J Hand Surg Am. 2022;47(7):611–20.
53. van Orten-Luiten AB, de Roos NM, Majait S, Witteman BJM, Witkamp RF. Effects of cannabidiol chewing gum on perceived pain and Well-being of irritable bowel syndrome patients: a placebo-controlled crossover exploratory intervention study with symptom-driven dosing. Cannabis Cannabinoid Res. 2022;7(4):436–44.
54. Huestis MA, Solimini R, Pichini S, Pacifici R, Carlier J, Busardò FP. Cannabidiol adverse effects and toxicity. Curr Neuropharmacol. 2019;17(10):974–89.
55. Food and Drug Administration. FDA approves first drug comprised of an active ingredient derived from marijuana to treat rare, severe forms of epilepsy. Published 2018. Accessed 20 Dec 2023.
56. VanDolah HJ, Bauer BA, Mauck KF. Clinicians' guide to cannabidiol and hemp oils. Mayo Clin Proc. 2019;94(9):1840–51.
57. Rapin L, Gamaoun R, El Hage C, Arboleda MF, Prosk E. Cannabidiol use and effectiveness: real-world evidence from a Canadian Medical Cannabis Clinic. J Cannabis Res. 2021;3(1):19.
58. Effects of U.S. State medical cannabis laws on treatment of chronic noncancer pain. Ann Intern Med. 2023;176(7):904–12.
59. VA/DoD Clinical Practice Guideline. Washington, DC: U.S. Government Printing Office; 2022.
60. Qaseem A, McLean RM, O'Gurek D, et al. Nonpharmacologic and pharmacologic management of acute pain from non-low back, musculoskeletal injuries in adults: a clinical guideline from the American College of Physicians and American Academy of Family Physicians. Ann Intern Med. 2020;173(9):739–48.
61. Dowell D, Ragan KR, Jones CM, Baldwin GT, Chou R. CDC clinical practice guideline for prescribing opioids for pain—United States, 2022. MMWR Recomm Rep. 2022;71(3):1–95.
62. Bhaskar A, Bell A, Boivin M, et al. Consensus recommendations on dosing and administration of medical cannabis to treat chronic pain: results of a modified Delphi process. J Cannabis Res. 2021;3(1):22.
63. Epidiolex. Package Insert. Greenwich Biosciences. Published 2018. Accessed.
64. Balachandran P, Elsohly M, Hill KP. Cannabidiol interactions with medications, illicit substances, and alcohol: a comprehensive review. J Gen Intern Med. 2021;36(7):2074–84.
65. Codeine. Package Insert. West-Ward Pharmaceuticals Corp. Published 2019. Accessed.
66. Sorkhou M, Singla DR, Castle DJ, George TP. Birth, cognitive and behavioral effects of intrauterine cannabis exposure in infants and children: a systematic review and meta-analysis. Addiction. 2023.
67. Evans DG. Medical fraud, mislabeling, contamination: all common in CBD products. Mo Med. 2020;117(5):394–9.
68. Moore A, Straube S, Fisher E, Eccleston C. Cannabidiol (CBD) products for pain: ineffective, expensive, and with potential harms. J Pain. 2023.

18 Individualized Medication Preparations: Considerations for Compounded Pharmaceutical Products

Justin P. Reinert and Cole Jerousek

Abbreviations

API	Active Pharmaceutical Ingredient
BAK	Baclofen, Amitriptyline, and Ketamine (compound formulation)
CIPN	Chemotherapy-Induced Peripheral Neuropathy
CRPS	Complex Regional Pain Syndrome
CTA	Compounded Topical Analgesic
FDA	U.S. Food and Drug Administration
HLT	Heated Lidocaine/Tetracaine
HPLC	High-Performance Liquid Chromatography
IV	Intravenous
NSAID	Nonsteroidal Anti-Inflammatory Drug
pH	Potential of Hydrogen (measure of acidity/alkalinity)
PLO	Pluronic Lecithin Organogel
PVC	Polyvinyl Chloride
RCT	Randomized Controlled Trial
USP <797>	U.S. Pharmacopeia General Chapter <797> for sterile compounding
USP <800>	U.S. Pharmacopeia General Chapter <800> for handling hazardous drugs
USP	United States Pharmacopeia
VAS	Visual Analog Scale

J. P. Reinert (✉)
The University of Toledo College of Pharmacy and Pharmaceutical Sciences, Toledo, OH, USA

C. Jerousek
Cleveland Clinic Akron General, Akron, OH, USA
e-mail: justin.reinert@utoledo.edu

Introduction

Topical analgesics offer a route of pain management that bypasses systemic circulation and directly targets localized areas of inflammation, neuropathy, or nociceptive pain [1, 2]. Compounded topical analgesics (CTAs) are customized formulations prepared in compounding pharmacies, typically involving combinations of multiple active pharmaceutical ingredients (APIs) such as lidocaine, ketamine, amitriptyline, gabapentin, baclofen, and nonsteroidal anti-inflammatory drugs (NSAIDs) [1, 3]. These formulations are often used in patients for whom conventional systemic therapy is contraindicated, poorly tolerated, or insufficient in providing relief.

CTAs appeal to prescribers and patients seeking individualized therapy. They may be prescribed for conditions such as complex regional pain syndrome (CRPS), peripheral neuropathy, musculoskeletal pain, and postherpetic neuralgia [1–3]. Advocates argue that these formulations provide additive or synergistic effects while minimizing systemic adverse events. However, their use has far outpaced the generation of high-quality clinical data supporting their efficacy and safety [4]. Regulatory oversight for compounded products is less stringent than that for FDA-approved drugs, which raises important considerations regarding consistency, sterility, stability, and therapeutic effectiveness [4, 5].

Formulaic Considerations

The therapeutic success of CTAs is highly dependent on formulation science [6–8]. Transdermal drug delivery is a complex process influenced by the physicochemical properties of the APIs (molecular weight, lipophilicity, ionization), the condition of the skin, the base formulation (e.g., liposomal, gel, cream), and the use of penetration enhancers. Lipophilic and low-molecular-weight drugs such as lidocaine and ketamine penetrate the stratum corneum, the outermost layer of the skin,

J. P. Reinert et al. (eds.), *Adjunctive Analgesic Strategies for the Bedside Clinician and Beyond*,
https://doi.org/10.1007/978-3-032-21675-5_18

more readily than hydrophilic molecules like gabapentin or baclofen, which may have negligible dermal absorption and thus may not be good candidates for topical formulations or may require higher doses formulated into the final product to achieve therapeutic benefit.

Maximizing the efficacy of topical analgesics depends heavily on the pharmaceutical formulation and delivery system used to facilitate percutaneous absorption and local tissue penetration. The stratum corneum serves as a major barrier to drug diffusion, and successful formulations must overcome this barrier while minimizing systemic exposure. Lipophilicity, low molecular weight (typically <500 Da), and low ionization are physicochemical characteristics that favor dermal absorption [9–11]. Among the most effective vehicles are liposomal, pluronic lecithin organogel (PLO), emulsion-based, and ethanol-based gels, which enhance solubility and penetration of both hydrophilic and lipophilic drugs [12]. Liposomes and PLO gels, for example, have been shown to encapsulate active ingredients such as lidocaine or ketamine, improving their ability to penetrate deeper skin layers and reach peripheral nociceptors and local nerves [10, 11].

Another promising approach involves thermosensitive hydrogels that change viscosity in response to skin temperature, enhancing retention and penetration. For example, a lidocaine–tetracaine patch embedded in a heated hydrogel (ZTlido®) has shown significantly improved absorption and faster onset of action compared to conventional lidocaine [13]. Additionally, penetration enhancers such as ethanol, propylene glycol, or surfactants are frequently incorporated to temporarily disrupt the lipid bilayer of the skin, though these may cause irritation or dermatitis in sensitive individuals [14].

Compounded preparations often involve multiple APIs in a single vehicle, which introduces challenges in drug-drug compatibility, stability, and solubility. Furthermore, compounding is not typically subjected to bioavailability or bioequivalence testing [15]. Variability in compounding practices across pharmacies may lead to differences in drug content and penetration potential, directly affecting therapeutic outcomes. Without rigorous pharmacokinetic profiling, it is difficult to ascertain whether sufficient drug concentrations are achieved in the target tissues, especially deeper structures like muscles or nerves [16].

Ultimately, the most effective topical analgesic formulations are those that strategically match drug characteristics with a delivery system tailored for targeted tissue penetration while balancing safety and patient tolerability. These limitations suggest that while some patients report benefit from CTAs, the current evidence base does not support widespread clinical use, especially when compared to FDA-approved topical agents like lidocaine 5% patches or diclofenac gel, which have demonstrated efficacy in rigorously controlled trials [17, 18]. Future development should focus on optimizing bioavailability through advanced carriers and validating these approaches through well-designed pharmacokinetic and pharmacodynamic trials.

Efficacy of Multimodal Topical Formulations

Compounded topical analgesics typically combine multiple agents targeting different pain mechanisms. Common ingredients include tricyclic antidepressants, NMDA receptor antagonists, anticonvulsants, and local anesthetics, though numerous other medications and drug classes may be eligible for inclusion in CTAs based upon patient requirements and prescriber preference. Medications that have been historically utilized as components of CTAs can be found in Table 18.1. The rationale for combination therapy stems from their synergistic potential and the poor penetration of many individual agents when applied topically.

Among commercially available topical analgesics, the *lidocaine 5% patch* is the most extensively studied and FDA-approved for postherpetic neuralgia [20, 21]. A randomized controlled trial by Galer et al. demonstrated that patients receiving lidocaine patches had significantly reduced pain scores and improved quality of life compared to placebo [20]. Evidence also supports off-label use in other localized neuropathic pain syndromes. A metaanalysis by Derry et al. found moderate-quality evidence for benefit in certain neuropathic conditions, albeit with varying effect sizes [1]. Capsaicin 8% patch, another FDA-approved agent, has shown efficacy in HIV-associated neuropathy and postherpetic neuralgia [22]. The ELEVATE trial showed the non-

Table 18.1 Medications commonly used in CTAs [19]

Medications	Drug Class
Amitriptyline Doxepin	Tricyclic antidepressants
Bupivacaine Lidocaine	Local anesthetics
Carbamazepine Gabapentin	Anticonvulsants
Dexamethasone	Corticosteroid
Meloxicam Naproxen	NSAID
Baclofen Cyclobenzaprine Orphenadrine	Muscle relaxant
Ketamine	NMDA antagonist
Clonidine	α_2 agonist
Tramadol	Opioid analgesic

inferiority of capsaicin to oral pregabalin with fewer systemic side effects, making it a suitable option for patients unable to tolerate oral therapies [23]. An additional formulation of lidocaine was studied by Gammaitoni et al. in 2013 [24]. This research explored the use of a heated lidocaine/tetracaine (HLT) patch in treating patellar tendinopathy, a common overuse injury in athletes [24]. The study reported significant pain reduction with the HLT patch, which was well-tolerated and did not result in systemic toxicity. The authors suggested that combining such topical analgesic therapy with eccentric training could enhance rehabilitation outcomes by improving compliance and reducing discomfort during exercise [24].

In cancer-related pain, topical preparations are often employed for localized cutaneous metastases, musculoskeletal pain near superficial tumors, or CIPN. While RCTs are fewer in this population, observational studies and case series support the utility of topical lidocaine and compounded formulations. One study by Barton et al. showed a modest improvement in CIPN symptoms using a compounded gel containing baclofen, amitriptyline, and ketamine (BAK) [25].

A randomized controlled trial by Popescu et al. in 2018 evaluated a compounded topical gel containing piroxicam (5 mg/g), lidocaine (20 mg/g), and cyclobenzaprine hydrochloride (5 mg/g) in 90 Romanian National rugby players with musculoskeletal injuries [26]. Participants applied the gel daily for 14 days. The study found that the multimodal gel led to a 70% reduction in pain scores by day 14, compared to a 45% reduction with piroxicam alone. Additionally, a higher percentage of participants in the multimodal group reported being pain-free during movement and pressure assessments. No adverse effects were reported, suggesting the formulation's safety and enhanced efficacy over monotherapy [26].

The Cochrane review by Derry et al. analyzed 61 studies involving over 8000 participants to assess the effectiveness of topical NSAIDs in acute musculoskeletal pain [1]. The review concluded that topical NSAIDs, particularly diclofenac and ketoprofen gels, provided significant pain relief compared to placebo. The incidence of local adverse events was low and comparable to placebo, highlighting the safety profile of topical NSAIDs in managing sports-related injuries [1]. Another systematic review and metaanalysis conducted by Nudo et al. focused on injured athletes and compared the efficacy of topical and oral analgesics [27]. The study found that topical medications had a significant effect size ($g = -0.64$) in pain reduction compared to placebo, whereas oral medications did not show a statistically significant difference ($g = -0.26$). These findings suggest that topical analgesics may be more effective than oral counterparts in the context of sports injuries, with the added benefit of reduced systemic side effects [27].

A randomized controlled trial conducted by Brutcher et al. evaluated the effectiveness of compounded topical pain creams in 399 patients with localized chronic pain, categorized into neuropathic, nociceptive, or mixed pain types [28]. Participants received creams compounded with agents such as ketamine, gabapentin, lidocaine, and NSAIDs, or a placebo cream, applied three times daily for 1 month. The study found no statistically significant differences in pain reduction between the active treatment and placebo groups across all pain categories. Reduction in average pain scores was minimal and comparable between groups, suggesting that these compounded formulations did not provide superior analgesia over placebo. The incorporation of analgesics with considerable data supporting their efficacy as monotherapy indicates potential issues with drug compatibility or tissue penetration that may have contributed to the results [28].

In a retrospective study, Somberg et al. evaluated the analgesic efficacy of two compounded topical creams compared to 1% diclofenac sodium gel in patients with chronic noncancer pain [29]. The compounded creams contained combinations of agents like flurbiprofen, tramadol, clonidine, cyclobenzaprine, baclofen, gabapentin, lidocaine, and bupivacaine. While the study reported greater pain reduction with the compounded creams compared to diclofenac gel, the lack of a placebo control and the retrospective design limit the strength of these findings. Additionally, the study's methodology does not allow for definitive conclusions about the efficacy of compounded formulations over standard treatments [29].

Another study by McCleane et al. assessed the efficacy of a combination cream containing 3.3% doxepin and 0.025% capsaicin, which was compounded from two commercially available products [30]. The study drug and its individual components were compared to a placebo for the treatment of chronic neuropathic pain as a three-times-daily application over a four-week period. Patients who received the combination cream experienced an average reduction in VAS pain scores by 1.07 ($p < 0.001$), which was similar to the reductions seen by doxepin (0.9 points) and capsaicin (1.12 points). Use of the doxepin/capsaicin combination product also led to a faster onset of its analgesic effects relative to the monotherapy formulations. The combination of manufactured topical analgesics, specifically doxepin and capsaicin, may be an effective and fast-acting multimodal treatment for chronic neuropathic pain [30].

Intravenous Multimodal Analgesic Combinations

In recent years, the strategic use of intravenously compounded adjunctive analgesic agents has expanded as part of multimodal pain management protocols, particularly in surgical, trauma, and intensive care settings [31]. These intravenous (IV) agents, often used off-label or in combination with one another, are designed to enhance analgesia while minimizing opioid exposure and its associated adverse effects. Commonly compounded agents include acetaminophen, dexmedetomidine, lidocaine, methocarbamol, orphenadrine, nalbuphine, and ketamine, among others. While these agents individually have demonstrated analgesic or opioid-sparing effects, their concurrent administration in compounded IV infusions raises important questions about safety, efficacy, compatibility, and clinical justification [31].

The compounded use of IV adjunctive analgesics introduces multiple safety concerns [31–33]. Physicochemical *compatibility and stability* data for these combinations are limited, and some agents, such as dexmedetomidine, are pH-sensitive and may precipitate when mixed with other drugs [32]. Furthermore, many compounded infusions are not prepared in compliance with USP <797> or <800> standards, raising the risk of contamination or degradation, particularly when beyond-use dating is not well established [34, 35].

A study by St-Jean et al. addressed the physical and chemical stability of compounded intravenous (IV) admixtures containing ketamine, lidocaine, and dexmedetomidine [36]. These combinations are increasingly utilized in perioperative and critical care settings to enhance analgesia while minimizing opioid consumption. However, the lack of standardized data on the stability and compatibility of such admixtures poses significant challenges for clinical implementation. In this investigation, the researchers prepared admixtures of the four drugs in various combinations and concentrations, simulating common clinical scenarios. The admixtures were stored in polyvinyl chloride (PVC) bags at room temperature and under refrigeration. Over a 14-day period, samples were analyzed at predetermined intervals using high-performance liquid chromatography (HPLC) to assess chemical stability, and visual inspections were conducted to detect any physical changes such as precipitation or color alteration. The findings revealed that all tested combinations remained physically and chemically stable for up to 7 days when stored under refrigeration, with no significant degradation of active pharmaceutical ingredients (APIs) or visual changes. However, at room temperature, certain combinations exhibited reduced stability, particularly those containing higher concentrations of ketamine and dexmedetomidine, which showed signs of precipitation and API degradation after 72 hours. These results underscore the importance of storage conditions in maintaining the integrity of compounded IV analgesic admixtures [36].

Similarly, a study by Senger et al. sought to determine the physical compatibility and chemical stability of a multimodal analgesic combination regimen including bupivacaine, epinephrine, and nalbuphine [37]. The study evaluated the compatibility and stability of these three agents in 0.45% sodium chloride, 0.9% sodium chloride, and Plasma-Lyte A. Using visual inspection, spectrophotometry, pH measurement, and HPLC analysis, the admixtures were monitored over 24 hours. Results demonstrated no physical incompatibility and confirmed the chemical stability of all three drugs throughout the study period under room temperature conditions. These findings provide essential evidence to support the safe preparation and use of this admixture in clinical settings, particularly for postoperative analgesia, and align with prior clinical studies demonstrating enhanced efficacy of these agents when used in combination; however, this data is in vitro and has not yet been deployed at the bedside [37].

Safety Considerations and Regulatory Oversight

Safety data on CTAs is also limited, primarily because compounded drugs are exempt from the FDA's rigorous approval process, including large-scale trials and post-marketing surveillance. This means adverse effects, interactions, and long-term outcomes may go undetected. While many practitioners perceive topical application to be safer due to reduced systemic exposure, this assumption may not hold true in all contexts.

Reports of systemic toxicity, such as CNS depression from topical ketamine or seizures from lidocaine, underscore the potential for percutaneous absorption at clinically significant levels, particularly when large surface areas are treated or skin integrity is compromised [20–25]. Although the presentation of safety data is rare in multimodal CTA studies, the inclusion of multiple APIs increases the likelihood of pharmacodynamic interactions, hypersensitivity reactions, and dermatologic side effects, including erythema, dermatitis, and ulceration [20–25].

Small studies have shown multimodal CTAs to be as safe as their individual components [30]. The previously mentioned trial by McCleane et al. suggests that some formulations of multi-agent topical analgesics can be utilized without a higher risk of adverse effects [30]. Study investigators observed similar rates of systemic adverse effects between the doxepin/capsaicin group and those receiving monotherapy. However, the doxepin/capsaicin group experienced a 20% lower rate of burning and discomfort after application compared to the capsaicin group.

The randomized study by Lynch et al. compared the use of a 2% amitriptyline and 1% ketamine cream to its individual components and a placebo in the treatment of neuropathic pain [38]. After applying 4 mL of the study medications three times daily for 3 weeks, no significant increase in adverse events was seen in the group receiving the combination cream. Four of the 80 total patients were found to have detectable levels of amitriptyline or ketamine, of whom none reported systemic effects [38].

Regulatory oversight for compounded medications falls under Sections 503A and 503B of the Federal Food, Drug, and Cosmetic Act, but enforcement is variable. Inspections have revealed inconsistencies in potency, contamination with endotoxins, and labeling errors. In the absence of USP <795> and <800> compliance, compounded topical products may lack stability and sterility assurance, particularly when produced in nonaccredited facilities. Thus, prescribers should exercise caution and select compounding pharmacies that meet the highest quality standards, such as accreditation by the Pharmacy Compounding Accreditation Board (PCAB) [34, 35].

Conclusions

Topical analgesics and specialty compounded topical preparations offer an attractive modality for localized pain management, particularly in patients who are unable to tolerate systemic therapies due to comorbidities or polypharmacy. Commercially available agents such as lidocaine patches, diclofenac gel, and high-concentration capsaicin patches are supported by robust clinical evidence and are approved for specific indications, including postherpetic neuralgia and musculoskeletal pain. Compounded topical analgesics, though increasingly used in clinical practice, lack consistent evidence for efficacy, and randomized controlled trials have generally failed to demonstrate superiority over placebo or standard topical treatments. While some observational and retrospective studies suggest potential benefit in niche populations such as cancer-related pain or chronic neuropathy, these findings are confounded by methodological limitations, inconsistent formulations, and the absence of pharmacokinetic validation. Moreover, compounded formulations carry risks related to variability in drug content, lack of regulatory oversight, and potential for systemic absorption and toxicity, particularly when involving multiple active ingredients. Clinicians must exercise careful judgment, balancing theoretical pharmacologic rationale with the available evidence, and ensure that compounded products are sourced from accredited pharmacies adhering to rigorous standards. Future research should prioritize high-quality, adequately powered trials to delineate the role of compounded topicals in multimodal analgesic strategies while also addressing critical safety, stability, and pharmacodynamic concerns.

References

1. Derry S, Wiffen PJ, Kalso EA, et al. Topical analgesics for acute and chronic pain in adults - an overview of cochrane reviews. Cochrane Pain, Palliative and Supportive Care Group, ed. Cochrane Database Syst Rev. 2017;2020(2).
2. Cline AE, Turrentine JE. Compounded topical analgesics for chronic pain. Dermatitis. 2016;27(5):263–27.
3. Leppert W, Malec-Milewska M, Zajaczkowska R, Wordliczek J. Transdermal and topical drug administration in the treatment of pain. Molecules. 2018;23(3):681.
4. Woodcock JW, Dohm J. Toward better-quality compounded drugs—an update from the FDA. N Engl J Med. 2017;377(26):2509–12.
5. Kim J, Konkel K, Jones SC, McCulley L. Systemic adverse events associated with compounded topical pain products. Drug Saf. 2020;43(5):497–501.
6. Richmond JM, Harris JE. Immunology and skin in health and disease. Cold Spring Harb Perspect Med. 2014;4(12):a015339.
7. Law RM, Ngo MA, Maibach HI. Twenty clinically pertinent factors/observations for percutaneous absorption in humans. Am J Clin Dermatol. 2020;21(1):85–95.
8. Ohman H, Vahlquist A. In vivo studies concerning a pH gradient in human stratum corneum and upper epidermis. Acta Derm Venereol. 1994;74(5):375–9.
9. Keurentjes AJ, Maibach HI. Percutaneous penetration of drugs applied in transdermal delivery systems: an in vivo based approach for evaluating computer generated penetration models. Regul Toxicol Pharmacol. 2019;108:104428.
10. Bassani AS, Banov D. Evaluation of the percutaneous absorption of ketamine HCL, gabapentin, clonidine HCL, and baclofen, in compounded transdermal pain formulations, using the Franz finite dose model. Pain Med. 2016;17(2):230–8.
11. Wang X, Black L. Ex vivo percutaneous absorption of ketamine, bupivacaine, diclofenac, gabapentin, orphenadrine, and pentoxifylline: comparison of versatile cream vs. reference cream. Int J Pharm Compd. 2013;17(6):520–5.
12. Pandey M, Belgamwar V, Gattani S, Surana S, Tekade A. Pluronic lecithin organogel as a topical drug delivery system. Drug Deliv. 2010;17(1):38–47.
13. Fudin J, Vought K, Patel K, Lissin D, Maibach H. Open-label adhesion performance study of a prescription lidocaine topical system 1.8% versus three lidocaine-containing over-the-counter patches in healthy subjects. J Pain Res. 2022;15:2051–65.
14. Mistry J, Notman R. Mechanisms of the drug penetration enhancer propylene glycol interacting with skin lipid membranes. J Phys Chem B. 2024;128(16):3885–97.
15. National Academies of Science, Engineering, and Medicine. There is a lack of evidence, transparency about ingredients to support use of compounded topical pain creams, says new report. 2020. Accessed 4 April 2025. Available at: https://www.nationalacademies.org/news/2020/05/there-is-a-lack-of-evidence-transparency-about-ingredients-to-support-use-of-compounded-topical-pain-creams-says-new-report.
16. Glinn MA, Lickteig AJ, Weber L, et al. Urinary concentrations of topically administered pain medications. J Anal Toxicol. 2016; https://doi.org/10.1093/jat/bkw110. Published online October 6, 2016.
17. Argoff CE, Galer BS, Jensen MP, Oleka N, Gammaitoni AR. Effectiveness of the lidocaine patch 5% on pain qualities in

three chronic pain states: assessment with the neuropathic pain scale. Curr Med Res Opin. 2004;20(sup2):S21–8.
18. Barthel HR, Haselwood D, Longley S, Gold MS, Altman RD. Randomized controlled trial of diclofenac sodium gel in knee osteoarthritis. Semin Arthritis Rheum. 2009;39(3):203–12.
19. National Academies of Sciences E, Division H and M, Policy B on HS, Creams C on the A of the ASDR the S and E of IU in CTP, Jackson LM, Schwinn DA. Science of compounded topical pain creams. National Academies Press (US); 2020.
20. Galer BS, Jensen MP, Ma T, Davies PS, Rowbotham MC. The lidocaine patch 5% effectively treats all neuropathic pain qualities: results of a randomized, double-blind, vehicle-controlled, 3-week efficacy study with use of the neuropathic pain scale. Clin J Pain. 2002;18(5):297–301.
21. Galer BS, Gammaitoni AR, Oleka N, Jensen MP, Argoff CE. Use of the lidocaine patch 5% in reducing intensity of various pain qualities reported by patients with low-back pain. Curr Med Res Opin. 2004;20(sup2):S5–S12.
22. Baranidharan G, Das S, Bhaskar A. A review of the high-concentration capsaicin patch and experience in its use in the management of neuropathic pain. Ther Adv Neurol Disord. 2013;6(5):287–97.
23. Viel E, Eerdekens M, Kandaswamy P. Treatment impact on patient-reported outcomes in peripheral neuropathic pain: comparing single intervention with topical high-concentration capsaicin to daily oral pregabalin. Pain Physician. 2021;24(6):453–63.
24. Gammaitoni A, Goitz H, Marsh S, Marriott T, Galer B. Heated lidocaine/tetracaine patch for treatment of patellar tendinopathy pain. JPR Published online. 2013:565.
25. Barton DL, Wos EJ, Qin R, et al. A double-blind, placebo-controlled trial of a topical treatment for chemotherapy-induced peripheral neuropathy: NCCTG trial N06CA. Support Care Cancer. 2011;19(6):833–841.s.
26. Popescu AN, Cotenescu E, Costandache B, et al. The benefits and risks of a tricomponent gel containing piroxicam, lidocaine, and cyclobenzaprine in musculoskeletal injuries in athletes. Farmacia. 2018;66(3):541–7.
27. Nudo S, Jimenez-Garcia JA, Dover G. Efficacy of topical versus oral analgesic medication compared to a placebo in injured athletes: a systematic review with meta-analysis. Scandinavian Med Sci Sports. 2023;33(10):1884–900.
28. Brutcher RE, Kurihara C, Bicket MC, et al. Compounded topical pain creams to treat localized chronic pain: a randomized controlled trial. Ann Intern Med. 2019;170(5):309–18.
29. Somberg JC, Molnar J. Retrospective evaluation on the analgesic activities of 2 compounded topical creams and voltaren gel in chronic noncancer pain. Am J Ther. 2015;22(5):342–9.
30. McCleane G. Topical application of doxepin hydrochloride, capsaicin and a combination of both produces analgesia in chronic human neuropathic pain: a randomized, double-blind, placebo-controlled study. Br J Clin Pharmacol. 2000;49(6):574–9.
31. Wilder AG, Foushee JA, Fox LM, Navalle J, Wright AM, Greer MA. Physical compatibility of medications used in critically ill patients with balanced fluid solutions. Int J Pharm Compd. 2020;24(3):238–41.
32. Marquis K, Hohlfelder B, Szumita PM. Stability of dexmedetomidine in 0. 9% sodium chloride in two types of intravenous infusion bags. Int J Pharm Compd. 2017;21(5):436–9.
33. American Society of Health-System Pharmacists. Handbook on injectable drugs. 20th ed. American Society of Health-System Pharmacists; 2018. p. vii–xi.
34. United States Pharmacopeia. Pharmaceutical compounding—sterile preparations <797>. In: USP-NF. Online. Rockville: USP; 2022.
35. United States Pharmacopeial Convention. Hazardous drugs—handling in healthcare settings <800>. In: USP-NF. Online. Rockville: USP; 2022.
36. St-Jean I, Hachemi D, Friciu M, et al. Stability of dexmedetomidine, ketamine and lidocaine combined injectable solution for analgesia. Eur J Hosp Pharm. Published online March 5, 2025:ejhpharm-2024-004177.
37. Senger Z, Mihigo GU, Howard MS, et al. Physical compatibility and chemical stability of bupivacaine, epinephrine, and nalbuphine in 0.45% sodium chloride, 0.9% sodium chloride, or plasma-lyte A. J Pharm Sci. 2024;113(12):3538–42.
38. Lynch ME, Clark AJ, Sawynok J, Sullivan MJ. Topical 2% amitriptyline and 1% ketamine in neuropathic pain syndromes: a randomized, double-blind, placebo-controlled trial. Anesthesiology. 2005;103(1):140–6.

Management of Adverse Drug Effects for Adjunctive Analgesics

19

Susan J. Lewis, Laura Sjoquist, and Mariann D. Churchwell

Introduction

According to the Centers for Disease Control and Prevention (CDC), there are approximately 1.3 million emergency visits per year attributed to adverse drug reactions (ADRs), with approximately 350,000 individuals requiring hospitalization. Patients 65 years of age and older are at an increased risk of an ADR, with almost 450,000 reported emergency department visits per year. The drugs most frequently identified with emergency department visits are anticoagulants, antiseizure medications, insulin, and prescription opioids [1].

A surveillance report from 60 hospitals reported that from 2016 to 2017, there were 267,020 emergency department visits for adverse effects related to opioids, of which 38.9% of visits were related to therapeutic use of opioids [2, 3]. Gastrointestinal effects were the most commonly reported adverse drug effect (ADE) for patients taking prescribed therapeutic use opioids (30.4%). Oxycodone was the drug identified in more than one-third of the cases. A more recent report of emergency rooms from 2017 to 2019 found analgesics (13.9%) and sedatives or hypnotics (12.2%) were the cause of medication harm of emergency room visits. Still, more than 90% of these visits were related to nontherapeutic uses [4]. A further breakdown of the information identified non-opioid-containing analgesics (2.9%), benzodiazepines (10.8%), antidepressants (6.5%), nonsteroidal anti-inflammatory drugs (3.6%), skeletal muscle relaxants (1.7%), anticonvulsant agents (3.4%), and other central nervous system agents (1.0%) associated with medication harm. Unsupervised exposure was highest with those less than 5 years of age, but self-harm, abuse, misuse, or overdose without indication of intent was highest in ages 15–24, followed by ages 25–44. For patients 65 years of age and older, the rate of emergency room visits for therapeutic and nontherapeutic medication harm when combined was higher compared to those less than 65 years of age, with 12.1 vs 5.0 visits per 1000 population [4].

Adverse drug effects (ADEs) for drugs utilized for the management of acute and chronic pain can range from itching, nausea, and constipation to fatigue, drowsiness, decreased respiratory rate, and death. Drugs prescribed for pain management need to be evaluated for drug-drug and drug-food interactions and ADEs, including fatal ADEs. The National Drug Council reported in 2021 that there were 98,268 deaths from preventable drug overdoses, which represent 92% of drug overdose deaths in the United States. Additionally, the American Geriatric Society (AGS) reports [5] that medications for managing pain in elderly patients should be used with caution. Many of the drugs discussed in this chapter are listed by the AGS as "avoid" because of enhanced sedation in elderly patients.

Depending on the ADR, the management of an ADR can range from stopping the drug to adjusting the dose or switching the patient to a different drug from the same drug class. A patient experiencing severe ADEs will need specific management for the reaction. Knowledge of adverse drug reaction management for adjunct analgesic agents is crucial for clinicians to provide optimal care for patients, especially those with complex pain management requirements. In this chapter, we examine the management of common adverse drug effects associated with adjunctive pain medications.

Acetaminophen, NSAIDs, and Topical Lidocaine

Acetaminophen

Acetaminophen (paracetamol or APAP) is an antipyretic analgesic used for fever, mild-to-moderate pain, or as an adjunctive therapy to opioids for moderate-to-severe pain. APAP is generally safe at recommended doses (4 g/day in adults and 50–75 mg/kg/day in children). Still, overdose can

S. J. Lewis · L. Sjoquist · M. D. Churchwell (✉)
Department of Pharmacy Practice, University of Findlay College of Pharmacy, Findlay, OH, USA
e-mail: mariann.churchwell@utoledo.edu

J. P. Reinert et al. (eds.), *Adjunctive Analgesic Strategies for the Bedside Clinician and Beyond*,
https://doi.org/10.1007/978-3-032-21675-5_19

result in dose-dependent acute hepatotoxicity and, in severe cases, acute hepatic failure. A single ingestion of greater than 7.5 g or 150 mg/kg is considered potentially toxic [6], while single doses less than 200 mg/kg in young children (age <6 years old) rarely cause toxicity [7–9]. The half-life of APAP is 2–2.5 h, but it can extend to 17 h with hepatic injury [10]. Peak serum concentrations occur within 4 h, although absorption may be delayed by co-ingestion with opioids or anticholinergics or the extended-release formulation [11].

APAP toxicity progresses through four clinical phases. In phase 1 (within 24 h), patients may be asymptomatic or experience nonspecific symptoms, including nausea, abdominal pain, and malaise. In phase 2 (24–48 h), hepatic injury becomes apparent with elevated liver enzymes [12–14]. Most patients do not progress beyond this stage, especially with prompt N-acetylcysteine (NAC) treatment [13, 14]. Stage 3 (3–5 days) marks peak hepatotoxicity [15], and in rare cases, fulminant hepatic failure and death [16]. Phase 4 represents recovery with no long-term consequences [12]. Risk factors for APAP hepatotoxicity include chronic alcohol use, malnutrition, prolonged fasting, and concomitant use of CYP2E1 inducers (e.g., carbamazepine, primidone, rifampin, and St. John's wort) [17].

For acute APAP overdose, a serum APAP concentration should be obtained at 4 h post-ingestion or as soon thereafter as possible and interpreted using the Rumack-Matthew nomogram to determine the risk of hepatotoxicity and the need for NAC treatment [15]. NAC provides cysteine for the replenishment of glutathione stores, enhances the sulfation metabolic pathway, and reduces N-acetyl-p-benzoquinone imine (NAPQI) back to APAP [16, 17]. NAC is protective against hepatotoxicity if administered within 8–10 h post-ingestion; however, patients with hepatic injury still benefit from NAC, as it may improve hepatic perfusion and oxygen delivery and extraction in patients with APAP-induced hepatic failure [18].

NAC is equally effective when administered orally or intravenously. The approved oral dosing regimen is a 140 mg/kg loading dose followed by 70 mg/kg every 4 h for a total of 18 doses over 72 h [19]. (Table 19.1) Patients with hepatic failure should receive intravenous NAC therapy. The recommended regimen is a 21-h continuous infusion of 150 mg/kg over 60 min, followed by 50 mg/kg over 4 h, and then 100 mg/kg over 16 h [20]. Treatment should be continued if APAP remains detectable or hepatic injury persists. Oral NAC commonly causes nausea and vomiting, which can be managed with antiemetics. Intravenous NAC can cause anaphylactoid reactions; however, a slower infusion (1 h vs. 15 min) of the loading dose reduces this risk. Minor anaphylactoid reactions (e.g., flushing, rash) can be managed with diphenhydramine, while serious reactions (e.g., angioedema, hypotension, wheezing) necessitate discontinuation of therapy [21].

Gastrointestinal decontamination with activated charcoal may be considered within 1–2 h of ingestion if the patient is alert and the airway is protected [22]. Hemodialysis is recommended in addition to NAC therapy if a patient has a highly elevated APAP level with metabolic acidosis and encephalopathy [23]. Transplantation should be considered in patients with full hepatic failure, encephalopathy, or multiorgan failure despite NAC therapy [24].

NSAIDs

Nonsteroidal anti-inflammatory drugs (NSAIDs) are widely used anti-inflammatory, antipyretic, and analgesic agents to treat mild-to-moderate pain, fever, and inflammatory conditions. NSAID-associated adverse effects primarily involve gastrointestinal (GI), cardiovascular (CV), renal, and central nervous system (CNS).

GI adverse effects are most common, ranging from mild dyspepsia, nausea, and abdominal pain to serious complications including ulceration, bleeding, and perforation. These effects result from reduced prostaglandin (PGE_2, PGI_2) synthesis, which impairs gastric mucosal protection. Although celecoxib, a COX-2 selective NSAID, is associated with fewer GI adverse effects than nonselective NSAIDs [25, 26], GI intolerance remains a concern, particularly in the elderly [27]. The risk increases with higher doses, longer duration, prior ulcers, untreated H. pylori, and concomitant use of corticosteroids, SSRIs, or anticoagulants [28]. Serious CV events such as myocardial infarction, stroke, and mortality are linked to selective COX-2 inhibition, which disrupts the balance between prothrombotic thromboxane A_2 (produced via COX-1) and antithrombotic prostacyclin (produced via COX-2) [29]. Rofecoxib and valdecoxib were withdrawn due to increased CV events [30, 31], whereas celecoxib has demonstrated comparable CV safety to ibuprofen or naproxen [32]. All NSAIDs carry box warnings for serious CV and GI risks [33].

Renal adverse effects result from vasodilatory prostaglandin inhibition, reducing renal perfusion and increasing the risk of acute kidney injury, especially in the elderly or those with kidney disease, heart failure, or dehydration. Additional effects include hyperkalemia and sodium-fluid retention, and rarely renal papillary necrosis, interstitial nephritis, and nephrotic syndrome [34]. CNS adverse effects include mood and cognition changes, drowsiness, dizziness, headaches, lethargy, hallucinations, and coma, and are more common with highly lipophilic NSAIDs (e.g., ibuprofen, naproxen, and ketoprofen). Seizures and aseptic meningitis have also been reported [35].

Table 19.1 Summary of adverse effects

Drug/class	Common adverse effects	Serious/toxic effects	Management strategies
Acetaminophen	Nausea, abdominal pain, malaise	Hepatotoxicity, encephalopathy, hepatic failure	Serum level and Rumack-Matthew nomogram, NAC (oral/IV), activated charcoal ($\leq$2 h), hemodialysis if severe, transplant if fulminant
NSAIDs	Dyspepsia, nausea, dizziness	GI bleeding, AKI, hyperkalemia, CV events, seizures, coma	Supportive care, activated charcoal ($\leq$2 h), no antidote, avoid chronic high doses, use lowest effective dose, add PPI/misoprostol
Topical lidocaine	Local rash, erythema, burning	LAST (seizures, arrhythmias), methemoglobinemia	Remove product, antihistamines/corticosteroids for rash, epinephrine for anaphylaxis, benzodiazepines + lipid emulsion for LAST, methylene blue for methemoglobinemia
Gabapentinoids (gabapentin, pregabalin)	Dizziness, drowsiness, edema, weight gain	Respiratory depression (esp. with opioids), withdrawal seizures	Dose reduction/taper, supportive care, hemodialysis if severe, manage withdrawal with benzos/haloperidol (case reports)
Carbamazepine	Ataxia, sedation, blurry vision, GI upset	SCARs (SJS/TEN/DRESS), aplastic anemia, agranulocytosis	Stop drugs, steroids for rash, HLA testing in at-risk groups, charcoal hemoperfusion/hemodialysis if severe overdose
Valproic acid	Tremor, somnolence, GI upset, weight gain	Hepatic failure, pancreatitis, teratogenicity, hyperammonemia	Stop drugs, supportive care, dialysis if severe toxicity, consider L-carnitine for hyperammonemia
Muscle relaxants	Drowsiness, dizziness, anticholinergic effects	Withdrawal (baclofen), seizures, serotonin syndrome, cardiotoxicity	Supportive care, restart/taper baclofen, flumazenil for carisoprodol (case), dialysis for renal impairment
Clonidine	Sedation, hypotension, dizziness	Bradycardia, CNS depression	Supportive care, atropine for bradycardia, fluids/vasopressors, naloxone sometimes helpful in pediatrics
Calcium channel blockers	Dizziness, hypotension	Severe bradycardia, shock, hyperglycemia	Supportive care, calcium IV, high-dose insulin, vasopressors, lipid emulsion if refractory
Ketamine	Nausea, dizziness, hallucinations	CV collapse, respiratory depression, dependence, withdrawal	Supportive care (airway, hemodynamics), charcoal if early ingestion, monitor for polysubstance toxicity
SNRIs/TCAs	Nausea, insomnia, sexual dysfunction, anticholinergic effects (TCAs)	Serotonin syndrome, suicidality, arrhythmias, hyponatremia	Stop offending drugs, supportive care, cyproheptadine for serotonin syndrome, taper to avoid withdrawal

APAP acetaminophen, *NAC* N-acetylcysteine, *IV* intravenous, *NSAID* nonsteroidal anti-inflammatory drug, *GI* gastrointestinal, *AKI* acute kidney injury, *CV* cardiovascular, *PPI* proton pump inhibitor, *LAST* local anesthetic systemic toxicity, *SCARs* severe cutaneous adverse reactions, *SJS* Stevens-Johnson syndrome, *TEN* toxic epidermal necrolysis, *DRESS* drug reaction with eosinophilia and systemic symptoms, *CNS* central nervous system, *SNRI* serotonin-norepinephrine reuptake inhibitor, *TCA* tricyclic antidepressant

Patients with acute NSAID overdose remain asymptomatic or present with mild GI symptoms (e.g., nausea, vomiting, abdominal pain). Ibuprofen ingestions of less than 100 mg/kg rarely causes toxicity; doses exceeding 400 mg/kg may lead to severe or life-threatening conditions [36]. Toxicity may manifest within hours and varies based on the pharmacokinetics of the ingested agent. NSAIDs are metabolized extensively via cytochrome P450 enzymes and glucuronidation with renal excretion. Clinicians should be aware that NSAID toxicity may be potentiated by concurrent use of antihypertensives, anticoagulants, antiplatelets, SSRIs, or any drugs known to injure GI mucosa. Furthermore, NSAIDS are highly protein-bound; thus, hypoalbuminemia and other highly protein-bound drugs can potentially increase the free serum concentrations. However, serum NSAID concentrations do not correlate with toxicity and should not guide treatment [37]. Clinicians should assess for renal dysfunction, acid-base and electrolyte abnormalities, GI bleeding, CNS changes, and other complications, including seizures, coma, hypotension, and anion gap metabolic acidosis.

Initial evaluation should focus on immediate life-threatening complications (e.g., airway, breathing, and circulation) and hemodynamic stability. If the patient presents within 1–2 h of ingestion and no contraindications are present, GI decontamination with a single dose of activated charcoal may be considered [38]. There is currently no antidote for NSAID toxicity; hence, supportive care focusing on correcting electrolyte and acid/base abnormalities and fluid replacement should be emphasized for acute toxicity. Hemodialysis is generally ineffective, given the high degree of protein binding of NSAIDs (Table 19.1).

Most NSAID-related toxicity occurs following chronic use. Prevention strategies include prescribing the lowest effective dose for the shortest duration, along with regular monitoring of blood pressure, renal function, and GI bleeding. Educating patients to recognize symptoms of toxicity is crucial for early detection and management. For individuals at risk of NSAID-related GI toxicity, concomitant use of gastroprotective agents such as proton pump inhibitors or misoprostol can be utilized to mitigate the risk.

Topical Lidocaine

Lidocaine is a local anesthetic with antiarrhythmic properties, widely used in topical formulations as an adjuvant analgesic for managing localized acute and chronic pain. It is available in various forms, including transdermal patches, creams, gels, ointments, sprays, and lotions.

Topical lidocaine preparations are generally well tolerated when used as directed. The most common adverse effects are localized cutaneous reactions such as transient erythema, burning, itching, or rash, which are typically mild and self-limiting [39, 40]. Management includes rotating application sites and, if needed, applying topical corticosteroids or emollients. Less commonly, patients may develop blistering, bruising, or irritant contact dermatitis due to the anesthetic or adhesive components. In such cases, the product should be removed to allow the skin to recover prior to reapplication. While true immune-mediated allergic reactions to lidocaine are rare, allergic contact dermatitis (a delayed Type IV hypersensitivity) has been reported [41, 42]. These are typically managed with topical corticosteroids. True IgE-mediated *anaphylaxis* to topical lidocaine is extremely rare, but anaphylactoid reactions with angioedema, hypersensitivity, bronchospasm, or urticaria can occur [43] and require prompt treatment with diphenhydramine, corticosteroids, or epinephrine, depending on severity.

Systemic toxicity is highly unlikely with topical lidocaine due to limited absorption. For example, a 5% lidocaine patch produces average plasma levels of ~0.13 μg/mL, far below the toxicity threshold of 5 μg/mL [44]. However, systemic exposure can increase with excessive dosing, prolonged application, use over broken or inflamed skin, or decreased drug elimination [45]. Once absorbed, lidocaine is widely distributed (Vd ~0.7–1.5 L/kg), approximately 65–80% protein-bound, metabolized hepatically via CYP1A2 and CYP3A4 to active metabolites, and renally excreted with a half-life of 1.5–2 h. Caution is warranted in vulnerable populations such as neonates, the elderly, or those with hypoalbuminemia or impaired hepatic or renal function [46].

Although rare, excessive systemic absorption of topical lidocaine can lead to local anesthetic systemic toxicity (LAST), a potentially life-threatening condition [47]. LAST typically begins with CNS symptoms such as perioral numbness, dizziness, tinnitus, or a metallic taste, and may progress to seizures, coma, or respiratory arrest. Cardiac toxicity, which typically follows CNS symptoms, can present as bradycardia, arrhythmias, hypotension, or cardiac arrest [39]. Management of LAST includes immediate discontinuation of lidocaine and supportive care [40]. The application site should be gently washed with mild, nontoxic soap and warm water [41]. Airway stabilization, oxygenation, and seizure control with benzodiazepines are critical initial steps. In severe cases, 20% intravenous lipid emulsion therapy should be administered promptly to reduce free circulating lidocaine and mitigate both neurologic and cardiovascular toxicity [40]. Methemoglobinemia is another rare but serious systemic adverse effect [48, 49], more likely when lidocaine is applied to mucous membranes or used in large amounts. It occurs when lidocaine or its metabolites oxidize hemoglobin, reducing its oxygen-carrying capacity. Patients may present with cyanosis, fatigue, and dyspnea unresponsive to oxygen therapy. Severe cases with symptoms or high methemoglobin levels above 20–30% should be treated with supplemental oxygen and intravenous methylene blue [40].

While these systemic toxicities are more commonly associated with injectable formulations, clinicians using topical lidocaine should remain vigilant for these rare but serious complications, especially in high-risk patients or scenarios of improper use.

Gabapentinoids

The gabapentinoids are FDA-approved for the treatment of some types of neuropathic pain, including the management of cancer and postherpetic neuralgia in adults. Pregabalin is FDA-approved for pain related to fibromyalgia [50, 51]. Additionally, pregabalin can be used as an adjuvant analgesic for the relief of chronic neuropathic pain in cancer survivors [50, 52]. The pharmacologic actions of gabapentinoids are dose-related, and higher doses can be associated with ADEs.

Gabapentinoid ADEs include nausea, swelling of the extremities, rash, and difficulty breathing. Patients taking gabapentinoids may also experience ADEs related to CNS depression, such as dizziness, drowsiness, weakness, or fatigue, which can increase the risk of falls and impaired mental abilities [53]. The risk of respiratory depression with gabapentinoids is increased with the use of concomitant CNS depressants (opioids). Patients at the highest risk of respiratory depression are those with an underlying respiratory impairment or older patients. The onset of adverse reactions is variable and impacted by concomitant use of medications known to cause CNS depression (e.g., opioids) [54]. Gabapentinoid ADEs can be exacerbated when gabapentin or pregabalin is taken with alcohol, antihistamines, benzodiazepines, muscle relaxants, opioids, and tricyclic antidepressants [55].

There is no definitive treatment for gabapentinoid ADEs, but a dose reduction, supportive care, and treatment or reversal of substances that were co-ingested are recommended

[56]. A dose reduction or taper is preferred for patients taking higher gabapentinoid doses to avoid gabapentinoid withdrawal symptoms such as mood swings, suicidal ideation, and sudden behavioral changes [57, 58]. For toxicity from gabapentin and pregabalin, the evidence for the use of extracorporeal treatment is inconclusive. Gabapentin is considered dialyzable, but clinicians must weigh the benefit versus the harm of initiating dialytic therapy. If the patient has kidney dysfunction and is receiving mechanical ventilation, intermittent hemodialysis or continuous renal replacement therapy (CRRT) may be beneficial in addition to supportive care [59]. For patients with kidney impairment receiving intermittent hemodialysis, treatment may be warranted. Patients with sudden stoppage of a gabapentinoid or those receiving dialytic therapy should be monitored for gabapentinoid withdrawal. If a patient experiences gabapentinoid withdrawal symptoms, consider reinstituting the drug at a lower dose to prevent serious ADEs such as akathisia from withdrawal [60]. Case reports have discussed administering a benzodiazepine or haloperidol for withdrawal symptoms, but the results are not conclusive [57, 61].

Gabapentinoids have been used to amplify the effect of illicit opioids. An overdose is associated with drowsiness, tachycardia, dizziness, hypotension, nausea, vomiting, and impaired coordination. Supportive care is the treatment for an overdose, but there is a seizure risk associated with gabapentinoid withdrawal. Phenytoin or phenobarbital has been used for seizures related to withdrawal [58, 61, 62].

Anti-Seizure Medications: Carbamazepine and Valproic Acid

Carbamazepine and valproic acid are sometimes prescribed for patients with intractable neuropathic pain. Common carbamazepine ADEs include ataxia, vertigo, blurry vision, sedation, weight gain, and osteoporosis [63]. Limitations to the use of carbamazepine beyond the 3–4 weeks until steady state is reached include challenging ADEs. Although carbamazepine may be beneficial in patients with chronic muscle pain [64, 65], a retrospective study of carbamazepine for chronic muscle pain reported that ADEs led to 17% of patients continuing treatment with carbamazepine for muscle pain and 44% of patients discontinuing treatment due to ADEs. The most common ADEs were elevated liver enzymes, nausea, and fatigue [64].

Carbamazepine should not be administered to patients with a history of bone marrow depression, hypersensitivity to carbamazepine or a tricyclic antidepressant [63, 66]. Carbamazepine has a boxed warning for aplastic anemia and agranulocytosis, as there is a five times greater risk compared to the general population. There is also a warning for the risk of severe cutaneous adverse reactions (SCARs), which are potentially fatal. These reactions include maculopapular exanthema (MPE), drug rash with eosinophilia and systemic symptoms (DRESS) syndrome, Stevens-Johnson Syndrome (SJS), and toxic epidermal necrolysis (TEN) [63, 67, 68]. The risk of dermatologic reactions is increased tenfold in individuals who self-identify as being of Asian descent, though such reactions have also been reported in individuals of African and Latin American descent [69, 70] Additionally, DRESS has been reported in patients with an *HLA-B*15:02* allele taking carbamazepine [71, 72]. The risk of carbamazepine-related SCARs has also been reported in patients with HLA-A*31:01 and HLA-B*15:11 [72]. Testing is recommended for at-risk populations, and carbamazepine avoidance is recommended if allele testing is positive [72, 73] (Table 19.2, CBZ/SCARs [69]). Depending on the severity of the rash, carbamazepine should be stopped, and patients can be treated with a topical or systemic corticosteroid.

Carbamazepine and valproic acid have an increased risk of suicidal ideation [74]. Suicide attempts in patients with bipolar disorders were listed as most likely with no treatment, followed by patients treated with carbamazepine, valproic acid, and lithium. Suicide deaths were associated with no treatment, followed by patients treated with valproic acid, lithium, and carbamazepine. The patients at greatest risk are those with underlying psychiatric disorders, but all patients receiving carbamazepine or valproic acid for an extended duration should be evaluated for suicidal ideation [74].

Depending on the dose, duration of therapy, and underlying reason for treatment with carbamazepine, abrupt discontinuation may lead to seizures, insomnia, dysphoria, hand fremitus, hallucinations, and severe headaches. Abrupt withdrawal should be avoided if possible, and a drug taper is suggested to minimize ADEs [75].

Carbamazepine overdose can result in death, so immediate management is imperative. This includes supportive care and activated charcoal if the airway is protected. Activated charcoal binds carbamazepine, decreases carbamazepine

Table 19.2 Carbamazepine severe cutaneous adverse reactions

Genotype	Populations at risk	Associated reaction	Clinical recommendation
HLA-B*15:02	Han Chinese, Thai, Malaysian, Filipino, Indian (2–15%)	SJS/TEN	Avoid carbamazepine; alternative therapy
HLA-A*31:01	Japanese, native American (15%); Han Chinese, Korean, European, Latin American (5–10%)	DRESS, SJS/TEN	Weigh risk vs benefit; avoid if positive
HLA-B*15:11	Korean (1.6%), Japanese (0.8%), Chinese (0.5%)	SJS/TEN	Avoid or use alternative therapy

HLA human leukocyte antigen, *SCARs* severe cutaneous adverse reactions, *SJS* Stevens-Johnson syndrome, *TEN* toxic epidermal necrolysis, *DRESS* drug reaction with eosinophilia and systemic symptoms absorption and enterohepatic drug circulation. Charcoal hemoperfusion has been beneficial, as the charcoal will compete with plasma proteins for carbamazepine binding [67]. For severe carbamazepine poisonings, extracorporeal treatment (EXTR) is suggested in cases of multiple refractory seizures life-threatening dysrhythmias, prolonged coma, or respiratory depression requiring mechanical ventilation. It is also recommended when toxicity persists, including when carbamazepine concentrations continue to increase or remain elevated. Intermittent hemodialysis is the preferred treatment and should continue until serum carbamazepine concentration is less than 10 mg/L (42.3 μmol/L) and clinical improvement is apparent [76]. If intermittent hemodialysis is not available or the patient is not able to use it, then continuous renal replacement therapy (CRRT) or intermittent hemoperfusion are extracorporeal options.

Valproate may offer a benefit to patients with chronic neuropathic pain or fibromyalgia, but it is contraindicated in patients with hepatic disease or severe hepatic dysfunction, urea cycle disorders, and mitochondrial disorders caused by DNA mutation [77]. Boxed warnings for valproate include the risk of hepatic failure, pancreatitis, and structural birth defects [77]. Additional precautions include patients with hyperammonemia (encephalopathy with combined topiramate use), urea cycle disorders, hypothermia, hypersensitivity reactions, dose-related thrombocytopenia and hematopoietic disorders, and suicidal behavior and ideation.

Common ADEs of valproic acid include CNS effects of tremor and somnolence, as well as weight gain, nausea, and rash. Specific valproate dose-related side effects include nausea, vomiting, dizziness, weight gain, reversible thrombocytopenia, and alopecia [77, 78]. Idiosyncratic reactions may also occur, including hepatotoxicity, idiopathic thrombocytopenia, and rash. Most ADEs associated with valproic acid are reported when the drug is initiated and can be managed with a dose reduction to minimize ADEs. Once the patient's ADEs have resolved, the valproic acid dose can be increased as tolerated. Patients reporting serious ADEs associated with valproic acid, such as hallucinations, hepatotoxicity, pancytopenia, or SJS/TEN, will require stoppage of the drug and supportive care. A sudden stoppage of the drug may trigger withdrawal seizures. Patients should be monitored for seizures and receive appropriate anti-seizure prophylaxis if warranted.

Pediatric patients receiving valproic acid have an increased risk of hyperammonemia. These patients may benefit from L-carnitine supplementation to lower ammonia concentrations [79]. Management of valproic acid overdose requires drug discontinuation and supportive care. This includes maintaining the patient's airway, IV fluids, and vasopressors to support blood pressure [80]. Hemodialysis or continuous renal replacement therapy can lower valproic acid serum concentrations [81, 82]. The preferred extracorporeal treatment (ECTR) for VPA poisonings is intermittent hemodialysis, but if this treatment is not available, intermittent hemoperfusion or continuous renal replacement therapy (CRRT) are suggested options. The Extracorporeal Treatments in Poisonings Workgroup (EXTRIP) recommends extracorporeal treatment (ECTR) if any of the following are present: VPA concentrations >1300 mg/L (9000 μmol/L), shock, or cerebral edema. The workgroup suggests initiating ECTR if any of the following are present: VPA concentrations >900 mg/L (6250 μmol/L), coma or respiratory depression requiring mechanical ventilation is present, acute hyperammonemia is present, or pH is <7.10 [82]. Cessation of EXTR is suggested when clinical improvement is apparent or VPA serum concentration is between 50 and 100 mg/L (350–700 μmol/L). If the patient has ingested an extended-release formulation, stopping dialytic therapy too soon can cause drug concentration rebound, and the patient may begin to exhibit drug toxicity signs and symptoms again. For these cases, restarting the dialytic therapy promptly is recommended [81, 82].

Administration of a carbapenem antimicrobial agent may be an option for patients with severe valproic acid overdose because of the significant drug-drug interaction, which lowers valproic acid concentrations [83]. The evidence is limited to case reports, but this may be an option for patients who do not respond to supportive care and renal replacement therapy.

Carbamazepine (CBZ) and valproic acid (VPA) have been linked to hyponatremia, although it is more common with CBZ. The highest-risk patients include the elderly or those taking a selective serotonin reuptake inhibitor (SSRI) concurrently. Carbamazepine-induced hyponatremia is usually associated with the syndrome of inappropriate antidiuretic hormone (SIADH) and should be managed conservatively if the patient has no symptoms [84]. Treatment options involve stopping carbamazepine and starting levetiracetam for seizures. If sodium regulation remains difficult, adding lacosamide as an additional anti-seizure medication may help stabilize serum sodium levels [84]. Correction of hyponatremia may require acute hospitalization if severe symptoms are present.

Idiosyncratic rashes can occur in patients taking CBZ or VPA; generally, the onset is within 2–8 days of initiation or dose increase [63, 77]. Any discovery of a rash with initiation of therapy, dose change, or throughout therapy warrants extreme caution and should result in acute evaluation to rule out SJS/TENs. Routine monitoring of basic metabolic parameters is recommended to reduce the risk of an electrolyte imbalance. Additionally, using vitamin D and calcium supplementation is prudent to prevent osteoporosis and fractures. Monitoring should include baseline complete blood counts and complete metabolic panels, then repeat every 3 months and annually, as well as medication levels. Signs and symptoms of CNS adverse reactions, such as dizziness, gait disturbance, intolerable or excessive somnolence, cognitive changes, and visual changes, should be evaluated and managed promptly. Management is likely dependent on the onset of symptoms, duration, laboratory workup, and medication blood concentrations, as well as other patient-specific variables such as age and past medical history.

Carbamazepine and valproate can cause acute toxicity [63, 77]. Harm with these medications is often derived from epilepsy research but remains relevant in the context of pain management. Valproic acid is associated with rare but serious adverse reactions, including hemorrhagic pancreatitis, coagulopathy, bone marrow suppression, encephalopathy, and hepatotoxicity. Teratogenicity has also been documented with valproate [85] (Table 19.3).

Skeletal Muscle Relaxants

Skeletal muscle relaxants are frequently prescribed for lower back pain as an alternative to opioids [86]. These agents are categorized as antispasmodics, nonbenzodiazepine antispasmodics, benzodiazepines, and miscellaneous.

The use of skeletal muscle relaxants should be avoided in elderly patients, given poor tolerance of anticholinergic adverse reactions, sedation, and increased risk of falls and fractures. (BEERS 2023) The 2023 American Geriatrics Society BEERs criteria update emphasizes caution when prescribing these medications to elderly patients [5]. Antispasticity muscle relaxants, such as baclofen and tizanidine, may be safe in older adults; however, substantial adverse reactions may still occur.

Table 19.3 Clinical pearls for overdose scenarios

Scenario	Key intervention
Acetaminophen overdose	NAC within 8–10 h most effective
NSAID overdose	Supportive only; dialysis ineffective
Lidocaine systemic toxicity	Stop drug + IV lipid emulsion
Gabapentinoid withdrawal	Taper slowly; consider benzos if severe
Carbamazepine overdose	Activated charcoal; hemodialysis if severe
Valproate overdose	Hemodialysis if VPA >900–1300 mg/L; consider L-carnitine
Baclofen withdrawal	Reinitiate baclofen; taper cautiously
Clonidine toxicity	Supportive; atropine for bradycardia
CCB overdose	High-dose insulin + IV calcium
Serotonin syndrome	Stop agent; cyproheptadine if moderate/severe

IV intravenous, *NAC* N-acetylcysteine, *NSAID* nonsteroidal anti-inflammatory drug, *VPA* valproic acid, *CCB* calcium channel blocker

Baclofen

Baclofen is used to treat muscle spasticity and musculoskeletal pain [86]. It is a gamma-aminobutyric acid (GABA-B) receptor agonist. Baclofen acts on the pre- and postsynaptic neurons in the central and peripheral nervous system by inhibiting synaptic reflexes to relax spasms [86, 87]. The adverse effects of drowsiness and dizziness are thought to be caused by GABA-B effects on the CNS and sympathetic nervous system [88]. Oral administration of baclofen is not reported to cross the blood-brain barrier effectively; however, intrathecal administration of baclofen achieves therapeutic cerebral fluid concentrations, making it suitable for treatments such as spasticity [86, 88].

In 2024, data from an Australian registry reported 102 deaths related to oral baclofen over a 2-year period, with 45.1% listed as unintentional or accidental [89]. There is variability in the presentation of baclofen toxicity as it can affect the cardiovascular, gastrointestinal, musculoskeletal, and neurological systems. A patient presenting with hypotonia, flaccid paralysis, hallucinations, or seizures may be experiencing baclofen toxicity [88, 90]. Treatment of toxicity is drug cessation and circulatory and respiratory supportive care. Baclofen clearance is dependent on kidney function, which may require patients with diminished kidney function to receive hemodialysis to decrease plasma concentrations [87]. Benzodiazepine treatment is recommended for baclofen toxicity-related seizures if the patient does not have baclofen-related metabolic encephalopathy. If metabolic encephalopathy is a concern, benzodiazepines should be used with caution and close monitoring. For the oral formulation, activated charcoal and gastric lavage may be beneficial in children; however, they have not shown a clear benefit in adults [88, 90]. Additionally, extracorporeal treatment (ECTR) is not recommended for baclofen toxicity unless the patient has kidney impairment and is in a coma or receiving mechanical ventilation. If ECTR is warranted, intermittent hemodialysis is recommended over other ECTR modalities [91].

Baclofen withdrawal syndrome is a complication of abruptly stopping baclofen or a significant dose reduction. This syndrome can progress rapidly and has a high risk of morbidity and mortality. Intrathecal baclofen withdrawal carries a higher risk of death than oral, but this syndrome has been reported in patients receiving either formulation [92]. The treatment is to reinitiate baclofen and slowly titrate the dose until withdrawal symptoms are manageable or cease. Additionally, patients will need supportive therapy and frequent monitoring.

Carisoprodol

Although the mechanism for carisoprodol's role in the relief of musculoskeletal pain is not fully understood, it is described as a centrally acting muscle relaxant that does not have a direct effect on skeletal muscle [93]. Carisoprodol's mechanism is partially attributed to its main active metabolite, meprobamate, which works at the GABA receptors. Carisoprodol is more lipophilic than meprobamate and will enter the central nervous system [93, 94]. Meprobamate has an extended half-life, and its effect on the GABA receptors is similar to the effects of benzodiazepines, which increase sedation and reduce anxiety. The recommended duration of treatment with carisoprodol is 3 weeks due to its high potential for abuse [95]. Prolonged use of carisoprodol can result in physical dependence similar to barbiturates, and withdrawal symptoms can mimic alcohol withdrawal [95].

Carisoprodol's adverse effects are CNS-related and include dizziness, headache, and drowsiness. Signs and symptoms of carisoprodol toxicity or overdose include ataxia, headaches, hallucinations, respiratory depression, and death. There is a risk of serotonin syndrome, which can manifest as agitation, confusion, fever, and tachycardia. Carisoprodol can accumulate in cardiac tissue, which increases the risk of cardiotoxicity [96, 97]. An examination of hypotension from carisoprodol self-poisoning reported a decrease in left ventricular function and cardiac index and an increase in the diameter of the vena cava. Patients with hypotension from carisoprodol required inotropic drugs and received mechanical ventilation for a longer duration [98].

Carisoprodol overdose requires supportive care. If the ingestion is within 1–2 h, activated charcoal and gastric lavage may decrease absorption of carisoprodol [94]. If the patient is identified several hours after ingestion, administration of flumazenil may be beneficial in reversing the effects of meprobamate at the GABA A receptor. Roberge RJ et al published a case report of a female patient who presented with a Glasgow Coma Score of 9 and a medication history including carisoprodol, clonidine, and buspirone [99]. The patient received intravenous (IV) naloxone 2 mg twice with no improvement. Her drug screen was positive for carisoprodol; serum concentrations for carisoprodol were 7.4 mcg/mL and for heprobamate 30.7 mcg/mL. Flumazenil 0.2 mg was administered intravenously over 2 min, 10 min after the last naloxone dose, and the patient became more alert within 2 min. After the second flumazenil dose was administered, all signs of intoxication were reversed [99]. Carisoprodol can accumulate in patients with kidney impairment, and it is easily removed during hemodialysis and peritoneal dialysis. Renal replacement therapy may provide an option for enhancing the clearance of carisoprodol for patients with decreased kidney clearance or prolonged overdose-related adverse effects [94].

Chlorzoxazone

Chlorzoxazone is a centrally acting muscle relaxant used for the short-term treatment of muscle pain and stiffness and may play a role in the treatment of spinocerebellar ataxia for its activation of calcium-activated potassium channels [100]. Chlorzoxazone may cause central nervous system depression, resulting in drowsiness, sedation, impairment of physical and mental abilities, and an increased fall risk in the elderly. There are reports of rare liver toxicity, which may be reversible on cessation of the chlorzoxazone [101, 102]. There is limited evidence on the treatment of chlorzoxazone overdose or toxicity. A case report described the use of flumazenil to reverse a coma induced by chlorzoxazone. The patient had a history of chronic back pain, seizures, and alcohol abuse for which he received disulfiram, diazepam, phenobarbital, and chlorzoxazone. After the patient received two doses of naloxone and awoke briefly after the second dose of naloxone, they became comatose again. There was a high suspicion of benzodiazepine overdose; therefore, flumazenil was administered. After the administration of flumazenil (0.10 mg), the patient rapidly awoke but was confused and groaning, then rapidly became comatose. Approximately 30 min after the first dose (approximately 5 h after chlorzoxazone ingestion), a second dose of flumazenil (0.25 mg) was administered, and the patient awoke without confusion. The patient remained awake and was able to answer questions [103].

Cyclobenzaprine

Cyclobenzaprine is a centrally acting skeletal muscle relaxant that is pharmacologically related to tricyclic antidepressants and may reduce muscle hyperactivity [104]. The onset of action for the immediate-release formulation is approximately 60 min, with a duration of 12–24 h. Cyclobenzaprine is hepatically metabolized via CYP 3A4, 1A2, and 2D6 and may undergo enterohepatic recirculation. It is excreted through the urine as glucuronide metabolites and in the feces as the unchanged drug [104].

Cyclobenzaprine should be used cautiously in elderly patients or those with mild liver impairment, and avoid use in patients with moderate to-severe liver impairment. A twofold increase in the steady-state concentration was reported in patients with mild liver impairment [105]. Common adverse effects of cyclobenzaprine include dry mucous membranes, dizziness, confusion, and somnolence. The adverse effects of xerostomia, confusion, mydriasis, ileus, urinary retention, hallucinations, and tachycardia are attributed to the drug's antagonizing effect on the muscarinic receptors, similar to tricyclic antidepressants.

Tachycardia has been attributed to vasodilation at the alpha-1 adrenergic receptor. Cyclobenzaprine is contraindicated in patients with a history of electrical conduction abnormalities (heart block, arrhythmias), patients recovering from a myocardial infarction or hyperthyroidism, or those taking a monoamine oxidase inhibitors (MAOI) [104–107].

Cyclobenzaprine should be avoided with serotonergic drugs such as duloxetine or phenelzine [104]. A report of two cases described serotonin syndrome in patients taking cyclobenzaprine with either duloxetine or phenelzine within hours of adding cyclobenzaprine to their medication regimen. The patient taking phenelzine experienced tremors, tachycardia, diaphoresis, and fever after three doses of cyclobenzaprine. Initially, the patient was alert and oriented but experienced delusions, hallucinations, and multifocal myoclonus. Cyclobenzaprine, opioids, and phenelzine were stopped. Haloperidol was initiated to help with agitation, but the haloperidol had a limited effect. After 3 days, the patient's serotonin syndrome subsided [108].

An overdose of cyclobenzaprine generally results in drowsiness and tachycardia. Rare but serious effects have been reported to cause cardiac arrest, cardiac dysrhythmia, hypotension, seizure, and neuroleptic malignant syndrome. For cases of suspected cyclobenzaprine toxicity, an electrocardiogram showing changes in the QRS duration or axis may aid in diagnosis. Ingestions of less than 100 mg can be treated with GI decontamination with activated charcoal [109]. A review of Poison Control data of adults and children who ingested cyclobenzaprine found that there were no seizures or deaths associated with the ingestions. The most frequent adverse effects were lethargy, sinus tachycardia, and agitation. The mean onset of symptoms was 4 h after ingestion, and the duration of adverse effects ranged from 2 to 36 h. Patients presenting with symptoms had ingested a mean dose of 184 mg (±165) and were generally treated with GI decontamination and supportive care. A minority of patients may require mechanical ventilation, dopamine, fluids, and sedation with serious toxicity from hypotension and respiratory depression. For children, serious toxicity was not seen in doses less than 100 mg [109].

Metaxalone

Metaxalone is a skeletal muscle relaxant that has been used for over 60 years to relieve pain associated with musculoskeletal issues [110]. Metaxalone's mechanism does not directly affect the contractility of striated muscle, nerve fiber, or the motor end plate, but its effects may be associated with depression of the nervous system [110].

The adverse effects of metaxalone are related to CNS depression and impairment of physical and mental abilities and can increase the risk of falls in the elderly [111]. The common adverse effects are dizziness, drowsiness, fatigue, headache, irritability, and nervousness. An examination of 142 cases reported to a Texas Poison Control Center identified lethargy as the most common adverse effect associated with doses greater than 2400 mg (mean dose, 7732.8 mg; range, 400–44,000 mg). Other findings include tachycardia, hypertension, muscle rigidity, seizure, mydriasis, diaphoresis, hyperthermia, and coma [112]. The treatments for metaxalone overdose in this report included activated charcoal, cathartic agents, drinking fluids, and IV fluids.

There is a rare, potentially life-threatening adverse effect of metaxalone that may be related to high doses and/or the concomitant use of serotonergic agents, including selective serotonin reuptake inhibitors, serotonin and norepinephrine reuptake inhibitors, tricyclic antidepressants, triptans, 5-HT_3 receptor antagonists, and monoamine oxidase inhibitors. Serotonin syndrome has been reported with metaxalone overdose [113] and in patients taking a combination of high-dose metaxalone with agents such as tramadol or paroxetine. Adverse effects of metaxalone can overlap with serotonin syndrome. Clinicians should be aware of the signs and symptoms and the risk of morbidity and mortality.

Methocarbamol

Methocarbamol is a centrally acting skeletal muscle relaxant used as an adjunctive treatment for muscle spasm and acute pain associated with musculoskeletal conditions. The adverse effects of methocarbamol are related to its effects on the CNS. These effects include confusion, dizziness, drowsiness, and sedation, which can impair physical and mental abilities and increase the risk of falls and fractures [114]. Concurrent use of alcohol or other CNS depressants increases the risk of impairment and injury [114, 115]. The commonly reported effects associated with overdose were drowsiness, tachycardia, vomiting, and slurred speech. Methocarbamol overdose requires supportive therapy, which includes intravenous fluids and gastric lavage with activated charcoal. Patients may also experience a change in the color of their urine with intoxication [116].

Orphenadrine

Orphenadrine is an anticholinergic agent prescribed as a skeletal muscle relaxant for skeletal muscle spasms or pain due to its action on the central nervous system and peripheral nervous system. Orphenadrine is usually prescribed with an NSAID or APAP. Orphenadrine is a derivative of diphenhydramine, and the main adverse effects are related to its anticholinergic properties, which include drowsiness, dizziness, dry mouth, and hallucinations. At therapeutic doses, patients can experience mild anticholinergic adverse effects such as drowsiness, dry mouth, and euphoria [117].

Non-sustained ventricular tachycardia was reported in a case of a patient with a history of paroxysmal atrial fibrillation taking propafenone. Orphenadrine citrate (35 mg) and paracetamol (450 mg) had been initiated twice daily for musculoskeletal pain. The patient experienced severe palpitations after 5 days of treatment. A 24-hour Holter recording revealed short-lasting atrial fibrillation and episodes of non-sustained ventricular tachycardia. The orphenadrine citrate and paracetamol were stopped, and within 1 week, the patient's heart rhythm and rate normalized [118].

The overdose signs and symptoms are related to the anticholinergic effect of orphenadrine and lead to anticholinergic syndrome. Generally, patients can be treated with supportive care until the drug's effect wanes. Physostigmine can be administered to relieve the anticholinergic effects of restlessness and hallucinations related to orphenadrine overdose [119]. Patients need to be monitored for the physostigmine adverse effects, including convulsions, bradycardia, and hypersalivation. Clinicians must be aware that the duration of action of physostigmine is approximately 60 min, and patients can relapse [120].

Physostigmine has also been used to reverse tachycardia in a pediatric patient who had accidentally ingested an unknown quantity of orphenadrine [119]. The patient was 3 years old, weighed 13 kg, and presented with confusion, seizure-like movements, and a heart rate of 160 bpm. The patient experienced two tonic-clonic seizures and was intubated and given two doses of lorazepam with no response, followed by two doses of diazepam, resulting in cessation of the seizure. The patient had a wide complex tachycardia for 20 min, for which physostigmine IV 0.02 mg/kg, two doses, was administered over 10 min. The patient converted to sinus tachycardia, which was sustained for 5 h. After 5 h, the patient's rhythm returned to wide complex tachycardia, and an additional dose of physostigmine was given [119].

Tizanidine

Tizanidine is a centrally acting alpha-2 receptor agonist that is approved for the management of muscle spasticity. This drug has several uses, which range from spasticity related to spinal cord injury or multiple sclerosis to migraine headaches and insomnia [121, 122].

Adverse effects include hepatotoxicity, hypotension, sedation, and withdrawal syndrome. Hypotension and sedation are related to the drug's pharmacologic action as an alpha-2 receptor agonist [121]. Hypotension can be dose-related and occur within 30 min, lasting up to 6 h, and be exacerbated by higher doses and/or a fast titration of tizanidine. Sedation may be dose-related and can occur within 60 min of ingestion. Sedation can be exacerbated by alcohol, CNS depressants, and concomitant use of CYP1A2 inhibitors such as ciprofloxacin and fluvoxamine, which can increase tizanidine serum concentrations by 10- and 33-fold, respectively [121]. Abrupt discontinuation of tizanidine can result in withdrawal syndrome, which can be life-threatening and include dysthermia, hallucinations, hypertension, nausea, tremor, tachycardia, increased spasticity, and potentially coma [122–124]. The effects of hypersecretion of catecholamines can be seen within 12–24 h after drug cessation. This reaction is generally seen in patients taking a high dose ($\geq$16 mg/day) or with prolonged use ($\geq$9 weeks). Tizanidine withdrawal can be managed with acetaminophen for hyperthermia, benzodiazepines for agitation and restlessness, beta-blockers for blood pressure, and mirtazapine and metoclopramide as needed, followed by reintroduction of tizanidine at a low dose with a planned dosing taper [123, 124].

Tizanidine overdose is associated with dizziness, depression, hypotension, and loss of consciousness, but bradycardia can occur from inhibition of presynaptic neurotransmitter release. For patients with bradycardia and hypotension, a recent case report found that cardiac pacing with initial vasopressor support of norepinephrine and adrenaline (epinephrine) helped to stabilize a 75-year-old female with suspected tizanidine overdose. Once stabilized, vasopressor support was changed to dopamine until the tizanidine effects were weaned off [125]. Overall, care for tizanidine overdose is supportive care with monitoring for withdrawal syndrome.

Antihypertensive Medications

Clonidine

Clonidine is a centrally acting alpha2 adrenergic agonist, which is used to treat hypertension and can be used to manage pain, intensive care sedation when transitioning from dexmedetomidine, opioid withdrawal, and reducing vasomotor symptoms. Clonidine can cause hypotension, dizziness, sedation, and somnolence. Some patients may experience irritability, aggressive behaviors, emotional disturbances, and nightmares or night terrors [126]. Clonidine has an orphan drug designation for use in epidurals with opioids for cancer pain [127]. Clonidine's toxicity in children is well-established, and the cause ranges from accidental ingestion to intentional overdose. It is listed as a dangerous drug, but clonidine is prescribed for children with behavioral disorders [127].

Clonidine's toxicity is attributed to its ability to reduce sympathetic outflow from the central nervous system, resulting in decreased peripheral and renal vascular resistance, blood pressure, and heart rate. Patients can experience hypotonia and muscle flaccidity due to the suppression of interneuron excitation in the spinal cord by excitatory amino acids, such as glutamate. Symptoms of clonidine toxicity may mimic those of opioids, with miosis and lethargy, but clonidine's cardiovascular effects are more severe. Patients with suspected clonidine toxicity will need to be evaluated for life-threatening airway, breathing, and circulatory complications. The most serious complications are hypotension, bradycardia, and CNS depression [128]. Patients may have delayed hemodynamic instability, so close monitoring is required. For patients who present with hypertension, avoid aggressively treating their blood pressure, as the blood pressure can quickly decrease, resulting in hypotension. If treatment for hypertension is necessary, use a low dose of a short-acting agent. Gastric lavage or a single dose of activated charcoal may be helpful if the patient presents within 1 h of ingestion. Gastric lavage is not routinely recommended due to its limited benefits and risk of complications. If the patient has ingested a transdermal patch, activated charcoal or whole bowel irrigation has been reported to eliminate the ingested patch [129].

No specific antidote exists for an overdose of clonidine. Administration of naloxone has not demonstrated clear evidence for successfully reversing clonidine's CNS depression, although it could be beneficial in pediatric ingestions. A naloxone dose has not been established for clonidine toxicity, but reports of naloxone 10 mg being administered without adverse effects exist and may be beneficial in pediatric patients with minimal response [130, 131].

For the treatment of bradycardia, atropine can be administered. Treatments for hypotension are dependent on the patient's response to the treatment with intravenous fluids, Trendelenburg positioning, and vasopressors. Patients who experience seizures should be treated with diazepam, lorazepam, or intramuscular or intranasal midazolam if IV access is not established. If additional agents are required, phenobarbital may be an option [128].

Calcium Channel Blockers

The inhibition of calcium channels by antagonism of the slow calcium channels may play a role in reducing pain. The transfer of calcium from the blood to the muscle is partially blocked by these agents, resulting in peripheral vasodilation and a decrease in blood pressure. Calcium channel antagonists target the L-type voltage-gated calcium channels in the heart, vascular smooth muscle, and the pancreas. This drug class, often referred to as calcium channel blockers (CCBs), is subdivided into two categories based on their primary effects: dihydropyridine and non-dihydropyridine [132–135]. The non-dihydropyridine CCBs (verapamil and diltiazem) reduce cardiac contractility through their effects on the sinoatrial (SA) and atrioventricular (AV) nodes and are associated with bradycardia and bradyarrhythmia. Diltiazem (a benzothiazepine), and verapamil (a phenylalkylamine,) are commonly prescribed for angina, atrial fibrillation or flutter rate control, hypertension, and tachycardia [132]. Verapamil is also prescribed for cluster headaches and migraine prevention [133]. Although both drugs suppress cardiac contractility, SA nodal automaticity, and AV conduction, verapamil has a stronger affinity for vascular smooth muscle, resulting in potent vasodilation. Diltiazem has a lesser vasodilator effect but exerts a stronger effect on chronicity. Diltiazem and verapamil should be avoided in patients who are also receiving a beta-blocker. have heart failure with reduced ejection fraction, or those with sinoatrial node dysfunction, or second- or third-degree AV block, unless the patient has a functioning pacemaker in place [132, 133].

Amlodipine, nifedipine, and nimodipine are dihydropyridine CCBs that exert their pharmacologic action on vascular smooth muscle and myocardium during depolarization. These actions relax the coronary vascular smooth muscle, leading to coronary vasodilation. These agents may be beneficial for patients with vasospastic angina, as an increase in myocardial oxygen delivery can help alleviate angina-related symptoms. Dihydropyridine CCBs reduce peripheral vascular resistance, which lowers arterial blood pressure and can help reduce Raynaud phenomenon attacks. As effective vasodilators, dihydropyridines will have a more pronounced effect on blood pressure with less impact on cardiac rate and myocardial contractility [134–136].

Bradycardia and/or hypotension are the primary cardiac-related symptoms of CCB overdose. Verapamil is associated with AV node block [137]. Hyperglycemia can be observed with CCB overdose from a reduction in pancreatic insulin secretion. Hypotension and bradycardia can progress to cardiogenic shock. Hypotension is caused by peripheral vasodilation and can be refractory to treatment, resulting in death. Other symptoms include confusion, metabolic acidosis, nausea, vomiting, and stupor. The toxicity related to CCB overdose can be more severe in patients who also take digoxin or a beta-adrenergic antagonist [136, 137].

The treatment of a CCB overdose relies on supportive care and reversal of hypotension and bradycardia. If a patient presents within 1 h of ingestion, single-dose activated charcoal or gastric lavage may be effective if the patient does not have a contraindication [138]. For a patient presenting more than 1 h after ingestion or who has ingested an extended-release formulation, an option is whole bowel irrigation with polyethylene glycol. If the patient is unable to drink the solution, it can be administered through a nasogastric tube. Ipecac and cathartics have not been shown to be effective for CCB overdose [139, 140].

A symptomatic patient with myocardial dysfunction will need supportive care and should receive IV calcium and insulin.. If the patient does not have myocardial dysfunction, treatment with IV fluids, calcium, and vasopressors is recommended [139, 140]. Fluids must be used with caution to avoid fluid overload in patients with inotropic failure. Calcium gluconate or chloride can be administered, but the amount needs to be large enough to create a concentration gradient to overcome the calcium channel blockade from the overdose. Serum ionized calcium concentrations may need to be 1.5–2 times the upper limit of normal to improve cardiac function. If a patient requires a third IV calcium bolus, an ionized calcium concentration needs to be checked after the third bolus. Patients who are in shock should receive norepinephrine or epinephrine, with norepinephrine preferred for vasodilatory shock. For cardiogenic shock, dobutamine or epinephrine may be initiated, and for symptomatic bradycardia, atropine should be considered as a first-line therapy [139, 140]. Unstable bradycardia or AV block may require the use of a pacemaker.

Calcium channel blockers are lipophilic and have a large volume of distribution (>2 liters/kg), which substantially limits the effectiveness of urine alkalinization and hemodialysis [141]. Due to the lipophilicity of CCBs, lipid emulsion therapy may be an option for patients who are refractory to standard treatments for CCB overdose. Lipid emulsion therapy has shown efficacy in adults and children, but it must be used with close monitoring, as this treatment can cause hypertriglyceridemia, pancreatitis, and acute kidney and lung injury [142, 143].

Anesthetics

Ketamine

Ketamine has multiple uses due to its antidepressant, dissociative, and general anesthetic properties [144, 145]. Adverse effects include cardiac effects, which range from increased blood pressure and heart rate to cardiac arrhythmia and cardiac decompensation. Ketamine is associated with drug dependence and drug tolerance, and sudden withdrawal may result in withdrawal syndrome. Symptoms of ketamine withdrawal syndrome include sweating, palpitations, delusions, and hallucinations, which can persist from 3 days up to 2 weeks. The mechanism of tolerance may be due to autoinduction of its metabolism, while dependence may be related to N-methyl-D-aspartate (NMDA) glutamate receptor blockade, which can produce alcohol-like and opioid effects [146]. Ketamine intoxication is dose-dependent, and the effects range from altered mental status and perceptions to psychological effects that include out-of-body experiences, hallucinations, and tactile distortions. Patients with toxicities associated with higher doses may have cardiovascular effects tachycardia, hypertension, palpitations, respiratory depression, extended sedation, and coma. Symptoms with parenteral formulation can begin within minutes and last up to 2 h, but the oral formulation can last 4–8 h.

There is no antidote for a ketamine overdose or toxicity. Treatment generally requires supportive care to correct and stabilize the airway, breathing, and circulation [147]. If the patient presents within 1 h of ingestion, gastric lavage may be beneficial, but overall, it is not recommended because of its limited effectiveness with a ketamine overdose. A single dose of activated charcoal may be beneficial if the patient presents within 1 h of ingestion, but it is contraindicated in patients with diminished consciousness unless they have airway protection [148]. Unfortunately, ketamine-related deaths have increased. An examination of Poison Control data from 2019 to 2023 identified 107 deaths, with approximately 82% of those deaths associated with polysubstance abuse, including illegally manufactured fentanyl, methamphetamine, and cocaine [149]. Clinicians may need to monitor and treat for multiple toxicities if ketamine toxicity is suspected.

Serotonin-Norepinephrine Reuptake Inhibitors and Tricyclic Antidepressants

Several medications commonly classified as antidepressants have a growing body of evidence in support of their use as co-analgesics or adjuvants [150]. Common antidepressant medications that have greater evidence include serotonin-norepinephrine reuptake inhibitors (SNRIs) such as duloxetine and venlafaxine [151–153], and tricyclic antidepressants (TCAs), including amitriptyline, nortriptyline, doxepin, and desipramine, among others. Many of these medications are also included in clinical guidelines for pain, particularly pain of neuropathic origins and fibromyalgia [154, 155]. Selective serotonin reuptake inhibitors are ineffective for chronic pain and will not be covered in this chapter.

Adverse drug effects can be expected across all SNRI and TCA agents given similar mechanisms of action. Most of the adverse effects are believed to be related to the ability of the drugs to block serotonin reuptake. Common side effects include acute anxiety, sleep disturbances (i.e., insomnia or sedation), headaches, nausea, weight gain, and sexual dysfunction (e.g., decreased libido) [156]. Less common side effects include bleeding events, hyponatremia, serotonin syndrome, and increased suicidality. Many of these ADEs are transient and may improve after a few weeks of routine therapy; however, some others, such as sexual adverse reactions, may not improve with time. Additionally, most of these reactions are rate-limiting and dose-dependent, meaning some may improve upon dose reduction [157].

Serotonin-Norepinephrine Reuptake Inhibitors

Serotonin-norepinephrine reuptake inhibitors have warnings or precautions for causing activation of mania/hypomania, abnormal bleeding, angle closure glaucoma, clinical worsening, suicidal risk, discontinuation syndrome, elevations in blood pressure, hyponatremia, serotonin syndrome, and seizures [158].

An increase in anticholinergic adverse effects, such as orthostatic hypotension and sedative effects, has been reported in older adults, and close monitoring is prudent [159]. Norepinephrine is known to stimulate sweat glands and may be a contributing factor to the development of hyperhidrosis reactions with these medications [160]. The risk of hyperhidrosis is approximately 10–12% with SNRIs, and treatments are discussed later in this chapter [161, 162].

Patients may experience eye dryness with SNRI usage due to a decrease in eye wetness. Clinicians should consider advising patients to use over-the-counter eye drops for dry eyes [163, 164].

The most common side effect documented in pediatric patients taking an SNRI is nausea. [165] Sleep disturbances such as insomnia have also been reported more commonly in pediatric patients taking SNRIs. Nausea can resolve with continued use, but slow dose titration may minimize nausea. If an over-the-counter anti-nausea medication is used, separate the administration timing by administering calcium carbonate or famotidine at least 30 min before administering the SNRI.

Hyponatremia linked to SNRIs has been attributed to changes in antidiuretic hormone secretion. A systematic review of the literature found that SNRIs accounted for 6.13% of hyponatremia cases, with venlafaxine posing the highest risk and duloxetine the lowest [166]. Treatment for hyponatremia should follow conservative management for chronic hyponatremia unless the patient is at high risk of seizure or coma [167]. Following correction, re-evaluation of the medication dose, dose reduction, or discontinuation of therapy may be appropriate to prevent recurrence [168].

The metabolic status of patients can be affected by venlafaxine and desvenlafaxine. Chronic usage can elevate cholesterol and triglycerides and lower HDL. Patients with SNRI-induced hyperlipidemia could be switched to another agent or initiate treatment based on the most recent guideline on the management of blood cholesterol [169]. Interstitial lung disease and eosinophilic pneumonia are rare but serious adverse reactions that have been documented with venlafaxine and desvenlafaxine. Treatment with the SNRI needs to be discontinued; patients will need to be referred to a pulmonary specialist for evaluation and a treatment plan, which can include corticosteroids, immunotherapy, antifibrotic therapy, and bronchodilators [151, 153].

Duloxetine has a warning of hepatotoxicity, orthostatic hypotension, falls and syncope, severe skin reactions, urinary hesitancy and retention, and sexual dysfunction. It also has a warning against use in patients with concomitant illnesses such as diabetes [152].

Duloxetine is associated with nausea and weight loss, which may limit its use. Nausea generally resolves with continued treatment, but proton pump inhibitors may be beneficial as a short-term therapy [170]. Administration of lansoprazole 30 mg before breakfast, followed by duloxetine 30 mg 2 hours after breakfast, was evaluated to determine whether lansoprazole improves symptom relief in patients requiring duloxetine therapy. There was an improvement in gastroesophageal reflux-related symptoms, including heartburn and nighttime awakening from heartburn, for patients receiving lansoprazole and duloxetine [171].

Hepatotoxicity, including severe elevations of liver enzymes (10× upper limit of normal), hepatitis, and jaundice, is a rare but serious reaction that has been documented with duloxetine that requires discontinuation of treatment. Onset typically occurs within 2 months of initiation. Patients with a history of preexisting chronic liver disease or alcohol misuse are at higher risk [172]. A case series of duloxetine-induced liver injury reported that liver enzymes normalized within a few weeks to months after duloxetine was stopped [173].

Urinary hesitation is another reaction that may occur with an SNRI and require dose reduction or switching to a medication with less noradrenergic activity. Duloxetine combined with tolterodine has been investigated for the treatment of mixed urinary incontinence (MUI). The combination therapy improved MUI symptoms and quality of life. The ADEs in this study were reported as constipation, dizziness, nausea, and dry mouth [174]. Venlafaxine-induced urinary incontinence (UI) has been reported in the literature. A recent case describes a patient with no previous history of UI who developed UI after an increase in the daily dose from 75 mg to 112.5 mg. After lowering the daily dose to 75 mg, the patient's UI symptoms ceased. Patients should be evaluated for dose reduction before the addition of a treatment for UI, since these agents work on muscarinic receptors and can increase ADEs [175].

Cardiovascular side effects are also common with both drugs. Increases in blood pressure, tachycardia, and/or orthostatic hypotensive reactions are more common with SNRIs and may require dose reduction or discontinuation [176]. Anticholinergic effects are of greater concern with TCAs, particularly with agents that exert more anticholinergic activity. Common presentations include cognitive changes or delirium, urinary retention, blurry vision, dry mouth, and constipation. Duplicate therapy within the same class should be avoided, given the lack of efficacy and safety at this time [177–179].

Serotonin syndrome, or serotonin toxicity, can be life-threatening and may occur with an SNRIs or TCAs alone or in combination with other medications with serotonergic activity. The risk appears to be highest when multiple serotonergic agents are used concomitantly. This condition presents with mental status changes or agitation, autonomic hyperactivity (e.g., hypertension, elevated heart rate, diaphoresis), and neuromuscular abnormalities such as hyperreflexia, clonus, and tremor [180]. Additional signs may include increased body temperature and gastrointestinal distress. Mild cases can be successfully managed by stopping the serotonergic agent(s) and providing supportive care. Moderate cases may require greater supportive care due to more pronounced autonomic instability and may necessitate administration of a 5-HT2A antagonist like cyproheptadine. Severe cases can be managed similarly but may also need intubation, neuromuscular paralysis, and sedation.

Discontinuation syndrome may also occur when SNRI or TCA therapy is suddenly stopped. This may result in flu-like symptoms, insomnia, nausea, irritability, sadness, headache, electric shock-like sensations, dizziness, and acute anxiety [181, 182]. Agents with shorter half-lives, such as venlafaxine, have a higher risk of causing this syndrome. The rapid reintroduction of stopped medication at the original dosage has the most documented success in alleviating acute symptoms. Tapering gradually or more slowly can reduce the likelihood of recurrence of these effects if a medication switch is warranted [181, 182].

SNRI overdose is rarely fatal; however, reduced consciousness, gastrointestinal upset, increased heart rate, and seizures may commonly occur. Case reports have been made of fatalities with venlafaxine overdose [183–185]. Aggressive supportive care is recommended [186]. Patients with venlafaxine overdose are at risk of seizure and cardiac collapse and may require extracorporeal life support (ECLS) in addition to gastrointestinal decontamination and supportive care such as intubation, IV fluids, and continuous renal replacement therapy (CRRT). Several case reports describe the use of ECLS, particularly for cases of large venlafaxine ingestions or ingestions greater than 8–10 grams [187, 188].

A patient requiring ECLS for cardiovascular collapse from a life-threatening venlafaxine overdose received ECLS with a hemadsorption device, the CytoSorb® filter. This device enhanced the removal of venlafaxine in addition to supportive care and treatments with gastric lavage and active charcoal. The quick removal of toxic venlafaxine concentrations aided in the neurological survival of this patient [189].

Delayed-onset cardiac and neurologic toxicities following overdose of bupropion and venlafaxine are well described. Such toxicity appears to be due to slow gut absorption from sustained release (SR) or extended-release (XR) formulations. For this reason, it is advisable to admit patients with such ingestions for a longer observation period (24 h is generally sufficient) with cardiac monitoring, especially if the formulation of the ingested drug is unknown. These patients typically need significant resources because serious toxicity (e.g., seizures, dysrhythmias) frequently occurs, and they are often admitted to intensive care units [190].

Early on in SNRI therapy, increased weight loss may happen in adolescents; however, the risk appears to decline with prolonged use [191, 192]. Weight gain may commonly occur in pediatric patients taking TCAs and may be more prevalent than weight changes with SNRI therapy. [193, 194] The pharmacologic mechanisms behind this phenomenon are unclear. Dry mouth is more commonly reported in pediatric patients undergoing TCA therapy [195]. Additional monitoring is warranted with both TCAs and SNRIs when used in pediatric patients for pain management. Pediatric patients may be at increased risk for side effects and overdose.

Tricyclic Antidepressants

Tricyclic antidepressants are included on the 2023 American Geriatric Society Beers criteria medication list of potentially harmful drugs for elderly patients [5]. Avoidance is recommended, and use of topical pain medications is encouraged as much as possible, or in low-doses (e.g., ≤6 mg/day) doxepin [5]. The anticholinergic effects related to TCAs are well-established and may be related to their receptor affinity. Amitriptyline has a high affinity for the muscarinic acetylcholine receptors compared with nortriptyline and desipramine, which have lower affinity [197, 200, 201]. Peripheral adverse effects of mydriasis, xerostomia, urinary retention, flushing, fever, tachycardia, and constipation, and central adverse effects of impaired concentration, confusion, attention deficit, and memory impairment can be managed initially by lowering the dose or by considering switching to a TCA with a lower affinity to muscarinic acetylcholine receptors [197, 200]. If a patient is receiving more than one drug with anticholinergic adverse effects, review the patient's medications and assess if one drug can be stopped or the dose lowered using a drug taper.

Peripheral ADEs can be difficult to manage and may decrease a patient's quality of life. For mydriasis, phentolamine ophthalmic solution 0.75% may alleviate symptoms because of its effects on the muscarinic receptors in the eye. However, its use can induce myopia and increase the risk of retinal detachment. Pilocarpine is contraindicated for patients with narrow-angle glaucoma and chronic obstructive pulmonary disorders (COPD) [202]. Xerostomia can be managed with increased water intake, ice chips, and saliva substitutes such as Biotene, Bioextra, or sialogogues such as pilocarpine. Patients should avoid routine use of hard candy or gum with sugar or juices to manage their dry mouth, as these patients are at an increased risk of dental caries and gum and buccal ulcerations. Sugarless candy or gum in moderation may help stimulate salivary flow [195, 200].

The risk of hyperhidrosis is approximately 12–15% with TCAs [161, 162]. For mild and severe cases of axillary, craniofacial, and palmar hyperhidrosis, topical agents with 20% aluminum chloride can be used as an initial treatment. If the topical treatment fails, consider injections of onabotulinumtoxin A. Other treatments for axillary hyperhidrosis include initiating an oral anticholinergic agent, microwave therapy, local surgery, or sympathetic denervation [203]. For axillary hyperhidrosis alone, topical agents containing 20% aluminum chloride hexahydrate have demonstrated effectiveness. Also, topical anticholinergics may be used, such as glycopyrrolate 2% spray or solution, glycopyrronium tosylate 2.4% cloth, and oxybutynin used as a 3% gel. If the topical treatment fails, consider injections of onabotulinumtoxin A or initiating clonidine 0.1 mg twice daily. Other treatments for axillary hyperhidrosis include initiating an oral anticholinergic agent, cryotherapy or laser therapy, local surgery, or sympathetic denervation [203, 204].

Common ADEs of TCAs include sedation, weight gain, orthostatic hypotension, tachycardia, arrhythmia, cardiac conduction abnormalities, and anticholinergic effects such as urinary retention and delirium [196, 197]. Anticholinergic effects can be especially serious and concerning in older adults, and the 2023 American Geriatric Society recommends that antidepressants with strong anticholinergic properties, such as amitriptyline and high-dose doxepin (>6 mg/day), be avoided or used with caution [5]. Elderly patients can have an increased sensitivity to TCAs and a decreased metabolism of the drug, especially extended-release formulations. All TCAs have the potential for cardiac toxicity and should be avoided in patients with heart disease [198]. All TCAs are contraindicated if there is a history of hypersensitivity and if a myocardial infarction has occurred recently. The definition of 'recent' is vague; it may be prudent to wait at least 6–12 months following a cardiac event before starting a TCA. Additional cardiac considerations are also relevant with TCAs, including the right bundle branch block. If present, TCA therapy should be avoided, and if it occurs, any TCA should be discontinued [199, 205].

Orthostatic hypotension is a common ADE that may lead to drug discontinuation. Patients with preexisting postural hypotension, receiving concomitant antihypertensive medications, or those with dehydration are at greatest risk of this ADE [180, 200]. Adjustments to antihypertensive medications, particularly agents that block alpha-adrenergic receptors and/or correction of dehydration, may help alleviate or minimize orthostatic hypotension. Patients taking TCAs may exhibit electrocardiogram changes, which can be benign, but QT interval prolongation needs close monitoring, particularly when coadministered with drugs that can prolong the QT interval. The use of a TCA should be avoided in patients with preexisting conduction delays because they are at an increased risk of TCA-induced heart block.

Decreased motility of the colon is a common ADE with TCAs, but immobility, sedentary lifestyle, dehydration, and poor dietary intake of fiber, fruits, and vegetables can contribute to this ADE [180, 200]. Treatment of constipation is best as a preventive treatment through appropriate patient counseling on diet, fluids, regular exercise, and a review of medications before initiating laxatives or enemas. Patients struggling with adding dietary fiber to their meals may benefit from daily intake of a fiber supplement such as psyllium or wheat dextrin, added to food or beverages. Additionally, stool softeners may be added for short-term relief of constipation but should be discontinued once the patient has regular bowel movements. Tricyclic antidepressants can block muscle contraction in the bladder through their effects on acetylcholine. Bethanechol can be administered to minimize urinary retention from nonobstructive causes, such as urinary muscle relaxation induced by a TCA. Flushing and fever induced by TCAs can be managed by stopping the drug. Patients should see improvement in symptoms within 72 h, although some cases may take 4–5 days for symptom resolution [206]. Some patients may improve with a reduction in the dose, but dosing needs to be tapered based on tolerability. Drugs to treat fever, such as APAP and NSAIDs, are not recommended for drug-related fever or flushing. If flushing is associated with itching, a topical corticosteroid could be applied to the affected area for a few days after drug stoppage or dose adjustment.

Secondary amines, such as nortriptyline, may be better tolerated than tertiary amines, like amitriptyline. Overall, desipramine may be better tolerated than other TCAs; however, this will vary from patient to patient, and therapy should be individualized. Hyponatremia is an independent and cumulative risk with TCAs; this electrolyte disorder may be caused by the TCA or when a TCA is combined with other medications that can cause hyponatremia. A careful evaluation of history, risk, and benefit is important when additional hyponatremia-inducing medications are used together [197].

The management of SNRI- or TCA-related serotonin syndrome requires that the offending agent be stopped and supportive care be provided. For agitation, benzodiazepine administration can induce sedation and lower mild increases in blood pressure and heart rate. The goal of therapy is sedation with normal vital signs, not somnolence. Large and rapid fluctuations of heart rate and blood pressure can be managed with short-acting agents such as esmolol, nicardipine, or nitroprusside, with doses titrated to maintain autonomic stability. Long-acting drugs should be avoided. Hyperthermia is related to muscular activity, so antipyretic agents should be avoided. Hyperthermia care is dependent on body temperature; patients with temperatures higher than 41.1 °C will require sedation, neuromuscular paralysis, and intubation. If patients continue to exhibit agitation, cyproheptadine can be administered as an antidote for serotonin syndrome [205, 207, 208].

There is a seizure risk related to TCA use, which increases with increasing doses. The TCA should be stopped, and the seizure should be managed with the administration of a benzodiazepine, such as diazepam or lorazepam, and antiseizure drugs, including levetiracetam [201].

Most ingestions of atypical antidepressants result in minimal toxicity and can be managed effectively with supportive care, including circulation, breathing, and a secure airway [205, 209]. Key factors to assess include the specific drug and dosage ingested, its formulation, the timing of ingestion, and any coingestants involved, such as TCAs, gabapentinoids, or opioids [201, 210]. In awake patients who are able to protect their airway, a single dose of activated charcoal (1 g/kg; the standard adult dose is 50 g) may be administered. It is important to avoid additional serotonergic agents to prevent exacerbation of toxicity. Seizures should be treated with benzodiazepines such as diazepam or lorazepam; for adults, an initial IV dose of 5–10 mg may be repeated every 5–10 min, while pediatric dosing varies by age. A prolonged QRS interval warrants treatment with sodium bicarbonate at 1 to 2 mEq/kg IV push (typically 50–100 mEq for adults), with repeat doses as needed until the QRS narrows or blood pH reaches 7.55. If narrowing occurs, a bicarbonate infusion may be initiated. Patients with prolonged QTc should be monitored for torsades de pointes, which is treated with magnesium sulfate—starting with 2 g IV over 2 min, repeatable after 10 min, with infusion as needed [208–211].

A toxic ingestion of TCA can present as altered mental status, tachycardia or bradycardia, and hypotension, with diminished bowel sounds that can lead to seizure, tachycardia, QRS prolongation, coma, and death if the patient is not appropriately managed. Early identification is important, as symptoms can appear 30 min to 2 h after toxic ingestion. Patients should receive supportive care, including IV fluids, airway protection, and ECG monitoring. If the ingestion is within 2 h and the patient's airway is protected, activated charcoal can be administered. Seizures can be treated with benzodiazepine, but refractory seizures may require phenobarbital, propofol, or general anesthesia.

Treatment for hypotension should include IV fluids and sodium bicarbonate, but if a patient does not respond adequately to this therapy, initiation of an alpha-1 adrenergic agonist such as norepinephrine should be considered. Patients with QRS prolongation more than 100 milliseconds should receive supportive care with IV crystalloid fluids, sodium bicarbonate, and magnesium sulfate to stabilize electrical conduction. Lipid emulsion therapy can be utilized for severe or refractory cases [212]. Alkalization increases the protein binding of TCAs, which decreases the free or active drug concentration in the blood and may mitigate cardiac and neurologic toxic effects. The goal of alkalization is to keep serum pH between 7.5 and 7.55 to stabilize cardiac conduction by narrowing the QRS complex [211, 213]. Administration of lipid emulsion infusions may inactivate the drug by binding the drug to the lipid molecule. Lipid emulsions have been effective in reversing ventricular arrhythmias in severe and refractory cases, including TCA ingestions of 5 mg/kg. Because TCAs have a long half-life and large volume of distribution [214], drug removal by hemodialysis or hemoperfusion is ineffective, although plasmapheresis following lipid emulsion therapy has been used in cases refractory to sodium bicarbonate [212]. Clinicians should avoid physostigmine, types 1A, 1C, and 3 antiarrhythmic agents, and flumazenil for TCA toxic injections [212].

Adverse bleeding events have been reported with SNRIs and TCAs [162, 197]. One proposed mechanism for the increased bleeding risk may be reduced serotonin reuptake on platelets, which in turn reduces platelet adhesion.

References

1. CDC. https://www.cdc.gov/medicationsafety/adult_adversedrugevents.html#:~:text=Adverse%20drug%20events%20cause%20approximately,visits%20for%20adverse%20drug%20events.
2. Lovegrove MC, Dowell D, Geller AI, et al. US emergency department visits for acute harms from prescription opioid use, 2016–2017. Am J Public Health. 2019;109(5):784–91. https://doi.org/10.2105/AJPH.2019.305007. PMID: 30896999; PMCID: PMC6459659.
3. Willy M, Kelly JP, Nourjah P, et al. Emergency department visits attributed to selected analgesics, United States, 2004-2005. Pharmacoepidemiol Drug Saf. 2009;18:188–95.
4. Budnitz DS, Lovegrove MC, Crosby AE. Emergency department visits for overdoses of acetaminophen-containing products. Am J Prev Med. 2011;40(6):585–92. https://doi.org/10.1016/j.amepre.2011.02.026.
5. By the 2023 American Geriatrics Society Beers Criteria® Update Expert Panel. American Geriatrics Society 2023 updated AGS Beers Criteria® for potentially inappropriate medication use in older adults. J Am Geriatr Soc. 2023;71(7):2052–81. https://doi.org/10.1111/jgs.18372.
6. Prescott LF. Paracetamol overdosage. Pharmacological basis and clinical management. Drugs. 1983;25(3):290–314.
7. Bond GR, Requa RK, Krenzelok EP, et al. Influence of time until emesis on the efficacy of decontamination using acetaminophen as a marker in a pediatric population. Ann Emerg Med. 1993;22(9):1403–7. https://doi.org/10.1016/s0196-0644(05)81986-9.
8. Caravati EM. Unintentional acetaminophen ingestion in children and the potential for hepatotoxicity. J Toxicol Clin Toxicol. 2000;38(3):291–6. https://doi.org/10.1081/clt-100100934.
9. Mohler CR, Nordt SP, Williams SR, et al. Prospective evaluation of mild to moderate pediatric acetaminophen exposures. Ann Emerg Med. 2000;35(3):239–44. https://doi.org/10.1016/s0196-0644(00)70074-6.
10. Wang YX, Du Y, Liu XF, et al. A hepatoprotection study of radix Bupleuri on acetaminophen-induced liver injury based on CYP450 inhibition. Chin J Nat Med. 2019;17(7):517–24. https://doi.org/10.1016/S1875-5364(19)30073-1.
11. Ye H, Nelson LJ, Gómez Del Moral M, et al. Dissecting the molecular pathophysiology of drug-induced liver injury. World

J Gastroenterol. 2018;24(13):1373–85. https://doi.org/10.3748/wjg.v24.i13.1373.
12. Chun LJ, Tong MJ, Busuttil RW, Hiatt JR. Acetaminophen hepatotoxicity and acute liver failure. J Clin Gastroenterol. 2009;43(4):342–9. https://doi.org/10.1097/MCG.0b013e31818a3854.
13. Schilling A, Corey R, Leonard M, Eghtesad B. Acetaminophen: old drug, new warnings. Cleve Clin J Med. 2010;77(1):19–27. https://doi.org/10.3949/ccjm.77a.09084.
14. Smilkstein MJ, Bronstein AC, Linden C, et al. Acetaminophen overdose: a 48-hour intravenous N-acetylcysteine treatment protocol. Ann Emerg Med. 1991;20(10):1058–63. https://doi.org/10.1016/s0196-0644(05)81352-6.
15. Rumack BH, Matthew H. Acetaminophen poisoning and toxicity. Pediatrics. 1975;55(6):871–6.
16. Larson AM. Acetaminophen hepatotoxicity. Clin Liver Dis. 2007;11(3):525–48. https://doi.org/10.1016/j.cld.2007.06.006. (Dahlin DC, Miwa GT, Lu AY, Nelson SD. N-acetyl-p-benzoquinone imine: a cytochrome P-450-mediated oxidation product of acetaminophen. Proc Natl Acad Sci USA. 1984;81(5):1327–31. https://doi.org/10.1073/pnas.81.5.1327).
17. Kalsi SS, Wood DM, Waring WS, Dargan PI. Does cytochrome P450 liver isoenzyme induction increase the risk of liver toxicity after paracetamol overdose? Emerg Med J. 2011;28(5):401–7. (Lin JH, Levy G. Sulfate depletion after acetaminophen administration and replenishment by infusion of sodium sulfate or N-acetylcysteine in rats. Biochem Pharmacol. 1981;30(19):2723–5. https://doi.org/10.1016/0006-2952(81)90547-5).
18. Heard KJ. Acetylcysteine for acetaminophen poisoning. N Engl J Med. 2008;359(3):285–92. https://doi.org/10.1056/NEJMct0708278.
19. Rumack BH, Peterson RC, Koch GG, Amara IA. Acetaminophen overdose: 662 cases with evaluation of oral acetylcysteine treatment. Arch Intern Med. 1981;141(3):380–5.
20. Prescott LF, Park J, Ballantyne A, et al. Treatment of paracetamol (acetaminophen) poisoning with N-acetylcysteine. Lancet. 1977;2(8035):432–4.
21. Bailey B, Blais R, McGuigan MA. Management of anaphylactoid reactions to intravenous N-acetylcysteine. Ann Emerg Med. 1998;31(6):710–5.
22. Yeates PJ, Thomas SH. Effectiveness of delayed activated charcoal administration in simulated paracetamol (acetaminophen) overdose. Br J Clin Pharmacol. 2000;49(1):11–4. https://doi.org/10.1046/j.1365-2125.2000.00107.x.
23. Gosselin S, Juurlink DN, Kielstein JT, et al. Extracorporeal treatment for acetaminophen poisoning: recommendations from the EXTRIP workgroup. Clin Toxicol (Phila). 2014;52(8):856–67. https://doi.org/10.3109/15563650.2014.946994.
24. Dart RC, Mullins ME, Matoushek T, et al. Management of acetaminophen poisoning in the US and Canada: a consensus statement. JAMA Netw Open. 2023;6(8):e2327739. https://doi.org/10.1001/jamanetworkopen.2023.27739.
25. McCormack PL. Celecoxib: a review of its use for symptomatic relief in the treatment of osteoarthritis, rheumatoid arthritis and ankylosing spondylitis. Drugs. 2011;71(18):2457–89. https://doi.org/10.2165/11208240-000000000-00000.
26. Jones P, Lamdin R. Oral cyclo-oxygenase 2 inhibitors versus other oral analgesics for acute soft tissue injury: systematic review and meta-analysis. Clin Drug Investig. 2010;30(7):419–37. https://doi.org/10.2165/11533350-000000000-00000.
27. Mallen SR, Essex MN, Zhang R. Gastrointestinal tolerability of NSAIDs in elderly patients: a pooled analysis of 21 randomized clinical trials with celecoxib and nonselective NSAIDs. Curr Med Res Opin. 2011;27(7):1359–66. https://doi.org/10.1185/03007995.2011.581274.
28. Hawkins C, Hanks GW. The gastroduodenal toxicity of nonsteroidal anti-inflammatory drugs: a review of the literature. J Pain Symptom Manag. 2000;20(2):140–51. https://doi.org/10.1016/s0885-3924(00)00175-5.
29. Caughey GE, Cleland LG, Penglis PS, et al. Roles of cyclooxygenase (COX)-1 and COX-2 in prostanoid production by human endothelial cells: selective up-regulation of prostacyclin synthesis by COX-2. J Immunol. 2001;167(5):2831–8. https://doi.org/10.4049/jimmunol.167.5.2831.
30. Baron JA, Sandler RS, Bresalier RS, et al. Cardiovascular events associated with rofecoxib in a colorectal adenoma chemoprevention trial. N Engl J Med. 2005;352(11):1092–102.
31. U.S. Food and Drug Administration. Information for clinicians: voluntary withdrawal of valdecoxib (Bextra®) from U.S. markets due to cardiovascular risks. 2005.
32. Nissen SE, Yeomans ND, Solomon DH, et al. PRECISION trial investigators. Cardiovascular safety of celecoxib, naproxen, or ibuprofen for arthritis. N Engl J Med. 2016;375(26):2519–29.
33. U.S. Food and Drug Administration. FDA advisory: all NSAIDs carry boxed warnings for cardiovascular and gastrointestinal risks. 2005–present.
34. Mobbs KJ, Tolwani AJ, Kamel KS. Nonsteroidal anti-inflammatory drugs and the kidney: adverse effects and mechanisms. Pharmacol Rev. 2010;62(2):136–52.
35. Hoppmann RA, Peden JG, Ober SK. Central nervous system side effects of nonsteroidal anti-inflammatory drugs: aseptic meningitis, psychosis, and cognitive dysfunction. Arch Intern Med. 1991;151(7):1309–13.
36. Volans G, Monaghan J, Colbridge M. Ibuprofen overdose. Int J Clin Pract Suppl. 2003;135:54–60.
37. McElwee NE, Veltri JC, Bradford DC, Rollins DE. A prospective, population-based study of acute ibuprofen overdose: complications are rare and routine serum levels not warranted. Ann Emerg Med. 1990;19(6):657–62. https://doi.org/10.1016/s0196-0644(05)82471-0.
38. Chyka PA, Seger D, Krenzelok EP, Vale JA. American Academy of clinical toxicology; European Association of Poisons Centres and Clinical Toxicologists. Position paper: single-dose activated charcoal. Clin Toxicol (Phila). 2005;43(2):61–87. https://doi.org/10.1081/clt-200051867.
39. Bahar E, Yoon H. Lidocaine: a local anesthetic, its adverse effects and management. Medicina (Kaunas). 2021;57(8):782.
40. Neal JM, Barrington MJ, Fettiplace MR, et al. The third American Society of Regional Anesthesia and Pain Medicine practice advisory on local anesthetic systemic toxicity: executive summary 2017. Reg Anesth Pain Med. 2018;43(2):113–23.
41. Amado A, Sood A, Taylor JS. Contact allergy to lidocaine: a report of sixteen cases. Dermatitis. 2007;18(4):215–20.
42. To D, Kossintseva I, de Gannes G. Lidocaine contact allergy is becoming more prevalent. Dermatologic Surg. 2014;40(12):1367–72. https://doi.org/10.1097/DSS.0000000000000190.
43. Ruffles SP, Gayres JG. Fatal bronchospasm after topical lignocaine before bronchoscopy. BMJ (Clin Res Ed). 1987;294(6588):1658–9.
44. Gammaitoni AR, Alvarez NA, Galer BS. Pharmacokinetics and safety of continuously applied lidocaine 5% patches. Am J Health Syst Pharm. 2002;59(22):2215–20.
45. Weinberg L, Peake B, Tan C, et al. Pharmacokinetics and pharmacodynamics of lignocaine: a review. World J Anesthesiol. 2015;4(1):17–29.

46. Reichel C, Skodra T, Nacke A, Spengler U, Sauerbruch T. The lignocaine metabolite (MEGX) liver function test and P-450 induction in humans. Br J Clin Pharmacol. 1998;46(6):535–9.
47. El-Boghdadly K, Pawa A, Chin KJ. Local anesthetic systemic toxicity: current perspectives. Local Reg Anesth. 2018;11:35–44.
48. StatPearls. Lidocaine toxicity. In: StatPearls [Internet]. Treasure Island, FL: StatPearls Publishing; 2022.
49. Gay HC, Amaral AP. Acquired methemoglobinemia associated with topical lidocaine administration: a case report. Drug Saf Case Rep. 2018;5(1):15. https://doi.org/10.1007/s40800-018-0081-4.
50. Wallach JD, Ross JS. Gabapentin approvals, off-label use, and lessons for Postmarketing evaluation efforts. JAMA. 2018;319(8):776–8. https://doi.org/10.1001/jama.2017.21897.
51. Rose MA, Kam PC. Gabapentin: pharmacology and its use in pain management. Anaesthesia. 2002;57(5):451–62. https://doi.org/10.1046/j.0003-2409.2001.02399.x.
52. Paice JA, Portenoy R, Lacchetti C, et al. Management of chronic pain in survivors of adult cancers: American Society of Clinical Oncology clinical practice guideline. J Clin Oncol. 2016;34(27):3325–45. https://doi.org/10.1200/JCO.2016.68.5206. PubMed 27458286.
53. Knowles GM, LaFleur GE, Churchwell MD. Evaluation of gabapentin and Pregabalin use in hospitalized patients with decreased kidney function. J Pharm Technol. 2024;40(1):30–6. https://doi.org/10.1177/87551225231217906. PMID: 38318261; PMCID: PMC10838538.
54. FDA Safety Alert. MedWatch. FDA warns about serious breathing problems with seizure and nerve pain medicines gabapentin (Neurontin, Gralise, Horizant) and pregabalin (Lyrica, Lyrica CR). Food and Drug Administration website. https://www.fda.gov/drugs/drug-safety-and-availability/fda-warns-about-serious-breathing-problems-seizure-and-nerve-pain-medicines-gabapentin-neurontin. Published December 19, 2019. Accessed 15 Dec 2024.
55. Smith RV, Havens JR, Walsh SL. Gabapentin misuse, abuse, and diversion: a systematic review. Addiction. 2016;111(7):1160–74. https://doi.org/10.1111/add.13324. PMID: 27265421; PMCID: PMC5573873.
56. Yasaei R, Katta S, Patel P, et al. Gabapentin. [Updated 2024 Feb 21]. In: StatPearls [Internet]. Treasure Island (FL): StatPearls Publishing; 2025. Available from: https://www.ncbi.nlm.nih.gov/books/NBK493228/.
57. Mersfelder TL, Nichols WH. Gabapentin: abuse, dependence, and withdrawal. Ann Pharmacother. 2016;50(3):229–33. https://doi.org/10.1177/1060028015620800.
58. Evoy KE, Peckham AM, Covvey JR, et al. Gabapentinoid pharmacology in the context of emerging misuse liability. J Clin Pharmacol. 2021;61(Suppl 2):S89–99. https://doi.org/10.1002/jcph.1833. PMID: 34396549.
59. Bouchard J, Yates C, Calello DP, EXTRIP Workgroup, et al. Extracorporeal treatment for gabapentin and Pregabalin poisoning: systematic review and recommendations from the EXTRIP Workgroup. Am J Kidney Dis. 2022;79(1):88–104. https://doi.org/10.1053/j.ajkd.2021.06.027. PMID: 34799138.
60. See S, Hendriks E, Hsiung L. Akathisia induced by gabapentin withdrawal. Ann Pharmacother. 2011;45(6):e31. https://doi.org/10.1345/aph.1Q057. PMID: 21652784.
61. Wood DM, Berry DJ, Glover G, et al. Significant pregabalin toxicity managed with supportive care alone. J Med Toxicol. 2010;6(4):435–7. https://doi.org/10.1007/s13181-010-0052-3. PMID: 20373065; PMCID: PMC3550463.
62. Reinert JP, Dunn RL. Management of overdoses of loperamide, gabapentin, and modafinil: a literature review. Expert Rev Clin Pharmacol. 2019;12(9):901–8. https://doi.org/10.1080/17512433.2019.1657830. Epub 2019 Aug 31. PMID: 31422705.
63. Tegretol prescribing information Novartis Pharmaceuticals Corporation East Hanover, NJ. www.accessdata.fda.gov/drugsatfda_docs/label/2007/016608s098lbl.pdf. Accessed 14 Aug 2025.
64. Dyong TM, Gess B, Dumke C, et al. Carbamazepine for chronic muscle pain: a retrospective assessment of indications, side effects, and treatment response. Brain Sci. 2023;13(1):123. https://doi.org/10.3390/brainsci13010123. PMID: 36672104; PMCID: PMC9857021.
65. Wiffen PJ, Derry S, Moore RA, et al. Carbamazepine for chronic neuropathic pain and fibromyalgia in adults. Cochrane Database Syst Rev. 2014;2014(4):CD005451. https://doi.org/10.1002/14651858.CD005451.pub3. PMID: 24719027; PMCID: PMC6491112.
66. Verrotti A, Scaparrotta A, Grosso S, et al. Anticonvulsant drugs and hematological disease. Neurol Sci. 2014;35(7):983–93.
67. Al Khalili Y, Sekhon S, Jain S. Carbamazepine toxicity. [Updated 2023 Jul 24]. In: StatPearls [Internet]. Treasure Island (FL): StatPearls Publishing; 2025. Available from: https://www.ncbi.nlm.nih.gov/books/NBK507852/.
68. Çetin M, Mis MD, Karaman K, et al. Carbamazepine-induced DRESS syndrome leading to reversible myocarditis in a child. Cent Eur J Immunol. 2019;44(1):102–5. https://doi.org/10.5114/ceji.2019.83700. PMID: 31114444; PMCID: PMC6526593.
69. Wong CSM, Yap DYH, Ip P, et al. HLA-B*15:11 status and carbamazepine-induced severe cutaneous adverse drug reactions in HLA-B*15:02 negative Chinese. Int J Dermatol. 2022;61:184–90. https://doi.org/10.1111/ijd.15792.
70. Puangpetch A, Koomdee N, Chamnanphol M, et al. HLA-B allele and haplotype diversity among Thai patients identified by PCR-SSOP: evidence for high risk of drug-induced hypersensitivity. Front Genet. 2015;5:478. https://doi.org/10.3389/fgene.2014.00478. PMID: 25657656; PMCID: PMC4302987.
71. Tonekaboni SH, Jafari N, Mansouri M, et al. HLA-B*1502 in Iranian children with anticonvulsant drugs-induced skin reactions. Iran. J Child Neurol. 2017 Spring;11(2):26–30.
72. Dean L. Carbamazepine therapy and HLA genotype. 2015 Oct 14 [Updated 2025 Jun 9]. In: Pratt VM, Scott SA, Pirmohamed M, et al., editors. Medical genetics summaries [Internet]. Bethesda: National Center for Biotechnology Information (US); 2012: https://www.ncbi.nlm.nih.gov/books/NBK321445/.
73. Mehta M, Shah J, Khakhkhar T, et al. Anticonvulsant hypersensitivity syndrome associated with carbamazepine administration: case series. J Pharmacol Pharmacother. 2014;5(1):59–62. https://doi.org/10.4103/0976-500X.124428. PMID: 24554914; PMCID: PMC3917170.
74. Caley CF, Perriello E, Golden J. Antiepileptic drugs and suicide-related outcomes in bipolar disorder: a descriptive review of published data. Ment Health Clin. 2018;8(3):138–47. https://doi.org/10.9740/mhc.2018.05.138. PMID: 29955559; PMCID: PMC6007633.
75. Chen MJ, Zhang WJ, Guo ZL, et al. Withdrawal reaction of carbamazepine after neurovascular decompression for trigeminal neuralgia: a preliminary study. J Neurol Sci. 2014;338(1–2):43–5. https://doi.org/10.1016/j.jns.2013.12.013. PMID: 24387898.
76. Ghannoum M, Yates C, Galvao TF, et al. EXTRIP workgroup. Extracorporeal treatment for carbamazepine poisoning: systematic review and recommendations from the EXTRIP workgroup. Clin Toxicol (Phila). 2014;52(10):993–1004. https://doi.org/10.3109/15563650.2014.973572. PMID: 25355482; PMCID: PMC4782683.
77. Depakote (valproic acid) [Package insert] Chicago, IL, AbbVie 2025. https://www.accessdata.fda.gov/drugsatfda_docs/label/2025/018723s070lbl.pdf.
78. Rahman M, Awosika AO, Nguyen H. Valproic acid. [Updated 2024 Mar 19]. In: In: StatPearls [Internet]. Treasure Island (FL):

StatPearls Publishing; 2025. Available from: https://www.ncbi.nlm.nih.gov/books/NBK559112/.
79. Hamed SA, Abdella MM. The risk of asymptomatic hyperammonemia in children with idiopathic epilepsy treated with valproate: relationship to blood carnitine status. Epilepsy Res. 2009;86(1):32–41. https://doi.org/10.1016/j.eplepsyres.2009.04.002.
80. Patel AR, Nagalli S. Valproate toxicity. [Updated 2024 May 6]. In: StatPearls [Internet]. Treasure Island (FL): StatPearls Publishing; 2025. Available from: https://www.ncbi.nlm.nih.gov/books/NBK560898/.
81. Johnson LZ, Martinez I, Fernández MC, et al. Successful treatment of valproic acid overdose with hemodialysis. Am J Kidney Dis. 1999;33(4):786–9. https://doi.org/10.1016/s0272-6386(99)70235-0. PMID: 10196025.
82. Ghannoum M, Laliberté M, Nolin TD, EXTRIP Workgroup, et al. Extracorporeal treatment for valproic acid poisoning: systematic review and recommendations from the EXTRIP workgroup. Clin Toxicol (Phila). 2015;53(5):454–65. https://doi.org/10.3109/15563650.2015.1035441. PMID: 25950372.
83. Muñoz-Pichuante D, Villa-Zapata L, Lolas R. Meropenem for management of valproic acid overdose: a case report. Drug Metab Pers Ther. 2020;35(2) https://doi.org/10.1515/dmpt-2019-0028. PMID: 32609645.
84. Morimoto M, Suzaki I, Shimakawa S, et al. Three cases in which drug-induced hyponatremia was improved by replacing carbamazepine with lacosamide. Clin Case Reports. 2020;8(7):1166–70. https://doi.org/10.1002/ccr3.2857. PMID: 32695350; PMCID: PMC7364071.
85. MotherToBaby | Fact Sheets [Internet]. Brentwood (TN): Organization of Teratology Information Specialists (OTIS); 1994. Valproic Acid 2023 Nov. Available from: https://www.ncbi.nlm.nih.gov/books/NBK583009/.
86. Baclofen prescribing information Teva Pharmaceuticals USA, Inc. North Wales PA. https://dailymed.nlm.nih.gov/dailymed/lookup.cfm?setid=5648c772-50cb-4961-996e-e68a8eb699ea. Accessed 15 Aug 2025.
87. Ghanavatian S, Derian A. Baclofen. [Updated 2024 Aug 11]. In: StatPearls [Internet]. Treasure Island (FL): StatPearls Publishing; 2025. Available from: https://www.ncbi.nlm.nih.gov/books/NBK526037/.
88. Romito JW, Turner ER, Rosener JA, et al. Baclofen therapeutics, toxicity, and withdrawal: a narrative review. SAGE Open Med. 2021;9:20503121211022197. https://doi.org/10.1177/20503121211022197. PMID: 34158937; PMCID: PMC8182184.
89. Zahra E, Darke S, Lappin J, et al. Baclofen-related deaths in Australia 2000–2022. Forensic Sci Int. 2024;365:112281. https://doi.org/10.1016/j.forsciint.2024.112281. PMID: 39486258.
90. Dease NM, Kershner EK, Wills BK. Baclofen toxicity. [Updated 2023 Mar 20]. In: StatPearls [Internet]. Treasure Island (FL): StatPearls Publishing; 2025. Available from: https://www.ncbi.nlm.nih.gov/books/NBK580550/.
91. Ghannoum M, Berling I, Lavergne V, Roberts DM, Galvao T, Hoffman RS, Nolin TD, Lewington A, Doi K, Gosselin S, EXTRIP workgroup. Recommendations from the EXTRIP workgroup on extracorporeal treatment for baclofen poisoning. Kidney Int. 2021;100(4):720–36. https://doi.org/10.1016/j.kint.2021.07.014. PMID: 34358487.
92. Coffey RJ, Edgar TS, Francisco GE, et al. Abrupt withdrawal from intrathecal baclofen: recognition and management of a potentially life-threatening syndrome. Arch Phys Med Rehabil. 2002;83(6):735–41. https://doi.org/10.1053/apmr.2002.32820. Erratum in: Arch Phys Med Rehabil 2002;83(10):1479. PMID: 12048649.
93. Carisoprodol prescribing information Nostrum Laboratories, Inc. Kansas City, MO. https://dailymed.nlm.nih.gov/dailymed/drugInfo.cfm?setid=ab22f1be-16c8-45b6-adaf-09e08bf7a545. Accessed 15 Aug 2025.
94. Conermann T, Christian D. Carisoprodol. In: StatPearls [Internet]. Treasure Island (FL): StatPearls Publishing; 2025. https://www.ncbi.nlm.nih.gov/books/NBK553077/.
95. Gonzalez LA, Gatch MB, Forster MJ, et al. Abuse potential of Soma: the GABA(A) Receptor as a target. Mol Cell Pharmacol. 2009;1(4):180–6.
96. Bramness JG, Mørland J, Sørlid HK, et al. Carisoprodol intoxications and serotonergic features. Clin Toxicol (Phila). 2005;43(1):39–45.
97. Kintz P, Tracqui A, Mangin P, et al. Fatal meprobamate self-poisoning. Am J Forensic Med Pathol. 1988;9(2):139–40.
98. Charron C, Mekontso-Dessap A, Chergui K, et al. Incidence, causes and prognosis of hypotension related to meprobamate poisoning. Intensive Care Med. 2005;31(11):1582–6. https://doi.org/10.1007/s00134-005-2816-9. PMID: 16217659.
99. Roberge RJ, Lin E, Krenzelok EP. Flumazenil reversal of carisoprodol (Soma) intoxication. J Emerg Med. 2000;18(1):61–4. https://doi.org/10.1016/s0736-4679(99)00177-8. PMID: 10645840.
100. Chlorzoxazone prescribing information. Camber Pharmaceuticals, Inc., Piscataway, NJ. https://dailymed.nlm.nih.gov/dailymed/drugInfo.cfm?setid=e9bb9ebf-fceb-4da8-950a-c4b1fd5a84f1. Accessed 15 Aug 2025.
101. Powers BJ, Cattau EL Jr, Zimmerman HJ. Chlorzoxazone hepatotoxic reactions. An analysis of 21 identified or presumed cases. Arch Intern Med. 1986;146(6):1183–6. https://doi.org/10.1001/archinte.146.6.1183. PMID: 3521519.
102. LiverTox: Clinical and research information on drug-induced liver injury [Internet]. Bethesda (MD): National Institute of Diabetes and Digestive and Kidney Diseases; 2012. Chlorzoxazone. [Updated 2017 Jan 30]. Available from: https://www.ncbi.nlm.nih.gov/books/NBK548137/.
103. Roberge RJ, Atchley B, Ryan K, et al. Two chlorzoxazone (Parafon forte) overdoses and coma in one patient: reversal with flumazenil. Am J Emerg Med. 1998;16(4):393–5. https://doi.org/10.1016/s0735-6757(98)90137-1. PMID: 9672460.
104. Cyclobenzaprine prescribing information. Teva Pharmaceuticals USA, Inc. Parsippany, NJ. https://dailymed.nlm.nih.gov/dailymed/drugInfo.cfm?setid=ca74d27a-f7c6-462d-a913-1cfa061bd8f3. Accessed 15 Aug 2025.
105. Winchell GA, King JD, Chavez-Eng CM, et al. Cyclobenzaprine pharmacokinetics, including the effects of age, gender, and hepatic insufficiency. J Clin Pharmacol. 2002;42(1):61–9. https://doi.org/10.1177/00912700022042001007. PMID: 11808825.
106. Chaffee DM. Cyclobenzaprine in the treatment of low back pain. Am Fam Physician. 2016;93(3):Online. PMID: 26926618.
107. Khan I, Kahwaji CI. Cyclobenzaprine. [Updated 2023 Aug 28]. In: StatPearls [Internet]. Treasure Island (FL): StatPearls Publishing; 2025. Available from: https://www.ncbi.nlm.nih.gov/books/NBK513362/.
108. Keegan MT, Brown DR, Rabinstein AA. Serotonin syndrome from the interaction of cyclobenzaprine with other serotoninergic drugs. Anesth Analg. 2006;103(6):1466–8. https://doi.org/10.1213/01.ane.0000247699.81580.eb. PMID: 17122225.

109. Spiller HA, Winter ML, Mann KV, et al. Five-year multicenter retrospective review of cyclobenzaprine toxicity. J Emerg Med. 1995;13(6):781–5. https://doi.org/10.1016/0736-4679(95)02019-5. PMID: 8747627.
110. Metaxalone prescribing information. Actavis Pharma, Inc., Parsippany, NJ. https://dailymed.nlm.nih.gov/dailymed/drugInfo.cfm?setid=b3a4f6bc-abd4-4b8e-970f-59b3aa6f17a0. Accessed 15 Aug 2025.
111. Spence MM, Shin PJ, Lee EA, et al. Risk of injury associated with skeletal muscle relaxant use in older adults. Ann Pharmacother. 2013;47(7–8):993–8. https://doi.org/10.1345/aph.1R735. PMID: 23821610.
112. Forrester MB. Adult metaxalone ingestions reported to Texas poison control centers, 2000–2006. Hum Exp Toxicol. 2010;29:55–62. https://doi.org/10.1177/0960327108098150.
113. Bosak AR, Skolnik AB. Serotonin syndrome associated with metaxalone overdose. J Med Toxicol. 2014;10(4):402–5. https://doi.org/10.1007/s13181-014-0404-5. PMID: 24805103; PMCID: PMC4252289.
114. Methocarbamol prescribing information. Actavis Pharma, Inc., Parsippany, NJ. https://dailymed.nlm.nih.gov/dailymed/drugInfo.cfm?setid=b3a4f6bc-abd4-4b8e-970f-59b3aa6f17a0. Accessed 15 Aug 2025.
115. Sibrack J, Patel P, Hammer R. Methocarbamol. In: StatPearls [Internet]. Treasure Island (FL): StatPearls Publishing; 2025. https://www.ncbi.nlm.nih.gov/books/NBK565868/.
116. Gangwani MK, Aziz M, Asif R, et al. Green urine and altered mental status: a case of intoxication. J Ayub Med Coll Abbottabad. 2019;31(2):278–81.
117. Orphenadrine prescribing information. Ammeal Pharmaceuticals, LLC, Bridgewater, NJ. https://dailymed.nlm.nih.gov/dailymed/drugInfo.cfm?setid=6e89e43d-a3fc-481e-8aed-d6955fa2a14b. Accessed 15 Aug 2025.
118. Dilaveris P, Pantazis A, Vlasseros J, et al. Non-sustained ventricular tachycardia due to low-dose orphenadrine. Am J Med. 2001;111(5):418–9. https://doi.org/10.1016/s0002-9343(01)00875-0. PMID: 11599527.
119. Danze LK, Langdorf MI. Reversal of orphenadrine-induced ventricular tachycardia with physostigmine. J Emerg Med. 1991;9(6):453–7. https://doi.org/10.1016/0736-4679(91)90217-4. PMID: 1787292.
120. Bennett NB, Kohn J. Case report: orphenadrine overdose cerebral manifestations treated with physostigmine. Anaesth Intensive Care. 1976;4(1):67. https://doi.org/10.1177/0310057X7600400113. PMID: 1251997.
121. Tizanidine prescribing information. Alembic Pharmaceuticals, Inc., Bedminister, NJ. https://dailymed.nlm.nih.gov/dailymed/drugInfo.cfm?setid=ee3e9813-a738-46d1-9c05-c931aee1495c. Accessed 15 Aug 2025.
122. Ghanavatian S, Derian A. Tizanidine. In: StatPearls [Internet]. Treasure Island (FL): StatPearls Publishing; 2025. https://www.ncbi.nlm.nih.gov/books/NBK519505/.
123. Escobar Gil T, McGeorge KJ, Jones AJ. A case of Tizanidine withdrawal and road to recovery. Cureus. 2024;16(2):e53444. https://doi.org/10.7759/cureus.53444. PMID: 38435197; PMCID: PMC10909376.
124. Morgom M, Sabir DM, Elbashir H, et al. A case of Tizanidine withdrawal syndrome: features and management in the emergency department. Cureus. 2023;15(11):e49248. https://doi.org/10.7759/cureus.49248. PMID: 38143690; PMCID: PMC10743202.
125. Morgom M, Anjum S, Elgassim MA, et al. Emergency response to Tizanidine overdose: a case report on critical care strategies. Cureus. 2024;16(10):e70696. https://doi.org/10.7759/cureus.70696. PMID: 39493159; PMCID: PMC11529801.
126. Clonidine hydrochloride prescribing information. Alembic Pharmaceuticals, Inc., Bedminster, NJ. https://dailymed.nlm.nih.gov/dailymed/drugInfo.cfm?setid=88a8db46-0fc9-48cd-b7cc-ac9c9cdea100. Accessed 15 Aug 2025. (Clonidine hydrochloride injection prescribing information. XGen Pharmaceuticals DJB, Inc., Big Flats, NY. https://dailymed.nlm.nih.gov/dailymed/drugInfo.cfm?setid=ada02f1f-ae78-4435-879e-492ae862d504. Accessed 15 Aug 2025).
127. Duong C, Lovett C, Downes MA, Isbister GK. Reality of clonidine poisoning in children and adolescents. J Paediatr Child Health. 2023;59(6):827–32. https://doi.org/10.1111/jpc.16399. PMID: 37036115; PMCID: PMC10946816.
128. Manzon L, Nappe TM, DelMaestro C, et al. Clonidine toxicity. [Updated 2023 Jun 26]. In: StatPearls [Internet]. Treasure Island (FL): StatPearls Publishing; 2025. Available from: https://www.ncbi.nlm.nih.gov/books/NBK459374/.
129. Horowitz R, Mazor SS, Aks SE, et al. Accidental clonidine patch ingestion in a child. Am J Ther. 2005;12(3):272–4.
130. Toce MS, Freiman E, O'Donnell KA, et al. Clinical effects of pediatric clonidine exposure: a retrospective cohort study at a single tertiary care center. J Emerg Med. 2021;60(1):58–66. https://doi.org/10.1016/j.jemermed.2020.09.018. PMID: 33036823.
131. Seger DL, Loden JK. Naloxone reversal of clonidine toxicity: dose, dose, dose. Clin Toxicol (Phila). 2018;56(10):873–9. https://doi.org/10.1080/15563650.2018.1450986. PMID: 29544366.
132. Diltiazem prescribing information. Alembic Pharmaceuticals, Inc., Bedminister, NJ. https://dailymed.nlm.nih.gov/dailymed/drugInfo.cfm?setid=04a85be5-f746-418e-8e37-292703f16934. Accessed 15 Aug 2025.
133. Verapamil hydrochloride prescribing information. Wilshire Pharmaceuticals, Inc., Atlanta, GA. https://dailymed.nlm.nih.gov/dailymed/drugInfo.cfm?setid=f9399858-fd7a-4b73-8759-3e5bf3af2666 Accessed 15 Aug 2025.
134. Nifedipine prescribing information. Alembic Pharmaceuticals, Inc., Bedminster, NJ. https://dailymed.nlm.nih.gov/dailymed/drugInfo.cfm?setid=63f062f6-5669-434c-8ded-9801d8486dbf. Accessed 15 Aug 2025.
135. Amlodipine prescribing information. Ammeal Pharmaceuticals, LLC., Bridgewater, NJ. https://dailymed.nlm.nih.gov/dailymed/drugInfo.cfm?setid=88a8db46-0fc9-48cd-b7cc-ac9c9cdea100. Accessed 15 Aug 2025.
136. McKeever RG, Patel P, Hamilton RJ. Calcium channel blockers. In: StatPearls [Internet]. Treasure Island (FL): StatPearls Publishing; 2025. https://www.ncbi.nlm.nih.gov/books/NBK537147/.
137. Talreja O, Cassagnol M. Diltiazem. [Updated 2023 Aug 28]. In: StatPearls [Internet]. Treasure Island (FL): StatPearls Publishing; 2025. Available from: https://www.ncbi.nlm.nih.gov/books/NBK532937/.
138. Ramoska EA, Spiller HA, Winter M, et al. A one-year evaluation of calcium channel blocker overdoses: toxicity and treatment. Ann Emerg Med. 1993;22(2):196–200. https://doi.org/10.1016/s0196-0644(05)80202-1. PMID: 8427431.
139. Chakraborty RK, Hamilton RJ. Calcium channel blocker toxicity. In: StatPearls [Internet]. Treasure Island (FL): StatPearls Publishing; 2023. https://www.ncbi.nlm.nih.gov/books/NBK482473/.
140. St-Onge M, Anseeuw K, Cantrell FL, et al. Experts consensus recommendations for the management of calcium channel blocker poisoning in adults. Crit Care Med. 2017;45(3):e306–15. PubMed 27749343.
141. Wong A, Hoffman RS, Walsh SJ, Roberts DM, Gosselin S, Bunchman TE, Kebede S, Lavergne V, Ghannoum M, EXTRIP workgroup. Extracorporeal treatment for calcium channel blocker poisoning: systematic review and recommendations from the EXTRIP workgroup. Clin Toxicol (Phila). 2021;59(5):361–75.

https://doi.org/10.1080/15563650.2020.1870123. Epub 2021 Feb 8. PMID: 33555964.
142. Sepulveda EA, Pak A. Lipid emulsion therapy. [Updated 2024 Feb 16]. In: StatPearls [Internet]. Treasure Island (FL): StatPearls Publishing; 2025. Available from: https://www.ncbi.nlm.nih.gov/books/NBK549897/.
143. Katlan B, Kesici S, Bayrakci B. Intravenous lipid emulsion treatment for Calcium-Channel blocker intoxication: pediatric case series and review of the literature. Pediatr Emerg Care. 2023;39(3):120–4. https://doi.org/10.1097/PEC.0000000000002703. Epub 2022 Mar 28. PMID: 35344530.
144. Ketamine hydrochloride Injection, prescribing information. Hikma Farmacêutica (Portugal), S.A. https://dailymed.nlm.nih.gov/dailymed/drugInfo.cfm?setid=58c86d9b-8694-4bd8-8254-f19ee3ad60b0. Accessed 15 Aug 2025.
145. Green SM, Roback MG, Kennedy RM, et al. Clinical practice guideline for emergency department ketamine dissociative sedation: 2011 update. Ann Emerg Med. 2011;57(5):449–61. https://doi.org/10.1016/j.annemergmed.2010.11.030. PMID: 21256625.
146. Garg A, Sinha P, Kumar P, et al. Use of naltrexone in ketamine dependence. Addict Behav. 2014;39(8):1215–6. https://doi.org/10.1016/j.addbeh.2014.04.004. PubMed 24813545.
147. Orhurhu VJ, Vashisht R, Claus LE, et al. Ketamine Toxicity. [Updated 2023 Jan 30]. In: StatPearls [Internet]. Treasure Island (FL): StatPearls Publishing; 2025. Available from: https://www.ncbi.nlm.nih.gov/books/NBK541087/.
148. Chyka PA, Seger D. Position statement: single-dose activated charcoal. American Academy of Clinical Toxicology; European Association of Poisons Centres and Clinical Toxicologists. J Toxicol Clin Toxicol. 1997;35(7):721–41. https://doi.org/10.3109/15563659709162569. PMID: 9482427.
149. Vivolo-Kantor AM, Mattson CL, Zlotorzynska M. Notes from the field: ketamine detection and involvement in drug overdose deaths – United States, July 2019–June 2023. MMWR Morb Mortal Wkly Rep. 2024;73(44):1010–2. https://doi.org/10.15585/mmwr.mm7344a4. PMID: 39509345; PMCID: PMC11542773.
150. Bonilla-Jaime H, Sánchez-Salcedo JA, Estevez-Cabrera MM, Molina-Jiménez T, Cortes-Altamirano JL, Alfaro-Rodríguez A. Depression and pain: use of Antidepressants. Curr Neuropharmacol. 2022;20(2):384–402. https://doi.org/10.2174/1570159X19666210609161447.
151. Pristiq [desvenlafaxine]. Package insert. Wyeth Pharmaceuticals LLC, a subsidiary of Pfizer Inc. 2008. Revised 2023.
152. Cymbalta [Duloxetine]. Package insert. Eli Lilly and Company 2004. Revised 2017.
153. Effexor ER [Venlafaxine]. Package insert. Wyeth Pharmaceuticals LLC, a subsidiary of Pfizer Inc. 1997. Revised 2017.
154. Ferreira GE, McLachlan AJ, Lin CC, et al. Efficacy and safety of antidepressants for the treatment of back pain and osteoarthritis: systematic review and meta-analysis. BMJ. 2021;372:m4825. https://doi.org/10.1136/bmj.m4825.
155. O'Malley PG, Balden E, Tomkins G, Santoro J, Kroenke K, Jackson JL. Treatment of fibromyalgia with antidepressants: a meta-analysis. J Gen Intern Med. 2000;15(9):659–66. https://doi.org/10.1046/j.1525-1497.2000.06279.x.
156. Rothmore J. Antidepressant-induced sexual dysfunction. Med J Aust. 2020;212(7):329–34. https://doi.org/10.5694/mja2.50522. PMID: 32172535.
157. Carvalho AF, Sharma MS, Brunoni AR, et al. The safety, tolerability and risks associated with the use of newer generation antidepressant drugs: a critical review of the literature. Psychother Psychosom. 2016;85(5):270–88. https://doi.org/10.1159/000447034. PMID: 27508501.
158. Sansone RA, Sansone LA. Serotonin norepinephrine reuptake inhibitors: a pharmacological comparison. Innov Clin Neurosci. 2014;11(3–4):37–42.
159. Nolan L, O'Malley K. Adverse effects of antidepressants in the elderly. Drugs Aging. 1992;2(5):450–8. https://doi.org/10.2165/00002512-199202050-00008.
160. Carvalho AF, Sharma MS, Brunoni AR, et al. Fava; the safety, tolerability and risks associated with the use of newer generation antidepressant 159. Drugs: a critical review of the literature. Psychother Psychosom. 2016;85(5):270–88. https://doi.org/10.1159/000447034.
161. Marcy TR, Britton ML. Antidepressant-induced sweating. Ann Pharmacother. 2005;39:748–52.
162. Peretti S, Judge R, Hindmarch I. Safety and tolerability considerations: tricyclic antidepressants vs. selective serotonin reuptake inhibitors. Acta Psychiatr Scand Suppl. 2000;403:17–25.
163. Koçer E, Koçer A, Özsütçü M, et al. Dry eye related to commonly used new antidepressants. J Clin Psychopharmacol. 2015;35(4):411–3. https://doi.org/10.1097/JCP.0000000000000356. PMID: 26075491.
164. Bet PM, Hugtenburg JG, Penninx BW, et al. Side effects of antidepressants during long-term use in a naturalistic setting. Eur Neuropsychopharmacol. 2013;23(11):1443–51. https://doi.org/10.1016/j.euroneuro.2013.05.001. Epub 2013 May 30. PMID: 23726508.
165. Mills JA, Strawn JR. Antidepressant tolerability in pediatric anxiety and obsessive-compulsive disorders: a Bayesian hierarchical modeling meta-analysis. J Am Acad Child Adolesc Psychiatry. 2020;59(11):1240–51.
166. Li Y, Du X, Wu H. The risk of hyponatremia induced by SSRIs and SNRIs antidepressants: a systematic review and meta-analysis. BMC Pharmacol Toxicol. 2025;26(1):144. https://doi.org/10.1186/s40360-025-00977-1. PMID: 40764948; PMCID: PMC12323117.
167. Adrogué HJ, Madias NE. The challenge of hyponatremia. J Am Soc Nephrol. 2012;23(7):1140–8. https://doi.org/10.1681/ASN.2012020128. PMID: 22626822.
168. Pinkhasov A, Xiong G, Bourgeois JA, et al. Management of SIADH-related hyponatremia due to psychotropic medications – an expert consensus from the Association of Medicine and Psychiatry. J Psychosom Res. 2021;151:110654. https://doi.org/10.1016/j.jpsychores.2021.110654.
169. Wilson PWF, Polonsky TS, Miedema MD, et al. Systematic review for the 2018 AHA/ACC/AACVPR/AAPA/ABC/ACPM/ADA/AGS/APhA/ASPC/NLA/PCNA Guideline on the Management of Blood Cholesterol: A Report of the American College of Cardiology/American Heart Association Task Force on Clinical Practice Guidelines. J Am Coll Cardiol. 2019;73(24):3210–27. https://doi.org/10.1016/j.jacc.2018.11.004. Erratum in: J Am Coll Cardiol. 2019;73(24):3242. 10.1016/j.jacc.2019.05.011. PMID: 30423394.
170. Greist J, McNamara RK, Mallinckrodt CH, et al. Incidence and duration of antidepressant-induced nausea: duloxetine compared with paroxetine and fluoxetine. Clin Ther. 2004;26(9):1446–55. https://doi.org/10.1016/j.clinthera.2004.09.010. PMID: 15531007.
171. Mokhtare M, Chaharmahali A, Bahardoust M, et al. The effect of adding duloxetine to lansoprazole on symptom and quality of life improvement in patients with gastroesophageal reflux diseases: a randomized double-blind clinical trial. J Res Med Sci. 2021;26:4. https://doi.org/10.4103/jrms.JRMS_300_19. PMID: 34084183; PMCID: PMC8103956.
172. Vuppalanchi R, Hayashi PH, Chalasani N, et al. Duloxetine hepatotoxicity: a case-series from the drug-induced liver injury network. Aliment Pharmacol Ther. 2010;32:1174–83.

173. Vuppalanchi R, Hayashi PH, Chalasani N, et al. Drug-induced liver injury network (DILIN). Duloxetine hepatotoxicity: a case-series from the drug-induced liver injury network. Aliment Pharmacol Ther. 2010;32(9):1174–83. https://doi.org/10.1111/j.1365--2036.2010.04449.x. PMID: 20815829; PMCID: PMC3773985.
174. Sobay R, Küçük EV. An investigation of the effect of combining Tolterodine and Duloxetine in the treatment of mixed-type urinary incontinence and the factors affecting success. J Clin Med. 2025;14(10):3575. https://doi.org/10.3390/jcm14103575. PMID: 40429567; PMCID: PMC12112282.
175. Yadav J, Manocha N, Yadav A, et al. Urinary retention: an uncommon adverse effect of venlafaxine. Prim Care Companion CNS Disord. 2023;25(6):23cr03605. https://doi.org/10.4088/PCC.23cr03605. PMID: 38134407.
176. Calvi A, Fischetti I, Verzicco I, et al. Antidepressant drugs effects on blood pressure. Front Cardiovasc Med. 2021;8:704281. https://doi.org/10.3389/fcvm.2021.704281. PMID: 34414219; PMCID: PMC8370473.
177. Millan MJ. On 'polypharmacy' and multi-target agents, complementary strategies for improving the treatment of depression: a comparative appraisal. Int J Neuropsychopharmacol. 2014;17(4):1009–37. https://doi.org/10.1017/S1461145712001496.
178. Rush AJ, et al. Combining antidepressant medications: a good idea? Am J Psychiatry. 2010;167(3):241–3. https://doi.org/10.1176/appi.ajp.2009.09121768.
179. Gelenberg AJ, Freeman MP, et al. Practice guideline for the treatment of patients with major depressive disorder. 3rd ed. Washington, DC: American Psychiatric Publishing; 2010.
180. Lieberman JA 3rd. Managing anticholinergic side effects. Prim Care Companion J Clin Psychiatry. 2004;6(Suppl 2):20–3. Erratum in: Prim Care Companion J Clin Psychiatry. 2012;14(1):PCC.12lcx01362. PMID: 16001097; PMCID: PMC487008.
181. Hosenbocus S, Chahal R. SSRIs and SNRIs: a review of the discontinuation syndrome in children and adolescents. J Can Acad Child Adolesc Psychiatry. 2011;20(1):60–7. PMID: 21286371; PMCID: PMC3024727.
182. Fornaro M, Cattaneo CI, De Berardis D, et al. Antidepressant discontinuation syndrome: a state-of-the-art clinical review. Eur Neuropsychopharmacol. 2023;66:1–10. https://doi.org/10.1016/j.euroneuro.2022.10.005. PMID: 36345093.
183. Banham ND. Fatal venlafaxine overdose. Med J Aust. 1998;169(8):445–8. https://doi.org/10.5694/j.1326-5377.1998.tb126848.x.
184. Bosse GM, Spiller HA, Collins AM. A fatal case of venlafaxine overdose. J Med Toxicol. 2008;4(1):18–20. https://doi.org/10.1007/BF03160945.
185. Höjer J, Hulting J, Salmonson H. Fatal cardiotoxicity induced by venlafaxine overdosage. Clin Toxicol. 2008;46(4):336–7. https://doi.org/10.1080/15563650701358755.
186. Sarko J. Antidepressants, old and new. A review of their adverse effects and toxicity in overdose. Emerg Med Clin North Am. 2000;18(4):637–54. https://doi.org/10.1016/s0733-8627(05)70151-6.
187. Murphy L, Rasmussen J, Murphy NG. Venlafaxine overdose treated with extracorporeal life support. CMAJ. 2021;193:E167.
188. Marquetand C, Langer HF, Klein JP, Graf T. The use of extracorporeal life support in a patient suffering from venlafaxine intoxication. A case report. J Crit Care Med (Targu Mures). 2020;6:120.
189. Hoffmann M, Akbas S, Kindler R, et al. Successful use of extracorporeal life support and hemadsorption in the context of venlafaxine intoxication requiring cardiopulmonary resuscitation: a case report. J Artif Organs. 2024;27(2):167–71. https://doi.org/10.1007/s10047-023-01399-8. PMID: 37115336; PMCID: PMC11126471.
190. McCabe DJ, Radke JB, Wilson BZ. Disposition, outcomes, and lengths of stay due to bupropion overdose at a tertiary care center with a medical toxicology service. Am J Emerg Med. 2022;54:269.
191. Strawn JR, Prakash A, Zhang Q, et al. A randomized, placebo-controlled study of duloxetine for the treatment of children and adolescents with generalized anxiety disorder. J Am Acad Child Adolesc Psychiatry. 2015;54(4):283–93.
192. Rynn MA, Riddle MA, Yeung PP, et al. Efficacy and safety of extended-release venlafaxine in the treatment of generalized anxiety disorder in children and adolescents: two placebo-controlled trials. Am J Psychiatry. 2007;164(2):290–300.
193. Salvi V, Mencacci C, Barone-Adesi F. H1-histamine receptor affinity predicts weight gain with antidepressants. Eur Neuropsychopharmacol. 2016;26(10):1673–7.
194. Blumenthal SR, Castro VM, Clements CC, et al. An electronic health records study of long-term weight gain following antidepressant use. JAMA Psychiaty. 2014;71(8):889–96.
195. Furness S, Worthington HV, Bryan G, et al. Interventions for the management of dry mouth: topical therapies. Cochrane Database Syst Rev. 2011;7(12):CD008934.
196. Uher R, Farmer A, Henigsberg N, et al. Adverse reactions to antidepressants. Br J Psychiatry. 2009;195(3):202–10. https://doi.org/10.1192/bjp.bp.108.061960. Erratum in: Br J Psychiatry. 2010;196(5):417. PMID: 19721108.
197. Pollock BG. Adverse reactions of antidepressants in elderly patients. J Clin Psychiatry. 1999;60(Suppl 20):4–8.
198. Arana GW, Rosenbaum JF. Antidepressant drugs. In: Handbook of psychiatric drug therapy. 4th ed. Philadelphia: Lippincott Williams & Wilkins; 2000. p. 53.
199. Roos JC. Cardiac effects of antidepressant drugs. A comparison of the tricyclic antidepressants and fluvoxamine. Br J Clin Pharmacol. 1983;15(Suppl 3):439S–45S. https://doi.org/10.1111/j.1365-2125.1983.tb02135.x.
200. Remick RA. Anticholinergic side effects of tricyclic antidepressants and their management. Progress Neuro-Psychopharmacol Biol Psychiatry. 1988;12(2–3):225–31. https://doi.org/10.1016/0278-5846(88)90039-5. ISSN 0278-5846. https://www.sciencedirect.com/science/article/pii/0278584688900395
201. Thour A, Marwaha R. Amitriptyline. [Updated 2023 Jul 18]. In: StatPearls [Internet]. Treasure Island (FL): StatPearls Publishing; 2025. Available from: https://www.ncbi.nlm.nih.gov/books/NBK537225/.
202. Phentolamine ophthalmic solution (POS) 0.75% Ocuphire Pharma, Inc. Farmington Hills, MI. https://www.ryzumvi.com/files/prescribing-information.pdf.
203. McConaghy JR, Fosselman D. Hyperhidrosis: management options. Am Fam Physician. 2018;97(11):729–34.
204. Arora G, Kassir M, Patil A, et al. Treatment of axillary hyperhidrosis. J Cosmet Dermatol. 2022;21(1):62–70. https://doi.org/10.1111/jocd.14378.
205. Khalid MM, Waseem M. Tricyclic antidepressant toxicity. [Updated 2023 Jul 17]. In: StatPearls [Internet]. Treasure Island (FL): StatPearls Publishing; 2025. Available from: https://www.ncbi.nlm.nih.gov/books/NBK430931/.
206. Tisdale JE. Drug-Induced Diseases 3rd Edition CH 54 p1185-1230. (Chapter authors Wilson SM, Ross IA.)
207. Graudins A, Stearman A, Chan B. Treatment of the serotonin syndrome with cyproheptadine. J Emerg Med. 1998;16(4):615–9. https://doi.org/10.1016/s0736-4679(98)00057-2. PMID: 9696181.
208. McDaniel WW. Serotonin syndrome: early management with cyproheptadine. Ann Pharmacother. 2001;35(7–8):870–3. https://doi.org/10.1345/aph.10203. PMID: 11485136.
209. Woolf AD, Erdman AR, Nelson LS, et al. Tricyclic antidepressant poisoning: an evidence-based consensus guideline for out-of-hospital management. Clin Toxicol (Phila). 2007;45(3):203–33.

210. Clark S, Catt JW, Caffery T. Rapid diagnosis and treatment of severe tricyclic antidepressant toxicity. BMJ Case Rep. 2015; https://doi.org/10.1136/bcr-2015-211428. PMID: 26468220; PMCID: PMC4612524.
211. Ramasubbu B, James D, Scurr A, Sandilands EA. Serum alkalinisation is the cornerstone of treatment for amitriptyline poisoning. BMJ Case Rep. 2016;11 https://doi.org/10.1136/bcr--2016-214685. PMID: 27068728; PMCID: PMC4840635.
212. Ahmadinejad A, Saeed A, Davoodi M. Successful outcome following intralipid emulsion and plasmapheresis in a patient with profound neurologic and cardiovascular manifestations due to nortriptyline poisoning: a case report. Int J Emerg Med. 2025;8:61. https://doi.org/10.1186/s12245-025-00824-4.
213. Nishimura T, Maruguchi H, Nakao A, et al. Unusual complications from amitriptyline intoxication. BMJ Case Rep. 2017; https://doi.org/10.1136/bcr-2017-219257. PMID: 29018010; PMCID: PMC5652553.
214. Yates C, Galvao T, Sowinski KM, et al. EXTRIP workgroup. Extracorporeal treatment for tricyclic antidepressant poisoning: recommendations from the EXTRIP Workgroup. Semin Dial. 2014;27(4):381–9. https://doi.org/10.1111/sdi.12227. PMID: 24712820; PMCID: PMC4282541.

Clinically Significant Drug-Drug Interactions

20

Mariann D. Churchwell and Justin P. Reinert

Abbreviations

ADE	Adverse drug event
ADH	Antidiuretic hormone
AKI	Acute kidney injury
AUC	Area under the concentration–time curve
BBB	Blood–brain barrier
CBZ	Carbamazepine
CI	Confidence interval
Cmax	Maximum plasma concentration
CNS	Central nervous system
COPD	Chronic obstructive pulmonary disease
CYP	Cytochrome P450 enzyme system
DHP-CCB	Dihydropyridine calcium channel blocker
DOAC	Direct oral anticoagulant
DRESS	Drug reaction with eosinophilia and systemic symptoms
ECG	Electrocardiogram
FDA	U.S. Food and Drug Administration
G6PD	Glucose-6-phosphate dehydrogenase
GI	Gastrointestinal
INR	International normalized ratio
IV	Intravenous
LAST	Local anesthetic systemic toxicity
MAOI	Monoamine oxidase inhibitor
MgO	Magnesium oxide
NMDA	N-methyl-D-aspartate
NSAID	Nonsteroidal anti-inflammatory drug
OR	Odds ratio
PD	Pharmacodynamic
P-gp	P-glycoprotein
PK	Pharmacokinetic
QTc	Corrected QT interval
SIADH	Syndrome of inappropriate antidiuretic hormone secretion
SNRI	Serotonin-norepinephrine reuptake inhibitor
SSRI	Selective serotonin reuptake inhibitor
TCA	Tricyclic antidepressant
THC	Tetrahydrocannabinol
UGT	Uridine 5′-diphospho-glucuronosyltransferase
VPA	Valproic acid

Introduction

A drug-drug interaction is described as a clinically significant modification in the pharmacological response of a primary agent, known as the object drug, resulting from the concurrent administration of a secondary agent, known as the precipitant drug. The interaction of concern may alter the efficacy or safety profile of the object drug [1].

It is plausible to recognize that, alongside increased prescriptions for analgesic medications, a corresponding increase in the number of drug interactions with these drug would also be anticipated. The percentage of prescriptions for pain in a Scottish community was 15.7% in 1995 and 17.9% in 2010 [2]. Although there was an increase in prescribing for pain, it was not equal across the drug classes. There was an increase in paracetamol, opioid, and gabapentin/pregabalin prescribing, but to a lesser extent than tramadol, fentanyl, morphine, or oxycodone.

A cross-sectional study of analgesic prescribing in Ireland from 2014 to 2022 observed a decrease in nonsteroidal anti-inflammatory drug (NSAID) prescribing from 29.4% in 2014 to 25.0% in 2022. However, an increase in the prevalence of other analgesic drug classes during the study period was noted for paracetamol from 29.7% in 2014 to 32.0% in 2022, topical analgesics from 14.0% to 14.9%, and other analgesics (low-dose amitriptyline, pregabalin, and gabapentin) from 7.6% in 2014 to 9.6% in

M. D. Churchwell (✉) · J. P. Reinert
Department of Pharmacy Practice, The University of Toledo College of Pharmacy and Pharmaceutical Sciences, Toledo, OH, USA
e-mail: Mariann.Churchwell@utoledo.edu

J. P. Reinert et al. (eds.), *Adjunctive Analgesic Strategies for the Bedside Clinician and Beyond*,
https://doi.org/10.1007/978-3-032-21675-5_20

2022. Opioids with the highest prevalence were codeine, with an increase from 12.8% to 14.9%; oxycodone prescribing increased from 1.2% to 2.1%, and tramadol decreased from 7.3% to 5.4% [3].

The focus of this chapter is to examine clinically significant drug-drug interactions for commonly used adjunctive analgesics for the management of pain. Most of the drugs discussed in this chapter have a long list of warnings and precautions listed in tertiary drug references. Some of the most frequent adverse drug effects reported are excess sedation, drowsiness, or increased central nervous system effects related to the precipitant drug or substance (i.e., alcohol, anti-seizure drugs, barbiturates, opioids, and tricyclic antidepressants).

Gabapentinoids

Gabapentin and pregabalin are mainly eliminated in urine as unchanged drugs, with a minor amount of the drugs undergoing metabolism [4]. Overall, gabapentinoids do not interact with other medications. Still, the most reported drug-drug interactions associated with the gabapentinoids are due to concomitant use of drugs affecting the central nervous system, which may increase sedation, drowsiness, confusion, and impaired coordination from the gabapentinoids [4].

In 2009 the American Geriatric Society recommended gabapentinoids as an adjuvant analgesic with or without opioids to manage chronic noncancer pain; Following this recommendation, the reported use of a gabapentinoid in patients ≥65 years old has significantly increased [5, 6]. A cross-sectional study was conducted among older Medicare beneficiaries (aged ≥65 years) with chronic noncancer pain who filled ≥1 opioid prescription within 3 months after a randomly selected chronic noncancer pain diagnosis (index date) in a calendar year between 2011 and 2018. 19.8% of the study sample had concurrent opioid–gabapentinoid use during their follow-up period between 2011 and 2018. The prevalence of concurrent use increased from 17.0% in 2011 to 23.5% in 2018 [6]. An examination of patients who received a prescription for an opioid and gabapentin found that there was a significant increase in the odds of opioid-related death (odds ratio [OR] 1.99, 95% CI 1.61 to 2.47, $p < 0.001$) when compared to patients who received only an opioid prescription. The authors also evaluated dosing using a dose-response analysis, which showed that the likelihood of death was higher with higher dosing, but patients receiving a moderate gabapentin dose were also at risk [moderate-dose (OR 2.05, 95% CI 1.46 to 2.87, $p < 0.001$) and high-dose (OR 2.20, 95% CI 1.58 to 3.08, $p < 0.001$)]. This analysis found that the combination of gabapentin with an opioid was associated with a nearly 60% increase in the odds of opioid-related death when compared to no gabapentin usage [7].

The combination of morphine and gabapentin resulted in a significant increase in pain tolerance compared to either drug administered alone with a placebo. The drug-drug interaction with morphine resulted in an increase in gabapentin AUC and a decrease in its clearance [8].

A decrease in gabapentin's effectiveness was reported when taken with antacids. Gabapentin 200 mg and magnesium oxide (MgO) 1 gram or omeprazole 20 mg were administered to healthy adults to determine if either drug influenced gabapentin concentrations [9]. Gabapentin concentrations were significantly decreased in those who received gabapentin and MgO compared to gabapentin alone or with omeprazole. Taking the antacid aluminum hydroxide/magnesium hydroxide and gabapentin at the same time results in a decrease in gabapentin bioavailability by 20%. If gabapentin is taken 2 hours after the antacid, the serum concentration is decreased by 10% [9]. Certizine may decrease gabapentin concentrations, resulting in a reduction in the effect of gabapentin on neuropathic pain [10]. The mechanism for this drug-drug interaction is not well-defined.

Gabapentin enacarbil, a prodrug of gabapentin, interacts with cimetidine, resulting in a 24% increase in gabapentin's area under the curve (AUC) and a decrease in the renal clearance of gabapentin when coadministered [11]. Administration of gabapentin enacarbil and morphine did not significantly alter the pharmacokinetics of either drug, but there was an increase in dizziness and somnolence when these drugs were coadministered [12].

The Federal Drug Administration (FDA) issued a Safety Alert for gabapentin and pregabalin when used with drugs that depress the central nervous system (CNS) in elderly patients and those with lung dysfunction, such as chronic obstructive pulmonary disease (COPD). The FDA warns about serious breathing problems with seizures when these agents are coadministered [13].

Pregabalin

Pregabalin is principally excreted unchanged in the urine, undergoes minimal metabolism, and does not bind to plasma proteins. Studies of pregabalin report that it is unlikely to have significant pharmacokinetic drug interactions and it does not interact with carbamazepine, valproic acid, lamotrigine, phenytoin, phenobarbital, and topiramate [4].

No pharmacokinetic interactions were seen with multiple oral doses of pregabalin when coadministered with oxycodone, lorazepam, or ethanol, but additive effects on cognitive and gross motor functioning were seen with coadministration. No clinically significant effects on respiration were seen [4].

Pregabalin, when combined with remifentanil, had additive analgesic effects. Still, respiratory depression was reported with an increase in end-tidal carbon dioxide of

16.4 mmHg (11.3 to 21.5, $P < 0.001$) when compared to the placebo of either drug separately [14]. Cognitive tests were also negatively affected when pregabalin and remifentanil were combined [14].

Carbamazepine

Carbamazepine is metabolized in the liver by cytochrome P450 3A4 into an active epoxide metabolite. With chronic use, it induces hepatic enzymes, accelerating the metabolism of itself and other drugs, thereby shortening its half-life over time. Approximately 18% of the drug is excreted via feces, with the remainder primarily eliminated in the urine [15]. Because carbamazepine is a CYP inducer, it can boost the metabolism of coadministered drugs that are processed by CYP 3A4, 2C9, and 2C19, leading to clinically relevant drug-drug interactions. For example, coadministration can lead to lower serum concentrations of clonazepam, felbamate, lamotrigine, levetiracetam, phenytoin, topiramate, valproate, and zonisamide. Monitoring and dosage adjustments are recommended if patients require treatment with carbamazepine and aripiprazole (increase dose), tacrolimus (monitoring), and lapatinib (avoid or careful titration).

The combination of carbamazepine with omeprazole, quinine, diltiazem, or verapamil may raise the risk of carbamazepine toxicity due to increased carbamazepine concentrations [16, 17]. Drugs that inhibit human microsomal epoxide hydrolase may increase carbamazepine-10,11 epoxide plasma concentrations and the risk of neurotoxicity. The list of drugs includes loxapine, quetiapine, valproic acid, and valproate, and dosage adjustments and carbamazepine monitoring are recommended when these drugs are coadministered [15].

Carbamazepine metabolism may be increased when coadministered with CYP3A4 inducers, resulting in decreased carbamazepine concentrations. CYP3A4 inducers include cisplatin, doxorubicin HCl, felbamate, fosphenytoin, rifampin, phenobarbital, phenytoin, primidone, methsuximide, theophylline, and aminophylline. Carbamazepine also affects the plasma concentrations of valproate, and it should be monitored when carbamazepine is introduced or withdrawn.

Carbamazepine-induced hyponatremia may occur independently at higher doses or additively with other medications such as serotonin-norepinephrine reuptake inhibitors, for example, duloxetine. An increase in carbamazepine serum concentrations and liver enzymes was reported with the coadministration of isoniazid. Liver enzymes continued to rise for 3 days after stopping isoniazid but returned to normal after 8 days post-isoniazid stoppage [16].

Other drug interactions include the inhibition of carbamazepine (CBZ) metabolism with verapamil administration, resulting in increased CBZ concentrations up to 46% (33% free plasma CBZ) during a dosing interval. Neurotoxicity was reported in several patients within a few days of coadministration [17]. Also, administration of direct oral anticoagulants such as rivaroxaban, apixaban, dabigatran, and edoxaban with carbamazepine may result in decreased plasma concentrations and reduced therapeutic efficacy. Rivaroxaban AUC_t decreased by 57.9%, and C_{max} decreased by 43.3% after administration of carbamazepine, resulting in a reduction of rivaroxaban efficacy [18].

The plasma concentrations of cannabinoid drugs containing tetrahydrocannabinol (THC) and its active metabolite 11-OH-THC can be decreased by strong CYP3A4 inducers such as carbamazepine [19].

Valproic Acid

Valproic acid (VPA) is mainly metabolized by the hepatic system via glucuronide conjugation (30–50%) and mitochondrial beta-oxidation (40%). Elimination in urine occurs as a glucuronide conjugate (30–50%) [20]. Valproic acid drug interactions are dependent on the perpetrator drug's pharmacokinetics and pharmacodynamics, for example, whether the interaction is enzyme-based or transporter-based.

Valproic acid is a weak CYP450 inhibitor, including CYP2C9 and CYP2C19, which results in enzyme-inducing drug interactions. These interactions include carbamazepine, phenytoin, and rifampin, which can increase the metabolism of VPA, resulting in reduced plasma concentrations that may require VPA dose adjustments or alternative treatment options for effective treatment [20].

Enzyme-inhibiting drug interactions with VPA occur because it is primarily metabolized via the glucuronidation pathway, mediated by uridine 5′-diphospho-glucuronosyltransferase (UGT) enzymes. Drugs that inhibit UGT can increase the plasma concentrations of VPA. Patients' VPA concentrations need to be monitored closely when coadministering drugs that inhibit the UGT enzyme, including aspirin, felbamate, and certain nonsteroidal anti-inflammatory drugs (NSAIDs). A study of felbamate and VPA administration observed a decrease in VPA clearance, resulting in a 28–54% increase in VPA concentrations [21]. An examination of naproxen and VPA revealed an increase in naproxen (10%) and VPA (20%) when administered together [22].

Valproic acid is highly bound to protein, mainly albumin [23]. The concurrent administration of VPA with other highly protein-bound medications (i.e., phenytoin, salicylates, and sulfonamides) may compete for albumin-binding sites, potentially increasing the free fraction of VPA. This interaction could increase adverse drug events (ADEs) associated with VPA; clinicians should monitor for signs of VPA toxicity and adjust VPA dosing as needed.

Cutaneous reactions have been reported with VPA and antiseizure therapies. One case report noted that within 3–4 days of adding lamotrigine, a patient experienced painful mouth ulcers, bleeding lips, rashes, and a fever. The patient was diagnosed with Stevens-Johnson Syndrome and was treated with IV fluids, prednisone, and cyclosporin [24]. This drug interaction is likely due to VPA's interference with lamotrigine clearance, resulting in higher concentrations of lamotrigine. A patient receiving serial administration of phenytoin, VPA, and phenobarbital developed a fever and maculopapular rash with erythema that was diagnosed as drug reaction with eosinophilia and systemic symptoms (DRESS). This drug-drug interaction resulted in fulminant liver failure requiring a transfer to a liver transplant center [25]. The interaction between VPA and anti-seizure medications can alter plasma concentrations, impacting efficacy and toxicity. Monitoring of drug concentrations is recommended, with dosing adjustments made as necessary.

Valproic acid serum concentrations can be reduced by administering a carbapenem antimicrobial agent. The reduction in VPA concentrations could potentiate a seizure and require monitoring [26]. The proposed mechanism involves the inhibition of a hepatic enzyme, acyl peptide hydrolase, which hydrolyzes VPA glucuronide, thereby increasing VPA elimination. This interaction appears to have a rapid onset and can reduce VPA concentrations by 60%. Ertapenem and meropenem appear to affect VPA concentrations more than imipenem/cilastatin [27].

Ritonavir coadministration with VPA may reduce VPA concentrations, possibly due to ritonavir's induction of glucuronidation. A report documents a patient receiving VPA with lopinavir/ritonavir, zidovudine, and lamivudine, which led to a reduction of VPA concentration by 48% and a recurrence of manic disease [28].

The risk for valproate-induced hyperammonemia with or without encephalopathy is increased when patients receive phenobarbital, phenytoin, or topiramate with VPA [29]. The pathway of this interaction is unknown, but excessive activation of N-methyl-D-aspartate (NMDA) receptors is suspected. A case of topiramate-VPA-induced hyperammonemia was attributed to an L-carnitine deficiency, as arginine is critical for ammonia detoxification into urea. The patient did not improve with L-carnitine supplementation, lactulose, and a reduction in the topiramate dose; therefore, VPA was stopped. L-carnitine supplementation, lactulose, and topiramate were continued as the patient improved after VPA was stopped [30].

Selective Serotonin Reuptake Inhibitors

SSRIs are well-known for their ability to inhibit hepatic cytochrome P450 (CYP) enzymes, particularly CYP2D6, CYP2C19, CYP1A2, and CYP3A4, depending on the agent [31–33]. Fluvoxamine, fluoxetine, and paroxetine are among the most potent inhibitors and are therefore most likely to precipitate drug-drug interactions via metabolic interference [34, 35]. These interactions can elevate serum concentrations of coadministered drugs, potentially resulting in adverse effects or toxicity. Coadministration with warfarin or clopidogrel can lead to increased bleeding risk or reduced antiplatelet efficacy, respectively, while interactions with drugs such as metoprolol, propranolol, clozapine, tamoxifen, and certain benzodiazepines may result in exaggerated pharmacologic effects [34, 35]. Clinicians should be especially cautious with fluvoxamine, which significantly inhibits CYP1A2, leading to notable increases in plasma concentrations of tizanidine and other CYP1A2 substrates [36, 37].

SSRIs impair platelet aggregation by depleting intraplatelet serotonin, a key mediator of platelet activation. [38] When used concomitantly with agents that also affect hemostasis, such as NSAIDs, aspirin, warfarin, or P2Y12 inhibitors, the bleeding risk is substantially magnified [39, 40]. Clinical data suggest a two- to sixfold increase in gastrointestinal bleeding risk, particularly in elderly patients and those with additional risk factors [41, 42]. Notably, combining SSRIs with NSAIDs poses a greater bleeding risk than either agent alone, and concurrent use with antiplatelet drugs like clopidogrel or prasugrel has been linked to an increased risk of upper GI and intracranial hemorrhage [39, 42, 43]. While the absolute risk may remain low in some populations, the relative risk increase is clinically relevant, warranting caution, monitoring, and in some cases, co-prescription of gastroprotective agents.

Serotonin syndrome is a potentially life-threatening condition resulting from overstimulation of central and peripheral serotonin receptors, particularly 5-HT1A and 5-HT2A [44]. SSRIs significantly increase serotonergic tone, and when used with other serotonergic agents, such as monoamine oxidase inhibitors (MAO) (e.g., linezolid, phenelzine), serotonergic opioids (e.g., tramadol, meperidine), triptans, mirtazapine, or herbal products like St. John's wort, the risk of serotonin syndrome increases substantially [45]. Clinically, this syndrome presents with autonomic instability, hyperthermia, agitation, neuromuscular hyperactivity (e.g., clonus, tremor), and altered mental status [44]. Fluoxetine's long half-life demands a particularly extended washout period before initiating an MAOI. Clinicians should be vigilant in avoiding serotonergic combinations and educating patients on early signs and symptoms of serotonin toxicity [44].

SSRIs are associated with an increased risk of hyponatremia, particularly in elderly patients or those concurrently using diuretics [46, 47]. This effect is thought to be mediated via inappropriate antidiuretic hormone secretion (SIADH), which may be potentiated by thiazide or loop diuretics. The onset is typically insidious, and symptoms may range from mild cognitive disturbances to seizures or coma in severe cases. Routine monitoring of serum sodium is recommended in at-risk populations, especially within the first few weeks of therapy or after dosage increases [46, 47].

Among SSRIs, citalopram and escitalopram carry the highest risk for QTc prolongation, particularly at higher doses or in the setting of coadministration with other QT-prolonging agents such as amiodarone, sotalol, or methadone. [48, 49] The mechanism involves inhibition of cardiac potassium channels, which can predispose patients to torsades de pointes and other life-threatening arrhythmias [49]. In clinical practice, this necessitates ECG monitoring, especially in patients with underlying cardiac disease, electrolyte disturbances, or those receiving interacting medications. Additionally, pharmacokinetic interactions may elevate SSRI levels and potentiate this risk further [48, 49].

Less common, but clinically significant, interactions include those between SSRIs and agents like sildenafil, where fluoxetine or fluvoxamine can inhibit CYP3A4 and increase sildenafil levels, occasionally resulting in cardiovascular events such as myocardial infarction or priapism [50, 51]. St. John's wort, a CYP inducer and serotonergic agent, may reduce SSRI efficacy and simultaneously increase the risk of serotonin syndrome when combined [31]. These examples underscore the importance of evaluating all prescription, over-the-counter, and herbal products for interaction potential when initiating or modifying SSRI therapy.

Selective Norepinephrine Reuptake Inhibitors

Venlafaxine and duloxetine are primarily metabolized via CYP2D6 and, to a lesser extent, CYP1A2/3A4 for duloxetine, making them vulnerable to pharmacokinetic interactions when co-prescribed with CYP inhibitors or inducers [52, 53]. Duloxetine specifically is inhibited by strong CYP2D6 and CYP3A4 inhibitors such as fluoxetine, paroxetine, fluvoxamine, ketoconazole, or itraconazole, leading to significantly elevated serum concentrations and potential toxicity or adverse effects [53, 54]. Additionally, venlafaxine bioavailability can be altered via drugs affecting CYP2D6, such as bupropion, raising venlafaxine levels at the expense of its active metabolite desvenlafaxine, which may change clinical response thresholds [52].

As with SSRIs, SNRIs impair platelet serotonin uptake, increasing bleeding risk in patients on concomitant anticoagulants, antiplatelet agents, or NSAIDs. A systematic review highlighted elevated risk for GI and intracranial hemorrhage when SNRIs are used with these agents, mediated primarily through pharmacodynamic synergy rather than metabolism [40].

SNRIs can precipitate hyponatremia by potentiating inappropriate ADH secretion, particularly in elderly patients or those taking diuretics [55, 56]. Although literature is more extensive for mirtazapine and SSRIs, duloxetine has also been implicated, and risk should be monitored early in therapy initiation or dose escalation, especially in vulnerable populations.

SNRIs increase norepinephrine levels, with corresponding effects on blood pressure and heart rate [57, 58]. Duloxetine's noradrenergic action may exacerbate hypertension and require monitoring, especially when combined with antihypertensive agents or stimulants [59]. Patients with uncontrolled hypertension or cardiac disease should be monitored closely, and combination with other agents raising norepinephrine is cautioned.

Various rare but clinically significant interactions include visual and auditory hallucinations reported with venlafaxine coadministered with propafenone and serotonin syndrome reported with combinations including weight reduction agents, trazodone, pethidine, dihydroergotamine, or herbal supplements like ginseng [44, 60, 61]. Furthermore, polypharmacy with agents such as calcineurin inhibitors or lithium has been associated with serotonin toxicity when combined with SNRIs like venlafaxine or desvenlafaxine [62, 63].

Tricyclic Antidepressants

Tricyclic antidepressants (TCAs), including tertiary agents such as amitriptyline, imipramine, and clomipramine, and secondary agents, including nortriptyline and desipramine, are metabolized by several CYP450 enzymes, primarily CYP2D6, CYP2C19, CYP1A2, and CYP3A4 [64]. While TCAs themselves are generally weaker inhibitors of CYPs compared to SSRIs, potent inhibitors such as fluoxetine, paroxetine, fluvoxamine, cimetidine, and ketoconazole can significantly increase TCA plasma concentrations, often two- to fourfold, elevating risks of anticholinergic effects, sedation, cardiovascular arrhythmias, or serotonin syndrome [65]. For example, fluoxetine added to amitriptyline therapy has been shown to double amitriptyline levels and elevate nortriptyline by 1.5-fold [65]. Conversely, CYP inducers such as carbamazepine, phenytoin, barbiturates or St. John's wort may reduce TCA levels and risk therapeutic failure [66].

Combining TCAs with other serotonergic drugs poses a risk of serotonin syndrome. This is especially pronounced with potent serotonergic TCAs such as clomipramine and imipramine, particularly when combined with MAOIs, which irreversibly block serotonin breakdown [67, 68]. Case series and controlled trials report rapid onset of severe autonomic, neuromuscular and mental status changes, and fatalities have been observed when clomipramine and MAOIs are combined [68, 69]. Moreover, even fluoxetine plus amitriptyline can increase TCA levels four- to fivefold and precipitate serotonin toxicity via both pharmacokinetic and pharmacodynamic synergy [65, 70].

TCAs share electrophysiological properties with class IA and III antiarrhythmic drugs, including QT prolongation and sodium-channel blockade, making combinations with other QT-prolonging agents particularly risky for ventricular arrhythmias or torsades de pointes [71, 72]. TCAs also have pronounced anticholinergic and antihistaminic effects; coadministration with other agents that depress CNS function, such as benzodiazepines, antihistamines, or antipsychotics, can produce additive sedation, risk of delirium, urinary retention and ileus [73].

Though direct evidence is limited, some TCAs may alter bleeding risk via interference with platelet serotonin uptake or displacement of plasma protein-bound anticoagulants. Occasional reports describe INR fluctuations when combined with warfarin; clinicians should monitor coagulation parameters when adding or withdrawing TCAs in patients on anticoagulants [74, 75].

TCAs blunt the antihypertensive efficacy of clonidine by blocking presynaptic alpha-2 receptors and may antagonize guanethidine. Conversely, TCAs potentiate the effects of sympathomimetic agents such as epinephrine and phenylephrine, increasing the risk of hypertensive episodes. Their noradrenergic effects may be compounded in combination with other stimulants or amphetamines [76, 77].

NSAIDs

NSAIDs significantly elevate bleeding risk when used with anticoagulants or antiplatelet agents [78]. Randomized and observational studies demonstrate approximately a twofold increase in gastrointestinal bleeding when NSAIDs are added to warfarin therapy compared with warfarin alone (OR $\approx$ 1.98 for GI bleeds; general bleeding OR $\approx$ 1.58) [79]. The pharmacodynamic interaction arises from NSAID-induced gastroduodenal mucosal injury and inhibition of platelet function. In patients also receiving SSRIs or aspirin, the risk is compounded further [80, 81]. Meta-analyses and cohort studies show that concurrent SSRI + NSAID use can increase GI bleeding risk 2–6× above baseline, yielding a small number needed to harm in high-risk populations [78, 81–83].

NSAIDs constrict afferent renal arterioles by inhibiting prostaglandin-mediated vasodilation, while angiotensin-converting enzyme inhibitors (ACE-Is) /angiotensinogen II receptor blockers (ARBs) dilate the efferent arteriole, and diuretics decrease intravascular volume [84, 85]. When all three classes are combined, renal autoregulation fails and acute kidney injury (AKI) risk rises significantly, up to approximately 31% increased among patients on all three agents, with most cases occurring within the first 30 days of combination therapy [84, 85]. This interaction is especially relevant in older adults and those with baseline renal impairment.

NSAIDs diminish the therapeutic effects of antihypertensive agents, including ACE inhibitors, ARBs, and beta-blockers, as well as diuretics, by promoting sodium and water retention and reducing renal perfusion. This pharmacodynamic antagonism often leads to diminished blood pressure control and possible volume overload or worsening heart failure [84, 86–88]. Epidemiologic studies corroborate a dose-dependent increase in myocardial infarction and stroke risk with prolonged NSAID therapy [88, 89].

NSAIDs reduce renal clearance of medications. Lithium is significantly implicated, leading to elevated serum lithium levels and risk of toxicity, including tremor, confusion, and ataxia. Case series document increases in lithium concentration by more than 50–400% when NSAIDs are coadministered [82]. NSAIDs can also interfere with the renal excretion of methotrexate, increasing the risk of hepatotoxicity and nephrotoxicity. While data are more limited than for other drugs, clinical reports warn against co-prescribing NSAIDs during methotrexate therapy without monitoring [82].

Acetaminophen

Acetaminophen, particularly when taken in moderate to high doses, defined as 2–4 grams/day over several days, has been linked to supratherapeutic INR and bleeding in patients on warfarin [90, 91]. One case-control study found acetaminophen was responsible for approximately 30% of INR elevations above 6 in warfarin users, even at typical analgesic doses [90]. Case reports describe patients developing gingival, GI, or retroperitoneal bleeding with INR values as high as 16 after 4–10 days of therapy (1–4 g/day) [92]. Reviews and randomized crossover trials confirm this dose-dependent INR elevation. Clinical guidance recommends keeping acetaminophen under 2 g/day in warfarin users and performing more frequent INR monitoring [93].

Chronic alcohol consumption induces CYP2E1 and depletes glutathione, significantly increasing production and accumulation of n-acetyl-p-benzoquinone imine (NAPQI), acetaminophen's hepatotoxic metabolite, thus elevating liver injury risk even at therapeutic doses [94]. Co-use of other CYP2E1 inducers like isoniazid, phenobarbital, or phenytoin may also enhance hepatotoxic risk via similar metabolic pathways [95, 96].

Chronic use of enzyme-inducing medications like phenytoin or phenobarbital can accelerate acetaminophen metabolism, increasing the formation of toxic NAPQI and potentially decreasing analgesic efficacy [97, 98]. Case reports have linked this combination with severe liver damage even at standard dosing. Routine liver function monitoring and dose caution are advised [97, 98].

Agents affecting gastric emptying may modestly alter acetaminophen absorption. Metoclopramide shortens the time to peak concentration, while opioids or anticholinergics may delay absorption [99, 100]. These changes generally lack well-established clinical repercussions for the overall analgesic effect. Acetaminophen also inhibits sulfation of ethinylestradiol, increasing its plasma concentration by 22%, which may have theoretical implications for combined oral contraceptive dosing or side effects, though clinical correlation remains limited [101].

Many over-the-counter and prescription combination products include acetaminophen, increasing the risk of unintentional overdose and hepatotoxicity if multiple products are used concurrently. When combined with codeine, there is additional risk of respiratory depression, especially with CNS depressants; opioid-sparing effects altered by CYP2D6 inhibitors or inducers; and heightened abuse potential or dependence [102].

Topical Analgesics

Topical NSAIDs have minimal systemic absorption, with approximately 1% of that seen with oral diclofenac [103]. This dramatically reduces but does not eliminate systemic interaction risk. Randomized crossover studies show that topical diclofenac does not meaningfully interfere with loop diuretic pharmacodynamics, unlike the oral NSAID forms [103]. Guidelines support topical NSAIDs as safer than oral formulations, especially in patients on ACE inhibitors, ARBs, beta-blockers, or other cardiovascular agents, with no evidence of significant interaction; however, case reports have described INR elevation and GI bleeding when topical methyl salicylate was used in warfarin-treated patients, likely via displacement or inhibition effects [104, 105], Similarly, topical NSAIDs combined with warfarin have yielded rare reports of increased anticoagulation, prompting recommendations for more frequent INR monitoring in such scenarios [106].

Topical counter-irritants and local anesthetic patches typically act locally with very low systemic exposure, and major drug interactions are rare. Tertiary drug information sources indicate that capsaicin, lidocaine, and menthol topical formulations have over 90 listed interactions, but only two are classified as major, with the remainder being listed as mild or theoretical [107, 108]. One clinically relevant interaction is the additive risk of methemoglobinemia when lidocaine patch use overlaps with other methemoglobin-inducing agents, particularly in vulnerable patient populations such as infants and those with G6PD deficiency due to systemic absorption even from topical use [109]. While capsaicin has been shown in vitro to induce CYP3A4 expression, typical topical use does not reach systemic levels high enough to alter CYP-mediated metabolism appreciably [110].

IV Lidocaine

Intravenous lidocaine is extensively metabolized in the liver by CYP3A4 and CYP1A2 into active and inactive metabolites [111]. In vitro studies using human liver microsomes demonstrate that midazolam noncompetitively inhibits lidocaine metabolism and thiamylal is a competitive inhibitor, suggesting potential for elevated plasma lidocaine levels and toxicity when coadministered with these agents [112]. Cimetidine, pancuronium, and vecuronium showed weaker inhibition, but still within therapeutic ranges, notably raising concern in sedated patients receiving combination therapies that affect CYP450 pathways [112].

IV lidocaine has a narrow therapeutic index with a target plasma range of 2.5–3.5 μg/mL [113]. Supratherapeutic lidocaine levels are associated with local anesthetic systemic toxicity (LAST) [114]. Neurologic toxicity such as perioral tingling, dizziness, and tinnitus occurs above 5 μg/mL, progressing to seizures or coma at higher concentrations [114–116]. Cardiotoxic effects, including bradycardia, conduction block, and arrhythmias, typically emerge at yet higher levels of 10–15 μg/mL and may be exacerbated by metabolic acidosis, hypoxia, hypoalbuminemia, or concurrent medications delaying metabolism [117]. Agents that impair hepatic function or reduce protein binding may further potentiate toxicity risks.

Lidocaine is often coadministered with sedatives like propofol or midazolam. Its synergistic sedative and respiratory depressant effects can enhance hypotension or bradycardia; studies recommend dose reductions of coadministered sedatives when using lidocaine infusions. Moreover, in vitro midazolam-mediated CYP inhibition may elevate lidocaine levels, compounding CNS-depressant effects and toxicity concern [112]. There are clinical reports and pharmacologic concerns that mixing lidocaine with propofol in the same syringe may alter solution pH and promote lipid emulsion stability issues, potentially forming precipitates or liposomes with embolic risk. These studies caution against routine mixing despite observed practices [118].

Skeletal Muscle Relaxants

Across the skeletal muscle relaxant class, the majority of clinically significant interactions are pharmacodynamic in nature, reflecting additive CNS or cardiorespiratory depression, anticholinergic load, or hemodynamic instability, rather than purely pharmacokinetic. Tizanidine and carisoprodol represent notable exceptions where defined metabolic pathways contribute to clinically consequential pharmacokinetic interactions. Awareness of these patterns is essential when designing pharmacotherapy regimens in patients with polypharmacy, hepatic or renal impairment, or advanced age. A review of specific interactions related to select skeletal muscle relaxant use is described below.

Baclofen

Clinically important interactions with baclofen primarily involve additive central nervous system (CNS) depression and altered anticoagulant response [119]. Coadministration with opioids, benzodiazepines, sedative-hypnotics, or alcohol potentiates sedation, confusion, and respiratory depression, particularly in older adults or those with impaired renal clearance [119]. Rare case reports have described potentiation of warfarin's anticoagulant effect during concurrent baclofen therapy, manifesting as elevated international normalized ratios and bleeding events. Although the mechanism remains uncertain, the interaction underscores the need for close INR monitoring when baclofen is introduced in patients stabilized on warfarin [120]. Clinicians should exercise caution when prescribing baclofen alongside any sedative or anticoagulant regimen and consider dose adjustments or enhanced surveillance in patients with renal impairment.

Tizanidine

Tizanidine is notable for pharmacokinetic interactions mediated by cytochrome P450 1A2 (CYP1A2) inhibition [121]. Concomitant administration with potent CYP1A2 inhibitors, most prominently ciprofloxacin and fluvoxamine, can result in several-fold increases in systemic tizanidine concentrations, leading to profound hypotension, bradycardia, and excessive somnolence [121, 122]. Because of these findings, these combinations are formally contraindicated in prescribing information and substantiated by clinical case data. Additive pharmacodynamic effects are also significant; concomitant use with antihypertensive drugs, sedatives, or other α_2-adrenergic agonists increases the likelihood of orthostatic hypotension, dizziness, and falls [123]. When tizanidine must be used in patients on potential CYP1A2 inhibitors or multiple antihypertensives, gradual titration from low doses and close monitoring of blood pressure and mental status are recommended.

Cyclobenzaprine

The interaction profile of cyclobenzaprine reflects its structural and pharmacologic similarity to tricyclic antidepressants. Concomitant use with other CNS-sedating medications or substances results in additive sedation and psychomotor impairment, substantially increasing fall and accident risk [119, 124]. Moreover, because cyclobenzaprine possesses serotonergic activity, concurrent administration with monoamine oxidase inhibitors (MAOIs), selective serotonin reuptake inhibitors (SSRIs), or other serotonergic agents can precipitate serotonin toxicity characterized by agitation, autonomic instability, and neuromuscular hyperactivity [125]. Case reports and postmarketing surveillance data describe such events, though they remain infrequent [126]. Cyclobenzaprine also contributes to anticholinergic burden when combined with first-generation antihistamines or tricyclic antidepressants, predisposing to confusion, urinary retention, or tachyarrhythmias in susceptible populations. Overall, clinicians should avoid overlapping serotonergic or strongly anticholinergic drugs and limit combined CNS depressant exposure.

Carisoprodol

Carisoprodol's interactions are dominated by additive CNS depression and metabolic concerns related to CYP2C19. Coadministration with opioids, benzodiazepines, barbiturates, or alcohol can lead to synergistic respiratory depression, excessive sedation, and fatal overdose [127]. These effects are particularly pronounced due to its active metabolite, meprobamate, a sedative-hypnotic with abuse potential [128, 129]. Patients who are poor metabolizers via CYP2C19 or who receive strong CYP2C19 inhibitors such as omeprazole may accumulate higher concentrations of carisoprodol and meprobamate, predisposing them to toxicity [128]. Clinicians should therefore avoid prescribing carisoprodol in combination with other CNS depressants, limit its use to short courses, and remain vigilant for signs of misuse or dependence.

Chlorzoxazone

Although used less frequently in contemporary practice, chlorzoxazone exhibits extensive interaction potential. It undergoes hepatic metabolism involving multiple oxidative pathways and has been demonstrated to alter the pharmacokinetics of other cytochrome P450 substrates in controlled studies. In one human trial, chlorzoxazone significantly increased the oral bioavailability of midazolam, suggesting inhibition of gastrointestinal CYP3A activity [130]. The drug's labeling also notes additive CNS depression when combined with alcohol, opioids, or sedative-hypnotics, as well as heightened hepatotoxic risk when coadministered with other hepatically metabolized or hepatotoxic agents such as isoniazid or acetaminophen. Given these findings, clinicians should perform comprehensive medication reconciliation before initiating chlorzoxazone and monitor liver function during combined therapy.

Methocarbamol

Methocarbamol interacts primarily through additive CNS depression. Concomitant administration with alcohol, opioids, benzodiazepines, or other sedatives produces enhanced somnolence, respiratory depression, and decreased psychomotor performance. These effects are magnified in geriatric patients and in those with hepatic or renal impairment. Case reports of overdose and fatal respiratory depression involving methocarbamol in combination with other depressants highlight the clinical relevance of this risk [131]. Although specific enzyme-mediated interactions are not well documented, prudent prescribing requires dose reduction or avoidance of polypharmacy involving multiple CNS depressants.

Metaxolone

Metaxolone shares a similar adverse interaction profile, characterized by additive CNS depression and hepatotoxic risk. Reports of excessive sedation and respiratory compromise have occurred when metaxolone is combined with ethanol, opioids, or benzodiazepines [131]. Serotonin syndrome may also be an implicated adverse effect when metaxolone interacts with a serotonergic medication [132]. Because metaxolone undergoes hepatic metabolism, concurrent administration with drugs that alter hepatic enzyme activity, such as carbamazepine, rifampin, or strong CYP inducers, may unpredictably modify plasma concentrations, although definitive interaction studies remain limited [121]. In patients receiving polypharmacy or chronic hepatotoxic medications, baseline and periodic liver function monitoring is advisable.

Orphenadrine

Clinically significant interactions with orphenadrine primarily arise from additive anticholinergic and CNS-depressant effects. Coadministration with other anticholinergic agents, including tricyclic antidepressants, first-generation antihistamines, or antipsychotics, can lead to urinary retention, blurred vision, tachycardia, and confusion, particularly in older adults [133]. In addition, the combination of orphenadrine with opioids or sedative-hypnotics enhances drowsiness and impairs coordination, increasing the risk of accidents and falls. Because orphenadrine is metabolized hepatically, potential interactions with enzyme inducers or inhibitors may alter systemic exposure, although these effects have not been systematically quantified [121]. Conservative dosing and avoidance of concurrent strong anticholinergics are recommended in patients receiving orphenadrine.

Calcium Channel Blockers

Across both classes of calcium channel blockers, the predominant mechanisms of clinically significant drug-drug interactions involve CYP3A4-mediated metabolic changes, P-gp transporter effects, and additive pharmacodynamic burdens such as hypotension and bradycardia [134]. The more predictable pharmacokinetic interactions of DHP-CCBs, chiefly via CYP3A4, contrast with the more complex precipitant-object dynamics of non-DHP-CCBs mediated by CYP3A4 + P-gp + conduction/chronotropic effects [134]. This chapter focuses on dihydropyridine calcium channel blockers as the most likely to be used in analgesic settings [135].

Dihydropyridine calcium channel blockers (DHP-CCBs) are widely used antihypertensive and anti-ischemic agents whose metabolism and interaction potential warrant careful attention in polypharmacy settings. One of the most extensively documented interaction risks involves the coadministration of DHP-CCBs with HMG-CoA reductase inhibitors, or statins as they are conventionally known, particularly those highly dependent on CYP3A4 metabolism [136]. In a comprehensive review of pharmacokinetic drug-drug interactions between 1,4-DHP-CCBs and statins, Zhou et al. found that concomitant use with simvastatin and other CYP3A4 substrates can significantly increase statin exposure, potentially increasing myopathy risk [137]. Clinically, this means that in patients treated with DHP-CCBs such as amlodipine or nifedipine who are also on statins, the choice of statin and its dose must be adjusted. For instance, because simvastatin has a greater intestinal first-pass effect and stronger CYP3A4 dependence, the interaction with DHP-CCBs poses a more significant myopathy risk than atorvastatin, which is less impacted [136, 137]. In addition to statins, DHP-CCBs are substrates of CYP3A4 and may be affected by strong inhibitors or inducers of CYP3A4, including macrolide antibiotics, azole antifungals, protease inhibitors and grapefruit juice, which can elevate DHP-CCB levels and thus increase the risk of hypotension and related adverse events [136].

Ketamine

Clinically meaningful pharmacokinetic interactions with ketamine are best documented for modulators of CYP-mediated N-demethylation to norketamine. In healthy-volunteer crossover studies with oral S-ketamine, the macrolide clarithromycin, a strong CYP3A inhibitor, increased ketamine exposure substantially with an approximately 3.6-fold higher C_{max} and 2.6-fold higher AUC. This led to a modest amplification of behavioral effects, underscoring the need to reduce oral doses or intensify monitoring when potent CYP3A inhibitors are co-prescribed [138]. In contrast, the strong CYP3A inhibitor itraconazole did not increase oral S-ketamine exposure in a randomized, blinded crossover study, whereas the CYP2B6 inhibitor ticlopidine increased S-ketamine AUC by 2.4-fold and reduced norketamine formation, highlighting a prominent role for CYP2B6 in first-pass metabolism [139]. With respect to enzymatic induction, rifampicin and derivatives markedly lower ketamine and norketamine concentrations: pretreatment decreased oral S-ketamine (and S-norketamine) exposure consistent with induced first-pass metabolism and reduced parent-drug AUC after intravenous dosing as well. Clinically, coadministration with rifamycins (or other strong inducers) can yield subtherapeutic effects, particularly with oral/esketamine regimens, and may warrant dose adjustment or alternative therapy [140]. Complementing these trials, PK modeling and pharmacogenetic work further corroborate CYP2B6 as a quantitatively important pathway influencing ketamine exposure and DDI magnitude [141].

Pharmacodynamic (PD) interactions are common in practice. Converging evidence indicates benzodiazepines attenuate the antidepressant response to ketamine: a systematic review of 24 studies found benzodiazepines repeatedly reduced the duration of benefit, and a secondary analysis of a randomized IV ketamine trial showed that higher benzodiazepine doses were associated with diminished antidepressant effect at 24 hours [142]. Interactions involving the opioid system remain debated. An early randomized, double-blind study reported that naltrexone pretreatment blocked ketamine's antidepressant but not dissociative effects, prompting early termination [143]. Subsequent evaluation suggests attenuation rather than complete blockade, indicating patient-specific and context-dependent variables. Clinicians should avoid routine coadministration of naltrexone at the time of ketamine dosing for mood disorders unless there is a compelling indication, and they should counsel that concurrent opioid antagonism may blunt benefit [144].
When ketamine is combined with other sedative-hypnotics, additive PD effects are expected, but respiratory outcomes vary by partner drug and dosing strategy. In emergency-department procedural sedation, ketamine in combination with propofol ("ketofol") has repeatedly shown no increase, and in some trials a reduction, in respiratory adverse events compared with propofol alone, presumably via dose-sparing and counterbalancing hemodynamic/airway effects; nevertheless, close monitoring is essential when any CNS depressant is coadministered [145]. Finally, limited human data hint that lamotrigine may attenuate ketamine's psychotropic/antidepressant effects in some studies, whereas MAOI coadministration (e.g., tranylcypromine) has not consistently provoked hemodynamic instability in case series—points that merit individualized risk–benefit assessment and vigilant vital-sign monitoring when these combinations are unavoidable [142].

Conclusion

Adjunctive analgesics play an essential role in modern pain management; however, their use is frequently complicated by clinically meaningful drug-drug interactions, particularly in patients with polypharmacy, advanced age, or comorbid organ dysfunction. As demonstrated throughout this chapter, most high-risk interactions arise not only from metabolic inhibition or induction but also from additive or synergistic pharmacodynamic effects, including sedation, respiratory depression, bleeding, cardiac arrhythmias, and renal injury. Agents such as gabapentinoids, antidepressants, antiepileptic drugs, NSAIDs, muscle relaxants, and emerging therapies like ketamine or intravenous lidocaine require careful consideration of both object and precipitant drug characteristics.

Effective mitigation of interaction-related harm depends on a thorough understanding of underlying mechanisms, vigilant patient assessment, and thoughtful regimen design. Clinicians must remain attentive to dose-dependent effects, timing of administration, and the cumulative burden of central nervous system depressants or serotonergic agents. Equally important is recognition that "low-risk" or topical therapies are not entirely free of interaction potential, particularly in vulnerable populations or when combined with anticoagulants and other narrow therapeutic index medications.

Ultimately, safe and effective pain management requires an individualized, evidence-based approach that integrates pharmacologic knowledge with clinical judgment. Ongoing education, routine medication review, and interprofessional collaboration are essential to identifying and managing drug-drug interactions, thereby improving therapeutic outcomes and reducing preventable adverse events in patients receiving adjunctive analgesic therapies.

References

1. Hines LE, Murphy JE. Potentially harmful drug-drug interactions in the elderly: a review. Am J Geriatr Pharmacother. 2011;9(6):364–77. https://doi.org/10.1016/j.amjopharm.2011.10.004.
2. Dumbreck S, Flynn A, Nairn M, et al. Drug-disease and drug-drug interactions: systematic examination of recommendations in 12 UK national clinical guidelines. BMJ. 2015;350:h949. https://doi.org/10.1136/bmj.h949.
3. Mattsson M, Hassan Ali A, Boland F, et al. Patterns of analgesic prescribing and high-risk prescribing in primary care in Ireland 2014-2022-A repeated cross-sectional study. Eur J Pain. 2025;29(9):e70115. https://doi.org/10.1002/ejp.70115.

4. Bockbrader HN, Wesche D, Miller R, Chapel S, Janiczek N, Burger P. A comparison of the pharmacokinetics and pharmacodynamics of pregabalin and gabapentin. Clin Pharmacokinet. 2010;49(10):661–9. https://doi.org/10.2165/11536200-000000000-00000.
5. Johansen ME. Gabapentinoid use in the United States 2002 through 2015. JAMA Intern Med. 2018;178(2):292–4. https://doi.org/10.1001/jamainternmed.2017.7856.
6. Chen C, Lo-Ciganic W-H, Winterstein AG, Tighe P, Wei Y-JJ. Concurrent use of prescription opioids and gabapentinoids in older adults. Am J Prev Med. 2022;62(4):519–28. https://doi.org/10.1016/j.amepre.2021.08.024.
7. Gomes T, Juurlink DN, Antoniou T, Mamdani MM, Paterson JM, van den Brink W. Gabapentin, opioids, and the risk of opioid-related death: a population-based nested case-control study. PLoS Med. 2017;14(10):e1002396. https://doi.org/10.1371/journal.pmed.1002396.
8. Eckhardt K, Ammon S, Hofmann U, Riebe A, Gugeler N, Mikus G. Gabapentin enhances the analgesic effect of morphine in healthy volunteers. Anesth Analg. 2000;91(1):185–91. https://doi.org/10.1097/00000539-200007000-00035.
9. Yagi T, Naito T, Mino Y, Umemura K, Kawakami J. Impact of concomitant antacid administration on gabapentin plasma exposure and oral bioavailability in healthy adult subjects. Drug Metab Pharmacokinet. 2012;27(2):248–54. https://doi.org/10.2133/dmpk.dmpk-11-rg-108.
10. Costa ACC, Yamamoto PA, Lauretti GR, et al. Cetirizine reduces gabapentin plasma concentrations and effect: role of renal drug transporters for organic cations. J Clin Pharmacol. 2020;60(8):1076–86. https://doi.org/10.1002/jcph.1603.
11. Lal R, Sukbuntherng J, Luo W, et al. Clinical pharmacokinetic drug interaction studies of gabapentin enacarbil, a novel transported prodrug of gabapentin, with naproxen and cimetidine. Br J Clin Pharmacol. 2010;69(5):498–507. https://doi.org/10.1111/j.1365-2125.2010.03616.x.
12. Chen C, Upward J, Arumugham T, Stier B, Davy M. Gabapentin enacarbil and morphine administered in combination versus alone: a double-blind, randomized, pharmacokinetic, and tolerability comparison. Clin Ther. 2015;37(2):349–57. https://doi.org/10.1016/j.clinthera.2014.10.015.
13. FDA warns about serious breathing problems with seizure and nerve pain medicines gabapentin (Neurontin, Gralise, Horizant) and pregabalin (Lyrica, Lyrica CR) | FDA. Accessed 18 Dec 2025. https://www.fda.gov/drugs/drug-safety-and-availability/fda-warns-about-serious-breathing-problems-seizure-and-nerve-pain-medicines-gabapentin-neurontin.
14. Myhre M, Diep LM, Stubhaug A. Pregabalin has analgesic, ventilatory, and cognitive effects in combination with remifentanil. Anesthesiology. 2016;124(1):141–9. https://doi.org/10.1097/ALN.0000000000000913.
15. Bertilsson L. Clinical pharmacokinetics of carbamazepine. Clin Pharmacokinet. 1978;3(2):128–43. https://doi.org/10.2165/00003088-197803020-00003.
16. Wright JM, Stokes EF, Sweeney VP. Isoniazid-induced carbamazepine toxicity and vice versa: a double drug interaction. N Engl J Med. 1982;307(21):1325–7. https://doi.org/10.1056/NEJM198211183072107.
17. Macphee GJ, McInnes GT, Thompson GG, Brodie MJ. Verapamil potentiates carbamazepine neurotoxicity: a clinically important inhibitory interaction. Lancet. 1986;1(8483):700–3. https://doi.org/10.1016/s0140-6736(86)91099-8.
18. Ngo LT, Yang S-Y, Tran QT, Kim SK, Yun H-Y, Chae J-W. Effects of carbamazepine and phenytoin on pharmacokinetics and pharmacodynamics of rivaroxaban. Pharmaceutics. 2020;12(11) https://doi.org/10.3390/pharmaceutics12111040.
19. Herdegen T, Cascorbi I. Drug interactions of tetrahydrocannabinol and cannabidiol in cannabinoid drugs. Dtsch Arztebl Int. 2023;120(49):833–40. https://doi.org/10.3238/arztebl.m2023.0223.
20. Ghodke-Puranik Y, Thorn CF, Lamba JK, et al. Valproic acid pathway: pharmacokinetics and pharmacodynamics. Pharmacogenet Genomics. 2013;23(4):236–41. https://doi.org/10.1097/FPC.0b013e32835ea0b2.
21. Wagner ML, Graves NM, Leppik IE, et al. The effect of felbamate on valproic acid disposition. Clin Pharmacol Ther. 1994;56(5):494–502. https://doi.org/10.1038/clpt.1994.170.
22. Addison RS, Parker-Scott SL, Hooper WD, Eadie MJ, Dickinson RG. Effect of naproxen co-administration on valproate disposition. Biopharm Drug Dispos. 2000;21(6):235–42. https://doi.org/10.1002/bdd.235.
23. Perucca E, Aldenkamp A, Tallis R, Krämer G. Role of valproate across the ages. Treatment of epilepsy in the elderly. Acta Neurol Scand. 2006;184:28–37. https://doi.org/10.1111/j.1600-0404.2006.00668.x.
24. Kavitha S, Anbuchelvan T, Mahalakshmi V, et al. Stevens-Johnson syndrome induced by a combination of lamotrigine and valproic acid. J Pharm Bioallied Sci. 2015;7(Suppl 2):S756–8. https://doi.org/10.4103/0975-7406.163545.
25. Brizendine CE, Naik PJ. Drug rash with eosinophilia and systemic symptoms syndrome associated with use of phenytoin, divalproex sodium, and phenobarbital. Am J Health Syst Pharm. 2013;70(6):507–10. https://doi.org/10.2146/ajhp120408.
26. Wen ZP, Fan SS, Du C, et al. Drug-drug interaction between valproic acid and meropenem: a retrospective analysis of electronic medical records from neurosurgery inpatients. J Clin Pharm Ther. 2017;42(2):221–7. https://doi.org/10.1111/jcpt.12501.
27. Wu C-C, Pai T-Y, Hsiao F-Y, Shen L-J, Wu F-LL. The effect of different carbapenem antibiotics (ertapenem, imipenem/cilastatin, and meropenem) on serum valproic acid concentrations. Ther Drug Monit. 2016;38(5):587–92. https://doi.org/10.1097/FTD.0000000000000316.
28. Sheehan NL, Brouillette M-J, Delisle M-S, Allan J. Possible interaction between lopinavir/ritonavir and valproic acid exacerbates bipolar disorder. Ann Pharmacother. 2006;40(1):147–50. https://doi.org/10.1345/aph.1G418.
29. Wu J, Li J, Jing W, Tian X, Wang X. Valproic acid-induced encephalopathy: a review of clinical features, risk factors, diagnosis, and treatment. Epilepsy Behav. 2021;120:107967. https://doi.org/10.1016/j.yebeh.2021.107967.
30. Nguyen P, Chevillard L, Gouda AS, et al. L-carnitine does not improve valproic acid poisoning management: a cohort study with toxicokinetics and concentration/effect relationships. Ann Intensive Care. 2022;12(1):7. https://doi.org/10.1186/s13613-022-00984-z.
31. DeVane CL. Antidepressant-drug interactions are potentially but rarely clinically significant. Neuropsychopharmacology. 2006;31(8):1594–604; discussion 1614. https://doi.org/10.1038/sj.npp.1301069.
32. Brøsen K. Differences in interactions of SSRIs. Int Clin Psychopharmacol. 1998;13(Suppl 5):S45–7.
33. Hemeryck A, Belpaire FM. Selective serotonin reuptake inhibitors and cytochrome P-450 mediated drug-drug interactions: an update. Curr Drug Metab. 2002;3(1):13–37. https://doi.org/10.2174/1389200023338017.
34. Spina E, Santoro V, D'Arrigo C. Clinically relevant pharmacokinetic drug interactions with second-generation antidepressants: an update. Clin Ther. 2008;30(7):1206–27. https://doi.org/10.1016/s0149-2918(08)80047-1.
35. Isoherranen N, Lutz JD, Chung SP, Hachad H, Levy RH, Ragueneau-Majlessi I. Importance of multi-p450 inhibition in drug-drug interactions: evaluation of incidence, inhibition mag-

nitude, and prediction from in vitro data. Chem Res Toxicol. 2012;25(11):2285–300. https://doi.org/10.1021/tx300192g.

36. Uno T, Akamine Y, Furukori NY, Hirano T. Effects of selective serotonin reuptake inhibitors on the pharmacokinetics of proton pump inhibitors. Neuropsychiatry. 2018;07(04) https://doi.org/10.4172/Neuropsychiatry.1000227.
37. Granfors MT, Backman JT, Neuvonen M, Ahonen J, Neuvonen PJ. Fluvoxamine drastically increases concentrations and effects of tizanidine: a potentially hazardous interaction. Clin Pharmacol Ther. 2004;75(4):331–41. https://doi.org/10.1016/j.clpt.2003.12.005.
38. Abdelmalik N, Ruhé HG, Barwari K, et al. Effect of the selective serotonin reuptake inhibitor paroxetine on platelet function is modified by a SLC6A4 serotonin transporter polymorphism. J Thromb Haemost. 2008;6(12):2168–74. https://doi.org/10.1111/j.1538-7836.2008.03196.x.
39. Labos C, Dasgupta K, Nedjar H, Turecki G, Rahme E. Risk of bleeding associated with combined use of selective serotonin reuptake inhibitors and antiplatelet therapy following acute myocardial infarction. CMAJ. 2011;183(16):1835–43. https://doi.org/10.1503/cmaj.100912.
40. Nochaiwong S, Ruengorn C, Awiphan R, et al. Use of serotonin reuptake inhibitor antidepressants and the risk of bleeding complications in patients on anticoagulant or antiplatelet agents: a systematic review and meta-analysis. Ann Med. 2022;54(1):80–97. https://doi.org/10.1080/07853890.2021.2017474.
41. Jiang H-Y, Chen H-Z, Hu X-J, et al. Use of selective serotonin reuptake inhibitors and risk of upper gastrointestinal bleeding: a systematic review and meta-analysis. Clin Gastroenterol Hepatol. 2015;13(1):42–50.e3. https://doi.org/10.1016/j.cgh.2014.06.021.
42. Anglin R, Yuan Y, Moayyedi P, Tse F, Armstrong D, Leontiadis GI. Risk of upper gastrointestinal bleeding with selective serotonin reuptake inhibitors with or without concurrent nonsteroidal anti-inflammatory use: a systematic review and meta-analysis. Am J Gastroenterol. 2014;109(6):811–9. https://doi.org/10.1038/ajg.2014.82.
43. Renoux C, Vahey S, Dell'Aniello S, Boivin J-F. Association of selective serotonin reuptake inhibitors with the risk for spontaneous intracranial hemorrhage. JAMA Neurol. 2017;74(2):173–80. https://doi.org/10.1001/jamaneurol.2016.4529.
44. Simon LV, Torrico TJ, Keenaghan M. Serotonin syndrome. In: StatPearls. StatPearls Publishing; 2025.
45. Elli C, Novella A, Elli C, Pasina L. Selective Serotonin Reuptake Inhibitors and Risk of Serotonin Syndrome as Consequence of Drug-Drug Interactions: Analysis of the FDA Adverse Event Reporting System. Med Princ Pract. 2025;34(5):456–63. https://doi.org/10.1159/000546109.
46. Rottmann CN. SSRIs and the syndrome of inappropriate antidiuretic hormone secretion. Am J Nurs. 2007;107(1):51–8; quiz 58. https://doi.org/10.1097/00000446-200701000-00022.
47. Rajiv S, Nandimath MK. Association between serum sodium levels and selective serotonin reuptake inhibitors in patients with depression. Int J Basic Clin Pharmacol. 2017;6(2):349. https://doi.org/10.18203/2319-2003.ijbcp20170328.
48. Rochester MP, Kane AM, Linnebur SA, Fixen DR. Evaluating the risk of QTc prolongation associated with antidepressant use in older adults: a review of the evidence. Ther Adv Drug Saf. 2018;9(6):297–308. https://doi.org/10.1177/2042098618772979.
49. Farhat H, Tlaiss Y, Nassif L, Gutlapalli SD, Abdulaal R. Citalopram & escitalopram: mechanisms of cardiotoxicity, toxicology predisposition and risks of use in geriatric & hemodialysis populations. Glob Cardiol Sci Pract. 2024;2024(4):e202434. https://doi.org/10.21542/gcsp.2024.34.
50. Hesse C, Siedler H, Burhenne J, Riedel K-D, Haefeli WE. Fluvoxamine affects sildenafil kinetics and dynamics. J Clin Psychopharmacol. 2005;25(6):589–92. https://doi.org/10.1097/01.jcp.0000186866.82665.29.
51. Sager JE, Lutz JD, Foti RS, Davis C, Kunze KL, Isoherranen N. Fluoxetine- and norfluoxetine-mediated complex drug-drug interactions: in vitro to in vivo correlation of effects on CYP2D6, CYP2C19, and CYP3A4. Clin Pharmacol Ther. 2014;95(6):653–62. https://doi.org/10.1038/clpt.2014.50.
52. Luecht UR, Scholz W, Geiben A-K, Haen E, Hempel G. Physiologically based pharmacokinetic model of CYP2D6 associated interaction between venlafaxine and strong inhibitor bupropion-the influence of age-relevant changes and inhibitory dose to classify therapeutical success and harm. Pharmaceutics. 2025;17(2) https://doi.org/10.3390/pharmaceutics17020179.
53. Skinner MH, Kuan H-Y, Pan A, et al. Duloxetine is both an inhibitor and a substrate of cytochrome P4502D6 in healthy volunteers. Clin Pharmacol Ther. 2003;73(3):170–7. https://doi.org/10.1067/mcp.2003.28.
54. Hoffelt C, Gross T. A review of significant pharmacokinetic drug interactions with antidepressants and their management. Ment Health Clin. 2016;6(1):35–41. https://doi.org/10.9740/mhc.2016.01.035.
55. Sun C-F, Chen Y-L, Li Y-H, Kumaraswamy M, Lo Y-C, Chen Y-T. Duloxetine-induced hyponatremia in an elderly male patient with treatment-refractory major depressive disorder. Case Rep Psychiatry. 2019;2019:1–3. https://doi.org/10.1155/2019/4109150.
56. Mori M, Koide T, Imanishi Y, Matsui Y, Matsuda T. Duloxetine-induced hyponatremia in an elderly patient treated with thiazide diuretics. Indian J Pharmacol. 2014;46(6):657–9. https://doi.org/10.4103/0253-7613.144947.
57. Yekehtaz H, Farokhnia M, Akhondzadeh S. Cardiovascular considerations in antidepressant therapy: an evidence-based review. J Tehran Heart Cent. 2013;8(4):169–76.
58. Calvi A, Fischetti I, Verzicco I, et al. Antidepressant drugs effects on blood pressure. Front Cardiovasc Med. 2021;8:704281. https://doi.org/10.3389/fcvm.2021.704281.
59. Cui Y, Abdi SAH, Wei J, Azhar G. The long-term cardiovascular risks of duloxetine use in older adults: a retrospective medical record-based adverse drug reaction assessment. J Clin Med. 2024;13(24) https://doi.org/10.3390/jcm13247595.
60. Gareri P, De Fazio P, Gallelli L, et al. Venlafaxine-propafenone interaction resulting in hallucinations and psychomotor agitation. Ann Pharmacother. 2008;42(3):434–8. https://doi.org/10.1345/aph.1K405.
61. Bucaretchi F, de Capitani EM, Mello SM, et al. Serotonin syndrome following sibutramine poisoning in a child, with sequential quantification of sibutramine and its primary and secondary amine metabolites in plasma. Clin Toxicol (Phila). 2009;47(6):598–601. https://doi.org/10.1080/15563650903018603.
62. Newey CR, Khawam E, Coffman K. Two cases of serotonin syndrome with venlafaxine and calcineurin inhibitors. Psychosomatics. 2011;52(3):286–90. https://doi.org/10.1016/j.psym.2010.12.007.
63. Adan-Manes J, Novalbos J, López-Rodríguez R, Ayuso-Mateos JL, Abad-Santos F. Lithium and venlafaxine interaction: a case of serotonin syndrome. J Clin Pharm Ther. 2006;31(4):397–400. https://doi.org/10.1111/j.1365-2710.2006.00745.x.
64. Gillman PK. Tricyclic antidepressant pharmacology and therapeutic drug interactions updated. Br J Pharmacol. 2007;151(6):737–48. https://doi.org/10.1038/sj.bjp.0707253.
65. El-Yazigi A, Chaleby K, Gad A, Raines DA. Steady-state kinetics of fluoxetine and amitriptyline in patients treated with a combination of these drugs as compared with those treated with amitriptyline alone. J Clin Pharmacol. 1995;35(1):17–21. https://doi.org/10.1002/j.1552-4604.1995.tb04740.x.

66. Henderson L, Yue QY, Bergquist C, Gerden B, Arlett P. St John's wort (Hypericum perforatum): drug interactions and clinical outcomes. Br J Clin Pharmacol. 2002;54(4):349–56. https://doi.org/10.1046/j.1365-2125.2002.01683.x.
67. Wilson M, Tripp J. Clomipramine. In: StatPearls. StatPearls Publishing; 2025.
68. Power BM, Pinder M, Hackett LP, Ilett KF. Fatal serotonin syndrome following a combined overdose of moclobemide, clomipramine and fluoxetine. Anaesth Intensive Care. 1995;23(4):499–502.
69. Gillman PK. Monoamine oxidase inhibitors, opioid analgesics and serotonin toxicity. Br J Anaesth. 2005;95(4):434–41. https://doi.org/10.1093/bja/aei210.
70. Mitchell PB. Drug interactions of clinical significance with selective serotonin reuptake inhibitors. Drug Saf. 1997;17(6):390–406. https://doi.org/10.2165/00002018-199717060-00005.
71. Khalid MM, Waseem M. Tricyclic antidepressant toxicity. In: StatPearls. StatPearls Publishing; 2025.
72. Yap YG, Camm AJ. Drug induced QT prolongation and torsades de pointes. Heart. 2003;89(11):1363–72. https://doi.org/10.1136/heart.89.11.1363.
73. Moraczewski J, Awosika AO, Aedma KK. Tricyclic antidepressants. In: StatPearls. StatPearls Publishing; 2025.
74. Cochran KA, Cavallari LH, Shapiro NL, Bishop JR. Bleeding incidence with concomitant use of antidepressants and warfarin. Ther Drug Monit. 2011;33(4):433–8. https://doi.org/10.1097/FTD.0b013e318224996e.
75. Schelleman H, Brensinger CM, Bilker WB, Hennessy S. Antidepressant-warfarin interaction and associated gastrointestinal bleeding risk in a case-control study. PLoS One. 2011;6(6):e21447. https://doi.org/10.1371/journal.pone.0021447.
76. Boakes AJ, Laurence DR, Teoh PC, Barar FS, Benedikter LT, Prichard BN. Interactions between sympathomimetic amines and antidepressant agents in man. Br Med J. 1973;1(5849):311–5. https://doi.org/10.1136/bmj.1.5849.311.
77. Fairbanks CA, Stone LS, Wilcox GL. Pharmacological profiles of alpha 2 adrenergic receptor agonists identified using genetically altered mice and isobolographic analysis. Pharmacol Ther. 2009;123(2):224–38. https://doi.org/10.1016/j.pharmthera.2009.04.001.
78. Villa Zapata L, Hansten PD, Panic J, et al. Risk of bleeding with exposure to warfarin and nonsteroidal anti-inflammatory drugs: a systematic review and meta-analysis. Thromb Haemost. 2020;120(7):1066–74. https://doi.org/10.1055/s-0040-1710592.
79. Dalgaard F, Mulder H, Wojdyla DM, et al. Patients with atrial fibrillation taking nonsteroidal anti-inflammatory drugs and oral anticoagulants in the ARISTOTLE trial. Circulation. 2020;141(1):10–20. https://doi.org/10.1161/CIRCULATIONAHA.119.041296.
80. Targownik LE. Are we worried enough about selective serotonin receptor inhibitors and upper gastrointestinal bleeding? Clin Gastroenterol Hepatol. 2015;13(1):51–4. https://doi.org/10.1016/j.cgh.2014.08.032.
81. Lanas A, Gargallo CJ. Management of low-dose aspirin and clopidogrel in clinical practice: a gastrointestinal perspective. J Gastroenterol. 2015;50(6):626–37. https://doi.org/10.1007/s00535-015-1038-3.
82. Masclee GMC, Valkhoff VE, Coloma PM, et al. Risk of upper gastrointestinal bleeding from different drug combinations. Gastroenterology. 2014;147(4):784–792.e9; quiz e13. https://doi.org/10.1053/j.gastro.2014.06.007.
83. Lee M, Cha JM. Real-world bleeding risk of anticoagulant and nonsteroidal anti-inflammatory drugs combotherapy versus anticoagulant monotherapy. Gut Liver. 2024;18(5):824–33. https://doi.org/10.5009/gnl230541.
84. Dreischulte T, Morales DR, Bell S, Guthrie B. Combined use of nonsteroidal anti-inflammatory drugs with diuretics and/or renin-angiotensin system inhibitors in the community increases the risk of acute kidney injury. Kidney Int. 2015;88(2):396–403. https://doi.org/10.1038/ki.2015.101.
85. Haręźlak T, Religioni U, Szymański FM, et al. Drug interactions affecting kidney function: beware of health threats from triple whammy. Adv Ther. 2022;39(1):140–7. https://doi.org/10.1007/s12325-021-01939-9.
86. Page RL, O'Bryant CL, Cheng D, et al. Drugs that may cause or exacerbate heart failure: a scientific statement from the american heart association. Circulation. 2016;134(6):e32–69. https://doi.org/10.1161/CIR.0000000000000426.
87. Varga Z, Sabzwari SRA, Vargova V. Cardiovascular risk of nonsteroidal anti-inflammatory drugs: an under-recognized public health issue. Cureus. 2017;9(4):e1144. https://doi.org/10.7759/cureus.1144.
88. Angiolillo DJ, Weisman SM. Clinical pharmacology and cardiovascular safety of naproxen. Am J Cardiovasc Drugs. 2017;17(2):97–107. https://doi.org/10.1007/s40256-016-0200-5.
89. Bally M, Dendukuri N, Rich B, et al. Risk of acute myocardial infarction with NSAIDs in real world use: bayesian meta-analysis of individual patient data. BMJ. 2017;357:j1909. https://doi.org/10.1136/bmj.j1909.
90. Hylek EM, Heiman H, Skates SJ, Sheehan MA, Singer DE. Acetaminophen and other risk factors for excessive warfarin anticoagulation. JAMA. 1998;279(9):657–62. https://doi.org/10.1001/jama.279.9.657.
91. Parra D, Beckey NP, Stevens GR. The effect of acetaminophen on the international normalized ratio in patients stabilized on warfarin therapy. Pharmacotherapy. 2007;27(5):675–83. https://doi.org/10.1592/phco.27.5.675.
92. Hughes GJ, Patel PN, Saxena N. Effect of acetaminophen on international normalized ratio in patients receiving warfarin therapy. Pharmacotherapy. 2011;31(6):591–7. https://doi.org/10.1592/phco.31.6.591.
93. Lopes RD, Horowitz JD, Garcia DA, Crowther MA, Hylek EM. Warfarin and acetaminophen interaction: a summary of the evidence and biologic plausibility. Blood. 2011;118(24):6269–73. https://doi.org/10.1182/blood-2011-08-335612.
94. Kim SH, Choi HJ, Seo H, Kwon D, Yun J, Jung Y-S. Downregulation of glutathione-mediated detoxification capacity by binge drinking aggravates acetaminophen-induced liver injury through IRE1α ER stress signaling. Antioxidants (Basel). 2021;10(12) https://doi.org/10.3390/antiox10121949.
95. Yue J, Peng R. Does CYP2E1 play a major role in the aggravation of isoniazid toxicity by rifampicin in human hepatocytes? Br J Pharmacol. 2009;157(3):331–3. https://doi.org/10.1111/j.1476-5381.2009.00173.x.
96. James L, Roberts D. Isoniazid hepatotoxicity: progress in understanding the immunologic component. Hepatology. 2014;59(3):746–8. https://doi.org/10.1002/hep.26707.
97. Brackett CC, Bloch JD. Phenytoin as a possible cause of acetaminophen hepatotoxicity: case report and review of the literature. Pharmacotherapy. 2000;20(2):229–33. https://doi.org/10.1592/phco.20.3.229.34774.
98. Kostrubsky SE, Sinclair JF, Strom SC, et al. Phenobarbital and phenytoin increased acetaminophen hepatotoxicity due to inhibition of UDP-glucuronosyltransferases in cultured human hepatocytes. Toxicol Sci. 2005;87(1):146–55. https://doi.org/10.1093/toxsci/kfi211.
99. Tokola RA. The effect of metoclopramide and prochlorperazine on the absorption of effervescent paracetamol in migraine. Cephalalgia. 1988;8(3):139–47. https://doi.org/10.1046/j.1468-2982.1988.0803113.x.

100. Halcomb SE, Sivilotti MLA, Goklaney A, Mullins ME. Pharmacokinetic effects of diphenhydramine or oxycodone in simulated acetaminophen overdose. Acad Emerg Med. 2005;12(2):169–72. https://doi.org/10.1197/j.aem.2004.10.014.
101. Rogers SM, Back DJ, Stevenson PJ, Grimmer SF, Orme ML. Paracetamol interaction with oral contraceptive steroids: increased plasma concentrations of ethinyloestradiol. Br J Clin Pharmacol. 1987;23(6):721–5.
102. Dean L. Codeine therapy andCYP2D6Genotype. In: Pratt V, McLeod H, Dean L, Malheiro A, Rubinstein W, editors. Medical genetics summaries. National Center for Biotechnology Information (US); 2020.
103. Paterson CA, Jacobs D, Rasmussen S, Youngberg SP, McGuinness N. Randomized, open-label, 5-way crossover study to evaluate the pharmacokinetic/pharmacodynamic interaction between furosemide and the non-steroidal anti-inflammatory drugs diclofenac and ibuprofen in healthy volunteers. Int J Clin Pharmacol Ther. 2011;49(8):477–90. https://doi.org/10.5414/cp201492.
104. Shi C, Ye Z, Shao Z, et al. Multidisciplinary guidelines for the rational use of topical non-steroidal anti-inflammatory drugs for musculoskeletal pain (2022). J Clin Med. 2023;12(4) https://doi.org/10.3390/jcm12041544.
105. Lan M-J, Zhou Q. Potential therapeutic hazards due to drug-drug interaction between topically and systemically coadministered medications. Ther Clin Risk Manag. 2013;9:313–7. https://doi.org/10.2147/TCRM.S50375.
106. Rannou F, Pelletier J-P, Martel-Pelletier J. Efficacy and safety of topical NSAIDs in the management of osteoarthritis: evidence from real-life setting trials and surveys. Semin Arthritis Rheum. 2016;45(4 Suppl):S18–21. https://doi.org/10.1016/j.semarthrit.2015.11.007.
107. De Crem N, Verleden GM, Godinas L, Vos R. Once in a blue moon: primaquine-induced methemoglobinemia - A case report. Respir Med Case Rep. 2022;38:101675. https://doi.org/10.1016/j.rmcr.2022.101675.
108. Coderre K, Faria C, Dyer E. Probable warfarin interaction with menthol cough drops. Pharmacotherapy. 2010;30(1):110. https://doi.org/10.1592/phco.30.1.110.
109. Elyassi AR, Rowshan HH. Perioperative management of the glucose-6-phosphate dehydrogenase deficient patient: a review of literature. Anesth Prog. 2009;56(3):86–91. https://doi.org/10.2344/0003-3006-56.3.86.
110. Han EH, Kim HG, Choi JH, et al. Capsaicin induces CYP3A4 expression via pregnane X receptor and CCAAT/enhancer-binding protein β activation. Mol Nutr Food Res. 2012;56(5):797–809. https://doi.org/10.1002/mnfr.201100697.
111. Wang JS, Backman JT, Taavitsainen P, Neuvonen PJ, Kivistö KT. Involvement of CYP1A2 and CYP3A4 in lidocaine N-deethylation and 3-hydroxylation in humans. Drug Metab Dispos. 2000;28(8):959–65.
112. Nagashima A, Tanaka E, Inomata S, Honda K, Misawa S. A study of the in vitro interaction between lidocaine and premedications using human liver microsomes. J Clin Pharm Ther. 2005;30(2):185–8. https://doi.org/10.1111/j.1365-2710.2004.00617.x.
113. Torp KD, Metheny E, Simon LV. Lidocaine toxicity. In: StatPearls. StatPearls Publishing; 2025.
114. Hasan B, Asif T, Hasan M. Lidocaine-induced systemic toxicity: a case report and review of literature. Cureus. 2017;9(5):e1275. https://doi.org/10.7759/cureus.1275.
115. Tierney KJ, Murano T, Natal B. Lidocaine-induced cardiac arrest in the emergency department: effectiveness of lipid therapy. J Emerg Med. 2016;50(1):47–50. https://doi.org/10.1016/j.jemermed.2015.07.035.
116. Ciechanowicz SJ, Patil VK. Association of anaesthetists of Great Britain and Ireland. Intravenous lipid emulsion - rescued at LAST. Br Dent J. 2012;212(5):237–41. https://doi.org/10.1038/sj.bdj.2012.187.
117. Aronowitz DI, Bocchieri KA, Hartman AR, Yu P-J. Serum lidocaine levels in adult patients undergoing cardiac surgery with del nido cardioplegia. Ann Thoracic Surg Short Rep. 2024;2(2):302–5. https://doi.org/10.1016/j.atssr.2023.12.014.
118. Tan L-H, Hwang N-C. The effect of mixing lidocaine with propofol on the dose of propofol required for induction of anesthesia. Anesth Analg. 2003;97(2):461–4. https://doi.org/10.1213/01.ANE.0000066357.63011.75.
119. Spence MM, Shin PJ, Lee EA, Gibbs NE. Risk of injury associated with skeletal muscle relaxant use in older adults. Ann Pharmacother. 2013;47(7–8):993–8. https://doi.org/10.1345/aph.1R735.
120. Ko HY, Park JH, Kim H. Probable interaction between warfarin and baclofen: a report of two cases. Ann Rehabil Med. 1998;22(3)
121. Hakkola J, Hukkanen J, Turpeinen M, Pelkonen O. Inhibition and induction of CYP enzymes in humans: an update. Arch Toxicol. 2020;94(11):3671–722. https://doi.org/10.1007/s00204-020-02936-7.
122. Granfors MT, Backman JT, Neuvonen M, Neuvonen PJ. Ciprofloxacin greatly increases concentrations and hypotensive effect of tizanidine by inhibiting its cytochrome P450 1A2-mediated presystemic metabolism. Clin Pharmacol Ther. 2004;76(6):598–606. https://doi.org/10.1016/j.clpt.2004.08.018.
123. Mahajan R, Kalita J. Tizanidine induced hypotension: report of a case and review of the literature. Curr Drug Saf. 2024;19(2):313–6. https://doi.org/10.2174/1574886318666230725113855.
124. Kouladjian O'Donnell L, Gnjidic D, Nahas R, Bell JS, Hilmer SN. Anticholinergic burden: considerations for older adults. J Pharm Pract Res. 2017;47(1):67–77. https://doi.org/10.1002/jppr.1303.
125. Manivannan A, Kabbani D, Levine D. Use of multiple anticholinergic medications can predispose patients to severe non-exertional hyperthermia. BMJ Case Rep. 2021;14(3) https://doi.org/10.1136/bcr-2020-239873.
126. Keegan MT, Brown DR, Rabinstein AA. Serotonin syndrome from the interaction of cyclobenzaprine with other serotonergic drugs. Anesth Analg. 2006;103(6):1466–8. https://doi.org/10.1213/01.ane.0000247699.81580.eb.
127. Bramness JG, Furu K, Engeland A, Skurtveit S. Carisoprodol use and abuse in Norway: a pharmacoepidemiological study. Br J Clin Pharmacol. 2007;64(2):210–8. https://doi.org/10.1111/j.1365-2125.2007.02847.x.
128. Dalén P, Alvan G, Wakelkamp M, Olsen H. Formation of meprobamate from carisoprodol is catalysed by CYP2C19. Pharmacogenetics. 1996;6(5):387–94. https://doi.org/10.1097/00008571-199610000-00002.
129. Lewandowski TA. Pharmacokinetic modeling of carisoprodol and meprobamate disposition in adults. Hum Exp Toxicol. 2017;36(8):846–53. https://doi.org/10.1177/0960327116672912.
130. Palmer JL, Scott RJ, Gibson A, Dickins M, Pleasance S. An interaction between the cytochrome P450 probe substrates chlorzoxazone (CYP2E1) and midazolam (CYP3A). Br J Clin Pharmacol. 2001;52(5):555–61. https://doi.org/10.1046/j.0306-5251.2001.01479.x.
131. Kemal M, Imami R, Poklis A. A fatal methocarbamol intoxication. J Forensic Sci. 1982;27(1):217–22.
132. Bosak AR, Skolnik AB. Serotonin syndrome associated with metaxalone overdose. J Med Toxicol. 2014;10(4):402–5. https://doi.org/10.1007/s13181-014-0404-5.
133. Salahudeen MS, Nishtala PS, Duffull SB. The influence of patient characteristics on anticholinergic events in older people. Dement Geriatr Cogn Dis Extra. 2015;5(3):530–41. https://doi.org/10.1159/000441718.

134. Opie LH. Calcium channel antagonists. Part IV: side effects and contraindications drug interactions and combinations. Cardiovasc Drugs Ther. 1988;2(2):177–89. https://doi.org/10.1007/BF00051233.
135. Reinert JP, Tiemann AR, Barlow ML, Veronin MA. Evaluating the efficacy and safety of calcium channel blockers as adjunctive analgesics to opioid therapy: a literature review. J Pharm Pract Res. 2022;52(1):7–18. https://doi.org/10.1002/jppr.1769.
136. Wiggins BS, Saseen JJ, Page RL, et al. Recommendations for management of clinically significant drug-drug interactions with statins and select agents used in patients with cardiovascular disease: a scientific statement from the American Heart Association. Circulation. 2016;134(21):e468–95. https://doi.org/10.1161/CIR.0000000000000456.
137. Zhou Y-T, Yu L-S, Zeng S, Huang Y-W, Xu H-M, Zhou Q. Pharmacokinetic drug-drug interactions between 1,4-dihydropyridine calcium channel blockers and statins: factors determining interaction strength and relevant clinical risk management. Ther Clin Risk Manag. 2014;10:17–26. https://doi.org/10.2147/TCRM.S55512.
138. Hagelberg NM, Peltoniemi MA, Saari TI, et al. Clarithromycin, a potent inhibitor of CYP3A, greatly increases exposure to oral S-ketamine. Eur J Pain. 2010;14(6):625–9. https://doi.org/10.1016/j.ejpain.2009.10.003.
139. Peltoniemi MA, Saari TI, Hagelberg NM, et al. Exposure to oral S-ketamine is unaffected by itraconazole but greatly increased by ticlopidine. Clin Pharmacol Ther. 2011;90(2):296–302. https://doi.org/10.1038/clpt.2011.140.
140. Peltoniemi MA, Saari TI, Hagelberg NM, et al. Rifampicin has a profound effect on the pharmacokinetics of oral S-ketamine and less on intravenous S-ketamine. Basic Clin Pharmacol Toxicol. 2012;111(5):325–32. https://doi.org/10.1111/j.1742-7843.2012.00908.x.
141. Ashraf MW, Peltoniemi MA, Olkkola KT, Neuvonen PJ, Saari TI. Semimechanistic population pharmacokinetic model to predict the drug-drug interaction between S-ketamine and ticlopidine in healthy human volunteers. CPT Pharmacometrics Syst Pharmacol. 2018;7(10):687–97. https://doi.org/10.1002/psp4.12346.
142. Veraart JKE, Smith-Apeldoorn SY, Bakker IM, et al. Pharmacodynamic interactions between ketamine and psychiatric medications used in the treatment of depression: a systematic review. Int J Neuropsychopharmacol. 2021;24(10):808–31. https://doi.org/10.1093/ijnp/pyab039.
143. Jelen LA, Lythgoe DJ, Stone JM, Young AH, Mehta MA. Effect of naltrexone pretreatment on ketamine-induced glutamatergic activity and symptoms of depression: a randomized crossover study. Nat Med. 2025;31(9):2958–66. https://doi.org/10.1038/s41591-025-03800-w.
144. Williams NR, Heifets BD, Blasey C, et al. Attenuation of antidepressant effects of ketamine by opioid receptor antagonism. Am J Psychiatry. 2018;175(12):1205–15. https://doi.org/10.1176/appi.ajp.2018.18020138.
145. David H, Shipp J. A randomized controlled trial of ketamine/propofol versus propofol alone for emergency department procedural sedation. Ann Emerg Med. 2011;57(5):435–41. https://doi.org/10.1016/j.annemergmed.2010.11.025.

Pain in the Older Adult

21

Sophie Mullins, Emma Thorman, and Miriam Thake

Keywords and Definitions

Acute pain	Pain of sudden onset, limited duration, and usually associated with a specific illness or injury.
Anticholinergic burden	The cumulative effect of taking multiple medications with anticholinergic properties.
Chronic pain	Pain that persists or recurs for over 3 months.
Comprehensive Geriatric Assessment	A multidisciplinary inquiry into the medical, psychological, functional, and social needs of the older person.
CYP2D6	*G*ene coding for the CYP2D6 enzyme, which is required for the metabolism of many commonly prescribed medications.
Frailty	Age-associated syndrome of physiological decline, characterized by loss of inbuilt reserve and ability to recover from physiological insult.
Multimorbidity	The presence of multiple or coexisting diseases or health conditions.
Non-pharmacological treatment	Healthcare interventions not involving the use of medications.
Older adult	Those over the age of 65 years.
Pain threshold	The lowest intensity at which a stimulus is perceived as painful by the individual.
Pain tolerance threshold	The maximum intensity of a painful stimulus an individual can endure.
Pharmacodynamics	The biological and physiological effects of drugs on the body.
Pharmacokinetics	How the body manages drugs from administration to elimination, including absorption, distribution, metabolism, and excretion.
Polypharmacy	Regular use of five or more medications daily.

Abbreviations

ADR	Adverse drug reaction
BGS	British Geriatrics Society
CBT	Cognitive behavioral therapy
CCF	Congestive cardiac failure
CGA	Comprehensive Geriatric Assessment
CKD	Chronic kidney disease
CNS	Central nervous system
COPD	Chronic obstructive pulmonary disease
COX	Cyclo-oxygenase
GI	Gastrointestinal
GFR	Glomerular filtration rate
GSFPIG	Gold Standards Framework Proactive Identification Guidance

S. Mullins (✉)
St. Peter's Hospice, Bristol, UK

E. Thorman
North Bristol NHS Trust, Bristol, UK

M. Thake
Department of Medicine, University of Ottawa, Ottawa, ON, Canada

Ottawa Hospital Research Institute, Ottawa, ON, Canada
e-mail: mthake@toh.ca

J. P. Reinert et al. (eds.), *Adjunctive Analgesic Strategies for the Bedside Clinician and Beyond*,
https://doi.org/10.1007/978-3-032-21675-5_21

INN	International Nonproprietary Name
IV	Intravenous
NSAID	Nonsteroidal anti-inflammatory drug
NMDA	N-methyl-D-aspartate
NNT	Number needed to treat
PAINAD	Pain Assessment in Advanced Dementia
PNS	Peripheral nervous system
PO	Per oral
PR	Per rectum
PRN	Pro re nata
QTc	Corrected QT interval
SNRI	Serotonin noradrenaline reuptake inhibitor
SSRI	Serotonin-specific reuptake inhibitor
TCA	Tricyclic antidepressant
TD	Transdermal
TENS	Transcutaneous electrical nerve stimulation
USAN	United States Adopted Names
WHO	World Health Organization

Introduction

The growth of the aging population and increased life expectancy mean that many clinicians will spend more time managing pain in older adults. This group may accrue comorbidities that contribute to the prevalence and complexity of pain. In addition, physiological changes associated with aging can affect pain perception, further complicating assessment and treatment.

Patterns of disease are changing, with more people living with chronic debilitating conditions such as diabetes, cardiovascular disease, chronic obstructive pulmonary disease (COPD), dementia, and cancer (with associated symptoms resulting from treatment). These conditions frequently coexist in the older adult, necessitating careful history-taking and examination to accurately identify different sources of pain and tailor effective management strategies. Such skills are important to develop, given the profound impact of mismanaged pain on quality of life and overall health outcomes in the elderly population.

Incidence and Prevalence of Pain in the Geriatric Population

Globally, the number of people aged 60 and older is projected to increase by approximately 30% before 2030 [66]. It is well recognized that older adults live with an increased prevalence of pain compared to their younger counterparts, and that longer life expectancy does not correspond to more pain-free years. However, accurately quantifying the prevalence of pain in those >65 years is challenging with significant heterogeneity in studies that have sought to examine it [1]. As the population ages, physicians will be increasingly required to appreciate and manage the complexities of pain in older adults [39].

This burden of increased pain is not distributed evenly across the aging population, with clear associations between social determinants of health and pain prevalence. Individuals from poorer socioeconomic backgrounds and with lower levels of educational attainment are disproportionately affected [31]. Older women are more likely to suffer from pain than men, as are those with a higher body mass index (BMI) and those residing in institutions [25].

The complexity of pain in older adults may be better understood when considering the frailty syndrome which is more prevalent in this group. Rockwood's *Accumulation of Deficits* model conceptualizes frailty as a syndrome arising from the progressive buildup of age-related deficits across various domains of health. This accumulation of deficits ("frailty") may explain why older adults are also more likely to experience multisite, complex, mixed-etiology pain than their younger counterparts, with up to 20% of older adults reporting pain in four or more sites on comprehensive assessment [16].

Despite its high prevalence and clinical significance, pain is often underreported and under-assessed in the older adult, with many perceiving pain as a normal part of aging; this increases the risk of under-recognition and suboptimal management [24].

Causes of Pain in Older Adults

Advancing age is associated with an increased prevalence of multimorbidity, and many common conditions seen in this group of patients include pain as a prominent symptom [3]. Musculoskeletal conditions are particularly common among older adults, with osteoarthritis representing a leading cause of chronic pain. The spine, hips, knees, and neck are frequent sites of involvement [27].

Neuropathic pain is also a significant concern in this population, often arising secondary to conditions such as diabetic neuropathy, postherpetic neuralgia, and medication-induced peripheral neuropathy. Diabetic neuropathy is of particular importance due to the increasing prevalence of diabetes worldwide; it is estimated that 10% of people aged over 75 years and 14% of those aged over 85 years live with diabetes in the UK, with anywhere between 6% and 51% of those suffering from diabetic neuropathy depending on factors such as age and duration of disease [9].

The incidence of cancer rises with age, contributing to a higher burden of cancer-related pain in older adults, both because of the primary disease as well as treatments including surgery, chemotherapy, and radiotherapy. Uncontrolled pain demonstrably worsens performance status and quality of life in older adults with cancer [22].

Neurodegenerative conditions commonly associated with older adults, such as Parkinson's disease and dementia, are also associated with significant pain symptoms. Estimates of pain prevalence in Parkinson's disease range from 45% to 75% and between 45% and 56% in dementia [49, 59].

While chronic pain accounts for a substantial proportion of the overall pain burden in older adults, acute pain is also common. Frailty brings an increased susceptibility to acute injury, and consequently, proficiency in the assessment and management of acute pain in this population is essential for physicians. Those aged 65 and over represent a growing proportion of trauma presentations (so-called "Silver Trauma"), with individuals in this age group accounting for over 25% of all major trauma cases in the UK [2]. Falls are the most frequent mechanism of injury, with neck of femur and rib fractures particularly common and associated with pain, significant morbidity, functional decline, and prolonged hospitalization if inadequately managed [14].

Pain Perception in Older Adults

Aging is a complex phenomenon that is incompletely understood and affects not only all organ systems but also an individual's perception of, and response to, pain. Although viewed as a negative phenomenon, it is important to remember the role of pain as a protective biological mechanism. The implications of altered or reduced perception of pain may include increased risk of injury and misdiagnosis.

Age-related changes have been observed in both the peripheral nervous system (PNS) and central nervous system (CNS), and these affect how older adults perceive pain. In the peripheral nervous system, reduced nerve conduction velocities have been observed in the last third of life, and in animal studies, loss of both myelinated and demyelinated nerve fibers alongside axonal atrophy is seen with advancing age [60]. Additionally, there is a loss of $A\delta$ nerve fibers, implicated in the detection of sharp, localized pain, and a proliferation of glial cells replacing degenerating nociceptive neurons, resulting in impaired ability to detect harmful signals [23]. Moreover, repair to damaged neurons is slower and incomplete in the older subject [60], meaning pain episodes may last for longer.

Age-associated changes are also seen within the central nervous system. Neuroplasticity, the ability to recover from injury and the resolution of pain, appears to be slowed with aging [23]. Older adults have longer periods of hyperalgesia following painful stimuli. Combined with slower healing after injury, this may lead to prolonged periods of discomfort and functional impairment. Central nervous system changes appear to be enhanced in the presence of dementia, with heightened pain perception observed [10]. Although the exact mechanisms underpinning this remain unclear, one hypothesis is that degeneration of the prefrontal cortex may lead to impairment of descending inhibitory control [10]. This is important, as traditionally it is felt that dementia is not an inherently painful condition.

Due to the changes outlined above, the threshold at which pain is perceived becomes higher with age, meaning that sensitivity to low-intensity pain is reduced [33]. This is particularly true of thermal noxious stimuli and is less pronounced for mechanically evoked pain stimuli [23], meaning older adults may be more susceptible to injuries from extremes of heat, as their protective responses may be blunted. Conversely, pain tolerance generally lowers with age, and the efficacy of descending pain inhibition mechanisms becomes impaired. As a result, older adults may be more likely to perceive pain later in disease progression but be more vulnerable to escalating pain over time [33].

Impact of Pain on Older Adults

Poorly managed pain has implications not only for the individual but also for their family, caregivers, and society.

Physical Impacts

Studies have shown significant excess all-cause mortality in chronic pain sufferers [34]. From a physical perspective, pain is associated with multiple poor prognostic indicators in the older adult, including decreased gait speed and weaker grip strength, and there is an enhanced risk of falling. There are effects on sleep duration and quality as well as nutritional intake [56]. The risk of delirium, a condition with a high morbidity and mortality, is doubled in the context of pain [63].

Frailty, a reduction in physiological reserve, is a syndrome commonly seen in older adults and has huge implications for well-being in later life. Pain is associated with a higher risk of developing frailty, and this risk is increased further with greater pain severity, frequency, and number of sites affected [61]. Correspondingly, frailty can negatively impact the ability of an individual to manage pain both physically and psychologically [37].

Psychological Impacts

Chronic pain in older adults is associated with increased rates of depression, anxiety, and cognitive impairment [40]. The relationship between pain and depression is multidirectional; while chronic pain can precipitate or exacerbate depressive symptoms, depression itself alters the perception of pain and makes it harder to treat successfully [44].

Social Impacts

In addition to the negative physical and psychological effects of pain, those living with chronic pain are more likely to be socially isolated and dependent for activities of daily living, with an associated loss of independence and need for support from healthcare and social services [48].

Assessment of Pain in Older Adults

Comprehensive and inquisitive consultation is needed to identify pain and search for the underlying cause in older adults. Correctly identifying the etiology of pain will improve the likelihood of effective treatment while minimizing the use of ineffective interventions and medications, which may carry burdensome side effects. This can be more challenging in older adults, particularly those who are cognitively impaired. Such patients may find it difficult to provide a comprehensive history, may be harder to examine, and may have challenges undergoing various investigations. Multidisciplinary involvement is likely to yield a more accurate assessment than a physician assessment in isolation [46].

For geriatricians, use of the Comprehensive Geriatric Assessment (CGA) can provide the framework for such an assessment and ensure a holistic review of pain and its management for older adults. An overview of the key domains of the CGA can be seen in Fig. 21.1 below. Using this approach in the older adult with pain is likely to yield a more accurate assessment and therefore improved outcomes.

Using a comprehensive assessment model as a guide to pain assessment is well established and within guidelines [46]. The most comprehensive assessment of pain in older people involves a mixture of quantitative tools, such as those listed below, alongside assiduous history-taking from both patient and caregiver. The collateral history required for pain assessment in older adults who might have cognitive or communication difficulties is critical.

Use of Pain Assessment Tools

A variety of assessment tools have been developed to facilitate the identification and quantification of pain. However, it is recognized that self-reported pain may be influenced by confounding factors, including mood disturbances, fatigue, and the use of sedative medications [7].

Self-reporting remains the gold standard for pain assessment. Useful tools to aid assessment include simple numeric rating scales (e.g., a 0–10 pain scale) or more comprehensive instruments such as the McGill Pain Questionnaire and the Brief Pain Inventory [13, 36]. Pain assessment tools and pain scales have been more thoroughly explored in previous chapters within this textbook, but we will consider some of those pertaining to older adults.

In patients who are unable to accurately self-report due to cognitive or communicative impairments—such as those with delirium, dementia, or aphasia—observational pain assessment tools may be used. These tools rely on the evaluation of nonverbal indicators (e.g., facial grimacing, restlessness) and physiological signs commonly associated with pain (e.g., tachycardia) to aid clinical judgment.

Among these, the Abbey Pain Scale is frequently employed in clinical settings with older adults owing to its simplicity and ease of use, despite limited evidence supporting its validity; see Fig. 21.2.

Alternative tools, such as the Facial Action Coding System, are more robust in pain assessment of patients living with dementia but may be less practical due to the time required for their administration [50]. The American Geriatrics Society recommends using scales such as the Pain Assessment in Advanced Dementia (PAINAD) scale. The British Geriatric Society guidelines support the use of the PAINAD and Doloplus2 scales [9].

Points to Consider in the History of Older Adults

- Maintain a low threshold to consider pain as the cause for the presenting complaint in patients with impaired cognition or communication, e.g., agitation or restlessness, reduced oral intake.
- Take a thorough history of previous injuries or surgery that may continue to have sequelae.
- Assess the effect of the pain on day-to-day function, e.g., restrictions on daily activity like the ability to get dressed, social isolation, etc.
- Assess the person's beliefs regarding the underlying cause and expectations for management of pain.
- A review of what has already been tried for management of pain and the efficacy/adverse effects of these approaches.
- Ensure other symptoms that may be mistaken for pain, e.g., nausea, constipation, and anxiety, have been considered and addressed as far as possible.
- Assess and identify other conditions that may affect which treatment options are available, e.g., presence of constipation, renal disease, hepatic disease, drug-drug interactions, etc.

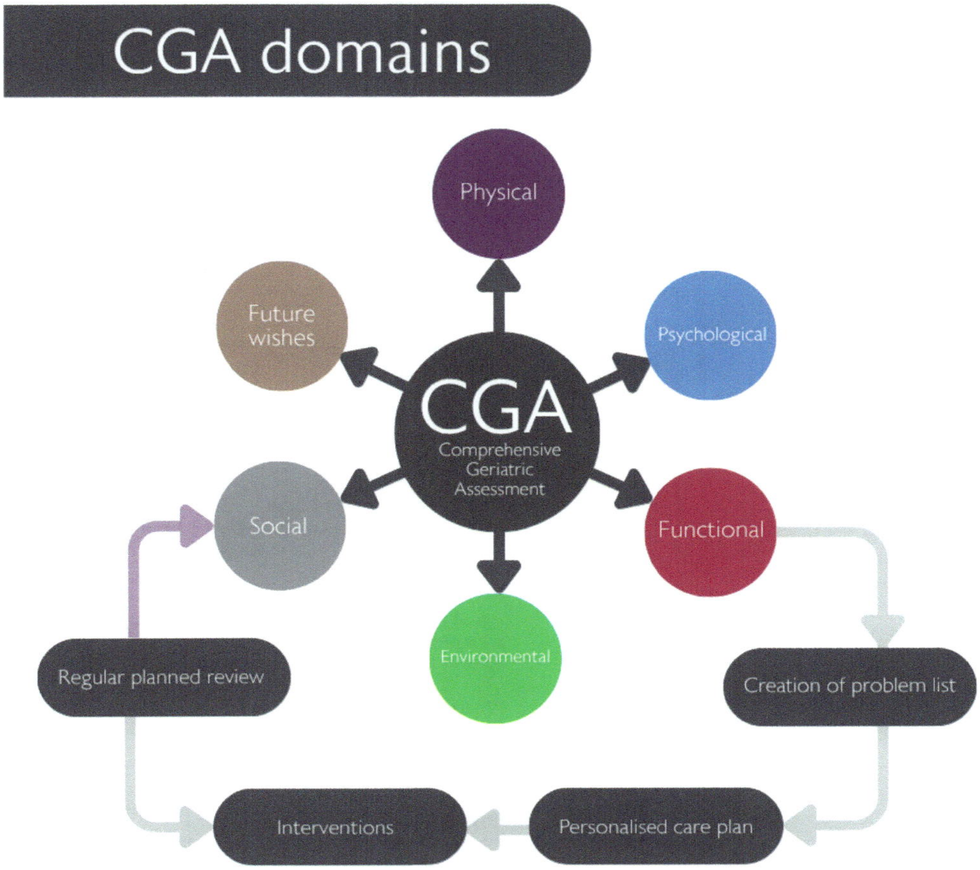

Fig. 21.1 Domains of the Comprehensive Geriatric Assessment. (Taken from British Geriatrics Society Good Practice Guideline)

Examination Considerations for Older Adults with Pain

Comprehensive assessment of discomfort in the older adult, particularly those who are unable to clearly describe symptoms due to impairment of cognition or communication, should include a review of common problem areas not usually included in the standard examination.

For example, failure to properly examine the mouth may lead to missed opportunities to relieve discomfort, with poor dentition, sores from ill-fitting dentures, and oral candidiasis as common findings. Similarly, it is crucial to examine the skin thoroughly, including inspection of the skin creases and pressure area assessment (requiring rolling the patient onto their side if less mobile)—pressure sores being a frequent cause of pain in the frailest frail or those who are less mobile.

Systematic examination of joints can reveal gout or previously unrecognized fractures following a fall. Older adults, particularly those with osteoporosis or low body weight, are at higher risk of fragility fractures even from low-impact events such as falls from standing height. The risk of missed injuries following such events was illustrated in a study reviewing a Silver Trauma Review clinic, which identified previously unrecognized injuries in 18% of the 137 patients seen [51]. This highlights the critical role of thorough secondary and tertiary assessment in older adults following trauma (Fig. 21.3).

Applications for Clinical Practice

Dosing Considerations

Pharmacokinetics

Older adults may experience the effects of analgesia differently for multiple reasons. There are several age-related metabolic changes that alter the pharmacokinetics of analgesic medications. These will be considered in the following Fig. 21.4, relevant to the related organ system.

Pharmacodynamics

Age-related changes in pharmacodynamics occur at the receptor and/or signal transduction level, and homeostatic mechanisms may be attenuated with more time required to regain the steady state [39, 57]. Differences in older adults are due to changes in drug-receptor interaction, post-receptor events, and homeostatic responses, and are also often due to pathologic changes in organs [45].

Fig. 21.2 The Abbey Pain Scale. Designed to assess pain for patients who cannot verbalize their pain. (Abbey et al. Abbey Pain Scale. Funded by the JH & JD Gunn Medical Research Foundation, 1998–2002)

Abbey Pain Scale

For measurement of pain in people with dementia who cannot verbalise.

How to use scale: While observing the resident, score questions 1 to 6

Name of resident: ....

Name and designation of person completing the scale: ....

Date: ....**Time:** ....

Latest pain relief given was..**at** ....**hrs.**

Q1. **Vocalisation**
eg. whimpering, groaning, crying **Q1** ☐
Absent 0 Mild 1 Moderate 2 Severe 3

Q2. **Facial expression**
eg: looking tense, frowning grimacing, looking frightened **Q2** ☐
Absent 0 Mild 1 Moderate 2 Severe 3

Q3. **Change in body language**
eg: fidgeting, rocking, guarding part of body, withdrawn **Q3** ☐
Absent 0 Mild 1 Moderate 2 Severe 3

Q4. **Behavioural Change**
eg: increased confusion, refusing to eat, alteration in usual patterns **Q4** ☐
Absent 0 Mild 1 Moderate 2 Severe 3

Q5. **Physiological change**
eg: temperature, pulse or blood pressure outside normal limits, perspiring, flushing or pallor **Q5** ☐
Absent 0 Mild 1 Moderate 2 Severe 3

Q6. **Physical changes**
eg: skin tears, pressure areas, arthritis, contractures, previous injuries. **Q6** ☐
Absent 0 Mild 1 Moderate 2 Severe 3

Add scores for 1 – 6 and record here ⇨ **Total Pain Score** ☐

Now tick the box that matches the Total Pain Score ⇨

0 – 2 No pain	3 – 7 Mild	8 – 13 Moderate	14+ Severe

Finally, tick the box which matches the type of pain ⇨

Chronic	Acute	Acute on Chronic

Dementia Care Australia Pty Ltd
Website: www.dementiacareaustralia.com

Abbey, J; De Bellis, A; Piller, N; Esterman, A; Giles, L; Parker, D and Lowcay, B.
Funded by the JH & JD Gunn Medical Research Foundation 1998 – 2002
(This document may be reproduced with this acknowledgment retained)

There is a significant heterogeneity of drug response in older adults, meaning the effects can vary vastly between individuals, and this may not always be predictable [39]. Cautious prescribing is therefore required for older adults, particularly those living with frailty, with careful choice of analgesic medication required and the potential need for lower starting doses, slower titration, and careful monitoring for side effects. Older adults frequently demonstrate exaggerated responses to CNS-active drugs such as benzodiazepines and opioids. This is partly because of changes described in CNS function but also because of increased pharmacodynamic sensitivity to these drugs [8].

Older adults are also more likely to experience multimorbidity and polypharmacy. This may alter the impact of medications prescribed for pain due to the increased risk of drug interactions and side effects. In clinical practice, this necessitates careful drug choice, dose adjustments, and close monitoring of the effects of analgesics when they are pre-

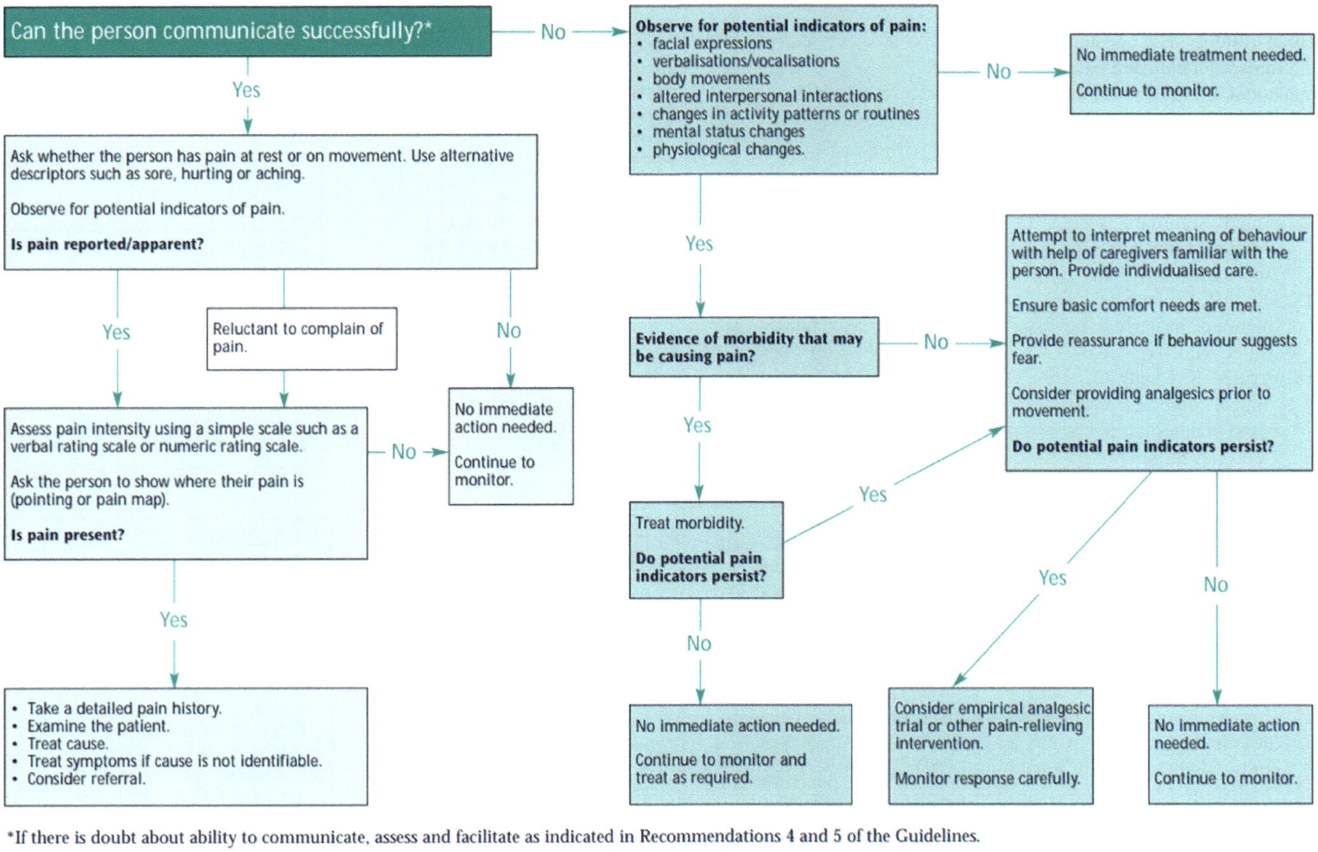

Fig. 21.3 Algorithm for the assessment of pain in older people taken from the 2007 NICE Guidelines from the British Pain Society, British Geriatrics Society, and Royal College of Physicians

scribed for older adults. Pharmacist involvement is often helpful.

Treatment of Pain in Older Adults

General Considerations for Treatment of Pain in Older Adults

Prior to commencing medication, consider any fears or misconceptions around medications. These may be more likely in older adults. There may be preconceptions, for example, that being on opiates indicates a shorter prognosis and more concerns about addiction. Opiates may be viewed as a final option for pain management, which might lead to delayed or inadequate pain relief. Patients may be less likely to take medication due to these beliefs, and it can affect compliance. Trying to ascertain what these beliefs are and alleviate fears is crucial when commencing medication and developing an analgesic strategy.

In addition, it is paramount to consider what the patients' goals of treatment are. Patients may prefer to have undertreated pain if this means they are not over-sedated and may prioritize their cognition; for others, treating pain may be their priority over other factors. A holistic approach and establishing goals of care prior to treatment strategies are therefore key.

Consider the impact of other comorbidities on the ability to take medication.

- Considering the physical ability of patients to take their medications is critical. Patients with cognitive impairment may require simplified regimens and/or devices or carers to prompt them if they are living and managing medications independently. Input from pharmacy colleagues can be invaluable here.
- Conditions affecting hand function and dexterity may impact patients' ability to draw up medication or remove it from packaging.
- Visual impairment may affect patients' ability to see the right dose, read instructions on packaging, or identify different medications. A common scenario is one in which a patient just takes a "swig" of liquid medication from a bottle rather than measuring it out; this has been shown to be of inconsistent volume and may be an important consideration when thinking about toxicity or responsiveness.

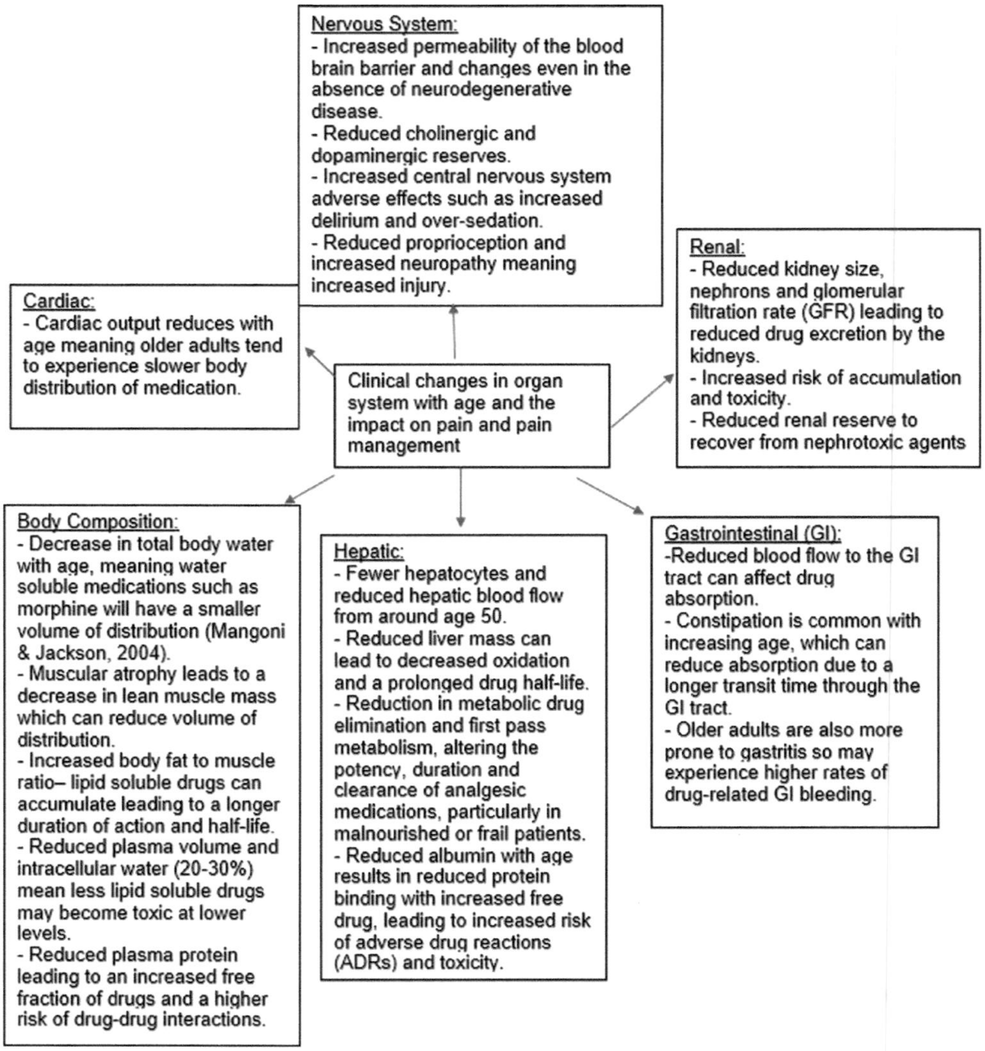

Fig. 21.4 Clinical changes in organ systems with age and the impact on pain and pain management. *ADR* adverse drug reaction, *GFR* glomerular filtration rate, *GI* gastrointestinal [35, 39]

- Swallowing difficulties are more common in older adults. Inability to swallow medication may lead to reduced concordance with the drug regimen as well as oral and/or esophageal ulcerations if taken and left in the mouth for too long. Consideration should be made as to the most appropriate medication form and instructions offered on how to take the medication (e.g., sitting upright and taking with a glass of water). It is worthwhile considering liquid or topical forms if available, whether the drug can be crushed and taken with, e.g., apple sauce or yogurt, or transdermal patches.

When initiating medication for older adults, it is usually recommended to start at lower doses and up-titrate carefully with frequent review. Care must be taken regarding cessation of ineffective medications (sometimes weaning in a similarly cautious manner to how they were initiated) to avoid significant polypharmacy, side effects, and drug-drug interactions. Care also needs to involve caregivers for those with cognitive impairment to ensure accurate review of efficacy and side effects. If possible, in older adults, new medications should be started one at a time, allowing the effect of individual medications to be monitored and side effects attributed to the correct causative drug.

Although increased caution is warranted when prescribing analgesia for the older adult, this should not preclude effective pain management. It should be remembered that most can take and tolerate analgesic medications safely when they are selected and monitored with care. Undertreatment of pain stemming from conservatism or excessive caution in prescribing can also lead to significant negative outcomes for the patient.

The timing of medication is important. Consider rapidly acting formulations with short half-lives for severe episodic pain in addition to background analgesia for more continuous pain [47]. Consider the cognitive ability of older adults to recognize the need for PRN medications or the ability to communicate this need, e.g., in the hospital or care home setting.

A prior assessment should be made for any preexisting voiding difficulties or constipation, which may be augmented by analgesic use. Opiates and anticholinergics commonly cause constipation and urinary retention in older adults.

It is worth considering other symptomatology or diseases when selecting analgesics in the context of multimorbidity. This can help to reduce tablet burden and increase the effectiveness of the treatment. For example, coexistent depression/anxiety may lead to choosing certain analgesics over others, e.g., using duloxetine as a neuropathic agent if there is concurrent depression to avoid polypharmacy.

Consider co-prescribed medication and polypharmacy likely to worsen cognition, e.g., anticholinergic burden. Anticholinergic burden refers to the overall effect of taking multiple medications that block the action of acetylcholine. This cumulative effect can lead to various adverse reactions, especially in older adults, particularly related to cognitive impairment. While opiates are generally not considered anticholinergics, they do interact with the cholinergic system, leading to classically anticholinergic side effects. Use of tools such as the Anticholinergic Burden (ACB) calculator [29] gives an overall anticholinergic burden score. If shown to be high, it may be prudent to consider if medications with a lower anticholinergic burden can be used or if other co-prescribed medications with a high anti-cholinergic effect can be stopped or reduced. Many medications display dose dependency regarding anticholinergic side effects.

Critical to the initiation of any analgesic plan is the reassessment. This can be increasingly difficult in the older adult, where impaired cognition may impact the ability to recall whether interventions have been effective. Encouraging carers and relatives to use tools such as pain diaries can be especially useful to gauge if treatments are working.

It is important to recognize that escalating pain may signal disease-specific progression or global physiological deterioration, potentially indicating a change in prognosis. This may provide a prompt to discuss the wider implications of this and to review patients' advanced care plans and goals of care. Tools such as the Gold Standards Framework Proactive Identification Guidance (GSFPIG) can be used to help identify patients who are nearing the end of their life [53]. The GSFPIG includes more general indicators of deterioration, such as complex symptom burden, as well as disease-specific indicators. Recognizing that time may be short helps to guide the clinician in determining the types of treatment that are likely to benefit the patient, while avoiding options that are highly burdensome or unlikely to produce a timely effect. For example, initiation of medication requiring slow titration (e.g., gabapentinoids) may not be appropriate for a patient with only days or short weeks to live.

Non-pharmacological Therapies

The use of non-pharmacological strategies such as physiotherapy, cognitive behavioral therapy (CBT), transcutaneous electrical nerve stimulation (TENS), orthotics, social prescribing, and acupuncture should be routinely considered in older adults with pain from any cause. This approach is a key point in the summary report produced by Schofield et al. in the update of evidence-based guidelines for the management of pain in older adults [47]. These treatments may reduce the need for medication(s), which, as outlined above, may have a greater negative impact on adults.

- Transcutaneous electrical nerve stimulation (TENS)

TENS can be an important adjunct to the management of pain. Chronic neuropathy and, less commonly, postfracture recovery are the leading indications for using the portable stimulative device, although it has also been applied successfully in relieving low-back pain, postherpetic neuralgia, myofascial pain, phantom-limb pain, and advanced, painful malignancies. TENS is rarely used alone for pain relief but instead should be part of a larger management program that may include other modalities.

There have been mixed reports for the use of TENS in older adults, with some studies suggesting that it can be an effective adjunct [54]. Other sources suggest TENS is not effective for experimental pain in older adults. Looking at high-frequency, low-frequency, and placebo TENS in a double-blind crossover study, Beregron-Vezina et al. found no difference in high- and low-frequency TENS compared to baseline and no difference compared to placebo TENS in pain reduction for older adults. A significant difference was found in this study for younger patients, where pain intensity diminished after high-frequency and low-frequency TENS [5]. Looking at the population of older adults assisted living with chronic musculoskeletal pain, Barr et al. found no difference in two different aged populations (55–75 and >76) on the impact TENS had on pain, or between conventional and pulse-burst TENS; however, both modalities reduced pain in comparison to control TENS. They concluded that treatment should be initiated with conventional TENS [4]. Elbiom-Gabyzon et al. conducted a randomized controlled trial looking at the use of TENS in older hip fracture patients. They found significantly reduced pain in the active TENS arm, as well as increased mobility and walking distance on day 5 postoperatively. This suggests TENS should be added to standard care [17].

Although there are mixed reports for efficacy, TENS is relatively safe, and so if available, it may be a useful tool to try.

- Social Prescribing

Social prescribing is a person-centered approach that links patients to community resources. Activities prescribed can include art, physical activity, social interaction, and personal development. These interventions have been shown to reduce isolation and enhance well-being. There have been positive benefits shown for people with chronic pain and other health issues [43]. Evidence suggests that social prescribing may reduce pain severity, medication use, and clinical appointments. More research is required to provide more robust evidence for the use of social prescribing for chronic pain in general and specifically in older adults.

- Psychological Therapies

CBT shows promise for managing chronic pain in older adults and is recommended for use as an adjunctive therapy in older adults [1].

- Occupational Therapy/Physiotherapy/Orthotics

Consideration of the optimization of the environment for older adults experiencing pain may include a seating assessment, profiling of beds and mattresses, assessment of correct walking aids, etc., depending on the type and location of pain. Therapists' assessments of environment and function are some of the pillars of the CGA and are critical in managing patients with pain. Even with treatment, in many cases, patients may be left with residual pain, and optimizing function despite this is crucial.

Orthoses should be considered and assessed for in patients with lower limb joint or back pain that may be related to poor alignment or biomechanical issues. Examples where orthotics can help include reducing heel pain in plantar fasciitis and using lateral wedge insoles to reduce medical knee joint loading in osteoarthritis. Evidence on using orthotics in older adults with chronic pain secondary to osteoarthritis is inconclusive, with some benefits for sub-talar strapping and insoles, but no benefit for lateral wedge insoles [62]. Orthotics with and/or without metatarsal pads were demonstrated to decrease pain and fear of falling in older adults [32]. The best results come with an individualized assessment, proper fitting, and follow-up.

Physical activity is important in managing chronic pain in older people; it helps to maintain independence and improve quality of life. Reviews of randomized controlled trials recommend programs that involve strengthening, endurance, and flexibility for patients regardless of age [11]. Tse et al. undertook a randomized controlled trial evaluating the effects of a physical exercise program on patients in nursing homes with chronic pain. 369 patients were recruited from ten nursing homes in Hong Kong and were randomized to an experimental group with a personalized exercise program or a control group without this. The intervention arm received an 8-week program with a physiotherapist and nurses; the control group received no training. The intervention group had significantly reduced pain intensity, as well as improved markers of psychological well-being [55].

Because older adults are generally more susceptible to side effects, there is the potential for much more to be gained from pursuing non-pharmacological strategies.

Pharmacological Therapies

- World Health Organization Pain Ladder

The World Health Organization (WHO) pain ladder was designed in 1986 as a guide to treating cancer pain (World Health Organization, 1996) Fig. 21.5. Current WHO guidelines for the management of cancer pain in adults and adolescents advise administering medication "by mouth," "by the clock," "for the individual," and "with attention to detail" [65]. New guidance recognizes and highlights that the pain management ladder is only a guide, and it is important to note that it is primarily designed for use in cancer patients [65]. For patients with pain from different etiologies, different approaches may be needed, but it remains a useful tool when considering escalation of pain management. It is important, particularly in older adults, to approach pain management in a stepwise manner, reassessing post-intervention. This should include deprescribing after an appropriate trial if the intervention has had minimal effect on pain management.

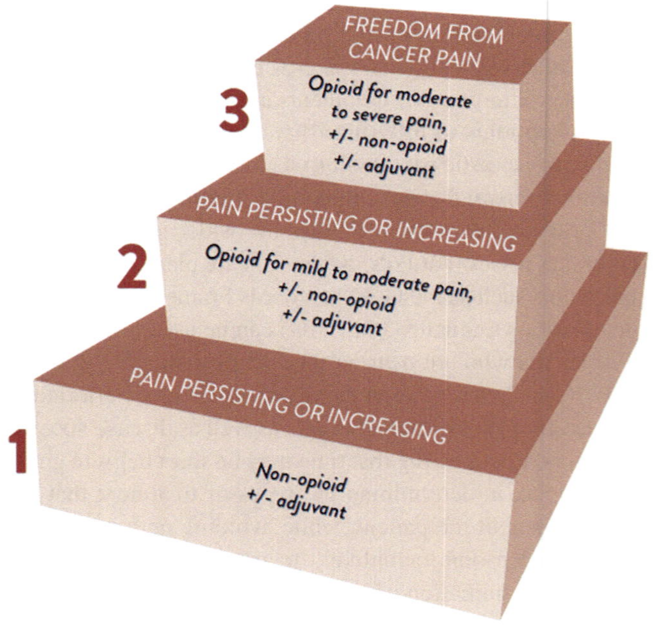

Fig. 21.5 The WHO Pain Ladder taken from the World Health Organization [64]

Acetaminophen

Acetaminophen is the generic name assigned using the United States Adopted Names (USAN) system and is the name used in the USA, Canada, etc., whereas paracetamol is the name assigned using the International Nonproprietary Name (INN) generic name system and is the generic name used in Europe, Australia, India, etc.

These drugs work by inhibiting prostaglandin synthesis, possibly via the inhibition of COX enzymes within the central nervous system. They are known to be an effective form of analgesia and have antipyretic properties, but do not have any anti-inflammatory properties.

In older adults, paracetamol/acetaminophen has been demonstrated to reduce total pain scores and the requirement for opioid analgesia. They can be administered intravenously (IV), orally (PO), or rectally (PR).

Evidence from the literature search suggests that paracetamol/acetaminophen should be considered as first-line treatment for the management of both acute and persistent pain [1]. There are a few contraindications to prescribing these drugs, but considerations are reducing the dose if body weight is less than 50 kg or in liver failure, and not prescribing over the maximum dose. However, these drugs do come with risks and side effects and should not be continually prescribed without rereview and consideration of effectiveness, tablet burden, and potential side effects [28]. Kaur et al. conducted a retrospective study looking at the safety of paracetamol in adults older than 65 years in which they defined exposure as two prescriptions within 6 months. Paracetamol prescriptions were associated with an increased risk of GI perforation, ulceration, or bleeding, along with several other conditions [28].

Nonsteroidal Anti-inflammatories (NSAIDs)

These drugs work by inhibiting cyclo-oxygenase (COX) enzymes, which produce prostaglandins, reducing the levels of prostaglandins that regulate pain, fever, and inflammation. There are two main types of COX enzyme—COX1 and 2. Nonsteroidal drugs can be either nonselective or selective, depending on whether they are more selective for COX2 inhibition. COX1 enzymes produce prostaglandins that regulate normal physiological processes such as gastric mucosal integrity and kidney function. Selective COX2 inhibitors are more likely to cause cardiovascular events, whereas nonselective inhibitors seem to be more likely to cause GI bleeding [6].

Older adults have a higher baseline risk of GI bleeding, myocardial infarction, stroke, and renal impairment [15], so increased caution should be applied when considering prescribing NSAIDs for older adults. NSAIDs also increase the risk of fluid retention and are associated with heart failure decompensation [58]. In general, because of these concerns, NSAIDs should be avoided for the treatment of chronic pain in older adults. If NSAIDs are required, this should be considered on an individual basis, balancing risks vs. benefits, and should be given at the lowest effective dose for as short a course as possible, with a definite stop date [46]. In older adults, co-prescription of a proton pump inhibitor is recommended to reduce the risk of bleeding. Consider other co-prescribed medications that can lead to drug-drug interactions, particularly those with an increased risk of GI bleeding, such as aspirin, serotonin-specific reuptake inhibitors (SSRIs), anticoagulants, etc.

Opioids

As suggested by the WHO analgesic ladder, opioids should be considered for use in mild to moderate pain when simple analgesics have proven insufficient. When initiating opioids for older adults, it is important to provide patients and relatives/carers with information about common side effects and co-prescribe as-needed medications in anticipation of these side effects (e.g., laxatives). Older adults are more vulnerable to all of the listed side effects of opioids, including constipation, nausea, respiratory depression, urinary retention, confusion, sedation, falls, and sleep disturbance [26]. While some side effects may diminish over time, others, such as constipation, often persist throughout treatment and should be actively assessed for and treated. Careful consideration of preexisting bladder and bowel function is necessary before initiation of opioids, as known problems will alert the prescriber to have increased vigilance in preemptively managing potential side effects such as constipation or urinary retention.

Weak opioids are such that they exhibit no further therapeutic effect at higher doses and only lead to increased adverse effects. If a patient has trialed and failed with a weak opiate and is moving to a strong opiate, then generally the weak opiate should be stopped. Tramadol, on occasion, may be continued for its cross-reactivity effects, as seen in Table 21.1.

Realistic treatment goals and a therapeutic plan should be made prior to commencing opioids, explaining to patients that opioids are often poorly effective for patients with chronic noncancer-related pain [19].

Due to the high fat-to-protein ratios in the older adult, it has been suggested that opioids should be started at 25–50% of the dose used in younger adults, with the as-needed (PRN) dose limited to 5% of the total daily dose every 4 hours. It is worth noting that due to dose preparations of some opioids, it is not always possible to start at these lower doses [18].

Opioids should be tapered or stopped if they are not providing useful pain relief and not just increased incrementally. Patients on large doses may need support from specialist services prior to reducing medications. Other events, which should trigger consideration of dose weaning, include improvement or resolution of the underlying condition, the

Table 21.1 Specific considerations for the use of certain opiates

Opiate/strength	Considerations in the older adult
Dihydrocodeine/ weak	Not affected by polymorphisms in *CYP2D6*. Similar side effect profile to codeine
Codeine	Polymorphisms in the *CYP2D6* gene can lead to poor metabolism and reduced efficacy, but ongoing adverse effects such as constipation [25]
Tramadol	Cross-reactivity at other receptor sites leads to increased neurocognitive complications, a common practice to avoid in the older adult if possible
Morphine	Caution in renal impairment
Oxycodone	Safer in renal impairment, but caution is still required in patients with chronic kidney disease (CKD) stage 4–5. Extensively metabolized by the liver Indications of an improved side effect profile when compared to morphine with respect to nausea, hallucinations, and pruritus [41]
Fentanyl	Not administered via the oral route due to extensive first-pass metabolism. The transdermal (TD) route may have lower absorption rates in older adults. Potentially lower clearance in the older adult due to lower plasma albumin, reduced hepatic blood flow, and renal clearance [30]
Buprenorphine	The half-life of the active drug and metabolites is not increased in the older adult. Available as transdermal patches, which are replaced every 5–7 days, making up-titration in acute pain difficult. Buprenorphine TD patches have been increasingly used in older adults for chronic noncancer pain and shown to be both effective and safe [21]
Methadone	Methadone has complex pharmacokinetics and a long and variable half-life (30–110 hours). The effect of dose increases can be noticeable up to 5 days after implementation. It is stored in multiple tissues, including subcutaneous fat, which can be relatively higher in the older adult; therefore, dose incrementations can be more likely to cause toxicity. There is an increased risk of accumulation in the older adult and with co-prescription of CYP450 inhibitors, as patients with preexisting renal or hepatic impairment would have altered drug metabolism. Preexisting cardiovascular conditions, e.g., congestive cardiac failure (CCF), can be at increased risk of arrhythmogenic properties (can prolong QTc)
Hydromorphone	Strength means that the minimal dose orally is equivalent to 5 mg oral morphine; this would often be a higher starting dose than recommended in the older adult

development of intolerable side effects, or the provision of definitive pain-relieving treatment, such as a joint replacement [18].

When converting from one opiate to another, accurate dose conversion is hugely important, typically using standardized conversion tables or calculators. To account for incomplete cross-tolerance, the initial dose of the new opioid should generally be reduced to 50–67% of the calculated equivalent dose. Fentanyl and methadone are exceptions to this. Cross-tolerance effects can potentiate both the analgesic properties and adverse effects of the new opioid [12]. In older adults with enhanced susceptibility to medication side effects, extra caution is warranted. Starting at the lower end of the dose conversion—or even lower—may be necessary to ensure safety and tolerability of the new opioid.

In addition to these pharmacological considerations, the risk of opioid misuse in older adults should not be overlooked. The use of prescription opioids is associated with an increased risk of opioid misuse disorder and harm or even death from toxicity or overdose [38]. There is an emerging body of evidence suggesting older adults are equally susceptible to opioid abuse, especially as newer cohorts of older adults may have had increased exposure to substance use earlier in life [20]. In patients with a history of addiction, prioritization of non-opioid pain relief strategies is particularly advisable.

Adjuvant Analgesics

Adjuvant analgesics encompass a broad range of medications from different classes that are not primarily designed to treat pain but can be of help in various painful conditions. This section will review some of these therapies, with considerations for prescribing in the older adult (Table 21.2).

Antidepressants

Antidepressants are the most prescribed form of adjuvant medication for pain management, with SSRIs generally preferred over TCAs in older adults due to side effect profiles. Despite this, prevalence data indicate TCAs are more frequently prescribed to older patients than SSRIs. TCAs can contribute to increasing the risk of injury and falls, orthostatic hypotension, and, at higher doses, the risk of cardiac death. Despite these concerns, they have demonstrated superior efficacy for neuropathic pain, with a lower number needed to treat (NNT) compared to SNRIs (4.6 vs 7.4), also outperforming opiates (NNT 5.9) [52]. Thus, TCAs may retain a role for neuropathic pain management for some older patients following a comprehensive assessment of individual risks and benefits.

Topical Treatments

Absorption of transdermal drugs may vary in frail older people with significant subcutaneous tissue loss, thereby creating difficulties in predicting drug efficacy. The RELIEF feasibility trial has shown promising initial results in the treatment of localized rib pain following rib fractures, indicating that patients who have lidocaine patches post-rib fracture have a reduced incidence of pulmonary complications compared to the control

Table 21.2 Consideration of some oral adjuvant analgesics, mechanism of action, side effects, and considerations in the older adult

Class of drug	Mechanism of action and indication	Common side effects	Considerations in the older person
Anticonvulsants	Gabapentin and Pregabalin: block voltage-gated calcium channels Carbamazepine: Blocks voltage-gated sodium channels All effective for neuropathic pain	Arthralgia Confusion Headache Drowsiness Dizziness Dry mouth	Central nervous system effects can lead to oversedation, which in turn can contribute to falls and delirium
Tricyclic Antidepressants (TCA)s	Amitriptyline: Blocks norepinephrine and serotonin transporters Effective for neuropathic pain	Cardiac arrhythmias Drowsiness	Risk of anticholinergic side effects such as urinary retention, blurred vision and dry mouth TCAs can potentiate cardiac arrhythmias via the prevention of norepinephrine reuptake
SSRI and SNRI antidepressants	SSRI (selective serotonin reuptake inhibitors) and SNRI (serotonin and norepinephrine reuptake inhibitors)	Nausea Dry Mouth Constipation Fatigue Sexual dysfunction	Interfere with sodium regulation and can cause hyponatremia, particularly in the elderly, who are more vulnerable to age-related changes in fluid regulation Risk of GI bleeding higher in older adults
Ketamine	NMDA receptor antagonist, an anesthetic agent with well-recognized analgesic properties	Drowsiness Dizziness	A higher prevalence of coronary artery disease, hypertension, and atherosclerosis in the older adult could present a risk with use
Duloxetine	Inhibits the reuptake of serotonin and noradrenaline in the CNS. Helpful in the treatment of neuropathic pain, e.g., diabetic neuropathy	Headache Diarrhea Dry mouth Insomnia	Can lead to drug-induced movement disorders, confusion, and hypertension as a result of noradrenergic effects [25]

Adapted from Hosseini et al. [25]

group (48% with lidocaine vs. 59% without). Similarly, capsaicin 8% patches have a moderate certainty of evidence in neuropathic pain [52]. Importantly, patches have been shown to be well tolerated in older adults, with a safety profile comparable to that in younger patients. The most common adverse effect is localized erythema at the application site [42].

Interventional Pain Therapies

Interventional pain procedures can be an important part of multimodal treatment for pain, depending on the condition and patient comorbidities. Interventional procedures vary in complexity, and a detailed discussion of individual techniques is beyond the scope of this chapter. However, in older adults, it is important to appraise the feasibility of such procedures considering mobility, frailty, and overall clinical condition. Regional anesthesia, in particular, may be technically more challenging due to age-related anatomical changes such as degenerative bone disease, vertebral joint degeneration, narrowing of intervertebral and epidural spaces, and calcification of the ligamentum flavum.

Despite these challenges, interventional therapies may offer significant benefits for older adults. While the burdens and risks may be higher than in younger, fitter patients, the potential to reduce reliance on systemic analgesics—thereby minimizing adverse effects and polypharmacy—can make these interventions especially valuable in carefully selected individuals.

Conclusion

Providing adequate analgesia for older adults can be challenging due to age-related physiological changes, polypharmacy, multimorbidity, and altered drug metabolism, along with common underreporting and under-recognition of pain in this population. Proactive inquiry, comprehensive and holistic assessment, and using appropriate supplementary assessment tools, especially for patients who have difficulty communicating, can improve pain detection and treatment. When analgesics are carefully selected, appropriately titrated, and closely monitored, the complex pain management needs of older adults can be met safely and effectively. Tailoring treatment to the individual, while considering their overall medical context, remains central to optimizing outcomes in this population.

References

1. Abdulla A, Adams N, Bone M, Elliott A, Gaffin J, Jones D, et al. Guidance on the management of pain in older people. Age Ageing. 2013;42:1–75.
2. Atinga A, Shekkeris A, Fertleman M, Batrick N, Kashef E, Dick E. Trauma in the elderly patient. Br J Radiol. 2018;
3. Barnett K, Mercer S, Norbury M, Wat G, Wyke S, Guhrie B. Epidemiology of multimorbidity and implications for health care, research, and medical education: a cross-sectional study. Lancet. 2012;380(7):37–43.

4. Barr J, Weissenbuehler S, Cleary C. Effectiveness and comfort of Transcutaenous Electrical Nerve Stimulation for older persons with chronic pain. J Geriatr Phys Ther. 2004;27(3):93–9.
5. Bergeron-vezina K, Corriveua H, Martel M, Harvey M-P, Leonard G. High- and low-frequency transcutaneous electrical nerve stimulation dose not reduce experimental pain in elderly individuals. Pain. 2015;156(10):2093–9.
6. Bing R, Lomnicka M. Why do cyclo-oxygenase-2 inhibitors cause cardiovascular events? J Am Coll Cardiol. 2002;39(3):521–2.
7. Boring B, Walsh K, Nanavaty N, Ng B, Mathur V. How and why patient concerns influence pain reporting: a qualitative analysis of personal accounts and perceptions of others' use of numerical pain scales. Front Psychol; 2021.
8. Bowie M, Slattum P. Pharmacodynamics in older adults: a review. Am J Geriatr Pharmacother. 2007;5(3):263–303.
9. British Geriatrics Society. Diabetes. Retrieved from British Geriatrics Society; 2018. https://www.bgs.org.uk/diabetes-0
10. Bunk S, Zuidema S, Koch K, Lautenbacher S, De Deyn P, Kunz M. Pain processing in older adults with dementia-related cognitive impairment is associated with frontal neurodegeneration. Neurobiol Aging. 2021;106:139–52.
11. Chan H, Chan C. Managing chronic pain in older people. Clin Med. 2022;22(4):292–4.
12. Chau D, Walker V, Pai L, Cho L. Opiates and elderly: uses and side effects. Clin Interv Aging. 2008;3(2):273–8.
13. Cleeland C, Ryan K. Pain assessment: global use of the Brief Pain Inventory. Ann Acad Med Singap. 1994;23:129–38.
14. Connolly KK. A silver lining: the identification of silver trauma at triage for older persons (>65) presenting to the emergency department. Age Ageing. 2023;52(Suppl 3)
15. Davis A, Robson J. The dangers of NSAIDs: look both ways. BR J General Pract. 2016;66:172–3.
16. Domenichiellio A, Ramsden C. The silent epidemic of chronic pain in older adults. Prog Neuro-Psychopharmacol Biol Psychiatry. 2019:284–90.
17. Elbiom-Gabyzon M, Andrawus Najar S, Shtarker H. Effects of transcutaneous nerve stimulation (TENS) on acute postoperative pain intensity andmobility after hip fracture: a double blinded, randomized trial. Clin Interv Aging. 2019;14:1841–50.
18. FacultyofPainMedicineoftheRoyalCollegeofAnaesthetists.A structured approach to opioid prescribing. Retrieved from Facult of Pain Medicine of the Royal College of Anaesthetists; 2025. https://www.fpm.ac.uk/opioids-aware-structured-approach-opioid-prescribing/tapering-and-stopping
19. Frieden T, Houry D. Reducing the risks of relief — the CDC opioid-prescribing guideline. N Engl J Med. 2016;374(16):1501–4.
20. Gazelka H, Leal J, Lapid M, Rummans T. Opioids in older adults: indications, prescribing, complications, and alternative therapies for primary care. Mayo Clin Proc. 2020;95(4):793–800.
21. Gianni W, Madaio M, Ceci M. Transdermal buprenorphine for the treatment of chronic noncancer pain in the oldest old. J Pain Symptom Manage. 2011;41(4):707–14.
22. Hachem G, Rocha F, Pepersack T, Jounblat Y, Drowart A, Lago L. Advances in pain management for older patients with cancer. Ecancermedicalscience. 2019;
23. Hadjistavropoulos T, Herr K, Prkachin K, Craig K, Gibson S, Lukas A, Smith J. Pain assessment in elderly adults with dementia. Lancet Neurol. 2014:1216–77.
24. Herr K, Garand L. Assessment and measurement of pain in older adults. Clin Geriatr Med. 2001;17(3):457–78.
25. Hosseini F, Mullins S, Gibson W, Thake M. Acute pain management of older adults. Clin Med. 2022;22(4):302–6.
26. Jassal M, Egan G, Dahri K. Opioid prescribing in the elderly: a systematic review. J Pharm Technol. 2020;36(1):28–40.
27. Jones M, Ehrherd K, Ripoll J. Pain in the elderly. Curr Pain Headach Rep. 2016:20–3.
28. Kaur J, Nakafero G, Abhishek A, Mallen C, Doherty M, Zhang W. Incidence of side effects associated with acetaminophen in people aged 65 years or more: a prospective cohort study using data from the clinical practice research datalink. Arthritis Care Res. 2024;77(5):666–75.
29. King R, Rabino S. ACB calculator. Retrieved from ACB Calculator; 2025. https://www.acbcalc.com/.
30. Kuip E, Zandvliet M, Koolen S, Mathijssen R, van der Rij C. A review of factors explaining variability in fentanyl pharmacokinetics; focus on implications for cancer patients. Br J Clin Pharmacol. 2016;83:294–313.
31. Lacey R, Belcher J, Croft P. Does life course socio-economic position influence chronic disabling pain in older adults? A Genral population study. Eur J Public Health. 2013;23(4):534–40.
32. Lacourse J, Sims J, Ampat G. Do Orthtoics with a metatarsal pad decrease pain and fear of falling in older adults? A randomised control trial. Phys Occup Ther Geriatr. 2023;41(4):596–612.
33. Lautenbacher S, Kunz M, Strate P, Nielsen J, Arendt-Nielsen L. Age effects on pain thresholds, temporal summation and spatial summation of heat and pressure pain. Pain. 2005;115(3):410–8.
34. Macfarlane G, Barnish M, Jones G. Persons with chronic widespread pain experience excess mortality: longitudinal results from UK biobank and meta-analysis. Ann Rhem Dis. 2017;76(11):1815–22.
35. Mangoni A, Jackson S. Age related changes in pharmacokinetics and pharmacodynamics basic principles and practical applications. Br J Clin Pharmacol. 2004;57(1):6–14.
36. Melzack R. The McGill pain questionnaire: from description to measurement. Anesthesiology. 2005;103:199–202.
37. Merrick M, Grange R, Rudd S, Shipway D. Evaluation and treatment of acute trauma pain in older adults. Drugs Aging. 2023:869–80.
38. Mullachery P, Lima-Costa M, de Loyloa Filho A. Prevalence of pain and use of prescription opioids among older adults: results from the Brazilian Longitudinal Study of Aging (ELSI-Brazil). Lancet Reg Health Am. 2023;
39. Mullins S, Hosseini F, Gibson W, Thake M. Physiological changes from ageing regarding pain perception and is impact on pain management for older adults. Clin Med. 2022;22(4):307–10.
40. Ord A, Coddington K, Sautter S, al, e. Neuropsychological symptoms and functional capacity in older adults with chronic pain. Gerontol Geriatr Med. 2024;
41. Ordonez Gallego A, Gonzalez Baron M, Espinosa Arranz E. Oxycodone: a pharmacological and clinical review. Clin Transl Oncol. 2007;9(5):298–307.
42. Pickering G, Engelen S, Stupar M, Ganry H, Eerdekens M. Is the Capsaicin 179mg (8%) cutaneous patch and appropriate treatment option for older patients wih peripheral neuropathic pain? J Pain Res. 2024;17:1327–44.
43. Pilkington G, Johnson M, Thomspon K. Social prescribing for adults with chronic pain in the U.K.: a rapid review. Br J Pain. 2025;19(3):176–86.
44. Rayner L, Hotopf M, Petkova H, Matcham F, Simpson A, McCracken LM. Depression in patients with chronic pain attending a specialised pain treatment centre: prevalence and impact on health care costs. Pain. 2016;157(7):1472–9. https://doi.org/10.1097/j.pain.0000000000000542.
45. Ruscin J, Linnebur S. MSD manuals: pharmacodynamics in older adults; 2025.
46. Schofield P. The assessment of pain in older people: UK National Guidelines. Age Ageing. 2018;47:i1–i22.
47. Schofield P, Dunham M, Martin D, Bellamy GF, Sookhoo D, Boncaro A, et al. Evidence-based clinical practice guidelines on the

management of pain in older people - a summary report. Br J Pain. 2022;16(1):6–13.
48. Simsek I, Simsek T, Yumin E, Sertel M, Ozturk A, Yumin M. The effects of pain on health-related quality of life and satisfaction with life in older adults. Top Geriatr Rehabil. 2010;26(4):361–7.
49. Skogar O, Kokk J. Pain management in patients with Parkinson's disease: challenges and solutions. J Multidisipl Healthc. 2016:469–79.
50. Smith T, Harvey K. Psychometric properties of pain measurements for people living with dementia: a COSMIN systematic review. Eur Geriatr Med. 2022;13(5):1029–45.
51. Smyth H, Breslin D, Mullany L, Ramiah V, Riches R, Laguna R, et al. Silver Trauma Review Clinic: a novel model of care to manage non-operative injuries in older patients. Emerg Med J. 2023;40:721–5.
52. Soliman N, Moisset X, Ferraro M, de Andrade D, Baron R, Belton J, et al. Pharacotherapy and non-invasive neuromodulation for neuropathic pain: a systematic review and meta-analysis. Lancet Neurol. 2025;25(5):413–28.
53. The Gold Standards Framework; Royal College of General Practitioners. The GSF Prognostic Indicator Guidance; 2011. Retrieved July 27, 2025, from https://www.futureplanning.org.uk/uploads/8/0/4/0/80407130/gsf_prognostic_indicator_guidance.pdf
54. Thorsteinsson G. Chronic pain: use of TENS in the elderly. Geriatrics. 1987;
55. Tse M, Tang S, Wan V, Vong S. The effectiveness of physical exercise training in pain, mobility, and psychological well being of older persons living in nursing homes. Pain Manag Nurs. 2014;15(4):778–88.
56. Turk D, Fillingim R, ohrbach, R., & Patel, K. Assessmen of psychosocial and functional impact of chronic pain. J Pain. 2016:21–49.
57. Turnheim K. When drug herapy gets old, pharamackinetics and pharmacodynamics in the elderly. Exp Gerontol. 2003;38:843–53.
58. Ungprasert P, Srivali N, Kittanamongkolchai W. Non-steroidal anti-inflammatory drugs and risk of heart failure exacerbation: a systematic review and meta-analysis. Eur J Intern Med. 2015;26(9):685–90.
59. van Kooten JBT. A review of pain prevalence in Alzheimer's, vascular, frontotemporal and Lewy body dementias. Dement Geriatr Cogn Disord. 2016;41(3–4):220–32.
60. Verdú E, Ceballos D, Vilches J, Navarro X. Influence of aging on peripheral nerve function and regeneration. J Peripher Nerv Syst. 2000;5:191–208.
61. Wade K, Marshall A, Vanhoute B, Wu F, O'Neill T, Lee D. Does pain predict frailty in older men and women? findings from the English longitudinal study of ageing. J Gerontol A Biol Med Sci. 2017;72(3):403–9.
62. Wagner A, Luna S. Effect of footwear on joint pain and function in older adults with lower exremity osteoartritis. J Geriatr Phys Ther. 2018;41(2)
63. White N, Bazo-Alvarez J, Koopsman M, Est E, Sampson E. Understanding the association between pain and delirium in older hospital inpatients: systematic review and meta-analysis. Age Ageing. 2024;
64. WHO Guidelines for the Pharmacological and Radiotherapeutic Management of Cancer Pain in Adults and Adolescents Geneva: World Health Organization; 2018.
65. World Health Organisation. WHO Guidelines for the pharmacological and radiotherapeutic management of cancer pain in adults and adolescents; 2019.
66. World Health Organisation. Ageing: global population; 2025. Retrieved from Wrold Health Orgnaisation: https://www.who.int/news-room/questions-and-answers/item/population-ageing#:~:text=The%20number%20of%20people%20aged%2060%20and%20older,demographic%20shift%20has%20significant%20implications%20for%20public%20health.

Pediatric Pain Management

22

Norman E. Fenn III

Abbreviations

CBD	cannabidiol
FLACC	face legs activity crying consolability
GVHD	graft-versus-host disease
IN	intranasal
IV	intravenous
JFM	juvenile fibromyalgia
NP	neuropathic pain
NRS	numerical rating scale
NSAID	nonsteroidal anti-inflammatory drug
SCD	sickle cell disease
SSRI	selected serotonin reuptake inhibitor
TCA	tricyclic antidepressant
THC	tetrahydrocannabinol

Introduction

The pediatric population is its own entity, comprised of several general life stages. Neonates are defined as the first 28 days of life, while an infant is defined as an age of 1 month to 2 years. Children are generally classified as two to 12 years of age, and adolescents are aged 13 to 21 years [46] and are supported by the FDA and U.S. Department of Health, though there is some variation in age ranges among scholars and in practice, as well as in clinical trials [37, 101]. The American Academy of Pediatrics (AAP) general consensus definitions of these staging categories are described in Table 22.1. Physiologic development varies in each of these life stages, including height and weight, as well as organ development, which can change dramatically over time. As an example, cytochrome P450 enzymes are immature at birth, with the exception of the CYP 3A7 enzyme. This particular enzyme function is markedly above adult levels at birth, with a functional peak by the first 7 days of life equating to a 15-fold increase compared to adult function, and can metabolize CYP 3A4 substrates, though to a lesser extent [58]. This enzyme then dramatically decreases to adult levels at about 1 month of age. Physiologic development of the CYP 2D6 pathway, relevant in opioid metabolism, also has an unclear maturation period. Studies have shown this isozyme to mature sometime between 2 and 5 years, though the evidence is divergent [20, 56, 57]. Pharmacogenomics also plays a significant role in isoenzyme expression and is continuing to be investigated. How medications are metabolized should be a consideration when prescribing adjunctive therapy for pain management, especially if it is not well understood or described.

Table 22.1 Classification of pediatric patients

Classification	Definition
Premature neonate	Born <37 weeks gestational age
Neonate	0 to 28 days of life
Infant	1 month to <2 years
Child	2 to 11 years
Adolescent	12 years and older

Evaluation of pain in pediatric patients is also different compared to adults. Babies and toddlers are unable to verbally communicate their discomfort effectively, so alternative assessment is needed. There are several validated nonverbal pain scales for pediatric patients. The FLACC (Face, Legs, Activity, Crying, and Consolability) scale utilizes a 0 to 2 score with an assessment for each of these components. The total points from this assessment also correlate to a 0 to 10 pain scale, facilitating a determination of mild, moderate, or severe pain. The Wong-Baker FACES scale utilizes images that correlate with a particular pain score akin to the patient's current visage, similar to the traditional 0 to 10 pain scale. Other pain assessment tools have been employed

N. E. Fenn III (✉)
Manchester University College of Pharmacy & Health Sciences, Manchester, UK

Parkview Women's and Children's Hospital, Fort Wayne, IN, USA
e-mail: nefenn@manchester.edu

J. P. Reinert et al. (eds.), *Adjunctive Analgesic Strategies for the Bedside Clinician and Beyond*,
https://doi.org/10.1007/978-3-032-21675-5_22

in the literature, further exacerbating the heterogeneity of available literature and its interpretation.

Pain management in the pediatric population depends on several factors, including age, weight, indication, and tolerance [100]. Opioids are the foundation of severe pain management in children and are used in many pain studies as a comparator and/or the standard of care. The non-opioid management of pain in the pediatric population beyond acetaminophen and ibuprofen remains challenging, as most studies involve small sample populations, single-center experiences, limited indications, and patient diversity. Most medications prescribed for adjunctive pain therapy rely on adult literature with scarce or no pediatric equivalent data. Included in this chapter is a comprehensive review of medications utilized to manage pain in pediatric patients.

Drug Class Evidence

Acetaminophen

Acetaminophen is the most commonly utilized analgesic in the pediatric population and is indicated for both the treatment of fever and pain at all ages [1]. It increased in popularity in the 1950s when it was marketed as an alternative to aspirin and gained over-the-counter status in the U.S. in the 1960s [41]. Much of the pharmacologic information on acetaminophen can be found in Chap. 3 of this textbook, though there is one difference in pediatrics to highlight. Pharmacokinetically, preterm neonates have underdeveloped metabolic pathways, including the primary CYP 2E1 pathway [70]. These patients metabolize the drug through secondary pathways, including glucuronidation and sulfation, which are saturated more quickly. As a result, lower doses and extended intervals are needed in this population.

Obesity is another factor that can influence acetaminophen serum concentrations and may reduce efficacy. In a pharmacokinetic study of 11 adolescent female patients with severe obesity, investigators explored the effect of a single, 1000 mg dose of IV acetaminophen [45]. Authors demonstrated undetectable serum acetaminophen concentrations at 2 hours after administration, indicating the established maximum dose of acetaminophen would be insufficient for pain control. Authors also noted that a dose of 2250 mg of acetaminophen would be needed for an adolescent with obesity to achieve similar serum concentrations to an adolescent without obesity [45].

Acetaminophen comes in a variety of formulations, including liquid, tablet, caplet, and suppository, and may be administered via oral, intravenous (IV), and rectal routes. Dosing for the rectal route is slightly higher compared to the other options, based on decreased absorption from the gastrointestinal tract. Liquid formulations of acetaminophen now come in one concentration. Acetaminophen liquid used to come in multiple concentrations until 2011, when the Consumer Healthcare Products Association collaborated with drugmakers to standardize the medication in order to avoid dosing errors [43]. As a result, the current acetaminophen liquid is only available in one strength (32 mg/mL). Table 22.2 provides the common pain indication dosing for this and other medications. Table 22.3 lists the medications based on route of administration.

Comparison between routes of administration of acetaminophen has been described in the literature to varying extents. A systematic review and meta-analysis published in 2024 by Osorio included children aged 1 month to 17 years who were postoperative status [69]. Fourteen randomized, controlled studies were included and compared rectal, IV, and oral formulations of acetaminophen administered during the pre-, peri-, and postoperative periods. Investigators reported no difference in pain control with rectal versus IV and oral versus IV routes but found that with rectal versus oral routes, there was slightly better pain improvement with oral administration [69]. The authors did note the evidence only warranted very low and low certainty of the route comparisons and highlighted the need for better study methodology to address this question. Noninferiority was evidenced between IV and oral acetaminophen in a randomized, double-blind, prospective study involving 66 pediatric patients undergoing tonsillectomy and adenoidectomy [53], though the IV dose was 15 mg/kg and the oral dose was 30 mg/kg. The authors noted no difference in opioid use or reported severe pain between cohorts.

Acetaminophen is not a powerful pain reliever, but it does have extensive documentation supporting both its safety and efficacy in managing mild pain in pediatric patients as well as its use as part of a multimodal approach for moderate and severe pain. It has been shown to reduce opioid consumption when coadministered with these agents [72, 78, 102], though other studies suggest otherwise (Dhebaria et al. 2020, [49, 89]). It is important to note that it is possible to exceed the maximum daily dose if following the approved dosing regimen in children—caution should be used when prescribing or instructing families on administration.

Postoperative pain often utilizes a multimodal approach and includes optimization of non-opioid medications, including acetaminophen. However, the literature has described mixed findings with acetaminophen inclusion in the pain management strategy. One study evaluated the effect of rectal acetaminophen administration in pediatric patients post-adenotonsillectomy [32]. The authors recruited 104 patients between 7 and 15 years of age who underwent adenotonsillectomy and compared acetaminophen 40 mg/kg administered rectally to placebo after standard anesthesia induction, which included midazolam, remifentanil, and sodium thiopental. Pain scores were significantly lower in the acetaminophen group at each interval over the 6 hours, and patients

Table 22.2 Medication table and dosing considerations

Medication	Initial dosing	Maximum dose	Clinical pain pearls
Acetaminophen	Neonate: dependent on gestational age *Children 1 month and older* PO/IV: 10–15 mg/kg/dose every 4 to 6 hours PR: 10–20mg/kg/dose	*Single dose*: 15 mg/kg/dose or 1000mg *Single day*: 75 mg/kg/day or 4000mg	Caution in mild/ moderate liver impairment Avoid in severe liver impairment
NSAIDs Ibuprofen Naproxen Ketorolac Celecoxib	PO/IV: Ibuprofen 5–10 mg/kg/dose every 6 to 8 hours Naproxen 5–7 mg/kg/dose po q8–12h Ketorolac: 0.5–1 mg/kg/dose IV q6–8h Celecoxib: 1-2 mg/kg/dose po BID	Ibuprofen: 40 mg/kg/day or 800mg Naproxen: 15 mg/kg/day or 500mg Ketorolac: 30mg Celecoxib: 100mg	Avoid use in infants <6 months of age Caution in mild/ moderate renal impairment Avoid in severe renal impairment Ketorolac should not be used for more than 5 days
Gabapentin	Neonate/infant: 2.5–5 mg/kg/day Child/adolescent: 5–10 mg/kg/day	Neonate/infant: 35 mg/kg/day Child/adolescent: 50–70 mg/kg/day	May cause sedation, drowsiness, or weight gain
Lidocaine	One patch applied topically	Maximum three patches applied for no more than 12 hours in a 24-hour period	To be used externally only
Ketamine	Bolus: 0.25–0.5 mg/kg/dose PO/IV q6–8h PRN Low-dose infusion: 0.1–0.3 mg/kg/hr		May cause hallucinations, hypotension
Muscle relaxants Methocarbamol Cyclobenzaprine Carisoprodol	Not studied in the pediatric population		
Antidepressants Duloxetine Amitriptyline Milnacipran	Not established in the pediatric population		

Table 22.3 Available routes of administration

Route of administration	Available agents
Oral	Acetaminophen, NSAIDs, gabapentin, ketamine, muscle relaxants, antidepressants
Rectal	Acetaminophen, naproxen, indomethacin
Intravenous	Acetaminophen, ibuprofen, ketorolac, ketamine
Intramuscular	Ketorolac
Transdermal	Lidocaine

required less rescue analgesic to manage postoperative pain [32]. In a study by Hiller et al., 36 pediatric patients aged 10 to 18 years underwent scoliosis surgery and were given IV acetaminophen 30 mg/kg every 8 hours or a placebo in addition to the standard of care (oxycodone as needed) [49]. Investigators noted better pain control in the acetaminophen group, but no difference in oxycodone use over the 24-hour study period. A similar study involving 57 pediatric patients aged 10 to 18 years undergoing posterior spinal fusion (PSF) compared IV acetaminophen plus standard of care to standard of care alone [78]. Patients randomized to the acetaminophen arm received 15 mg/kg of IV acetaminophen intraoperatively and every 6 hours for 42 hours postoperatively. Investigators noted a statistically significant decrease in opioid use at 24 hours in the acetaminophen cohort compared to standard of care, as well as reduced duration of opioid patient-controlled analgesia (PCA) use by 17 hours [78]. Of note, there was no difference in time to mobilization, hospital discharge, or adverse events between groups.

Another study evaluated single-dose IV acetaminophen compared to placebo in 239 pediatric patients aged 2 to 8 years of age who underwent adenotonsillectomy [89]. All patients also received a single dose of morphine as standard of care. Pain was assessed in the postanesthesia care unit (PACU) five times over the first hour with no significant difference in pain scores between groups at any interval. No difference was seen between groups and the use of breakthrough pain medication, suggesting IV acetaminophen made no difference in pain control post-adenotonsillectomy [89].

Vaso-occlusive crisis (VOC) is a painful, acute-on-chronic manifestation associated with sickle cell disease (SCD), often requiring extensive opioid administration. Two studies have evaluated the use of IV acetaminophen with VOC secondary to SCD [11, 34]. A retrospective analysis of 46 pediatric patients with a mean age of 9.6 years evaluated administration of IV acetaminophen dosed between 12.5 mg/kg IV every 4 hours to 15 mg/kg IV every 6 hours and evaluated at 24-hour intervals [11]. Authors noted an overall decrease in pain scores by 2.3/10 in the acetaminophen group, along with nonstatistically significant decreases in opioid dosing, opioid administration, and opioid-related adverse events. In a prospective study, 71 patients aged 4 to 16 years in the emergency department with VOC secondary to SCD were randomly assigned to receive IV acetaminophen 15 mg/kg or placebo in addition to standard of care, defined as IV morphine 0.1 mg/kg/dose and/or IV ketorolac 0.5 mg/kg/dose [34]. Pain scores were slated to be assessed every 30 minutes for 2 hours and again at discharge. Authors reported no difference in pain scores, morphine use, admission rates, return visits within 72 hours, or adverse events between groups, indicating no short-term benefit with IV acetaminophen administration in the emergency department for VOC management [34].

In a large comparative effectiveness study, investigators evaluated data from 274 U.S. hospitals on pediatric inpatients who were administered IV acetaminophen prior to administration of IV opioids [72]. In their analysis, the authors noted an estimated reduction of IV opioid use of 15.5% with an absolute IV opioid reduction of 7.5 hours in the IV acetaminophen group, suggesting a modest decrease in opioid exposure with IV acetaminophen use. Two cost-effective studies evaluating IV acetaminophen have also been published, evaluating postoperative pain. A 2014 study analyzed the cost-effectiveness of IV acetaminophen use in the PACU for pain management associated with tonsillectomy [87]. The authors' assessment showed the combination of IV acetaminophen with opioids was both modestly cheaper and more effective compared to opioid-only use. Authors noted the combined medication costs were higher in the acetaminophen cohort, but overall costs were lower due to fewer adverse events and time spent in the unit [87]. The second cost-effectiveness study evaluated IV acetaminophen and ketorolac in 36 adolescents who underwent PSF [26]. Authors compared IV acetaminophen and IV acetaminophen with ketorolac to an opioid regimen (morphine PCA). Results of the study demonstrated less opioid utilization in both the IV acetaminophen and IV acetaminophen with IV ketorolac cohorts, along with shorter time to eating and less constipation. The IV acetaminophen approach was considered intermediate in both cost and effectiveness, while the IV acetaminophen with IV ketorolac approach was the most cost-effective. The interpreted cost savings of these outcomes were $510 and $947 U.S. dollars, respectively (cost based on 2015 value), supporting IV acetaminophen as an adjunct to pain management for postoperative pain secondary to PSF [26].

One of the common practices for non-opioid pain management, especially postoperative pain, is to alternate acetaminophen with NSAIDs such as ibuprofen and ketorolac. A review article published in 2010 evaluated these practices in adult and pediatric populations [67]. Though the authors collectively concluded that alternating these medications was potentially superior to either agent alone, the data were overwhelmingly from adult studies. In the two pediatric studies in this review, the alternating practice was generally no better at managing pain than giving either agent independently [48, 97]. A clinical update reiterated that the common clinical practice is without sufficient evidence supporting either efficacy or safety [85]. A subsequent review published in 2014 evaluated IV acetaminophen and ketorolac for surgical pain in pediatric patients and described mixed results individually and in comparison to each other [12]. Newer literature evaluating IV acetaminophen to IV ketoprofen as part of a postoperative multimodal pain regimen noted no benefit of IV acetaminophen, though patients returned to baseline oral intake quicker after general surgery in the acetaminophen group [80].

NSAIDs

NSAIDs are also acceptable for adjunctive pain management in pediatric patients. Information on individual NSAIDs can be found in Chap. 4. There are four NSAID medications that are included in this chapter due to their reasonable evidentiary support and use in everyday clinical practice ibuprofen, naproxen, celecoxib, and ketorolac.

The most commonly utilized NSAID in children is ibuprofen, which is available over the counter like acetaminophen. It is recommended for use in infants 6 months of age and older for both fever and pain (ibuprofen package insert). Use in infants younger than 6 months for pain is generally not recommended due to an increased risk of gastrointestinal (GI) bleed as well as acute kidney injury, excluding medically specific indications unrelated to pain. It has been shown to be equivalent in pain reduction when compared to oral morphine for fractures. Poonal et al. [73] described no difference in analgesic effect between these agents in children with an extremity fracture, with ibuprofen having fewer adverse effects compared to oral morphine.

Naproxen can be used in pediatric patients 4 years of age and older. One benefit of naproxen is its duration of action, which is longer than that of ibuprofen. It comes in tablet form over the counter, but the liquid formulation of naproxen currently requires a prescription. Naproxen has shown efficacy as a single intervention or as part of a multimodal pain strategy. Studies have shown benefit in several indications, including general pain, surgical/traumatic pain, and orthopedic pain. Adverse effects mirror those of the NSAID drug class, including stomach upset, renal function impairment, and, rarely, GI bleeding.

Celecoxib is indicated in children 2 years of age and older, specifically for juvenile idiopathic arthritis, though it can be used off-label for other pain-related indications. The only remaining COX-2 inhibitor on the market has not shown the same serious adverse effects that were observed with other medications in the drug class. Celecoxib is a potent NSAID with a longer duration of action compared to other NSAIDs and can be given once or twice daily. It comes in both capsule and liquid forms, though the latter is specifically indicated for migraine use in adults only.

Celecoxib's benefit has been observed in several studies for post-tonsillectomy pain. Giordano and colleagues demonstrated an overall reduction in pain from the procedure with a notable reduction in opioid consumption in patients with prolonged pain [44]. Of note, the authors administered a higher dose of celecoxib (6 mg/kg/day) for the 10-day study duration. When compared to acetaminophen, celecoxib exhibited lower pain scores on the first day, with no noticeable difference in subsequent days, and improved oral intake postoperatively [39]. A larger study showed a smaller difference in pain reduction and lower consumption of as-needed acetaminophen [65].

Ketorolac is a potent NSAID for pain management in pediatric patients, though it is almost exclusively used in the inpatient setting and given via the IV route. Of note, ketorolac should be prescribed for a duration not to exceed 5 days in length, as it carries an increased risk of kidney injury. Additionally, oral ketorolac should not be prescribed without a patient first receiving at least one IV or intramuscular (IM) dose beforehand.

An analysis of collective NSAID use in pediatric patients status post cardiac surgery found no increased incidence of renal dysfunction or increased chest tube output [83]. Ketorolac specifically had a statistically significant reduction in both FLACC pain scoring and morphine requirements. Clinically, the morphine reduction was significant, with a decrease of 0.2 mg/kg/day within 24 hours of ketorolac initiation [83]. A newer study compared the impact of a single dose of ketorolac IV 0.5 mg/kg on postoperative pain in 142 pediatric patients aged 3 to 12 years who underwent adenotonsillectomy [109]. Investigators reported a decrease in pain score of approximately 2/10 points, but no difference was noted between cohorts on opioid usage or postoperative nausea and vomiting.

A subsequent review of NSAID use in perioperative and emergency department settings found opioid consumption reductions in 10 of 13 studies that evaluated this metric, as well as improvements or at least equivalent pain score reductions in 24 studies [27].

Adult studies have shown similar pain reduction between ketorolac IV 30 mg and morphine IV 4 mg [18, 96]. Though not studied to the same extent in children, ketorolac has shown a decreased need for opioids in this population. A Cochrane review evaluating ketorolac for postoperative pain reported a mean decrease in morphine equivalents in the PACU (−0.17 mg) and 4 hours postoperatively (−1.58 mg) [64]. Subsequent studies have shown that a lower capped dose of ketorolac, 10 to 15 mg, reduces pain roughly the same as a 30 mg dose with less renal dysfunction and overall toxicity [16, 55].

Gabapentinoids

Gabapentin and pregabalin are therapeutic agents utilized for adjunctive pain management in pediatric patients. The pharmacologic profile of these agents can be found in Chap. 6. An in-depth summary of available literature can be found in Table 22.4.

Gabapentin's use as adjunct therapy for pain management in children is somewhat controversial. Adult literature began exploring its use for neuropathic pain (NP) in the early 2000s, and pediatric patients soon followed. Its use in neonatal and infant populations is limited and described for multiple indications, including pain, though evidence remains sparse. In a retrospective study from 2019, investigators described the use of gabapentin for agitation and pain [22]. Patients were started on gabapentin at 2.5 to 5 mg/kg/day and titrated every 3 to 5 days as tolerated to a daily maximum of 35 mg/kg/day. After 14 days, authors reported reductions in neurosedative medications and pain/agitation scoring, with only one patient experiencing oversedation and no serious adverse effects [22].

Gabapentin has shown mixed results in small studies for several indications, including postoperative pain, phantom limb pain (PLP), and more. Gabapentin is used for pre-, peri-, and postsurgical procedures as part of a multimodal pain regimen. Investigators gave a 15 mg/kg preoperative dose of gabapentin followed by a postoperative regimen dosed at 5 to 10 mg/kg/day for 3 days [5, 40, 81, 90]). In an evaluation of postspinal fusion, Rusy and colleagues showed a statistically significant reduction in morphine use 48 hours postoperatively but not beyond 2 days in a cohort of 59 pediatric patients [81]. The clinical difference between these groups was less notable, with a difference in morphine use of less than 0.02 mg/kg/hr. Also, for postspinal fusion, Anderson et al. showed lower pain scores with the gabapentin cohort in the anesthesia recovery unit as compared to placebo, but not in the subsequent postoperative days [5]. Average opioid consumption was statistically significantly lower on postoperative days 1 and 2, though the difference was less than two morphine equivalents between groups. Fenikowski and colleagues evaluated gabapentin use for pain after a Ravitch procedure for pectus excavatum. The authors reported statistically significant decreases in average and maximal pain associated with the day of surgery, but not with coughing or deep breathing [40]. However, the score difference between groups was 1 point on a 10-point scale, limiting clinical significance. Tomaszek et al. also studied perioperative gabapentin use

Table 22.4 Summary of gabapentinoid studies

Study author, year	Study design, N, mean age (range)	Indication	Dosing (maximum)	Comparator	Primary outcome	Key takeaways
[22]	Case series 16 44 weeks (36–75 weeks)	Pain, movement disorders, irritability	Gabapentin 2.5–5 mg/kg/day (35 mg/kg/day)	None	Describe gabapentin use in neonates	Gabapentin reduced concurrent neurosedative medications by 0.8 after 14 days Gabapentin reduced pain scores by 0.6 after 3 days
[81]	Prospective RCT 59 14 years (9–18 years)	Post-op PSF pain	Gabapentin 15 mg/kg/day × 5 days	SOC (Morphine PCA, PRN diazepam)	Gabapentin effect on pain score	Morphine consumption was lower in the gabapentin cohort for post-op Days 1 and 2 Pain scores were lower in the gabapentin cohort on post-op Day 1
[5]	Prospective RCT 50 14 years (10–19 years)	Pre- and post-op PSF pain	Gabapentin 30 mg/kg/day (+SOC)	SOC (SCH ketorolac, hydromorphone PCA, PRN acetaminophen and oxycodone)	Gabapentin effect on pain score	Gabapentin cohort had reduced pain scores (1 out of 10) on Day 0 of procedure; no statistical difference on post-op Days 1–5 Gabapentin cohort used slightly less hydromorphone on post-op Day 1
[40]	Single-center RCT 56 14 years (9–17 years)	Post-op Ravitch procedure on pain, anxiety	Gabapentin 15 mg/kg/day orally × 3 days (+SOC)	SOC (continuous IV morphine, IV acetaminophen, ketoprofen or ibuprofen)	Gabapentin effect on pain score	Gabapentin cohort had reduced pain scores (0.5–1 out of 10) on Day 0 of procedure; no statistical difference on post-op Days 1–3 Gabapentin cohort used slightly less morphine overall on post-op Day 1
[90]	Single-center RCT 40 14 years (10–16 years)	Post-op Ravitch procedure on pain, anxiety	Gabapentin 15 mg/kg/day × 3 days (+SOC)	SOC (ropivacaine + fentanyl epidural, acetaminophen, NSAIDs, metamizol)	Gabapentin effect on pain score	No difference in median pain scores between cohorts No difference in analgesic use between cohorts
[88]	Retrospective review 101 14 years	Physical therapy goal after PSF surgery	Gabapentin 15 mg/kg/day × 3 days (300 mg/dose) (+SOC)	SOC (SCH acetaminophen, ketorolac, opioid PCA, PRN hydrocodone or oxycodone)	Perioperative gabapentin effect on physical therapy goals	Patients achieved completion of physical therapy goal on Day 1 more frequently in the gabapentin cohort No difference in LOS between cohorts
[62]	Single-center RCT 35 15 years	Post-op corrective spinal surgery	Gabapentin 600 mg (+SOC)	SOC (SCH acetaminophen, morphine PCA)	Morphine use 24 hr post-op	No difference in morphine use between cohorts No difference in time to rescue analgesia between cohorts
[14]	Retrospective review 87 11 years	Post-op appendectomy	Gabapentin 10 mg/kg/day (30 mg/kg/day) (+SOC)	SOC (SCH ketorolac, PRN acetaminophen, opioids)	Gabapentin effect on pain score	Time to pain score ≤ 3 similar in both cohorts (12 vs 17 hr) Gabapentin cohort used less opioids postoperatively

(continued)

Table 22.4 (continued)

Study author, year	Study design, N, mean age (range)	Indication	Dosing (maximum)	Comparator	Primary outcome	Key takeaways
[54]	Retrospective review of PHIS database 29,467 (236 with gabapentin) 10 years (2–18 years)	Post-op perforated appendectomy	Gabapentin dose not described	Opioid, acetaminophen, ketorolac, ibuprofen	Post-op opioid use with gabapentin	The gabapentin cohort used opioids 0.4 days less than the control cohort No difference in LOS between cohorts
[7]	Single-center RCT 25 (1–18 years)	Vincristine-related neuropathic pain	Gabapentin 20 mg/kg/day	Placebo	Reduction of opioid use with gabapentin	Patients in the gabapentin cohort used more morphine equivalents compared to placebo No difference in pain scores was noted between cohorts
[103]	Case report 1 4 years	Phantom pain post-amputation	Pregabalin 1.25 mg/kg (2.5 mg/kg)	Initial pain regimen (acetaminophen, ibuprofen, metamizol, morphine, fentanyl, ketamine)	Describe pregabalin use for phantom limb pain in a 4-year-old patient	Pregabalin was initiated on Day 13 prior to amputation and tolerated well Patient was discharged pain-free on pregabalin daily with PRN ibuprofen and metamizol
[47]	Single-center RCT 64 15 years (10–21 years)	Post-op PSF pain	Pregabalin 2 mg/kg × 2 doses pre-op, then × 5 days post-op (150mg) (+SOC)	SOC (SCH acetaminophen, oxycodone PCA, PRN etoricoxib)	Reduction of post-op opioid use with pregabalin	No difference in opioid consumption between cohorts at 48 hr No difference in pain scores between cohorts at 6 months, 1 year and 2 years post-op
[82]	Case report 1 15 years	Complex regional pain syndrome	Pregabalin 150mg/day	Failed NSAIDs, sertraline, mirtazepine, gabapentin	Pregabalin use after gabapentin failure	Pain and edema decreased within 24 hours of pregabalin inititation Pain recurred after stopping pregabalin and improved after restarting
[99]	Open-label prospective pilot trial 28 13.5 years (10–17)	Neuropathic pain in oncology pediatric patients	Pregabalin 150–300 mg/day × 8 weeks	None	Pregabalin efficacy, safety, and tolerability for chemotherapy-induced pain	Pain scores decreased by 58% in the pregabalin cohort at 8 weeks Adverse effects, described as mild/moderate intensity were reported in 4/28 patients

IV intravenous; *LOS* length of stay; *NSAID* non-steroidal anti-inflammatory drug; *PCA* patient-controlled analgesia; *PHIS* Pediatric Health Information System; *PRN* as needed; *PSF* posterior spinal fusion; *RCT* randomized controlled trial; *SCH* scheduled; *SOC* standard of care

for the Ravitch procedure. Investigators reported no statistical differences in postoperative median maximal pain, nor pain at rest, during coughing, or during deep breathing [90]. No differences between groups were observed with analgesic use.

Single-dose regimens also showed mixed findings. One study utilized a fixed dose of 400 mg preoperatively followed by 400 mg three times daily for 3 days in patients aged 10 to 18 years [88]. This regimen was shown to reduce the time to achieve physical therapy goals after spinal fusion compared to placebo, though morphine use was only reduced on the first postoperative day and pain scores on the second postoperative day. Mayell and colleagues studied a single preoperative gabapentin dose of 600 mg in children 10 to 17 years old [62]. They reported no change in postoperative morphine use or pain scores over the first three postoperative days.

Other studies evaluating gabapentin for postoperative indications show conflicting results. A 2018 retrospective study of 87 pediatric patients who underwent appendectomy was matched 2:1, no gabapentin to gabapentin [14]. Investigators reported a significant decrease in morphine equivalent use in the gabapentin cohort compared to the no-gabapentin cohort, the latter of which required three times more opioids. A larger retrospective analysis from the Pediatric Health Information System reported 0.8% of almost 30,000 retrieved cases from 50 hospitals received gabapentin for postoperative pain after perforated appendix [54]. Authors reported that patients who received gabapentin were more likely to have their pain managed through a multimodal strategy and were less likely to receive an opioid postoperatively. Though there was a statistically significant difference between groups for the mean number of days prescribing an opioid, this difference was less than half a day total, rendering the outcome less clinically impactful. In a perioperative review article evaluating gabapentin use, authors described similar findings of statistical significance in several studies with limited clinical significance, highlighting the lack of clinical evidence to support routine prescribing of gabapentin [25].

Although studied for neuropathic pain (NP) and prescribed clinically for varying pain indications, gabapentin's benefit remains unclear and unestablished with mixed study results. Its use to mitigate drug-related NP has not shown benefit with either prevention or treatment. One prospective randomized trial evaluated gabapentin combined with an opioid versus an opioid combined with a placebo to treat NP associated with vincristine in 49 children aged 1 to 18 years [7]. Gabapentin was dosed at 20 mg/kg/day in three divided doses, and all participants had open-label oral morphine ordered for breakthrough pain. Investigators reported increased pain scores and higher opioid consumption in the gabapentin arm compared to the placebo arm [7]. An earlier study by Anghelescu and colleagues evaluated gabapentin for the prevention and treatment of chemotherapy-induced neuropathic pain [6]. At a daily dose of 15 mg/kg, investigators noted that gabapentin did not prevent recurrence of NP after the initial episode; its effect on treating drug-induced NP was not described.

Pregabalin has been evaluated in a handful of studies for pain management, including pain associated with amputation, PSF, complex regional pain syndrome, and NP [47, 82, 99, 103]. A modest pain reduction benefit was reported in three of the studies, though significant confounders cloud these findings, including concurrent opioid and sedation infusions and undiagnosed psychiatric issues [82, 103]. Helenius and colleagues reported no difference in postoperative opioid consumption or persistent pain [47].

Ultimately, gabapentinoids have demonstrated generally well-tolerated profiles in the studied populations with mixed beneficial findings. Due to the conflicting data, a careful evaluation of risks and benefits should be performed before prescribing these agents for these and other described pain conditions.

Ketamine

Ketamine is a relatively underutilized medication for pain management despite reasonable evidence supporting its benefit in SCD, postoperative, and chronic conditions, among others. It can be administered through various routes, including IV, oral, and intranasal. The primary concern with this medication is the adverse effect profile, which includes sedation, hypotension, hallucinations, and respiratory depression. More detail on the pharmacology of ketamine is provided in Chap. 13. Table 22.5 provides additional details on available ketamine literature for pain in pediatric patients.

Ketamine has demonstrated positive outcomes in pediatric patients with various oncologic indications as well as graft-versus-host disease. In an analysis of low-dose ketamine for oncologic, hematologic, and pain diagnoses, 58 children received 82 separate ketamine infusions over a 10-year period [8]. The median infusion rate was 0.15 mg/kg/hr over a period of 3 days. Authors reported significant decreases in opioid consumption in the oncologic cohort over all 3 days; the same changes were not observed in the hematologic and end-of-life pain cohorts. Adverse effects were frequently reported but minimal in nature, with the most common complaints being drowsiness, lethargy, nausea, and vomiting; these did not vary between groups [8]. A pilot study out of France evaluated low-dose ketamine infusions for refractory pain in pediatric and young adult patients with cancer [30]. Patients were on a combination of opioid and opioid-like medications prior to ketamine initiation. Investigators reported that 38 patients were started on a ketamine infusion at a rate of 0.01 to 0.2 mg/kg/hr. Pain scores decreased by a mean of 2.5 points on a 10-point scale by day 3 of treatment. Thirty patients also received a nonstatistically significant dose increase of their morphine infusion from 7.08 to 8.25 mg/kg/hr from day 1 to day 3. Nine patients reported poor tolerance of ketamine, defined as two or more adverse effects, though the rate of the ketamine infusion was less than 0.05 mg/kg/hr. No serious adverse effects were described in the study. Oral ketamine use has been described in a case report out of Turkey [92]. A 4-year-old male with terminal cancer received oral ketamine 3 mg/kg/day divided three times daily after reporting persistent uncontrolled pain with acetaminophen and morphine. Upon initiation, perceived pain by both patient and caregiver was significantly reduced by several points on a 10-point scale. Opioid consumption was also decreased by more than half with no reported adverse effects. Effects lasted for 2 weeks prior to disease progression, resulting in increased management with IV morphine and midazolam. In a separate case report, a 5-year-old male was initiated on long-term ketamine infusion for severe graft-versus-host disease (GVHD) secondary to a matched unrelated bone marrow transplant [23]. The patient was not controlled on 1 mg/kg/day of hydromorphone

Table 22.5 Summary of ketamine studies

Study author, year	Study design, N, mean age (range)	Indication	Dosing (maximum)	Comparator/ concurrent meds	Primary outcome	Key takeaways
[8]	Retrospective review 58 16 years (2–23 years)	Oncologic, SCD pain	(Median) Ketamine IV 0.15 mg/kg/hr (0.29 mg/kg/hr)	Opioid infusions, intermittent opioids, NSAIDs, gabapentinoids, TCAs, duloxetine, acetaminophen, muscle relaxants	Describe opioid-sparing effect of ketamine	No significant difference in mean opioid consumption from Day 1 to 3 Adverse effect described in 75.6% of patients including drowsiness, lethargy, N/V
[30]	Prospective, multicenter, observational trial 38 15 years (2–24 years)	Oncologic pain	Ketamine IV 0.01–0.2 mg/kg/hr	Morphine, methadone, nalbuphine, tramadol, acetaminophen	Ketamine effect on pain score	Pain scores decreased 2.4/10 points from Day 1 to 3 23% of patients experienced two or more adverse effects with ketamine including hallucinations, drowsiness, mood disorder
[92]	Case report 1 4 years	Oncologic pain	Ketamine oral 3 mg/kg/day	Morphine, acetaminophen	Describe oral ketamine use in terminal cancer in a 4-year-old	Morphine use decreased from 16mg to 6 mg daily Pain scores reduced from 8–9 to 0–1 No adverse effects reported
[23]	Case report 1 5 years	GVHD pain	Ketamine IV 0.54 mg/kg/hr	Hydromorphone PCA	Describe oral ketamine use in a 5-year-old with grade 4 GVHD	Pain was well controlled over several months with ketamine Adverse effects may have been caused by ketamine or concurrent medications including tacrolimus and corticosteroids
[108]	Case series 5 13 years (10–18 years)	Vaso-occlusive pain	Ketamine IV 0.06–0.1 mg/kg/hr (0.2 mg/kg/hr) +/− 0.1 mg/kg IV bolus	Opioid PCA	Describe low-dose ketamine infusion in SCD	No significant difference in opioid use with ketamine infusions Two of five patients experienced adverse events (dysphoria, nystagmus, HTN, unresponsiveness)
[56, 57]	Case series 8 (2–17 years)	Acute pain crisis	Ketamine IV 0.1 mg/kg/hr (0.3 mg/kg/hr)	Acetaminophen, NSAIDs, gabapentin, opioids, NSAIDs cyclobenzaprine, duloxetine, gabapentin	Describe low-dose ketamine infusion in acute pain crisis	Pain scores dropped a median of 3/10 points after initiation of ketamine infusion Opioid consumption was reduced in most patients
[106]	Retrospective review 19 14.6 years	Refractory pain in SCD and oncology	Ketamine IV 0.06–0.6 mg/kg/hr	Opioid PCA or intermittent, ketorolac,	Ketamine low-dose infusion on pain scores	No significant change in pain scores or opioid utilization with initiation of ketamine infusion Adverse effects reported included dysphoria, drowsiness, and blurred vision
[68]	Retrospective review 22 15 years (9–20 years)	SCD pain	Ketamine IV 0.02–0.15 mg/kg/hr (0.5 mg/kg/hr)	Acetaminophen, NSAIDs, morphine, hydromorphone, hydrocodone, oxycodone, gabapentin, methocarbamol	Ketamine effect on pain scores	34 of 46 admissions reported improved pain scores post-ketamine infusion Opioid use decreased from a mean of 173mg/day to 50mg/day
[66]	Retrospective review 85 15 years	SCD pain	Ketamine IV 0.05–0.4 mg/kg/hr (1 mg/kg/hr)	Not described	Ketamine effect on pain scores	Pain scores decreased from 7.5 to 4.6 after first ketamine initiation Opioid use was reduced by 1.3 mg/kg/day of oral ME
[15]	Double-blind, sequential trial 37 (0.5–5 years)	Post-op urologic pain	Ketamine IV 0.15 mg/kg × 1 + 0.08 mg/kg/hr	Nalbuphine, morphine, midazolam, acetaminophen	Ketamine effect on pain scores	No difference in pain scores up to 24 hours post-op between cohorts No difference in adverse effects between cohorts

(continued)

Table 22.5 (continued)

Study author, year	Study design, N, mean age (range)	Indication	Dosing (maximum)	Comparator/ concurrent meds	Primary outcome	Key takeaways
[74]	Retrospective study 112 15.5 years	Non-surgical pain	Ketamine IV 0.05–0.1 mg/kg/hr (0.3 mg/kg/hr)	Not described	Ketamine effect on pain scores	Ketamine reduced median pain scores by 2.5 points at 48 hours Opioid use was reduced by 57 mg/kg of oral ME
[31]	Single-center RCT 90 (5–7 years)	Tonsillectomy	Group 1: Placebo Group 2: Pre-op ketamine IV 0.5 mg/kg × 1 Group 3: Post-op ketamine IV 0.5 mg/kg × 1	Diclofenac, acetaminophen, dexamethasone, morphine	Ketamine effect on pain scores	Patients in the ketamine groups had small, statistically significant differences in pain reported post-op Patients in group 3 did not require rescue analgesia post-op
[3]	Prospective, pilot study 10 (3–8 years)	Adenoidectomy	Ketamine IV 0.5 mg/kg × 1	Administered concurrently: DM, acetaminophen, midazolam, dexmedetomidine	Efficacy of multimodal pain regimen including ketamine	No patients required opioid intervention Pain was well controlled 72 hours post-op on PRN acetaminophen and ibuprofen
[10]	Single-center RCT 98 6 years (3–12 years)	Adenoidectomy	Ketamine IV 0.25 mg/kg × 1	IV acetaminophen, PRN meperidine	Ketamine effect on pain scores	Pain scores were not clinically different at any time point post-op No difference between cohorts for rescue opioid administration or adverse effects
[36]	Single-center RCT 75 11 years (7–16 years)	Appendectomy	Group 1: Placebo Group 2: Ketamine IV 0.5 mg/kg × 1 Group 3: ketamine IV 0.5 mg/kg × 1 + 0.25 mg/kg/hr	Morphine PCA, NSAIDs, acetaminophen	Ketamine effect on opioid use post-op	No difference between cohorts on opioid consumption No difference in pain scores between cohorts Ketamine infusion group required more analgesia management compared to other cohorts
[13]	Single-center RCT 25 8 years (3–14 years)	Emergency orthopedic procedure	Ketamine IV 2 mg/kg × 1 (70mg)	(Comparator) Morphine 0.1 mg/kg × 1 + 0.05 mg/kg PRN (up to 5 mg total)	Ketamine effect on pain scores	No difference in pain scores or LOS between cohorts No difference in reported adverse effects
[75]	Meta-analysis 528 (7–12 years)	Emergency orthopedic procedure	Ketamine IN/IV 0.5–1.5 mg/kg	(Comparator) Fentanyl IN/IV 0.5–2 mcg/kg	Ketamine effect on pain scores	No difference in pain scores between cohorts at 15–20 and 30-minute intervals Ketamine had no described impact on rescue analgesia need
[76]	Single-center RCT 52 8 years (4–15 years)	Procedural analgesia for LP	Ketamine oral 0.8 mg/kg × 1 + topical analgesia	Placebo + topical analgesia	Ketamine effect on pain scores	Oral ketamine cohort had 2 point difference in pain scores compared to placebo Adverse effects were minimal in both groups
[105]	Prospective, open-label pilot study 28 9 years (3–13 years)	Emergency orthopedic procedure	Ketamine IN 0.85 mg/kg × 1; repeat 0.5 mg/kg × 1 PRN	None	Ketamine effect on pain scores	36% of patients required a second dose of ketamine due to higher pain scores Sedation was reported as mild and transient in 43% of patients

(continued)

Table 22.5 (continued)

Study author, year	Study design, N, mean age (range)	Indication	Dosing (maximum)	Comparator/ concurrent meds	Primary outcome	Key takeaways
[77]	Case series 5 15 years (10–16)	Musculoskeletal pain in the ED	Ketamine INH 0.75–1.5 mg/kg	Acetaminophen	Describe nebulized ketamine in the ED	Nebulized ketamine decreased pain scores by an average of 4 points within 60 minutes of administrationReported adverse effects included dizziness, mood change, and altered perception

DM dextromethorphan; *ED* emergency department; *GVHD* graft-versus-host disease; *HTN* hypertension; *IN* intranasal; *INH* inhaled; *IV* intravenous; *LOS* length of stay; *LP* lumbar puncture; *ME* morphine equivalent; *N/V* nausea/vomiting; *NSAIDs* non-steroidal anti-inflammatory drugs; *PCA* patient-controlled analgesia; *PRN* if needed; *SCD* sickle cell disease; *TCA* tricyclic antidepressants

administered via patient-controlled analgesia and was started on a ketamine infusion titrated to a rate of 0.54 mg/kg/hr over 4 months. Attempts to decrease the ketamine infusion resulted in significant increases in pain. Over the 6-week admission and after successful improvement of GVHD, the patient was titrated off both hydromorphone and ketamine on alternating days with minimal withdrawal reported, though the patient was using a clonidine patch for unrelated hypertension.

In SCD, ketamine has been studied with both bolus and continuous infusion dosing. A case series of five pediatric patients received a low-dose ketamine infusion at an initial dose of 0.06 to 0.17 mg/kg/hr with a maximum rate of 0.21 mg/kg/hr [108]. Two of the five patients achieved adequate pain reduction, though one of the patients only reported mild (3/10) pain at initiation. The other three patients in the series reported no improvement in their pain, and two patients experienced significant adverse effects resulting in therapy discontinuation. Another case series of eight patients received low-dose ketamine infusions at a mean starting dose of 0.1 mg/kg/hr titrated to a maximum of 0.3 mg/kg/hr for the management of acute pain crisis [56, 57]. The indications included SCD as well as palliative care, neuropathic pain, and cancer-related pain. Only one patient required bolus doses above the infusion. Pain scores decreased from a median of 6 at infusion initiation to 3 at discontinuation. Three patients experienced notable adverse effects, including hallucinations and emotional outbursts [56, 57]. A study of 19 pediatric patients with a low-dose ketamine infusion showed nonsignificant outcomes during admission [106]. Patients had either SCD and/or an oncologic diagnosis and were initiated on a median ketamine dose of 0.06 mg/kg/hr over 6 days on average. No differences were noted in pain scores or opioid consumption. Larger pediatric studies involving 22 and 85 patients, respectively, noted decreased pain scores and opioid consumption with low-dose ketamine infusions [66, 68]. Onyebuchi and colleagues reported on 46 admissions with 22 different patients who received ketamine at a mean starting infusion dose of 0.09 mg/kg/hr with a maximum rate of 0.21 mg/kg/hr [68]. Approximately 75% of patient visits had improvement in pain management and required less opioid administration during their stay with the ketamine infusion. Eleven encounters reported an adverse effect, with four instances requiring discontinuation [68]. Nobrega et al. also reported significant decreases in pain scores and opioid consumption with ketamine infusions on first and subsequent visits for acute pain [66]. Of note, investigators reported greater improvement in males and older patients. Dosing was not specifically reported, though initial rates were potentially higher than the low-dose regimens, with dosing between 0.05 to 0.4 mg/kg/hr titrated to a maximum rate of 1 mg/kg/hr as determined by the pain specialty team.

An older randomized, prospective study compared the addition of low-dose ketamine infusion to standard of care pain management (acetaminophen, nalbuphine, morniflumate) in predominantly urologic surgery [15]. The 38 patients included in the study were randomized to receive either a ketamine bolus of 0.15 mg/kg perioperatively followed by a 24-hour continuous infusion at 1.4 mcg/kg/min (0.084 mg/kg/hr) or saline. The study was ended at the third sequential analysis due to an observed lack of impact on pain scores and nalbuphine utilization. Notably, this study used lower doses than those previously mentioned. A subsequent retrospective study analyzed low-dose ketamine infusions over a 10-year period [74]. In the 115 patients, the median starting rate was 0.08 mg/kg/hr with a median maximum rate of 0.09 mg/kg/hr. The median duration of the infusion was 85 hours. Median pain reduction was approximately 2.5 points on a 10-point scale. Adverse effects were reported in nearly 30% of cases, with most being mild and including dysphoria, irritability, and hallucinations. Seven patients discontinued therapy due to intolerable adverse effects.

Ketamine has been studied for the management of postoperative pain, though its benefit largely depends on the type of procedure. It has shown mixed results when treating pain post-tonsillectomy and adenoidectomy. In a single-dose study from Brazil, 90 pediatric patients between 5 and 7 years of age received a 0.5 mg/kg bolus dose of ketamine either before or after the procedure [31]. Most patients in the control group (standard pain regimen) required rescue analgesia more frequently. Minimal adverse events were reported. A pilot study involving ten children between 3 and 8 years of age evaluated ketamine as part of a non-opioid analgesic regimen that included dextromethorphan, acetaminophen, and midazolam preoperatively, with ketamine and dexmedetomidine administered perioperatively [3]. Propofol and isoflurane were also given for sedation. The authors reported pain scores of 5 or lower using the FLACC assessment tool on the day of the procedure and the following 3 days. Patients' pain was controlled at home with acetaminophen and/or ibuprofen as needed. A randomized, triple-blinded clinical trial comparing ketamine with acetaminophen to acetaminophen alone was conducted in 2016 [10]. Ninety-eight patients were equally divided into the two cohorts, with the ketamine group receiving a single 0.25 mg/kg bolus dose just prior to the end of the surgery. Although the authors reported statistically significant differences in pain scores between the control and intervention groups at 0.5, 6, and 12 hours postoperatively, the differences were less than a point on a 13-point scale. No differences were observed between groups for rescue narcotics or adverse effects [10].

In a 2003 study evaluating ketamine in pediatric appendectomy, 75 pediatric patients received either standard analgesia plus a saline infusion or a 0.5 mg/kg bolus dose preoperatively followed by either a 0.004 mg/kg/min infusion or a saline placebo postoperatively [36]. The authors noted no significant differences in morphine requirements between the three groups, with similar pain scores at each evaluation point. The ketamine infusion group also had a higher incidence of headaches. Multiple review articles have evaluated ketamine in the role of spinal surgery. Park and colleagues reviewed the use of perioperative ketamine at varying doses for spinal procedures [71]. Only one retrieved study involved pediatrics, and it showed no difference in efficacy, defined as cumulative morphine consumption, or safety, including pain and adverse effect reports. A subsequent review by Zhou et al. evaluating low-dose ketamine infusions also remarked on no changes in pain scores, though their analysis showed opioid consumption was significantly less than the control group at 24 hours [110]. However, this characteristic was not observed at 12 or 48 hours.

Ketamine has shown promising use in pediatric orthopedic emergencies. A small study of 25 patients randomized to receive midazolam 0.2 mg/kg (up to 10 mg) in conjunction with either morphine 0.1 mg/kg with subsequent 0.05 mg/kg bolus doses at provider discretion (maximum 5 mg) or ketamine 2 mg/kg (maximum 70 mg) with no additional bolus doses [13]. Treatment was initiated immediately prior to the procedure. Authors reported no significant differences in most outcomes, including pain, recollection of procedure, or adverse effects. Only the duration of the procedure was statistically different (morphine: 3 minutes versus ketamine: 5 minutes). A subsequent meta-analysis evaluated ketamine versus fentanyl via intranasal or IV routes for either fracture, extremity, or musculoskeletal injury [75]. Ketamine was dosed between 0.5 mg/kg and 1.5 mg/kg, while fentanyl dosing was between 0.5 and 2 mcg/kg. Authors reported similar pain scores between agents within 15, 20, and 30-minute intervals. Ketamine was found to have statistically significant increases in nausea, vomiting, and dizziness.

Ketamine's use for procedural pain has been intermittently assessed. In a study of 52 pediatric patients with cancer, oral ketamine was administered at a dose of 0.8 mg/kg 30 minutes prior to lumbar puncture [76]. Patients in the placebo arm received mango juice only. Both cohorts also had lidocaine/prilocaine cream applied as per standard protocol. Pain scores were two points lower on a 10-point scale in the ketamine cohort, with a slightly smaller difference perceived by caregivers. Two patients reported mild adverse effects.

Other routes of ketamine have been documented for pain management. Intranasal (IN) ketamine is an agent often employed in emergency settings due to its quick onset and ease of administration. A pilot study evaluated IN ketamine administration for pain associated with limb injury in 28 pediatric patients [105]. The authors administered a mean initial dose of 0.84 mg/kg with an as-needed mean secondary dose of 0.57 mg/kg administered at least 15 minutes later. Ten patients required more than one dose in the 60-minute assessment window. Pain scores post-ketamine administration were reduced by about 17%. No significant adverse effects were reported. A subsequent review of IN ketamine literature for acute pain highlighted three studies that compared 1 to 2 mcg/kg IN fentanyl to 1.5 mg/kg IN ketamine [79]. No difference in pain reduction was noted between the two agents at the 60-minute mark, though mild adverse events were more commonly reported in the ketamine cohorts. In all three studies, ketamine was deemed noninferior to fentanyl for acute pain control. A case series of five male pediatric patients studied the administration of nebulized ketamine for acute pain secondary to extremity injury [77]. Patients received between 0.75 and 1.5 mg/kg of ketamine via nebulizer. Pain scores were reduced by 2 to 6 points on a 10-point pain scale at 60 minutes. Adverse effects were reported as mild in nature. The authors concluded that nebulized ketamine could be a viable option for pain relief if other avenues are not readily available.

In summary, ketamine has generally favorable data supporting its use in a variety of pain scenarios. It consistently demonstrated reductions in pain scores and opioid consumption at varying dosages and routes of administration. Additionally, it has demonstrated noninferiority to opioids in terms of short-term pain control. Adverse effects were experienced by a significant portion of patients studied, though most were mild in nature and tolerated. It is reasonable to consider ketamine as part of a multimodal pain strategy, either as an adjunctive agent to opioid pain management or in place of opioids. Appropriate monitoring should be in place while giving ketamine.

Alpha-2 Adrenergic Agonists

Dexmedetomidine and clonidine are centrally acting alpha-2 adrenergic receptor agonists more traditionally utilized for sedation, blood pressure management, and attention-deficit hyperactivity disorder. Their effects on pain are not as well established as these other indications, with limited and mixed outcomes. The pharmacologic profile of these agents can be found in greater detail in Chap. 10.

Since the introduction of dexmedetomidine to the market, it has been extensively ordered for the management of sedation in pediatric patients due in part to presumed lower withdrawal effects, a better safety profile, and acceptable efficacy as compared to opioids and benzodiazepines, and is recommended in the PANDEM guidelines as a primary sedation agent [86]. In addition, its inclusion in caudal nerve blocks has shown promising and consistent outcomes of prolonging the effect of these blocks and reducing opioid consumption [4, 38, 60, 91, 104].

Several postoperative studies described reduced opioid consumption in the dexmedetomidine cohorts as compared to opioids or other anesthetics [2, 21, 84, 95, 98]. However, other studies have provided alternative, conflicting data refuting its impact on pain reduction and opioid consumption [42, 51], while others still suggest no difference between dexmedetomidine and opioids for pain management [33].

Clonidine has been described in two pain studies. A systematic review and meta-analysis of oral and IV clonidine use as premedication for pediatric ophthalmic surgery described a small but statistically significant reduction in pain scores and pain-free occurrences while reducing analgesic need as compared to placebo [50]. An evaluation of epidural bupivacaine with fentanyl or clonidine showed no difference between groups in pediatric patients with cerebral palsy undergoing orthopedic surgery [24]. Clonidine did demonstrate less postoperative vomiting and oxygen desaturation compared to fentanyl, though systolic blood pressure and heart rate were both lower in the clonidine group.

The effect of dexmedetomidine and clonidine for pediatric pain management remains unclear and warrants further exploration. At present, a strong recommendation cannot be made either for or against prescribing these therapies for a pain indication in children. However, their use in this population for prolonging caudal nerve blocks and reducing opioid consumption via this mechanism is encouraging, with a favorable benefit versus risk profile.

Antidepressants

Antidepressants such as amitriptyline and duloxetine have been utilized as part of multimodal pain strategies in adults for years. However, their use in pediatric patients is described much less frequently and for diverse conditions. Greater detail on antidepressant use for adjunctive pain management can be found in Chaps. 7, 8, and 9.

A Cochrane review of antidepressant use for noncancer pain in pediatrics highlighted this paucity of evidence, noting only four retrieved studies [28, 29]. In their analysis, the investigators noted none of the studies met their primary outcome of either a 30% or 50% reduction of participant-reported pain. The secondary outcome highlighted generally good tolerability and minimal adverse events of the study medications; no serious adverse events were reported. Further analysis was not possible due to the small sample sizes and insufficient data.

In a retrospective analysis of antidepressants used for functional abdominal pain, 75% (63/84) of pediatric patients reported some level of improvement in their pain with selective serotonin reuptake inhibitor (SSRI) medication and 61% (56/92) on a tricyclic antidepressant (TCA), though pain was not quantified in the study [107]. Adverse effects and discontinuation rates were similar between groups. A subsequent systematic review evaluated and discussed the use of TCAs and SSRIs for functional abdominal pain [17]. Authors reported no notable differences in pain scores with amitriptyline and limited improvement with SSRIs, and ultimately concluded that, based on available evidence, antidepressants are not efficacious in pain management for functional abdominal pain.

An international clinical trial of duloxetine compared to placebo for juvenile fibromyalgia (JFM) showed no statistically significant changes in pain severity over 13 weeks of treatment [94]. Patients in the duloxetine cohort also had an increase in reported adverse events. Milnacipran was also evaluated in the treatment of pain associated with JFM [9]. The study was originally supposed to be a double-blinded control, but ended early due to poor enrollment after only recruiting 20 participants. In the open-label arm and subsequent extension, pain scores were reduced by an average of 1.1 on a 10-point scale, leading authors to conclude milnacipran was not beneficial for pain in JFM.

Two studies compared an antidepressant to gabapentin. Brown et al. compared amitriptyline 10 mg at bedtime to gabapentin 300 mg three times daily for the treatment of complex regional pain syndrome (CRPS) type I or NP over a 6-week period [19]. The authors reported a decrease in pain scores of 1.16 to 1.50 for amitriptyline and 1.56 to 1.77 for gabapentin on a standard 10-point scale; the differences were not statistically significant.

Though antidepressants are sometimes used as adjunctive pain medications, the evidence does not support their consideration for functional abdominal pain or JFM. Use as part of a multimodal pain strategy for other conditions should be carefully considered, as the benefit has not been clearly established in children.

Additional Agents

Anticonvulsants can be used in adults for adjunctive pain management and are described in greater detail in Chap. 12. However, beyond the gabapentinoid class described previously, the use of anticonvulsants for pain management in children is extremely limited and rather controversial. A 2017 Cochrane review seeking to describe anticonvulsant use for chronic noncancer pediatric pain only yielded two studies, both of which evaluated gabapentinoids [28, 29]. An evaluation of anticonvulsants prescribed to Swedish children and adolescents displayed a diverse pattern of these agents ordered specifically for pain despite no evidence supporting their use for non-migraine pain management [59]. Some of the more regularly prescribed agents included oxcarbazepine, carbamazepine, phenobarbital, and valproic acid. A case report from 2005 assessed oxcarbazepine for complex regional pain syndrome in a 12-year-old male who was uncontrolled despite multimodal pain strategies [52]. Only after oxcarbazepine was added to a regimen that included multiple opioids, amitriptyline, gabapentin, ketorolac, and topical lidocaine did the patient's pain become controlled enough to participate in physical therapy and engage in more weight-bearing activities [52]. Melatonin has also been discussed as a potential therapy for adjunctive pain management in more theoretical terms and evaluated in animal studies; human studies are lacking [61].

The consideration of medical cannabis as a potential adjunctive pain agent is early in its development. There are challenges with using this medication, including the diversity of and subsequent standardization of available products, inadequate oversight and regulation from governing bodies, and the transition from an illicit substance. As of 2024, cannabis and marijuana were still considered Schedule 1 drugs, meaning they have no accepted medical use and a high likelihood of abuse [93]. Cannabidiol has also been briefly studied for chronic pain management in children. A case report from France involving a 15-year-old with sickle cell disease was initiated on pure synthetic CBD without THC after multiple hospitalizations for acute pain crisis [63]. The patient was titrated to 22 mg/kg/day in three divided doses over a month. Improvement was noted at 2 weeks through pain regression in affected areas, including the spine, chest, and knee. Interestingly, due to a drug shortage, the patient experienced an interruption in treatment that caused a recurrence of pain in the aforementioned areas. This was resolved within a week of restarting the medication. In another study out of Italy, six pediatric palliative care patients were prescribed a medical cannabis product containing 5–8% THC and 7.5–12% CBD for pain management [35]. The dose was titrated at weekly intervals up to 1 mg/kg/day in three divided doses. Pain was reduced in four patients, somewhat reduced in one patient, and no change was described for one patient.

Though anticonvulsants are often considered part of a multimodal pain strategy in adults, the evidence supporting these agents in pediatrics is inadequate, with small sample sizes and inconsistent results. Subsequently, the use of anticonvulsants for adjunctive pain management cannot be recommended at this time due to a paucity of evidence. Further study with these medications is needed.

Key Themes

- Considerable heterogeneity exists in the current literature involving adjunctive pain management in pediatric patients
- Beyond acetaminophen and NSAIDs, adjunctive therapies for pediatric pain management have limited data to support routine prescribing
- Gabapentin, despite its regular use in practice, does not regularly demonstrate clinically significant improvement in pain scores
- Ketamine appears to have a place in adjunctive pain management, but adverse effects may limit its use to supervised administration
- Most studies have limited applicability due to their short duration and/or limited benefit profile

Conclusions

Evidence supporting adjunctive pain management in pediatric patients is generally conflicting, with insufficient data to strongly support the use of most medications. Most of the literature addresses pain in older children and adolescents, with fewer studies evaluating pain in infants and young children. Acetaminophen and NSAIDs have the strongest body of evidence for all pediatric patients and have demonstrated benefit in pain score reduction and as part of a multimodal strategy in most situations. Ketamine, dexmedetomidine, and clonidine show promise as alternative agents to treat pain, though further study is required. Gabapentin, despite being commonly prescribed, shows limited clinical significance in the management of most forms of acute pain. Drug classes used to treat pain in adults, such as anticonvulsants and antidepressants, are sparsely studied and should be carefully evaluated to assess the risk and benefit of prescribing these agents for pain management.

References

1. Acetaminophen [package insert]. Lake Zurich: Fresenius Kabi; 2015.
2. Adler AC, Daszkowski A, Tan JC, et al. The association of dexmedetomidine on perioperative opioid consumption in children undergoing adenotonsillectomy with and without obstructive sleep apnea. Pediatr Anesth. 2021;133(5):1260–8. https://doi.org/10.1213/ANE00000000000054110.
3. Alghamdi F, Roth C, Jatana KR, et al. Opioid-sparing anesthetic technique for pediatric patients undergoing adenoidectomy: a pilot study. J Pain Res. 2020;13:2997–3004. https://doi.org/10.2147/JPR.S281275.
4. Al-Zaben KR, Qudaisat IY, Aja'bari AN, et al. The effects of caudal or intravenous dexmedetomidine on postoperative analgesia produced by caudal bupivacaine in children: a randomized controlled double-blinded study. J Clin Anesth. 2016;33:386–94. https://doi.org/10.1016/j.jclinane.2016.04.049.
5. Anderson DE, Duletzke NT, Pedigo EB, Halsey MF. Multimodal pain control in adolescent posterior spinal fusion patients: a double-blind, randomized controlled trial to validate the effect of gabapentin on postoperative pain control, opioid use, and patient satisfaction. Spine Deformity. 2020;8:177–85. https://doi.org/10.1007/s43390-020-00038-z.
6. Anghelescu DL, Faughnan LG, Jeha S, et al. Neuropathic pain during treatment for childhood acute lymphoblastic leukemia. Pediatr Blood Cancer. 2011;57(7):1147–53. https://doi.org/10.1002/pbc.23039.
7. Anghelescu DL, Tesney JM, Jeha S, et al. Prospective randomized trial of interventions for vincristine-related neuropathic pain. Pediatr Blood Cancer. 2020;67(9):e28539. https://doi.org/10.1002/pbc.28539.
8. Anghelescu DL, Ryan S, Stritch C, et al. Low-dose ketamine infusions reduce opioid use in pediatric and young adult oncology patients. Pediatr Blood Cancer. 2022;69(9):e29693. https://doi.org/10.1002/pbc.29693.
9. Arnold LM, Bateman L, Palmer RH, Lin Y. Preliminary experience using milnacipran in patients with juvenile fibromyalgia: lessons from a clinical trial program. Pediatr Rheumatol. 2015;13:Article 27. https://doi.org/10.1186/s12969-015-0025-9.
10. Asadi HK, Nikooseresht M, Noori L, Behnoud F. The effect of administration of ketamine and paracetamol versus paracetamol singly on postoperative pain, nausea, and vomiting after pediatric adenotonsillectomy. Anesth Pain Med. 2016;6(1):e31210. https://doi.org/10.5812/aapm.31210.
11. Baichoo P, Asuncion A, El-Chaar G. Intravenous acetaminophen for the management of pain during vaso-occlusive crises in pediatric patients. P T. 2019;44(1):5–8.
12. Baley K, Michalov K, Kossick MA, McDowell M. Intravenous acetaminophen and intravenous ketorolac for management of pediatric surgical pain: a literature review. AANA J. 2014;82(1):53–64.
13. Barcelos A, Garcia PCR, Portela JL, et al. Comparison of two analgesia protocols for the treatment of pediatric orthopedic emergencies. Rev Assoc Med Bras (1992). 2015;61(4):362–7. https://doi.org/10.1590/1806-9282.61.04.362.
14. Baxter KJ, Hafling J, Sterner J, et al. Effectiveness of gabapentin as a postoperative analgesic in children undergoing appendectomy. Ped Surg Int. 2018;34:769–74. https://doi.org/10.1007/s00383-018-4274-9.
15. Bazin V, Bollot J, Asehnoune K, et al. Effects of perioperative intravenous low dose of ketamine on postoperative analgesia in children. Eur J Anaesthesiol. 2010;27(1):47–52.
16. Bindseil I, Soderstrom R, Balmat R. Evaluation of ketorolac ceiling dose effects in pediatric patients in the emergency department. Am J Emerg Med. 2025;89:139–43. https://doi.org/10.1016/j.ajem.2024.12.011.
17. Bonilla S, Nurko S. Focus on the use of antidepressants to treat pediatric functional abdominal pain: current perspectives. Clin Exp Gastroenterol. 2018;11:365–72. https://doi.org/10.2147/CEG.S146646.
18. Brown CR, Moodie JE, Wild VM, Bynum LJ. Comparison of intravenous ketorolac tromethamine and morphine sulfate in the treatment of postoperative pain. Pharmacothersapy. 1990;10(6(Pt2)):116–21S.
19. Brown SC, Johnston BC, Amaria K, et al. A randomized controlled trial of amitriptyline versus gabapentin for complex regional pain syndrome type I and neuropathic pain in children. Scand J Pain. 2016;13:156–63. https://doi.org/10.1016/j.sjpain.2016.05.039.
20. Buck ML. Drug metabolism via cytochrome P450 2D6: ontogeny and variation in children. Pediatr Pharmacother. 2007;13(10).
21. Burns J, Jackson K, Sheehy KA, et al. The use of dexmedetomidine in pediatric palliative care: a preliminary study. J Palliat Med. 2017;20(7):779–83. https://doi.org/10.1089/jpm.2016.0419.
22. Burnsed JC, Heinan K, Letzkus L, Zanelli S. Gabapentin for pain, movement disorders, and irritability in Dashti neonates. Dev Med Child Neurol. 2020;62(3):386–9. https://doi.org/10.1111/dmcn.14324.
23. Busse J, Phillips L, Schecter W. Long-term intravenous ketamine for analgesia in a child with severe chronic intestinal graft versus host disease. Case Rep Anesthesiol. 2015;2015:834168. https://doi.org/10.1155/2015/834168.
24. Chalkiadis GA, Sommerfield D, Low J, et al. Comparison of lumbar epidural bupivacaine with fentanyl or clonidine for postoperative analgesia in children with cerebral palsy after single-event multilevel surgery. Dev Med Child Neurol. 2016;58(4):402–8. https://doi.org/10.1111/dmcn.12930.
25. Chen O, Cadwell JB, Matsoukas K, et al. Perioperative gabapentin usage in pediatric patients: a scoping review. Pediatr Anesth. 2023;33:598–608. https://doi.org/10.1111/pan.14674.
26. Chidambaran V, Subramanyam R, Ding L, et al. Cost-effectiveness of intravenous acetaminophen and ketorolac in adolescents undergoing idiopathic scoliosis surgery. Paediatr Anaesth. 2018;28(3):237–48. https://doi.org/10.1111/pan.13329.
27. Cooney MF. Pain management in children: NSAID use in the perioperative and emergency department settings. Pediatr Drug. 2021;23:361–72. https://doi.org/10.1007/s40272-021-00449-z.
28. Cooper TE, Heathcote LC, Clinch J, et al. Antidepressants for chronic non-cancer pain in children and adolescents. Cochrane Database Syst Rev. 2017a;8:CD012535. https://doi.org/10.1002/14651858.CD012535.pub2.
29. Cooper TE, Wiffen PJ, Heathcote LC, et al. Antiepileptic drugs for chronic non-cancer pain in children and adolescents. Cochrane Database Syst Rev. 2017b;8(8):CD012536. https://doi.org/10.1002/14651858.CD012536.pub2.
30. Courade M, Bertrand A, Guerrini-Rousseau L, et al. Low-dose ketamine adjuvant treatment for refractory pain in children, adolescents, and young adults with cancer: a pilot study. BMJ Support Palliat Care. 2022;12(e5):e656–63. https://doi.org/10.1136/bmjspcare-2018-001739.
31. Da Conceicao MJ, Da Conceicao DB, Leao CC. Effect of an intravenous single dose of ketamine on postoperative pain in tonsillectomy patients. Pediatr Anesth. 2006;16:932–7. https://doi.org/10.1111/j.1460-9592.2006.01893.x.
32. Dashti GA, Amini S, Zanguee E. The prophylactic effect of rectal acetaminophen on postoperative pain and opioid requirements after adenotonsillectomy in children. Middle East J Anaesthesiol. 2009;20(2):245–9.
33. Dewhirst E, Fedel G, Raman V, et al. Pain management following myringotomy and tube placement: intranasal dexmedetomi-

dine versus intranasal fentanyl. Int J Pediatr Otorhinolaryngol. 2014;78(7):1090–4. https://doi.org/10.1016/j.ijporl.2014.04.014.
34. Dhebaria T, Sivitz A, Tejani C. Does intravenous acetaminophen reduce opioid requirement in pediatric emergency department patients with acute sickle cell crisis? Acad Emerg Med. 2021;28(6):639–46. https://doi.org/10.1111/acem.14149.
35. Divisic A, Avagnina I, De Tommasi V, et al. The use of medical cannabis in pediatric palliative care: a case series. Ital. J Pediatr. 2021;47:Article 229. https://doi.org/10.1186/s13052-021-01179-1.
36. Dix P, Martindale S, Stoddart PA. Double-blind randomized placebo-controlled trial of the effect of ketamine on postoperative morphine consumption in children following appendicectomy. Paediatr Anaesth. 2003;13:422–6. https://doi.org/10.1046/j.1460-9592.2003.01090.x.
37. Eiland LS, Meyers RS. Caring for and assessing pediatric patients: aspects to consider as a pharmacy practitioner. Am J Health-Syst Pharm. 2019;76(19):1463–71. https://doi.org/10.1093/ajhp/zxz160.
38. El-Hennawy AM, Abd-Elwahab AM, Abd-Elmaksoud AM, et al. Addition of clonidine or dexmedetomidine to bupivacaine prolongs caudal analgesia in children. Br J Anaes. 2009;103(2):268–74. https://doi.org/10.1093/bja/aep159.
39. Faramarzi M, Roosta S, Eghbal MH. Comparison of celecoxib and acetaminophen for pain relief in pediatric day case tonsillectomy: a randomized double-blind study. Laryngosc Investig Otolaryngol. 2021;6(6):1307–15. https://doi.org/10.1002/lio2.685.
40. Fenikowski D, Tomaszek L, Mazurek H, et al. The effects of gabapentin on post-operative pain and anxiety, morphine consumption and patient satisfaction in pediatric patients following the Ravitch procedure – a randomized, double-blind, placebo-controlled, Phase 4 trial. J Clin Med. 2022;11:4695. https://doi.org/10.3390/jcm11164695.
41. Food and Drug Administration. Drug therapeutics and regulation in the US. 2023 Jan 31. Available at: https://www.fda.gov/about-fda/fda-history-exhibits/drug-therapeutics-regulation-us. Accessed 18 Apr 2025.
42. Franz AM, Dahl JP, Huang H, et al. The development of an opioid sparing anesthesia protocol for pediatric ambulatory tonsillectomy and adenotonsillectomy surgery – a quality improvement project. Pediatr Anesth. 2019;29:682–9. https://doi.org/10.1111/pan.13662.
43. Gever J. No more infant dose of OTC acetaminophen. Medpage Today. 2011 May 5. Available at https://www.medpagetoday.com/pediatrics/generalpediatrics/26297. Accessed 4 Feb 2024.
44. Giordano T, Durkin A, Simi A, et al. High-dose celecoxib for pain after pediatric tonsillectomy: a randomized controlled trial. Otolaryngol Head Neck Surg. 2023;168(2):218–26. https://doi.org/10.1177/01945998221091695.
45. Hakim M, Anderson BJ, Walia H, et al. Acetaminophen pharmacokinetics in severely obese adolescents and young adults. Paediatr Anaesth. 2019;29(1):20–6. https://doi.org/10.1111/pan.13525.
46. Hardin AP, Hackell JM, Committee on Practice and Ambulatory Medicine, et al. Age limit of pediatrics. Pediatrics. 2017;140(3):e20172151. https://doi.org/10.1542/peds.2017-2151.
47. Helenius L, Yrjala T, Oksanen H, et al. Pregabalin and persistent postoperative pain following posterior spinal fusion in children and adolescents: a randomized clinical trial. J Bone Joint Surg Am. 2021;103:2200–6. https://doi.org/10.2106/JBJS.21.00153.
48. Hiller A, Meretoja OA, Korpela R, et al. The analgesic efficacy of acetaminophen, ketoprofen, or their combination for pediatric surgical patients having soft tissue or orthopedic procedures. Anesth Analg. 2006;102(5):1365–71. https://doi.org/10.1213/01.ane.0000204278.71548.bf.
49. Hiller A, Helenius I, Nurmi E, et al. Acetaminophen improves analgesia but does not reduce opioid requirement after major spine surgery in children and adolescents. Spine. 2012;37(20):e1225–31. https://doi.org/10.1097/BRS.0b013e318263165c.
50. Hsu YP, Chu KCW, Bai CH, et al. Safety and efficacy of clonidine on postoperative vomiting and pain in pediatric ophthalmic surgery: a systematic review and meta-analysis. Paediatr Anaesth. 2019;29(10):1011–23. https://doi.org/10.1111/pan.13712.
51. Jones JS, Cotugno RE, Singhal NR, et al. Evaluation of dexmedetomidine and postoperative pain management in patients with adolescent idiopathic scoliosis: conclusions based on a retrospective study at a tertiary pediatric hospital. Pediatr Crit Care Med. 2014;15(6):e247–52. https://doi.org/10.1097/PCC.0000000000000119.
52. Lalwani K, Shoham A, Koh JL, McGraw T. Use of oxcarbazepine to treat a pediatric patient with resistant complex regional pain syndrome. J Pain. 2005;6(10):704–6. https://doi.org/10.1016/j.jpain.2005.05.005.
53. Lammers CR, Schwinghammer AJ, Hall B, et al. Comparison of oral loading dose to intravenous acetaminophen in children for analgesia after tonsillectomy and adenoidectomy: a randomized clinical trial. Anest Analg. 2021;133(6):1568–76. https://doi.org/10.1213/ANE.0000000000005678.
54. Lascano D, Zamora AK, Mahdi E, et al. Gabapentin is associated with decreased postoperative opioid use and length of stay after appendectomy in children with perforated appendicitis: a propensity score-matched analysis. J Pediatr Surg. 2023;58:1935–41. https://doi.org/10.1016/j.jpedsurg.2023.03.009.
55. Lefchak B, Morgan D, Finch M, et al. Ketorolac dose ceiling effect for pediatric headache in the emergency department. J Pediatr Pharmacol Ther. 2024;29(5):494–500. https://doi.org/10.5863/1551-6776-29.5.494.
56. Li C, Doellner C, Leis A, et al. Low-dose ketamine infusion as adjuvant therapy during an acute pain crisis in pediatric patients. J Pain Palliat Care Pharmacother. 2021a;35(1):31–7. https://doi.org/10.1080/15360288.2021.1873216.
57. Li Q, Wu Y, Wang K, et al. Developmental pharmacogenetics of CYP2D6 in Chinese children: loratadine as a substrate drug. Front Pharmacol. 2021b;12:657287. https://doi.org/10.3389/fphar.2021.657287.
58. Lim SY, Pettit RS. Pharmacokinetic considerations in pediatric pharmacotherapy. Am J Health-Syst Pharm. 2019;76(5):1472–80. https://doi.org/10.1093/ajhp/zxz161.
59. Lind LK, Wide K, Wettermark B, von Euler M. Utilization of antiepileptic medicines in Swedish children and adolescents with different diagnoses. Basic Clin Pharmacol Toxicol. 2018;123(1):94–100. https://doi.org/10.1111/bcpt.12981.
60. Lundblad M, Trifa M, Kaabachi O, et al. Alpha-2 adrenoceptor agonists as adjuncts to peripheral nerve blocks in children: a meta-analysis. Pediatr Anesth. 2016;26:232–8. https://doi.org/10.1111/pan.12825.
61. Marseglia L, D'Angelo G, Manti S, et al. Analgesic, anxiolytic, and anaesthetic effects of melatonin: new potential uses in pediatrics. Int J Mol Sci. 2015;16:1209–20. https://doi.org/10.3390/ijms16011209.
62. Mayell A, Srinivasan I, Campbell F, Peliowski A. Analgesic effects of gabapentin after scoliosis surgery in children: a randomized controlled trial. Pediatr Anaesth. 2014;24:1239–44. https://doi.org/10.1111/pan.12524.
63. Mayrand L, Tarbe de Sait Hardouin AL, Maciel TT, et al. Dramatic efficacy of cannabidiol on refractory chronic pain in an adolescent with sickle cell disease. Am J Hematol. 2023;98(11):e295–7. https://doi.org/10.1002/ajh.27049.
64. McNicol ED, Rowe E, Cooper TE. Ketorolac for postoperative pain in children. Cochrane Database Syst Rev. 2018;7(7):CD012294. https://doi.org/10.1002/14651858.CD012294.pub2

65. Murto K, Lamontagne C, McFaul C, et al. Celecoxib pharmacogenetics and pediatric adenotonsillectomy: a double-blinded randomized controlled study. Can J Anaesth. 2015;62(7):785–97. https://doi.org/10.1007/s12630-015-0376-1.
66. Nobrega R, Sheehy KA, Lippold C, et al. Patient characteristics affect the response to ketamine and opioids during the treatment of vaso-occlusive episode-related pain in sickle cell disease. Pediatr Res. 2018;83(2):445–54. https://doi.org/10.1038/pr.2017.197.
67. Ong CKS, Seymour RA, Lirk P, Merry AF. Combining paracetamol (acetaminophen) with nonsteroidal anti-inflammatory drugs: a qualitative systematic review of analgesic efficacy for acute postoperative pain. Pain Med. 2010;110(4):1170–9. https://doi.org/10.1213/ANE.0b013e3181cf9281.
68. Onyebuchi CO, Chumpitazi CE, Placencia JL, et al. Ketamine for pain in sickle cell disease reduces opioid usage. J Pain Sympt Manage. 2023;S0885-3924(23):00785–6. https://doi.org/10.1016/j.jpainsymman.2023.11.012.
69. Osorio D, Maldonado D, Rijs K, et al. Efficacy of different routes of acetaminophen administration for postoperative pain in children: a systematic review and network meta-analysis. Can J Anesth. 2024;71:1103–16. https://doi.org/10.1007/s12630-024-02760-y.
70. Pacifici GM, Allegaert K. Clinical pharmacology of paracetamol in neonates: a review. Curr Ther Res Clin Exp. 2014;77:24–30. https://doi.org/10.1016/j.curtheres.2014.12.001.
71. Park PJ, Makhni MC, Cerpa M, et al. The role of perioperative ketamine in postoperative pain control following spinal surgery. J Spine Surg. 2020;6(3):591–7. https://doi.org/10.21037/jss-19-306.
72. Patel AK, Gai J, Trujillo-Rivera E, et al. Association of intravenous acetaminophen administration with the duration of intravenous opioid use among hospitalized pediatric patients. JAMA Netwe Open. 2021;4(12):e2138420. https://doi.org/10.1001/jamanetworkopen.2021.38420.
73. Poonal N, Bhullar G, Lin K, et al. Oral administration of morphine versus ibuprofen to manage postfracture pain in children: a randomized trial. CMAJ. 2014;186(18):1358–63.
74. Pribonic AP, Brancolini SA, Brea F, Cladis FP. Expanded indications of ketamine infusions for pediatric non-surgical pain: a 10-year, single-center experience. Pain Med. 2023;24:1111–3. https://doi.org/10.1093/pm/pnad052.
75. Qiu J, Xie M. Influence of ketamine versus fentanyl on pain relief for pediatric orthopedic emergencies: a meta-analysis of randomized controlled studies. Medicine (Baltimore). 2021;100(42):e27409. https://doi.org/10.1097/MD0000000000027409.
76. Rayala S, Backdahl T, Reddy N, et al. Low-dose oral ketamine for procedural analgesia in pediatric cancer patients undergoing lumbar puncture at a resource-limited cancer hospital in India. J Palliat Med. 2019;22(11):1357–63. https://doi.org/10.1089/jpm.2018.0667.
77. Rhodes AJ, Fagan MJ, Motov SM, Zerzan J. Nebulized ketamine for managing acute pain in the pediatric emergency department: a case series. Turk J Emerg Med. 2021;21(2):75–8. https://doi.org/10.4103/2452-2473.313334.
78. Rizkalla N, Zane NR, Prodell JL, et al. Use of intravenous acetaminophen in children for analgesia after spinal fusion surgery: a randomized clinical trial. J Pediatr Pharmacol Ther. 2018;23(5):395–404. https://doi.org/10.5863/1551-6776-23.5.395.
79. Rocchio RJ, Ward KE. Intranasal ketamine for acute pain. Clin J Pain. 2021;37:295–300. https://doi.org/10.1097/AJP.0000000000000918.
80. Rugyte D, Gudaityte J. Intravenous paracetamol in adjunct to intravenous ketoprofen for postoperative pain in children undergoing general surgery: a double-blinded randomized study. Medicina (Kaunas). 2019;55(4):86. https://doi.org/10.3390/medicina55040086.
81. Rusy LM, Hainsworth KR, Nelson TJ, et al. Gabapentin use in pediatric spinal fusion patients: a randomized, double-blind, controlled trial. Anesth Analg. 2010;110(5):1393-8. https://doi.org/10.1213/ANE.0b013e3181d41dc2.
82. Saltik S, Sozen HC, Basgul S, et al. Pregabalin treatment of a patient with complex regional pain syndrome. Pediatr Neurol. 2016;54:88–90.
83. Savva DA, Kishk OA, Morgan JA, et al. Post-operative nonsteroidal anti-inflammatory drug use for pain in infant and paediatric cardiac surgery patients. Cardiol Young. 2019;29(12):1440–4. https://doi.org/10.1017/S1047951119002312.
84. Sheehy KA, Finkel JC, Darbari DS, et al. Dexmedetomidine as an adjuvant to analgesic strategy during vaso-occlusive episodes in adolescents with sickle cell disease. Pain Pract. 2015;15(8):e90–7. https://doi.org/10.1111/papr.12336.
85. Smith C, Goldman RD. Alternating acetaminophen and ibuprofen for pain in children. Can Fam Physician. 2012;58(6):645–7.
86. Smith HA, Besunder JB, Betters KA, et al. 2022 Society of Critical Care Medicine clinical practice guidelines on prevention and management of pain, agitation, neuromuscular blockade, and delirium in critically ill pediatric patients with consideration of the ICU environment and early mobility. Pediatr Crit Care Med. 2022;23(2):e74–110. https://doi.org/10.1097/PCC.0000000000002873.
87. Subramanyam R, Varughese A, Kurth CD, Eckman MH. Cost-effectiveness of intravenous acetaminophen for pediatric tonsillectomy. Paediatr Anaest. 2014;24(5):467–75. https://doi.org/10.1111/pan.12359.
88. Thomas JJ, Levek C, Quick HD, et al. Utility of gabapentin in meeting physical therapy goals following posterior spinal fusion in adolescent patients with idiopathic scoliosis. Pediatr Anesth. 2018;28:558–63. https://doi.org/10.1111/pan.13398.
89. Thung AK, Elmaraghy CA, Barry N, et al. Double-blind randomized placebo-controlled trial of single-dose intravenous acetaminophen for pain associated with adenotonsillectomy in pediatric patients with sleep-disordered breathing. J Pediatr Pharmacol Ther. 2017;22(5):344–51. https://doi.org/10.5863/1551-6776-22.5.344.
90. Tomaszek L, Fenikowski D, Maciejewski P, et al. Perioperative gabapentin in pediatric thoracic surgery patients – randomized, placebo-controlled, Phase 4 trial. Pain Med. 2020;21(8):1562–71. https://doi.org/10.1093/pm/pnz207.
91. Tu Z, Tan X, Li S, Cui J. The efficacy and safety of dexmedetomidine combined with bupivacaine on caudal epidural block in children: a meta-analysis. Med Sci Monit. 2019;25:165–73. https://doi.org/10.12659/MSM.913098.
92. Ugur F, Gulcu N, Boyaci A. Oral ketamine for pain relief in a child with abdominal malignancy. Pain Med. 2009;10(1):120–1. https://doi.org/10.1111/j.1526-4637.2008.00424.x.
93. United States Drug Enforcement Administration DEA. United States. Available at: https://www.dea.gov/drug-information/drug-scheduling#:~:text=Schedule%20I%20drugs%2C%20substances%2C%20or,)%2C%20methaqualone%2C%20and%20peyote. Accessed 29 Jan 2024.
94. Upadhyaya HP, Arnold LM, Alaka K, et al. Efficacy and safety of duloxetine versus placebo in adolescents with juvenile fibromyalgia: results from a randomized controlled trial. Pediatr Rheumatol Online J. 2017;17(1):Article 27. https://doi.org/10.1186/s12969-019-0325-6.
95. Vaughns JD, Martin C, Nelson J, et al. Dexmedetomidine as an adjuvant for perioperative pain management in adolescents undergoing bariatric surgery: an observational cohort study. J Pediatr Surg. 2017;52:1787–90. https://doi.org/10.1016/j.jpedsurg.2017.04.007.
96. Vetter TR, Heiner EJ. Intravenous ketorolac as an adjuvant to pediatric patient-controlled analgesia with mor-

phine. J Clin Anesth. 1994;6(2):110–3. https://doi.org/10.1016/0952-8180(94)90006-x.
97. Viitanen H, Tuominen N, Vaaraniemi H, et al. Analgesic efficacy of rectal acetaminophen and ibuprofen alone or in combination for paediatric day-case adenoidectomy. Br J Anaesth. 2003;91(3):363–7. https://doi.org/10.1093/bja/aeg196.
98. Vivekanandaswamy AN, Shetty AP, Kanna RM, Shanmuganathan R. An analysis of the safety and efficacy of dexmedetomodine in posterior spinal fusion surgery for adolescent idiopathic scoliosis: a prospective randomized study. Eur Spine J. 2021;30:698–705. https://doi.org/10.1007/s00586-020-06539-9.
99. Vondracek P, Oslejskova H, Kepak T, et al. Efficacy of pregabalin in neuropathic pain in paediatric oncological patients. Eur J Paediatr Neurol. 2009;13:332–6. https://doi.org/10.1016/j.ejpn.2008.06.011.
100. Webb TL, Sanders JE. Chapter 12 – Pediatric pain. In: Cisewski DH, Motov SM, editors. EMRA pain management guide. 1st ed. Minneapolis: Emergency Medicine Residents' Association; 2020.
101. Williams K, Thomson D, Seto I, et al. Standard 6: age groups for pediatric trials. Pediatrics. 2012;129(supp3):S153–60. https://doi.org/10.1542/peds.2012-0055I.
102. Wong I, St John-Green C, Walker SM. Opioid-sparing effects of perioperative paracetamol and nonsteroidal anti-inflammatory drugs (NSAIDs) in children. Paediatr Anaesth. 2013;23(6):475–95. https://doi.org/10.1111/pan.12163.
103. Wossner S, Weber K, Steinbeck AC, et al. Pregabalin as adjunct in a multimodal pain therapy after traumatic foot amputation – a case report of a 4-year-old girl. Scand J Pain. 2017;17:146–9. https://doi.org/10.1016/j.sjpain.2017.09.001.
104. Yao Y, Yu C, Zhang X, et al. Caudal and intravenous dexmedetomidine similarly prolong the duration of caudal analgesia in children: a randomized controlled trial. Pediatr Anesth. 2018;28:888–96. https://doi.org/10.1111/pan.13469.
105. Yeaman F, Oakley E, Meek R, Graudins A. Sub-dissociative dose intranasal ketamine for limb injury pain in children in the emergency department: a pilot study. Emerg Med Australas. 2013;25:161–7. https://doi.org/10.1111/1742-6723.12059.
106. Yu H, Chen A, Chen E, et al. Low-dose ketamine infusion for pediatric hematology/oncology patients: case series and literature review. J Pediatr Hematol Oncol. 2022;44:e188–93. https://doi.org/10.1097/MPH.0000000000002290.
107. Zar-Kessler CAM, Belkind-Gerson J, Bender S, Kuo BM. Treatment of functional abdominal pain with antidepressants: benefits, adverse effects, and the gastroenterologist's role. J Pediatr Gastroenterol Nutr. 2017;65(1):16–21. https://doi.org/10.1097/MPG.0000000000001416.
108. Zempsky WT, Loiselle KA, Corsi JM, Hagstrom JN. Use of low-dose ketamine infusion for pediatric patients with sickle cell disease-related pain. Clin J Pain. 2010;26:163–7. https://doi.org/10.1097/AJP.0b013e3181b511ab.
109. Zepeda AG, Childers AL, Thornton L, et al. Impact of intraoperative ketorolac on postoperative pain in children undergoing adenotonsillectomy: a double-blind, placebo-control trial. J Anesth. 2025. Published online April 25, 2025. https://doi.org/10.1007/s00540-025-03505-x
110. Zhou L, Yang H, Hai Y, Cheng Y. Perioperative low-dose ketamine for postoperative pain management in spine surgery: a systematic review and meta-analysis of randomized controlled trials. Pain Res Manag. 2022;2022:1507097. https://doi.org/10.1155/2022/1507097.

23 Analgesic Approaches and Considerations in the Transgender Patient Population

Kellyn Engstrom, Nathan Smith, Kyle A. Schofield, Fiona Emrys Fonseca, Kharmene Sunga, and Caitlin S. Brown

Background

Transgender and gender-diverse (TGD) people identify differently from the sex assigned to them at birth and, as a result, face unique psychosocial, societal, and systemic stressors that have clearly documented impacts on health and well-being [1, 2]. In the United States, TGD people have been shown to have fewer "good health" days and more experiences with poor mental and physical health compared to cisgender (non-TGD) people [3, 4]. Previous research has explained these health disparities using the minority stress model, which posits that experiencing additional life stress related to one's gender or sexual minority status can be proximal (such as internalized homophobia or transphobia, expectations of rejection, or expectations for threats and associated hypervigilance) or distal (for example, actual experiences with violence and abuse or anti-LGBTQ—lesbian, gay, bisexual, transgender, queer—laws) [5]. Cumulative effects of TGD minority stress can result in worse mental health (e.g., depression, suicidality, anxiety, substance use, or trauma) and physical health (e.g., cardiovascular disease, cancer, obesity, or poor nutrition) [6–11].

K. Engstrom (✉) · C. S. Brown
Department of Pharmacy, Mayo Clinic, Rochester, MN, USA

Department of Emergency Medicine, Mayo Clinic, Rochester, MN, USA
e-mail: engstrom.kellyn@mayo.edu; Brown.caitlin1@mayo.edu

N. Smith
Department of Pharmacy, Mayo Clinic, Rochester, MN, USA

Division of Pain Medicine, Mayo Clinic, Rochester, MN, USA

K. A. Schofield · F. E. Fonseca
Division of Endocrinology, Transgender and Intersex Specialty Care Clinic, Mayo Clinic, Rochester, MN, USA

Department of Psychiatry and Psychology, Mayo Clinic, Rochester, MN, USA

K. Sunga
Department of Emergency Medicine, Mayo Clinic, Rochester, MN, USA

Despite being at risk for poorer health compared to cisgender populations, TGD people face significant barriers to accessing healthcare. In the 2022 US Trans Survey, the largest survey to date on TGD people in the United States with a sample size of 92,329, participants reported that they were unable to obtain care due to cost (28%), avoided healthcare due to fears of being mistreated (24%), and had negative experiences when they did engage with healthcare providers (47%) or tried to obtain coverage for healthcare through insurance (26%) [4].

While previous research has reported increased prevalence of chronic pain among sexual minority (e.g., gay, lesbian, bisexual) individuals, research on pain and chronic pain conditions among TGD individuals is still in its infancy [12]. However, existing literature shows some evidence of disparities in pain experiences and chronic pain in this population. Previous work has identified several pain-related conditions for which TGD people show a higher prevalence, including fibromyalgia, endometriosis, migraine, hypermobile Ehlers-Danlos syndrome, and pelvic pain [13–17]. Related to pediatric populations, in a nationally representative sample, children aged 6–17 whose caregivers reported that they had experienced discrimination based on their sexual orientation or gender identity were twice as likely to also experience chronic pain in the past 12 months [18]. While many authors have discussed that minority stress factors play a role in the heightened prevalence of chronic pain conditions among TGD people, the specific mechanisms behind these health disparities are not presently fully understood. However, some literature has pointed to the impact of chronic hypothalamic-pituitary axis activation related to chronic stress, increased allostatic load, and associated metabolic and inflammatory changes, such as those related to health and aging [19, 20].

Disparities in pain management among TGD individuals are not well studied or documented in the literature, although based on studies of other minority populations, they likely exist. Research on pain management demonstrates that racial

J. P. Reinert et al. (eds.), *Adjunctive Analgesic Strategies for the Bedside Clinician and Beyond*,
https://doi.org/10.1007/978-3-032-21675-5_23

and ethnic minorities, such as non-Hispanic, Black, and Hispanic patients, are less likely to receive opioids for the management of acute pain than non-Hispanic White patients [21]. Similar disparities have been shown to exist in the management of chronic pain, as non-Hispanic, Black, and Hispanic populations exhibit significantly higher pain scores than white patients with chronic pain at the 1-year follow-up of chronic pain management [22]. When seen for acute pain in the emergency department (ED), older adults are less likely to receive pain medication than younger individuals [23]. Additionally, it has been shown that women are less likely to have pain medication prescribed to them for musculoskeletal pain than men, even though women experience higher rates of musculoskeletal pain [24]. In one study of pediatric patients in an intensive chronic pain treatment program, TGD patients were less likely to complete the program compared to non-TGD patients, though patients who completed the program showed similar rates of improvement [25].

While there are likely several reasons for a lack of literature evaluating disparities in pain management among TGD populations, the small size of this population, along with a lack of established methodology for identifying TGD patients in the electronic health record, likely serve as barriers to meaningful research in this area. A recent study successfully validated a methodology for identifying TGD patients in the electronic health record, which hopefully will serve as a model for further study and research in this area [26].

A gender-affirming approach to analgesia must begin with the acknowledgment of structural and interpersonal barriers. Such an approach involves creating a clinical environment that validates patients' gender identities, utilizes inclusive language, and actively addresses prior trauma (Table 23.1). A gender-affirming clinician acknowledges and respects the patient, using the patient's chosen name, pronouns, and terminology for their body both in the presence and absence of the patient (Table 23.2). Pain assessment should be conducted with attention to anatomical variation and medical history that may differ significantly from cisgender norms. However, it is essential for clinicians to adopt a balanced and individualized approach. It is important for clinicians to acknowledge that pain is not psychological by default and that quality care involves more than symptomatic management [27]. They must avoid the "trans broken arm syndrome"—engaging in an overt focus on the patient's gender identity when this is not pertinent to their presentation [28].

Table 23.1 Terminology

Term	Definition
Sex	A description of physiological/biological characteristics (such as hormone levels, gonads, chromosomes, genitalia, and secondary sex characteristics) that determine an individual as male, female, intersex, etc. Definitions of sex in the United States vary across settings, including level of government (e.g., state vs. federal), commercial organizations (e.g., policies around bathroom access and sex-segregated group membership), etc.
Intersex [91]	People with chromosomal, hormonal, and physiological variations that lie outside the male/female binary. Medical definitions have varied over time, and individuals with sex variations may or may not identify themselves as intersex. Examples of human sex variations that have been classified as intersex include Turner and Klinefelter syndromes, genitalia that are not subjectively defined as male or female, the presence of both ovarian and testicular tissues, etc.
Sex assigned at birth	The sex an individual is first labeled, typically based on the configuration of genitalia on a newborn infant
Gender	A socially defined categorization of an individual as a man, woman, nonbinary person, Two Spirit, etc. Definitions of gender and gender roles vary by culture and time. Socially accepted gender roles outside of the binary predate colonial times in North America among Native peoples. [92]
Gender identity	An individual's personal understanding of their gender, which may or may not correspond with outward appearance
Gender expression	Outward characteristics that communicate an individual's gender, such as clothing, makeup, mannerisms, and style of speech. Gender expression, like gender, shows variation by time and culture (e.g., the acceptability of long hair on men, the colors of clothing associated with a particular gender).
Transgender	An umbrella term for individuals whose sex and/or gender identity differs from sex and/or gender labels assigned at birth. Some, but not all, intersex individuals identify as transgender
Nonbinary	An individual who identifies their gender as being outside the categorization of man/woman. Nonbinary individuals may identify as both male and female, agender (no gender), genderfluid, etc., and may also combine this term with other gender categories (such as labeling oneself as a nonbinary transgender man).
Transgender man	An individual who was labeled female at birth, who identifies as a man
Transgender woman	An individual who was labeled male at birth, who identifies as a woman
Sexual orientation	The gender(s) that an individual is attracted to sexually and/or romantically. Sexual orientation is different from gender identity but may be influenced by one's gender (e.g., a lesbian is typically defined as a woman who is attracted to women).

In this chapter, we aim to provide an overview of areas of consideration specific to TGD populations. We will discuss drug information considerations, efficacy and safety of medications, and selection of analgesics, including those related to changes in metabolism that may occur for patients on gender-affirming hormone therapy (GAHT). We will also discuss several specific pain conditions that commonly occur among TGD populations, such as migraine, fibromyalgia, abdominal pain, postsurgical pain, and endometriosis.

Table 23.2 Pronouns

Pronoun	Description	Examples
He/him/his	Typically used to refer to men and boys, including transgender men, and sometimes used by nonbinary people	He is going to a concert tomorrow night His follow-up appointment will need to be scheduled for next month
She/her/hers	Typically used to refer to women and girls, and sometimes used by nonbinary people	She is hoping you can come visit us next year Her pain medication needs to be adjusted
They/them/theirs	Typically associated with nonbinary individuals as well as referring to a group of people Note that when referring to one person with these pronouns, grammatical structure remains plural, for the most part	My genderfluid friend got a new jacket, and they are very happy with it My nonbinary patient did not come to their appointment today; I am going to call them They were able to dress themself up this morning That group of clinicians is busy; they work very hard *Incorrect:* My nonbinary patient canceled their appointment; they is not coming
Ze/hir/hirs Ze/zir/zirs Pronunciation: Ze: "Zee" Hir: "Hear" Hirs: "Hears" Zir: "Zeer" Zirs: "Zeers"	Newer forms of pronouns, also called neopronouns, do not label gender and use a singular grammatical structure [93]. Other forms of neopronouns exist and may be used by patients. In our clinical experience, it is less common for patients to use these pronouns in medical settings, and the majority of TGD patients use he, she, or they pronouns; however, it is important to know that some patients may request you use neopronouns. If a patient indicates usage of pronouns that are unfamiliar to you, it is socially acceptable to politely ask the patient to clarify spelling and/or state an example sentence to help you adjust your language	Ze had a long day yesterday. I heard hir mowing the lawn late into the evening. That pile of lawn clippings is hirs. My patient left zir water bottle in the exam room; it is zirs. I hope ze comes back to get it soon.

Finally, we will discuss how providers can engage in gender-affirming and culturally aware practices with TGD patients.

Approaches to Practice

Pain is a subjective, personal, and often very private experience impacted by biological, psychological, and social factors. Holistic management of pain must begin with a whole-person approach to care [27, 29]. For TGD individuals, this means approaching pain as one piece of the picture. Healthcare, including pain management, often occurs within a context of systemic marginalization and stigmatization. Individuals who are TGD are at higher risk for being undertreated for pain or, conversely, being subjected to unwarranted scrutiny when seeking pain relief, due to pervasive stigma regarding both gender identity and substance use [19]. Research has shown that there are gaps in training for clinicians when it comes to working with the TGD population [30]. The mistrust that TGD patients have of medical advances and the medical profession is reflective of these very real historical and ongoing injustices [31]. Gender-affirming approaches to analgesia and pain management are responsive to the unique physiological, psychological, and social needs of TGD patients, aiming not only to control pain effectively but also to promote dignity and trust.

Studies suggest that marginalized and specifically TGD individuals experience higher rates of pain than the general population, with this phenomenon more marked in transmasculine individuals than transfeminine individuals when compared to cisgender counterparts [32]. Several studies appear to indicate that following initiation of GAHT, however, transfeminine individuals experience a worsening of pain phenomena, while transmasculine individuals may experience some improvement [14, 33–35]. Estrogens are generally considered to increase nociception and potentially modulate serotonergic, noradrenergic, dopaminergic, endocannabinoid, and endogenous opioid pathways. It is hypothesized that estrogenic impact on pain depends on the extent of involvement of various organ systems, as estrogens may influence each system in different ways [35–37]. Androgens are considered more protective from a nociceptive standpoint, with hypotheses including androgen receptor distribution throughout the limbic system and the effects of down-regulation of estrogen receptor expression, as well as androgenic reduction of inflammation [37]. This is despite some potential increase in pelvic pain for transmasculine individuals following initiation of testosterone, likely related to tissue atrophy [32]. This difference is particularly noted in studies involving musculoskeletal pain and headaches, including migraines [35, 38]. It is unknown whether these observations are due to peripheral or central actions of sex steroids, with the majority of these studies focusing on cisgender individuals. However, further studies are warranted as these findings may not be generalizable to TGD individuals. The elevated prevalence of mental health conditions such as depression, anxiety, and posttraumatic stress disorder (PTSD)—which can exacerbate pain perception—further complicates the clinical picture [39].

Despite these elevated risks, TGD patients frequently report negative healthcare experiences, including misgendering, denial of care, and providers' lack of knowledge regarding needs unique to the community [40]. These experiences contribute to avoidance of medical care, which may delay pain assessment and appropriate interventions. In addition to these differences, approaches to pain management must consider the surgical interventions that many TGD individuals receive [36].

Assessing pain may be more straightforward when it comes to acute pain or pain as a symptom of trauma or disease. However, even with such pain, in addition to pain intensity at rest, other factors, such as pain with movement (dynamic pain) or neuropathic components, for example, need to be defined and measured more accurately. Assessment of chronic pain is much more challenging, regardless of the cause [29]. The long list of published instruments indicates that pain assessment continues to be a challenge. Assessing pain in patients with whom there might be difficulties in communication poses further challenges because of the nature of pain itself. This is most noted for TGD patients who might have cognitive impairment or decline [41]. Verbal descriptions are but one way to assess pain, and an inability to communicate does not negate the possibility of pain [42].

Furthermore, clinicians must remain vigilant to the potential for biased prescribing practices. Pain management protocols must include considerations for patients undergoing gender-affirming surgeries, with preoperative and postoperative care plans designed to optimize comfort, healing, and long-term functional outcomes. An astute clinician must inquire about the patient's previous experiences of surgery and their experience with pain [27]. When pain persists, they must ask the questions: Is there an ongoing physical disease (e.g., infection, cancer)? Is there a problem with the use or misuse of analgesics? Is there a psychiatric condition complicating the pain (e.g., depression, anxiety, somatic symptom disorder, psychosis)? Is there another pain condition involving the central nervous system (e.g., allodynia)? Is this a pain behavior syndrome? What might we be missing that is unique to this patient, which impacts their experience of pain?

Non-pharmacological interventions are vital components of gender-affirming pain care. Cognitive-behavioral therapy (CBT), mindfulness-based stress reduction (MBSR), physical therapy, and complementary approaches such as acupuncture can be effective but should be offered in a manner that respects gender identity [43]. For TGD patients with a history of trauma, trauma-informed care frameworks can be especially important. These frameworks emphasize safety, trustworthiness, collaboration, and empowerment—principles that are particularly relevant when treating pain using both physical and psychological approaches [44].

Importantly, gender-affirming care is not limited to individual clinicians; it also involves institutional policies that protect and affirm TGD patients. This includes the use of chosen names and pronouns in medical records, the availability of gender-inclusive facilities, staff training on trans-specific care, and access to gender-affirming medical interventions as part of comprehensive pain management. For example, denying access to hormone therapy due to unrelated medical procedures may exacerbate psychological distress and thereby increase pain experiences, a phenomenon supported by biopsychosocial models of pain [45, 46]. Part of providing holistic pain management as a clinician working with TGD individuals can therefore involve advocating on the patient's behalf at the institutional or larger level.

Holistic and gender-affirming approaches to analgesia and pain management require an integration of clinical expertise, cultural competence, and institutional support. Individuals who are TGD face unique challenges in accessing and receiving adequate pain care, rooted in both physiological factors and broader social determinants of health. By centering the lived experiences of TGD patients, tailoring treatments to their medical and psychological contexts, and eliminating systemic barriers to care, healthcare providers can significantly improve pain outcomes and advance health equity. Continued research is essential to further elucidate the most effective gender-affirming pain management practices, as is the incorporation of TGD voices in the design and delivery of care.

Pharmacokinetic and Pharmacodynamic Considerations in Transgender Patients

It is important to consider possible impacts on pharmacokinetics and pharmacodynamics when selecting medications for pain management; however, there is limited evidence that potential changes in TGD patients' pharmacokinetics and pharmacodynamics impact clinical outcomes [47]. Gender-affirming therapy may affect body composition in TGD patients based on known differences with cisgender men and women, leading to alterations in the volume of distribution of medications [47]. Typically, cisgender women have higher total body fat than cisgender men, and cisgender men have higher lean body mass than cisgender women. This may lead to an increase in the volume of distribution of lipophilic drugs in cisgender women and an increase in the volume of distribution of hydrophilic drugs in cisgender men [47]. These changes in pharmacokinetics should be considered in TGD patients undergoing gender-affirming therapies. Figure 23.1 describes the impact of hormone therapy on body composition [47, 48].

Although there are limited specific models or studies evaluating differences in cytochrome P450 (CYP) metabolism among TGD patients, there are some specific CYP enzymes that play a role in GAHT metabolism that are worth noting. Estrogen may inhibit CYP1A2 metabolism, and oral contraceptives may increase the metabolism of uridine glucuronosyltransferase (UGT) substrates (acetaminophen) [47]. Estrogens, including injectable estradiol valerate used by transgender women, are metabolized at least partially through cytochrome P450 3A4; thus, any potent inducers and inhibitors of CYP3A4 should also be used with caution [49]. Testosterone is also metabolized through the liver via CYP3A4, and levels could be affected significantly in the presence of potent inducers and inhibitors of CYP3A4 or in the presence of significant liver dysfunction [50]. Common CYP3A4 inhibitors include azole antifungals, ritonavir (e.g., nirmatrelvir-ritonavir combination anti-viral for COVID-19), and grapefruit juice. On the other hand, common inducers include rifampin, St. John's Wort, phenytoin, and carbamazepine [51].

It is unlikely that there are significant changes in renal drug metabolism in TGD patients. A retrospective study found that there were serum creatinine changes in TGD patients after GAHT, and clinicians can use creatinine values approximately 6 months after initiating GAHT therapy as a patient's new baseline [52]. When determining glomerular filtration rate for medication dosing, clinicians can begin using the gender to which TGD patients have transitioned after being on GAHT therapy for approximately 6 months to 1 year. It is important to note that race-free estimations should be used [53].

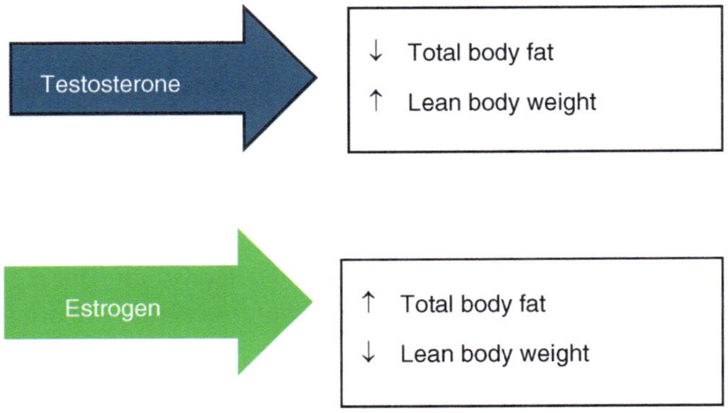

Fig. 23.1 Hormone therapy and drug disposition changes [47, 48]

Review of Evidence

Medication Efficacy and Safety

Individuals assigned male and female at birth have been shown to experience pain and develop chronic pain to a varying degree. Those in gender minority and sex minority groups are frequently underrepresented or unrepresented in research associated with the development of chronic pain [19]. It is well established that cisgender women are at an increased risk of pain-related conditions like fibromyalgia and migraine headaches [54, 55]. This may be complicated in the transgender population, as transgender individuals are also subject to gender minority stress, psychosocial factors, and complicating psychological comorbidities. TGD people frequently receive GAHT, which may be tied with worsening acute pain episodes and lead to the development of chronic pain conditions. Additionally, it has been suggested that gender role expectations and cultural influence on pain perception also play a role, possibly by delaying presentation for, and thus treatment of, acute pain, leading to the development of chronic pain [56].

Migraines

When compared with cisgender individuals, a higher incidence of migraine has been associated with TGD persons compared to cisgender men, but similar to cisgender women [15]. Patients on GAHT may be associated with the increased rates of migraine headaches, as transgender youths have a higher odds of developing migraines compared to those not receiving GAHT [57].

Psychiatric comorbidities, trauma, and discrimination are factors frequently associated with the development of chronic headache and migraine headache conditions. Given the commonality of these psychosocial comorbidities among the TGD population, a heightened risk of migraine headaches among them may be assumed [58]. Clinicians should aim to mitigate this risk through nonpharmacologic techniques aiming to improve psychosocial goals of care. Nonpharmacologic therapies may include cognitive behavioral therapy (CBT), behavioral activation, problem-solving therapy, interpersonal therapy, psychodynamic therapy, and mindfulness-based therapy [59].

The use of pharmacotherapeutic agents in the treatment of migraine headaches among transgender persons should be individualized and initiated in an approach, like that of cisgender persons. Detailed medication information is discussed separately under migraine treatment options. The American Headache Society recommends evidence-based acute treatment options such as nonsteroidal anti-inflammatory drugs (NSAIDs), acetaminophen, triptans, CGRP receptor antagonists, 5-HT1F agonists, and neuromodulation devices utilized in a stepwise approach based on therapeutic efficacy and severity of the attack [60]. While evidence is limited, clinicians should consider the potential vascular risk factors associated with GAHT and avoid the use of triptans and ergot alkaloids in patients with significant vascular risk factors due to the potential for vasoconstrictive complications [61].

Fibromyalgia

Fibromyalgia is a chronic pain condition characterized by widespread pain and fatigue, and it is associated with an increased prevalence among cisgender women [62]. It is a central pain syndrome that is thought to be the result of biological predisposition as well as emotional and physical etiologic factors, including stress and trauma. TGD persons have a significantly increased prevalence of fibromyalgia compared to cisgender individuals [63]. The increased risk observed in the TGD population is likely multifactorial and similarly impacted by the increased rates of trauma, minority stress, discrimination, and mood disorders discussed previously.

The perception of pain experienced by an individual is significantly impacted by sex hormones. Higher testosterone levels are associated with increased pain thresholds, while variations in estrogen levels may be associated with increased sensitivity to pain stimuli [37]. Therefore, it may be extrapolated that GAHT may play a role in the development and/or expression of fibromyalgia. While this has not been clearly demonstrated in currently available literature, limited evidence suggests that GAHT may influence fibromyalgia expression and severity of symptoms [37]. This should not deter clinicians from appropriately providing GAHT to TGD patients but rather serve as additional points of consideration when designing an individualized fibromyalgia therapy plan.

Evidence to guide the treatment of fibromyalgia in TGD individuals is severely limited [64]. Despite increased rates of fibromyalgia as well as common factors associated with the development of fibromyalgia in the TGD population, these individuals are frequently excluded from clinical trials. Thus, further research is needed to outline evidence-based recommendations for individualized treatment. Given the lack of study in TGD patients, treatment should follow the same algorithmic approach as recommended for cisgender patients. Providers should utilize the AAPT 2019 Diagnostic Criteria for Fibromyalgia and recommend nonpharmacologic interventions as first-line therapy prior to initiating pharmacologic treatments [65]. Nonpharmacologic interventions may include patient education, exercise, CBT, and complementary and alternative medicines [65]. Evidence-based treatments for the pharmacologic management of fibromyalgia in the general population include amitriptyline, cyclobenzaprine, duloxetine, milnacipran, and pregabalin [65]. Additional medications from other therapeutic classes may be utilized as well, with the primary goal of treating the most problematic symptoms for the individual. Fibromyalgia treatment should be personalized for each individual patient, and this is true for cisgender and transgender patients alike. Currently, no evidence suggests GAHT alters the safety or efficacy of standard treatment options for fibromyalgia. Thus, transgender individuals receiving GAHT may be initiated on therapy and titrated accordingly based on analgesic response and tolerability.

Abdominal Pain

Abdominal pain is an extremely common presentation and the leading gastrointestinal (GI) cause of presentation to ambulatory clinics in the United States (US) [66]. Additionally, it is the most common emergency department (ED) chief complaint, comprising 5–10% of all ED visits in the US [67]. A recent survey of adult patients with a history of abdominal pain reported that over half of adults had experienced recurrent abdominal pain, with 81% of these patients experiencing an episode of pain within the past week. However, only 61.5% of these patients reported seeking care for their symptoms due to lack of access, lack of pain severity, and additional socioeconomic factors [68].

As with the general population, abdominal pain is a common presentation and complaint among TGD patients. TGD patients experience the same gastrointestinal disorders as cisgender patients, but with notably different patterns [69]. The Centers for Disease Control and Prevention has noted that TGD patients are at a higher risk for sexually transmitted infections (STIs) secondary to reduced access to treatment and prevention [70]. Extrapolating from existing data, TGD individuals are less likely to have obtained routine cancer screenings, including those for colorectal and other abdominal cancers, which should be considered in those presenting with concerning abdominal symptoms [71]. Rates of inflammatory bowel disease (IBD) appear to be similar for TGD and cisgender populations, but a recent review notes a significant lack of literature regarding the effects of GAHT, lack of access, and stigma on the incidence and outcomes of IBD in TGD patients [72]. A recent study found that over 70% of transgender men experience abdominal pain after initiation of GAHT with unclear etiology, again demonstrating the significant gaps in knowledge regarding optimization of abdominal pain in TGD patients [73].

Biopsychosocial abdominal pain is an increasingly common presentation in both cisgender and TGD populations, and further research into the etiology and optimal treatment of this type of abdominal pain is ongoing [74]. While there are no high-quality comparative studies, given the prevalence of mental health conditions within the TGD population, it is worth considering that biopsychosocial abdominal pain could be more common in TGD patients. This is also supported by the observation that TGD college-age students report high rates of eating disorders, even higher than rates observed among cisgender women [75].

A recent study evaluating disparities in pain management among TGD patients presenting to the ED found that TGD patients were much less likely to receive opioids than cisgender patients, particularly cisgender men, despite similar reported pain scores [78]. A study examining symptoms in patients with IBD noted sex and gender differences, with higher associated rates of depression among TGD patients. The study also found differences in symptom presentation among cisgender men and cisgender women, but did not examine these further in TGD patients [79]. These disparities in abdominal pain management are consistent with many health disparities among TGD individuals, and these studies both demonstrate that there is a significant amount of work to be done to both identify and eliminate these disparities.

Postsurgical Pain Management

An important consideration for TGD patients who may undergo gender-affirming surgery is the need to ensure adequate pain management postoperatively. There are various forms of surgery, and each patient may select a different one based on their own needs. Forms of feminizing surgery include orchiectomy, vaginoplasty (which may include penectomy), breast augmentation, facial feminization surgery, abdominoplasty, liposuction, gluteal augmentation, tracheal shave, and hair transplantation or removal [80]. Masculinizing surgeries include mastectomy, chest contouring, hysterectomy, oophorectomy, vaginectomy, phalloplasty, metoidioplasty, scrotoplasty, and penile prosthesis implantation [81].

As with many surgical procedures, complications include significant postoperative pain. When considering pain management strategies for TGD patients after gender-affirming surgery, it is important to consider that biological, social, and psychological factors may play into pain experience [82]. Estrogen and testosterone have been shown to impact pain perception, with fluctuating and low levels of estrogen and testosterone contributing to increased pain perception [37]. This is especially important to consider postoperatively with patients on GAHT, especially if there is any disruption to therapy. Given the known increased prevalence of substance use disorder among TGD patients, consideration should be given to the duration of opioids when prescribed postoperatively [83]. One study showed increased opioid consumption for gender-affirming mastectomy compared to oncologic mastectomy, but it was limited by a small sample size [84]. Overall, there is insufficient evidence evaluating the interplay of many factors on postoperative pain in TGD patients to inform specific recommendations for pain management in the setting of gender-affirming surgery [85].

The specific type and location of gender-affirming surgery will likely determine the optimal strategies for pain management. For example, facial surgeries are unlikely to be amenable to regional anesthesia and may require oral medications such as nonsteroidal anti-inflammatory drugs (NSAIDs), acetaminophen, and/or opioids if necessary [86]. Regional nerve blocks, such as an erector spinae plane or pectoralis nerve block, may be particularly useful in chest surgery [85, 87]. A transversus abdominus plane block or quadratus lumborum nerve block may be effective in patients undergoing genital surgery [85, 88]. Additional multimodal options for pain management include topical agents (e.g., lidocaine patches, analgesic ointments), neuropathic agents (gabapentin, pregabalin), muscle relaxants (methocarbamol, diazepam, tizanidine, cyclobenzaprine), and opioids [89]. While evidence has not been established, acupuncture could also provide some relief and target the complex interplay of factors affecting pain [85].

Endometriosis

Endometriosis can affect all patients with a uterus and ovaries; however, a recent systematic review found TGD patients suffer from endometriosis at a prevalence of 25% compared to 5–10% in cisgender patients [13]. Given the high rate of endometriosis in TGD patients, it is imperative that appropriate treatment be considered in this patient population. It is also important to consider that patients on testosterone therapy may still experience endometriosis [13].

Endometriosis is characterized by chronic and cyclic pelvic pain and is estrogen-dependent. Treatment is usually based on hormonal suppression and surgical incision and requires shared decision-making [13]. Progestins, selective estrogen receptor modulators, or combined oral contraceptives are options for treating endometriosis; however, patients on testosterone therapy might be hesitant to initiate these medications [90]. Consultation with a patient's endocrinology provider is imperative before initiating hormonal therapy. Beyond medication treatment, surgical intervention can be considered.

Conclusion

There is a complex interplay of biological, psychological, and social factors that impact the pain experience in TGD patients. The treatment of pain in this population necessitates a thoughtful evaluation of these factors, including potential altered pharmacokinetics/pharmacodynamics, considerations for medication interactions, and unique considerations for specific disease states that may be more common or present differently in TGD patients. Unfortunately, it is clear that disparities in pain management likely contribute to the health inequity seen among TGD populations, and there is a significant need for targeted research to identify optimal strategies for safe and effective pain management.

References

1. Scheim AI, Baker KE, Restar AJ, Sell RL. Health and health care among transgender adults in the United States. Annu Rev Public Health. 2022;43:503–23. https://doi.org/10.1146/annurev-publhealth-052620-100313.
2. Kokka I, Bacopoulou F, Chrousos GP, et al. Allostatic load and psychological characteristics of transgender individuals. Preliminary case-control findings. Psychoneuroendocrinology. 2025;173:107277. https://doi.org/10.1016/j.psyneuen.2024.107277.
3. Azagba S, de Silva GSR, Ebling T. Examining general, physical, and mental health disparities between transgender and cisgender adults in the U.S. Int J Equity Health. 2025;24(1):37. https://doi.org/10.1186/s12939-024-02364-4.
4. Rastogi A, Menard L, Miller GH, et al. Health and wellbeing: a report of the 2022 U.S. transgender survey.
5. Hoy-Ellis CP. Minority stress and mental health: a review of the literature. J Homosex. 2023;70(5):806–30. https://doi.org/10.1080/00918369.2021.2004794.
6. Valentine SE, Shipherd JC. A systematic review of social stress and mental health among transgender and gender non-conforming people in the United States. Clin Psychol Rev. 2018;66:24–38. https://doi.org/10.1016/j.cpr.2018.03.003.
7. Transgender and Gender-Diverse Minority Stress and Substance Use Frequency and Problems: Systematic Review and Meta-Analysis | Transgender Health. Accessed June 22, 2025. https://www.liebertpub.com/doi/10.1089/trgh.2023.0025
8. Poteat TC, Divsalar S, Streed CG, Feldman JL, Bockting WO, Meyer IH. Cardiovascular disease in a population-based sample of transgender and cisgender adults. Am J Prev Med. 2021;61(6):804–11. https://doi.org/10.1016/j.amepre.2021.05.019.
9. Leone AG, Trapani D, Schabath MB, et al. Cancer in transgender and gender-diverse persons: a review. JAMA Oncol. 2023;9(4):556–63. https://doi.org/10.1001/jamaoncol.2022.7173.
10. Current status of breast cancer screening in transgender and gender-diverse populations | European Radiology. Accessed June 22, 2025. https://link.springer.com/article/10.1007/s00330-025-11355-0
11. Bishop A, Overcash F, McGuire J, Reicks M. Diet and physical activity behaviors among adolescent transgender students: school survey results. J Adolesc Health. 2020;66(4):484–90. https://doi.org/10.1016/j.jadohealth.2019.10.026.
12. Zajacova A, Grol-Prokopczyk H, Liu H, Reczek R, Nahin RL. Chronic pain among U.S. sexual minority adults who identify as gay, lesbian, bisexual, or "something else". Pain. 2023;164(9):1942. https://doi.org/10.1097/j.pain.0000000000002891.
13. Giacomozzi M, Bouwens J, Aubin SG, Pastoor H, Verdonk P, Nap A. Transgender and gender diverse individuals embodying endometriosis: a systematic review. Front Med. 2024;11:1430154. https://doi.org/10.3389/fmed.2024.1430154.
14. Levit D, Yaish I, Shtrozberg S, Aloush V, Greenman Y, Ablin JN. Pain and transition: evaluating fibromyalgia in transgender individuals. Clin Exp Rheumatol. 2021;39 Suppl 130(3):27–32. https://doi.org/10.55563/clinexprheumatol/pq0qp6.
15. Trovão, Diniz E, Rocha Leite JB, Ribeiro Coutinho Madruga C, Maia Arca V, Macedo Cavalcanti Albuquerque JA, Sampaio Rocha-Filho PA. Headache in transgender men using gender-affirming hormone therapy: a case-control study. Headache. 2025; https://doi.org/10.1111/head.14944.
16. Stein T, Collins S, St LJ. The prevalence of hypermobile Ehlers-Danlos syndrome at a gender-affirming primary care clinic. SAGE Open Med. 2025;13:20503121251315021. https://doi.org/10.1177/20503121251315021.
17. Zwickl S, Burchill L, Wong AFQ, et al. Pelvic pain in transgender people using testosterone therapy: a national survey. Published online May 30, 2022. https://doi.org/10.22541/au.165388691.10496458/v1.
18. Weiss KE, Li R, Chen D, Palermo TM, Scheurich JA, Groenewald CB. Sexual orientation/gender identity discrimination and chronic pain in children: a National Study. Am J Prev Med. 2024;67(2):175–83. https://doi.org/10.1016/j.amepre.2024.03.010.
19. Stocking SQ, Webb CK, Miller GH, Thomeer MB, Goodin BR, Sorge RE. Understanding Risk of Chronic Pain Development and Related Mental Health Disparities Among Transgender People: A Review of Current Literature and Future Directions. J Pain. 2024:104681. https://doi.org/10.1016/j.jpain.2024.104681.
20. Fiselier A, Narendran G, Raiche J, et al. From discrimination and dis-ease to aging and disease-an epigenetic connection. Lancet Reg Health Am. 2022;12:100282. https://doi.org/10.1016/j.lana.2022.100282.
21. Boley S, Sidebottom A, Stenzel A, Watson D. Racial disparities in opioid administration practices among undifferentiated abdominal pain patients in the emergency department. J Racial Ethn Health Disparities. 2024;11(1):416–24. https://doi.org/10.1007/s40615-023-01529-1.
22. Perez LG, Schell TL, Richmond TS, et al. Racial and ethnic disparities in chronic pain following traumatic injury. Pain Med Off J Am Acad Pain Med. 2022;24(6):716–9. https://doi.org/10.1093/pm/pnac177.
23. Platts-Mills TF, Esserman DA, Brown DL, Bortsov AV, Sloane PD, McLean SA. Older US emergency department patients are less likely to receive pain medication than younger patients: results from a national survey. Ann Emerg Med. 2012;60(2):199–206. https://doi.org/10.1016/j.annemergmed.2011.09.014.
24. Leresche L. Defining gender disparities in pain management. Clin Orthop. 2011;469(7):1871–7. https://doi.org/10.1007/s11999-010-1759-9.
25. Scheurich JA, Sim LA, Gonzalez CA, et al. Gender diversity among youth attending an intensive interdisciplinary pain treatment program. J Clin Psychol Med Settings. 2024;31(3):560–70. https://doi.org/10.1007/s10880-023-09997-7.
26. Engstrom K, Bellolio F, Jeffery MM, et al. Validation of a methodology to investigate care inequities for transgender patients. West J Emerg Med Integrating Emerg Care Popul Health. 2025;26(3) https://doi.org/10.5811/westjem.21279.
27. Nejad S, Alpay M. Massachussetts general hospital handbook of. Gen Hosp Psychiatry. 2010;17
28. Trans broken arm syndrome. In: Wiktionary, the free dictionary; 2025. Accessed July 8, 2025. https://en.wiktionary.org/w/index.php?title=trans_broken_arm_syndrome&oldid=85398060
29. Breivik H, Borchgrevink PC, Allen SM, et al. Assessment of pain. Br J Anaesth. 2008;101(1):17–24. https://doi.org/10.1093/bja/aen103.
30. Morris M, Cooper RL, Ramesh A, et al. Training to reduce LGBTQ-related bias among medical, nursing, and dental students and providers: a systematic review. BMC Med Educ. 2019;19(1):325. https://doi.org/10.1186/s12909-019-1727-3.

31. Jaiswal J, Halkitis PN. Towards a more inclusive and dynamic understanding of medical mistrust informed by science. Behav Med. 2019;45(2):79–85. https://doi.org/10.1080/08964289.2019.1619511.
32. Goetsch MF, Ribbink PJA. Penetrative genital pain in transgender men using testosterone: a survey study. Am J Obstet Gynecol. 2022;226(2):264–70. https://doi.org/10.1016/j.ajog.2021.09.019.
33. Craig KD, Holmes C, Hudspith M, et al. Pain in persons who are marginalized by social conditions. Pain. 2020;161(2):261–5. https://doi.org/10.1097/j.pain.0000000000001719.
34. Motmans J, Meier P, Ponnet K, T'Sjoen G. Female and male transgender quality of life: socioeconomic and medical differences. J Sex Med. 2012;9(3):743–50. https://doi.org/10.1111/j.1743-6109.2011.02569.x.
35. Aloisi AM, Bachiocco V, Costantino A, et al. Cross-sex hormone administration changes pain in transsexual women and men. Pain. 2007;132(Suppl 1):S60–7. https://doi.org/10.1016/j.pain.2007.02.006.
36. Anger JT, Case LK, Baranowski AP, et al. Pain mechanisms in the transgender individual: a review. Front Pain Res. 2024;5:1241015. https://doi.org/10.3389/fpain.2024.1241015.
37. Athnaiel O, Cantillo S, Paredes S, Knezevic NN. The role of sex hormones in pain-related conditions. Int J Mol Sci. 2023;24(3):1866. https://doi.org/10.3390/ijms24031866.
38. Migraine prevalence in male to female transsexuals on hormone therapy - PubMed. Accessed July 8, 2025. https://pubmed.ncbi.nlm.nih.gov/15304612/
39. White Hughto JM, Reisner SL, Pachankis JE. Transgender stigma and health: a critical review of stigma determinants, mechanisms, and interventions. Soc Sci Med. 1982;2015(147):222–31. https://doi.org/10.1016/j.socscimed.2015.11.010.
40. Safer JD, Coleman E, Feldman J, et al. Barriers to healthcare for transgender individuals. Curr Opin Endocrinol Diabetes Obes. 2016;23(2):168–71. https://doi.org/10.1097/MED.0000000000000227.
41. Achterberg WP, Pieper MJC, van Dalen-Kok AH, et al. Pain management in patients with dementia. Clin Interv Aging. 2013;8:1471–82. https://doi.org/10.2147/CIA.S36739.
42. Raja SN, Carr DB, Cohen M, et al. The revised International Association for the Study of Pain definition of pain: concepts, challenges, and compromises. Pain. 2020;161(9):1976–82. https://doi.org/10.1097/j.pain.0000000000001939.
43. Geziry AE. Non-pharmacological pain management. In: Pain management in special circumstances. https://doi.org/10.5772/INTECHOPEN.79689.
44. Tidmarsh LV, Harrison R, Ravindran D, Matthews SL, Finlay KA. The influence of adverse childhood experiences in pain management: mechanisms, processes, and trauma-informed care. Front Pain Res. 2022;3:923866. https://doi.org/10.3389/fpain.2022.923866.
45. Puckett JA, Cleary P, Rossman K, Newcomb ME, Mustanski B. Barriers to gender-affirming care for transgender and gender nonconforming individuals. Sex Res Soc Policy. 2018;15(1):48–59. https://doi.org/10.1007/s13178-017-0295-8.
46. Institute of Medicine (US) Committee on Advancing Pain Research, Care, and Education. Relieving pain in America: a blueprint for transforming prevention, care, education, and research. National Academies Press (US); 2011. Accessed July 8, 2025. http://www.ncbi.nlm.nih.gov/books/NBK91497/
47. Cirrincione LR, Huang KJ. Sex and gender differences in clinical pharmacology: implications for transgender medicine. Clin Pharmacol Ther. 2021;110(4):897–908. https://doi.org/10.1002/cpt.2234.
48. Klaver M, Dekker MJHJ, de Mutsert R, Twisk JWR, den Heijer M. Cross-sex hormone therapy in transgender persons affects total body weight, body fat and lean body mass: a meta-analysis. Andrologia. 2017;49(5):e12660. https://doi.org/10.1111/and.12660.
49. Tsuchiya Y, Nakajima M, Yokoi T. Cytochrome P450-mediated metabolism of estrogens and its regulation in human. Cancer Lett. 2005;227(2):115–24. https://doi.org/10.1016/j.canlet.2004.10.007.
50. Usmani KA, Tang J. Human cytochrome P450: metabolism of testosterone by CYP3A4 and inhibition by ketoconazole. Curr Protoc Toxicol. 2004.;Chapter 4:Unit4.13; https://doi.org/10.1002/0471140856.tx0413s20.
51. Bauters T, Dadkhah A. Table 31.1, [CYP3A4 substrates, inhibitors, and inducers...]. April 11, 2024. Accessed June 23, 2025. https://www.ncbi.nlm.nih.gov/books/NBK608254/table/ch31.Tab1/
52. Maheshwari A, Dines V, Saul D, Nippoldt T, Kattah A, Davidge-Pitts C. The effect of gender-affirming hormone therapy on serum creatinine in transgender individuals. Endocr Pract. 2022;28(1):52–7. https://doi.org/10.1016/j.eprac.2021.08.009.
53. St. Peter WL, Bzowyckyj AS, Anderson-Haag T, et al. Moving forward from Cockcroft-Gault creatinine clearance to race-free estimated glomerular filtration rate to improve medication-related decision-making in adults across healthcare settings: A consensus of the National Kidney Foundation Workgroup for Implementation of Race-Free eGFR-Based Medication-Related Decisions Accessed June 17, 2025. https://doi.org/10.1093/ajhp/zxae317
54. Vetvik KG, MacGregor EA. Sex differences in the epidemiology, clinical features, and pathophysiology of migraine. Lancet Neurol. 2017;16(1):76–87. https://doi.org/10.1016/S1474-4422(16)30293-9.
55. Siracusa R, Paola RD, Cuzzocrea S, Impellizzeri D. Fibromyalgia: pathogenesis, mechanisms, diagnosis and treatment options update. Int J Mol Sci. 2021;22(8):3891. https://doi.org/10.3390/ijms22083891.
56. Pieretti S, Di Giannuario A, Di Giovannandrea R, et al. Gender differences in pain and its relief. Ann Ist Super Sanita. 2016;52(2):184–9. https://doi.org/10.4415/ANN_16_02_09.
57. Hranilovich JA, Millington K. Headache prevalence in transgender and gender diverse youth: a single-center case-control study. Headache. 2023;63(4):517–22. https://doi.org/10.1111/head.14493.
58. Pace A, Barber M, Ziplow J, Hranilovich JA, Kaiser EA. Gender minority stress, psychiatric comorbidities, and the experience of migraine in transgender and gender-diverse individuals: a narrative review. Curr Pain Headache Rep. 2021;25(12):82. https://doi.org/10.1007/s11916-021-00996-7.
59. Simon GE, Moise N, Mohr DC. Management of depression in adults: a review. JAMA. 2024;332(2):141. https://doi.org/10.1001/jama.2024.5756.
60. Ailani J, Burch RC, Robbins MS, Board of Directors of the American Headache Society. he American headache society consensus statement: update on integrating new migraine treatments into clinical practice. Headache. 2021;61(7):1021–39. https://doi.org/10.1111/head.14153.
61. Robbins MS. Diagnosis and management of headache: a review. JAMA. 2021;325(18):1874. https://doi.org/10.1001/jama.2021.1640.
62. Jones GT, Atzeni F, Beasley M, Flüß E, Sarzi-Puttini P, Macfarlane GJ. The prevalence of fibromyalgia in the general population: a comparison of the American College of Rheumatology 1990, 2010, and modified 2010 classification criteria. Arthritis Rheumatol. 2015;67(2):568–75. https://doi.org/10.1002/art.38905.
63. Rosendale N, Wong JO, Flatt JD, Whitaker E. Sexual and gender minority health in neurology: a scoping review. JAMA Neurol. 2021;78(6):747–54. https://doi.org/10.1001/jamaneurol.2020.5536.
64. Godbout-Parent M, Julien N, Nguena Nguefack HL, et al. Changing society, changing research: integrating gender to better understand physical and psychological treatments use in chronic pain man-

agement. Pain. 2024;165(3):674–84. https://doi.org/10.1097/j.pain.0000000000003072.
65. Winslow BT, Vandal C, Dang L. Fibromyalgia: diagnosis and management. Am Fam Physician. 2023;107(2):137–44.
66. Peery AF, Crockett SD, Murphy CC, et al. Burden and cost of gastrointestinal, liver, and pancreatic diseases in the United States: update 2018. Gastroenterology. 2019;156(1):254–272.e11. https://doi.org/10.1053/j.gastro.2018.08.063.
67. Broder JS, Oliveira J, e Silva L, Bellolio F, et al. Guidelines for Reasonable and Appropriate Care in the Emergency Department 2 (GRACE-2): low-risk, recurrent abdominal pain in the emergency department. Acad Emerg Med. 2022;29(5):526–60. https://doi.org/10.1111/acem.14495.
68. Lakhoo K, Almario CV, Khalil C, Spiegel BMR. Prevalence and characteristics of abdominal pain in the United States. Clin Gastroenterol Hepatol. 2021;19(9):1864–1872.e5. https://doi.org/10.1016/j.cgh.2020.06.065.
69. Vélez C, Newman KL, Paul S, Berli JU, Tangpricha V, Targownik LE. Approaching digestive health care in transgender and gender-diverse communities. Gastroenterology. 2024;166(3):369–375.e2. https://doi.org/10.1053/j.gastro.2024.01.011.
70. Transgender and Gender Diverse Persons. July 21, 2022. Accessed June 23, 2025. https://www.cdc.gov/std/treatment-guidelines/trans.htm
71. Sterling J, Garcia MM. Cancer screening in the transgender population: a review of current guidelines, best practices, and a proposed care model. Transl Androl Urol. 2020;9(6):2771–85. https://doi.org/10.21037/tau-20-954.
72. Newman KL, Chedid VG, Boden EK. A systematic review of inflammatory bowel disease epidemiology and health outcomes in sexual and gender minority individuals. Gastroenterology. 2023;164(6):866–71. https://doi.org/10.1053/j.gastro.2022.11.048.
73. Zwickl S, Burchill L, Wong AFQ, et al. Pelvic pain in transgender people using testosterone therapy. LGBT Health. 2023;10(3):179–90. https://doi.org/10.1089/lgbt.2022.0187.
74. Drossman DA. Functional abdominal pain syndrome. Clin Gastroenterol Hepatol. 2004;2(5):353–65. https://doi.org/10.1016/S1542-3565(04)00118-1.
75. Diemer EW, Grant JD, Munn-Chernoff MA, Patterson DA, Duncan AE. Gender identity, sexual orientation, and eating-related pathology in a national sample of college students. J Adolesc Health. 2015;57(2):144–9. https://doi.org/10.1016/j.jadohealth.2015.03.003.
76. Grasso C, Goldhammer H, Thompson J, Keuroghlian AS. Optimizing gender-affirming medical care through anatomical inventories, clinical decision support, and population health management in electronic health record systems. J Am Med Inform Assoc. 2021;28(11):2531–5. https://doi.org/10.1093/jamia/ocab080.
77. Coleman E, Radix AE, Bouman WP, et al. Standards of care for the health of transgender and gender diverse people, version 8. Int J Transgender Health. 2022;23(Suppl 1):S1–S259. https://doi.org/10.1080/26895269.2022.2100644.
78. Engstrom K, Bellolio F, Jeffery MM, et al. Disparities in pain management among transgender patients presenting to the emergency department for abdominal pain. Acad Emerg Med. 2025;32(2):130–6. https://doi.org/10.1111/acem.15027.
79. Kamp K, Yang PL, Tsai CS, et al. Gender and sex differences in abdominal pain, fatigue, and psychological symptoms among adults with inflammatory bowel disease: a network analysis. Inflamm Bowel Dis. 2025;31(2):442–9. https://doi.org/10.1093/ibd/izae279.
80. Gender-affirming surgery: Feminizing procedures - UpToDate. Accessed June 23, 2025. https://www.uptodate.com/contents/gender-affirming-surgery-feminizing-procedures
81. Gender-affirming surgery: Masculinizing procedures - UpToDate. Accessed June 23, 2025. https://www.uptodate.com/contents/gender-affirming-surgery-masculinizing-procedures?search=masculinizing%20surgery&source=search_result&selectedTitle=1~150&usage_type=default&display_rank=1
82. Strand N, Gomez DA, Kacel EL, et al. Concepts and approaches in the management of transgender and gender-diverse patients. Mayo Clin Proc. 2024;99(7):1114–26. https://doi.org/10.1016/j.mayocp.2023.12.027.
83. Kecojevic A, Wong CF, Schrager SM, et al. Initiation into prescription drug misuse: differences between lesbian, gay, bisexual, transgender (LGBT) and heterosexual high-risk young adults in Los Angeles and New York. Addict Behav. 2012;37(11):1289–93. https://doi.org/10.1016/j.addbeh.2012.06.006.
84. Robinson KA, Duncan S, Austrie J, et al. Opioid consumption after gender-affirming mastectomy and two other breast surgeries. J Surg Res. 2020;251:33–7. https://doi.org/10.1016/j.jss.2019.12.043.
85. Patel A, Palayeker V, Shekane P. Optimal perioperative pain management of the transgender patient for gender affirming surgery: a scoping review. Curr Pain Headache Rep. 2024;28(7):663–71. https://doi.org/10.1007/s11916-024-01219-5.
86. Sanchez KJ, Sanchez RA, Ben Khallouq B, Ellis DB. Perioperative care of transgender and gender-diverse patients: a biopsychosocial approach. Anesth Analg. 2023;137(1):234. https://doi.org/10.1213/ANE.0000000000006480.
87. Aquino NJ, Boskey ER, Staffa SJ, et al. A single center case series of gender-affirming surgeries and the evolution of a specialty anesthesia team. J Clin Med. 2022;11(7):1943. https://doi.org/10.3390/jcm11071943.
88. Bosinci EŠ, Stević MM, Simić DM, Kupeli I, Spasic SM, Simić IR. A combination of bilateral pectoral nerve block and bilateral erector spinae plane block for one-stage female-to-male gender affirmation surgery: a report of two cases. J Clin Anesth. 2021;72:110298. https://doi.org/10.1016/j.jclinane.2021.110298.
89. Joshi GP, Kehlet H. Postoperative pain management in the era of ERAS: an overview. Best Pract Res Clin Anaesthesiol. 2019;33(3):259–67. https://doi.org/10.1016/j.bpa.2019.07.016.
90. Kaltsas A, Stavropoulos M, Symeonidis EN, et al. Endometriosis in transgender men: bridging gaps in research and care—a narrative review. Biomedicine. 2024;12(7):1481. https://doi.org/10.3390/biomedicines12071481.
91. Intersex: What Is Intersex, Intersex Surgery. Cleveland Clinic. Accessed July 1, 2025. https://my.clevelandclinic.org/health/articles/16324-intersex
92. Wolf-Gould C, Denny D, Green J, Lynch K. A history of transgender medicine in the United States: from margins to mainstream. SUNY Press; 2025.
93. Ze/Hir and Ze/Zir Pronouns. Pronouns.org Resources on Personal Pronouns. Accessed July 6, 2025. https://pronouns.org/ze-hir

Ethics and Analgesia

24

Thomas J. Papadimos

Introduction

Pain is a primary reason that patients visit the hospital [1, 2], and pain has been defined as "an unpleasant sensory and emotional experience associated with actual or potential tissue damage" [3]. From 2006 to 2014, hospital visits increased 18.4% in the USA, from 89.6 million to 106.0 million, and continue to increase [4]. Up to 70% of these visits are due to pain [5]. Untreated/undertreated pain is termed oligo--analgesia (the Greek word for inadequate treatment of pain) and may lead to poor overall health, as well as the possibility of chronicity [6–9]. Pain undertreatment is an international problem.

Ethics examines right and wrong actions [10]. In many instances, difficult choices need to be made [11]. Historically, healthcare providers (HPs) have limited pain medications in order to make a diagnosis, fearing that alleviation of pain would hinder diagnostic efforts. Therefore, ethical frameworks for pain treatment have become important [12, 13], especially in view of the ongoing opioid crisis [14, 15]. It is the ethical duty of physicians, pharmacists, and other HPs to treat pain.

Bioethics

The problem of inappropriate pain treatment goes back to the 1973 landmark paper by Marks and Sachar [16]. Six years later, Beauchamp and Childress published their work on biomedical ethics [17]. This was followed by the reintroduction of the term "oligo-analgesia" to medicine [18]; Notably, over 50% of the patients studied received no pain medication despite having acute medical conditions. Despite this evidence of the need for appropriate pain relief for patients, the first part of the twenty-first century continued to find reports of inadequate efforts to treat pain [19–21]. The concept of pain treatment as a human right has been previously highlighted [22–26]. It had become evident by 2013 that the inability to manage pain adequately was an important ethical issue [12]. This was again reiterated in the American Journal of Public Health in 2019 [27].

Concern for ethically adequate treatment of pain can be traced back to three sources: [1] The World Medical Association's Declaration of Helsinki-Ethical Principles for Medical Research Involving Human Subjects [28]; The Belmont Report: Ethical Principles and Guidelines for the Protection of Human Subjects of Research [29]; and in *Principles of Biomedical Ethics* by Beauchamp and Childress, where the authors argue for autonomy, beneficence, nonmaleficence, and justice [17].

While the Declaration of Helsinki is aimed at the ethical principles of medical research in humans, it has areas applicable also to those who seek pain treatment, i.e., patients not involved in research [28]. The preamble states that physicians are bound by two statements: "The health of my patient will be my first consideration" and "A physician shall act in the patient's best interest when providing medical care [28]." It goes on further to address the need for protection of vulnerable groups and the need for informed consent. The Belmont Report was released by the Office of the Secretary of the Department of Health, Education, and Welfare [29]. This report summarized basic ethical principles that the Commission found important and had three basic ethical principles. The first was *respect for persons*. The second basic ethical principle was *beneficence*. The third basic ethical principle espoused is that of *justice*. Thomas Beauchamp and James Childress are two internationally recognized medical philosophers whose book, *Principles of Biomedical Ethics*, has become mandatory

T. J. Papadimos (✉)
Departments of Surgery and Anesthesiology, University of Toledo College of Medicine and Life Sciences, Toledo, OH, USA
e-mail: Thomas.Papadimos@UToledo.edu

J. P. Reinert et al. (eds.), *Adjunctive Analgesic Strategies for the Bedside Clinician and Beyond*,
https://doi.org/10.1007/978-3-032-21675-5_24

reading in academic circles. Beauchamp and Childress present four principles: respect for autonomy, nonmaleficence, beneficence, and justice. Their work was directed toward the individual's healthcare setting, not research. Their work was akin to The Belmont Report; however, they added nonmaleficence [30]. Nonmaleficence can be viewed as "first do no harm [31]." Even though medications can do harm, there is an emphasis on unjustifiable/unnecessary acts that create risk. In regard to beneficence, they indicate that such a person will try to make more than the minimum effort to be charitable. Regarding justice, they emphasize its meaning to be more than a fair distribution of resources in an equitable fashion, understanding scarcity and prioritization of the "what or who."

Many HPs are familiar with the aforementioned sources of bioethical principles because the Belmont Report and other biomedical works are required reading if anyone endeavors to be part of any research project; this usually occurs through the Collaborative Institutional Training Initiative (CITI) program in the USA [32].

Management of Pain Undertreatment

Many reasons exist for the undertreatment of pain. Some surgeons have traditionally withheld pain medication to make a diagnosis, but Fosnocht et al., Zohar et al., and Wolfe et al. make a point that relief of pain should take precedence over a diagnosis [33–35]. We must also acknowledge that there is a socioeconomic status and race difference between many patients and the treating physician, and this can cause a problem with the assessment and treatment of pain [36–38]. A third perspective involves the physician's suspicion concerning drug-seeking behavior and its motivation [13]. Lack of training in medical school and a dearth of evidence-based continuing medical education courses may also allow the continued of oligo-analgesia [39]. Carter et al. argue that physicians may be showing an "epistemic preference for signs over pain" [39]. In other words, HPs are assigning a ranking, or rating, based on what they observe in the patient's behavior vis-à-vis the pain that is not based on their analysis and judgment of the patient's pain or the patient's self-report. This argument is supported by Bijur et al. and Marquie et al., who report that physicians are giving more weight to observable features as opposed to what the patient is reporting [40, 41]. The second argument of Carter et al. is the manner in which a physician approaches a patient in the ED. This second argument has four parts: [1] pain and anxiety contribute to an altered perpetuation of pain, [2] a physician who dismisses someone's report of pain causes distrust, thereby increasing fear/anxiety, [3] HPs may not provide enough information to calm or decrease the anxiety a patient has, and [4] the patient is objectified in a Foucauldian manner. Foucault coined the term "the medical gaze," in which a practitioner considers a patient only as a complex cluster of mechanisms and parts, and the patient can perceive this [42]. It is not only physicians who can be barriers to effective pain management, but an examination of nursing and its relationship to the oligo-analgesia must be studied and addressed.

Nursing input could be better handled by putting protocols in place, providing more training in pain management, and appointing a "pain champion" [43]. A significant conflict for nurses is caring for patients with serious pain while at the same time having a second patient with a life-threatening problem [43]. Additionally, some nurses do not believe in using pain as a fifth vital sign or in even taking an acceptable pain history [19, 43–46]. In addition to more and better pain training, protocols, champions, and scheduling appropriate workload and assignments, allowing more nursing autonomy in pain medication administration can be helpful. Hatherley et al. made five recommendations to improve acute pain management: mandate pain score documentation, pain should be assessed and reassessed, provide analgesia within 30 minutes, use time to analgesia as an ED-performance indicator, and implement nurse-led analgesia protocols [47]. Of special note, triage led by nursing teams in 50 French emergency departments demonstrated improved pain response to patients nationwide [48]. Nurse-led teams are well supported by the pain literature [43, 44, 49, 50]. Nurse-led teams can be vital because pain management can be influenced by a nurse's relationship with the treating HP [51]. In this study, the physicians were a problem for the nurses. The nurses reported that the physicians they knew well and with whom they had a long-term working relationship responded well, but they felt as if they had to exert pressure to get the medication the patient needed from HPs they did not know well. Many nurses in this study bypassed the HP by changing the dose on their own. Nurse-led analgesia teams may mitigate this problem. Another problem is that nurses outside of the English-speaking world, as indicated by a study from Poland, must read the medical literature in English [52]. Not being able to communicate with a patient in their native language can also be a hindrance to good pain control [53–56].

Delaying pain treatment more than 30 min should be justified, medically and morally. The barriers discussed show a lack of respect for patient autonomy because the patient who is seeking care is vulnerable and surrounded by many HPs who react paternalistically. Not treating pain is harmful. In so doing, the HP or nurse does not embrace nonmaleficence because any harm (oligo-analgesia) is unjustifiable.

Healthcare Disparities

Healthcare disparities in the USA are quite evident. Black patients have been subjected to poor interactions with physicians, and they are also prescribed opioids less often than White patients with the same diagnosis; in anesthesiology, they receive fewer regional anesthetics for joint surgery, as do all the underinsured [57, 58]. In Europe, things are no better [59, 60]. The Institute of Medicine (IOM), a nonprofit, independent institute of the National Academy of Sciences, was directed by the US Congress to report any racial or ethnic disparities related to healthcare. The IOM reported that, indeed, racial and ethnic barriers to care were demonstrable [61]. Cone et al. highlighted the need for workforce diversity and cultural competence in the healthcare workforce to improve the delivery of care and highlighted pain management [38]. As far back as 1993, Todd et al. reported that Hispanics were twice as likely to receive no pain medications in the ED when compared to Whites. After controlling for gender, language, insurance, type of injury, and healthcare provider profile, ethnicity remained the strongest factor. Shah et al. analyzed 6710 ED visits of nontraumatic acute abdomens over 5 years using the Centers for Disease Control--National Hospital Ambulatory Care Survey (CDC-NHAMCS) database regarding analgesic access of non-Hispanic Whites vs. non-Hispanic Blacks and reported the presence of racial/ethnic disparities nationally [62]. Additionally, a meta-analysis study in 2019 by Lee et al. demonstrated analgesic prescribing disparities according to race [36]. Many times, these disparities also extended to the treatment of chronic pain patients [63] and those with intellectual disabilities [64]. These racial and ethnic disparities also affect the treatment of pain in children (see section below on children) [65].

Health disparities are also gender related. Gender biases regarding pain can obstruct effective care [66]. There is evidence that HPs are more likely to send women with pain for psychological treatment than men [67, 68] and prescribe opioids more frequently for men [69–72]. A report by Safdar et al. was of interest because they studied 842 patients, of which 56% were women, to study age, race, and ethnicity [73]. Their results showed that male physicians prescribed opioids to male patients more often than females, and female physicians prescribed opioids more often to females than males (although females presenting with severe pain were more likely to be treated with an adequate opioid dose overall).

The elderly are also at high risk for oligo-analgesia [74]. They are less likely to be able to express themselves and represent a large portion of the population [75]. A major problem that they present to HPs is their inability to communicate well [74, 76]. As much as a quarter of elderly patients have an impairment in their ability to express themselves, especially with pain [77–79]. Allione et al. report that the patient's status, the physician attending the patient, and the etiology of the pain play major roles [74]. Although elderly patients with trauma were likely to receive opioids, Quattromani et al. found that while 70% of those >65 years old with blunt trauma received pain medications, those 18–64 years old received pain medication 84% of the time [80]. Also, it took longer for the older patient group to receive their medications. Again, cognitive problems, an inability to report pain, or a lack of documentation or rating of pain by HPs continue to be a problem with older patients. It is noteworthy that half of emergency department physicians are uncomfortable with treating the pain of the elderly, and this discomfort seems not to have changed in nearly 30 years [81, 82]. In the elderly, documenting pain scores is very important, and while the elderly do have a sensitivity to opioids, effective treatment of pain can be provided through cautious prescribing [83].

There is a dearth of scholarly work regarding the lesbian, gay, bisexual, transgender, and queer (LGBTQ) community and pain treatment, but it does not take much to understand that this community suffers healthcare disparities. It is an underserved, poorly recognized, and poorly understood group [84]. Patients with disabilities may have trouble presenting themselves to the ED. Disabled citizens may have cognitive disorders, mobility limits, blindness, or intellectual difficulties [85]. About 20% of children and 26% of adults in the USA are disabled [86]. The disabled often have less education, lower incomes, less housing and food security, less computer or Internet access, and have a more difficult time becoming employed [87].

There is an exhaustive array of scholarly works that encompass race, ethnicity, age, disabilities, gender, and the LGBTQ community in all aspects of bioethics. Through the above-mentioned discourse on health disparities, it can be appreciated that the threads of autonomy/respect for persons, beneficence, nonmaleficence, and justice are relevant and evident throughout this discussion and can easily be applied to an ED.

The Ethical Impact of the Opioid Epidemic and Pandemics

Baruch and Springs highlighted that patients who have pain are always suspected of opioid abuse in their quest for pain relief because, "to have pain is certainty, to hear about pain is doubt [88]." It is true that "Pain is a narrative challenge as well as a medical one, and narrative plays an instrumental role in how clinicians understand and respond to pain at the bedside [89]." This presents a problem. Are HPs listening as providers of relief, or are they looking for opioid seekers?

This was a problem during the COVID-19 pandemic because the number of opioid-seeking/addicted patients had globally increased. It is important to recognize that individuals with substance use disorders may also develop painful conditions that require appropriate analgesic management [15, 89–91]. Stratton et al. make it clear that patients and healthcare providers are in this dilemma because of large pharmaceutical companies and unscrupulous HPs [15, 92, 93]. There has been a moral failing [15]. Pharmacists have also found this entire crisis ethically challenging and confusing [15]. It is important to be careful in prescribing and filling medication prescriptions, but when prescriptive authority becomes strict and limiting, without considering the patient context, then adverse ethical events may occur [94]. The misfortunes of the opioid epidemic and the COVID-19 pandemic have contributed to the ongoing problem of oligo-analgesia. Many ethical challenges have arisen during COVID-19, and many can affect pain treatment in the ED. While the leading challenge has been the rationing of scarce resources (this can differ among hospitals, regions, and states), many other challenges have presented themselves during COVID-19 that have been enumerated by the Association of Bioethics Program Directors (ABPD) task force [95].

Children and Oligo-Analgesia

Children are a vulnerable population [96]. This vulnerability is threefold: [1] children do not have the cognitive skills to determine their needs, [2] even if they can recognize their healthcare needs, they cannot acquire what they need because of their dependency on adults, and [3] society and government give parents autonomy, though not unlimited, to care for their children as they see fit [96]. In the third aspect above, children are vulnerable to poor decisions, possible violence, and neglect, and are dependent on adults for food and shelter. Furthermore, generally, the most vulnerable come from the poorer corners of society and may have the poorest health. "For children, access is not enough; we have a moral responsibility to ensure that children receive needed healthcare services in ways that reflect their special vulnerabilities [96]."

As stated previously, oligo-analgesia occurs frequently in the emergency department and other outpatient settings, but this can be especially true for children [97–99]. Children, generally, do not have their pain treated appropriately [97, 100, 101]. Focusing on a child's diagnosis or source of pain and ignoring treatment of the pain occurs on a regular basis [97, 102]. Children can indicate their pain by 18 months of age, and by age 3, some children can express the intensity of their pain [97, 103, 104].

Bromberg et al. found that children with appendicitis were only treated for their pain about one-half of the time, and one in four were undertreated for their pain [105]. Additionally, Goyal et al. reported that Black children seen in the emergency department with appendicitis were less likely to receive analgesia than their White counterparts, and those Black children with severe pain were less likely to receive opioids [106]. Again, children may not be able to verbalize their pain and may not demonstrate the same physical signs as adults. Therefore, the use of pain scales can be important, but the scales used by pediatric providers should be standardized to ensure consistency [107]. Appropriate pain assessment in children should become mandatory [108]. In addition to abdominal pain and headaches, oligo-analgesia has also been a problem with the treatment of trauma in children [109–112]. Additionally, Sahyoun et al. have voiced a concern that in many institutions around the world, there is a shortage of appropriate medications, staff, and space in which to perform procedures when it comes to supporting the care of children [113].

Other matters of concern involve the role that language barriers play in timely and adequate pain control in pediatric practice, especially concerning the prompt administration of pain medications [53]. Furthermore, race and ethnicity are associated with longer pediatric waiting times to be seen by an HP [114]. These concerns are in addition to those of shortages of medications, staff, and space mentioned above.

One final important point to make in the ethical care of children is to *ensure that healthcare providers ask children if they have pain.* Bergeron et al. concluded that "children who requested analgesia had higher pain scores on the verbal numeric scale (VNS) and the visual analog scale (VAS) than those who did not request analgesia [115]." These authors suggest that all children who have pain should be asked whether they wish to receive analgesia.

Conclusion

The field of bioethics may not have a scientific basis for the treatment of pain, but it gives the practitioner a scope of practice from which to approach the treatment of pain. Suffering is a manifestation of the human condition. Ethical considerations provide a window to our compassion for the sufferer.

References

1. McLeod D, Nelson K. The role of the emergency department in the acute management of chronic or recurrent pain. Australas Emerg Nurs J. 2013;16(1):30–6.
2. Moceri JT, Drevdahl DJ. Nurses' knowledge and attitudes toward pain in the emergency department. J Emerg Nurs. 2014;40(1):6–12.
3. Pain terms: a list with definitions and notes on usage. Recommended by the IASP Subcommittee on taxonomy. Pain. 1979;6(3):249.

4. Lin MP, Baker O, Richardson LD, Schuur JD. Trends in emergency department visits and admission rates among US acute care hospitals. JAMA Intern Med. 2018;178(12):1708–10.
5. Cordell WH, Keene KK, Giles BK, Jones JB, Jones JH, Brizendine EJ. The high prevalence of pain in emergency medical care. Am J Emerg Med. 2002;20(3):165–9.
6. Sinatra R. Causes and consequences of inadequate management of acute pain. Pain Med. 2010;11(12):1859–71.
7. van der Leeuw G, Ayers E, Leveille SG, Blankenstein AH, van der Horst HE, Verghese J. The effect of pain on major cognitive impairment in older adults. J Pain. 2018;19(12):1435–44.
8. Lang AC, Igler EC, Defenderfer EK, Uihlein J, Brimeyer CT, Davies WH. Evaluating differential effects of specific pain dismissal interactions with physicians. Clin J Pain. 2018;34(7):664–9.
9. Vijayvargiya M, Panchal S, Asawale K, Desai A. Oligoanalgesia in the emergency setting – an Indian review. J Clin Orthop Trauma. 2021;18:38–43.
10. Fieser J. Ethics. Available from: https://iep.utm.edu/ethics/.
11. Allen K. What is an ethical dilemma? 2008. Available from: https://www.socialworker.com/feature-articles/ethics-articles/What_Is_an_Ethical_Dilemma%3F/.
12. Venkat A, Fromm C, Isaacs E, Ibarra J, Committee SE. An ethical framework for the management of pain in the emergency department. Acad Emerg Med. 2013;20(7):716–23.
13. Johnson SH. The social, professional, and legal framework for the problem of pain management in emergency medicine. J Law Med Ethics. 2005;33(4):741–60.
14. A time of crisis for the opioid epidemic in the USA. Lancet. 2021;398(10297):277.
15. Stratton TP, Palombi L, Blue H, Schneiderhan ME. Ethical dimensions of the prescription opioid abuse crisis. Am J Health Syst Pharm. 2018;75(15):1145–50.
16. Marks RM, Sachar EJ. Undertreatment of medical inpatients with narcotic analgesics. Ann Intern Med. 1973;78(2):173–81.
17. Beauchamp TL, Childress JF. Principles of biomedical ethics. 8th ed. New York: Oxford University Press; 2019. 496 p.
18. Wilson JE, Pendleton JM. Oligoanalgesia in the emergency department. Am J Emerg Med. 1989;7(6):620–3.
19. Rupp T, Delaney KA. Inadequate analgesia in emergency medicine. Ann Emerg Med. 2004;43(4):494–503.
20. Todd KH, Ducharme J, Choiniere M, Crandall CS, Fosnocht DE, Homel P, et al. Pain in the emergency department: results of the pain and emergency medicine initiative (PEMI) multicenter study. J Pain. 2007;8(6):460–6.
21. Karwowski-Soulie F, Lessenot-Tcherny S, Lamarche-Vadel A, Bineau S, Ginsburg C, Meyniard O, et al. Pain in an emergency department: an audit. Eur J Emerg Med. 2006;13(4):218–24.
22. Lohman D, Schleifer R, Amon JJ. Access to pain treatment as a human right. BMC Med. 2010;8:8.
23. Jansen RM. Inadequate treatment of pain: time for the South African courts to redress this human rights violation? Med Law. 2010;29(4):497–522.
24. Cousins MJ. Relief of acute pain: a basic human right? Med J Aust. 2000;172(1):3–4.
25. Cousins MJ, Brennan F, Carr DB. Pain relief: a universal human right. Pain. 2004;112(1–2):1–4.
26. Johnson SH. Relieving unnecessary, treatable pain for the sake of human dignity. J Law Med Ethics. 2001;29(1):11–2.
27. Brennan F, Lohman D, Gwyther L. Access to pain management as a human right. Am J Public Health. 2019;109(1):61–5.
28. Declaration of Helsinki. Recommendations guiding medical doctors in biomedical research involving human subjects. Ugeskr Laeger. 1976;138(7):399–400.
29. Protection of human subjects; Belmont Report: notice of report for public comment. Fed Regist. 1979;44(76):23191–23197.
30. Big Thinkers: Thomas Beauchamp and James Childress: The Ethics Centre; 2017. Available from: https://ethics.org.au/big-thinkers-thomas-beauchamp-james-childress/.
31. Sokol DK. "First do no harm" revisited. BMJ. 2013;347:f6426.
32. Initiative CIT. The trusted Standart in research, ethics, and compliance training Fort Lauderdale, FL: CITI Program; 2022. Available from: https://about.citiprogram.org/.
33. Fosnocht DE, Swanson ER, Barton ED. Changing attitudes about pain and pain control in emergency medicine. Emerg Med Clin North Am. 2005;23(2):297–306.
34. Zohar Z, Eitan A, Halperin P, Stolero J, Hadid S, Shemer J, et al. Pain relief in major trauma patients: an Israeli perspective. J Trauma. 2001;51(4):767–72.
35. Wolfe JM, Lein DY, Lenkoski K, Smithline HA. Analgesic administration to patients with an acute abdomen: a survey of emergency medicine physicians. Am J Emerg Med. 2000;18(3):250–3.
36. Lee P, Le Saux M, Siegel R, Goyal M, Chen C, Ma Y, et al. Racial and ethnic disparities in the management of acute pain in US emergency departments: meta-analysis and systematic review. Am J Emerg Med. 2019;37(9):1770–7.
37. Green CR, Anderson KO, Baker TA, Campbell LC, Decker S, Fillingim RB, et al. The unequal burden of pain: confronting racial and ethnic disparities in pain. Pain Med. 2003;4(3):277–94.
38. Cone DC, Richardson LD, Todd KH, Betancourt JR, Lowe RA. Health care disparities in emergency medicine. Acad Emerg Med. 2003;10(11):1176–83.
39. Carter D, Sendziuk P, Eliott JA, Braunack-Mayer A. Why is pain still under-treated in the emergency department? Two new hypotheses. Bioethics. 2016;30(3):195–202.
40. Marquie L, Sorum PC, Mullet E. Emergency physicians' pain judgments: cluster analyses on scenarios of acute abdominal pain. Qual Life Res. 2007;16(7):1267–73.
41. Bijur PE, Berard A, Esses D, Nestor J, Schechter C, Gallagher EJ. Lack of influence of patient self-report of pain intensity on administration of opioids for suspected long-bone fractures. J Pain. 2006;7(6):438–44.
42. Foucault M. The birth of the clinic: an archaeology of medical perception. London: Rutledge; 1989.
43. Pretorius A, Searle J, Marshall B. Barriers and enablers to emergency department nurses' management of patients' pain. Pain Manag Nurs. 2015;16(3):372–9.
44. Sardo S, Galletta M, Coni E, Aviles Gonzalez CI, Piras I, Pia G, et al. Nurses' behavior regarding pain treatment in an emergency department: a single-center observational study. J Pain Res. 2020;13:2355–9.
45. Corradi-Dell'Acqua C, Foerster M, Sharvit G, Trueb L, Foucault E, Fournier Y, et al. Pain management decisions in emergency hospitals are predicted by brain activity during empathy and error monitoring. Br J Anaesth. 2019;123(2):e284–e92.
46. van Zanden JE, Wagenaar S, Ter Maaten JM, Ter Maaten JC, Ligtenberg JJM. Pain score, desire for pain treatment and effect on pain satisfaction in the emergency department: a prospective, observational study. BMC Emerg Med. 2018;18(1):40.
47. Hatherley C, Jennings N, Cross R. Time to analgesia and pain score documentation best practice standards for the emergency department – a literature review. Australas Emerg Nurs J. 2016;19(1):26–36.
48. Gueant S, Taleb A, Borel-Kuhner J, Cauterman M, Raphael M, Nathan G, et al. Quality of pain management in the emergency department: results of a multicentre prospective study. Eur J Anaesthesiol. 2011;28(2):97–105.
49. Ridderikhof ML, Schyns FJ, Schep NW, Lirk P, Hollmann MW, Goslings JC. Emergency department pain management in adult patients with traumatic injuries before and after implementation

of a nurse-initiated pain treatment protocol utilizing fentanyl for severe pain. J Emerg Med. 2017;52(4):417–25.
50. Butti L, Bierti O, Lanfrit R, Bertolini R, Chittaro S, Delli Compagni S, et al. Evaluation of the effectiveness and efficiency of the triage emergency department nursing protocol for the management of pain. J Pain Res. 2017;10:2479–88.
51. Blondal K, Halldorsdottir S. The challenge of caring for patients in pain: from the nurse's perspective. J Clin Nurs. 2009;18(20):2897–906.
52. Medrzycka-Dabrowska W, Dabrowski S, Gutysz-Wojnicka A, Basinski A. Polish nurses' perceived barriers in using evidence-based practice in pain management. Int Nurs Rev. 2016;63(3):316–27.
53. Gaba M, Vazquez H, Homel P, Likourezos A, See F, Thompson J, et al. Language barriers and timely analgesia for long bone fractures in a pediatric emergency department. West J Emerg Med. 2021;22(2):225–31.
54. Showstack R. Patients don't have language barriers; the healthcare system does. Emerg Med J. 2019;36(10):580–1.
55. Carrasquillo O, Orav EJ, Brennan TA, Burstin HR. Impact of language barriers on patient satisfaction in an emergency department. J Gen Intern Med. 1999;14(2):82–7.
56. van Rosse F, de Bruijne M, Suurmond J, Essink-Bot ML, Wagner C. Language barriers and patient safety risks in hospital care. A mixed methods study. Int J Nurs Stud. 2016;54:45–53.
57. Mills AM, Shofer FS, Boulis AK, Holena DN, Abbuhl SB. Racial disparity in analgesic treatment for ED patients with abdominal or back pain. Am J Emerg Med. 2011;29(7):752–6.
58. Strand NH, Mariano ER, Goree JH, Narouze S, Doshi TL, Freeman JA, et al. Racism in pain medicine: we can and should do more. Mayo Clin Proc. 2021;96(6):1394–400.
59. Ahlberg BM, Hamed S, Thapar-Bjorkert S, Bradby H. Invisibility of racism in the global neoliberal era: implications for researching racism in healthcare. Front Sociol. 2019;4:61.
60. Cloos P, Bilsen J. Editorial commentary: public mental health and racism in Europe. Arch Public Health. 2021;79(1):200.
61. Smedley BDSA, Nelson A. Unequal treatment; confronting racial and ethnic disparities in health care. Washington, DC: National Academies Press; 2002.
62. Shah AA, Zogg CK, Zafar SN, Schneider EB, Cooper LA, Chapital AB, et al. Analgesic access for acute abdominal pain in the emergency department among racial/ethnic minority patients: a nationwide examination. Med Care. 2015;53(12):1000–9.
63. Morales ME, Yong RJ. Racial and ethnic disparities in the treatment of chronic pain. Pain Med. 2021;22(1):75–90.
64. Magana S, Parish S, Morales MA, Li H, Fujiura G. Racial and ethnic health disparities among people with intellectual and developmental disabilities. Intellect Dev Disabil. 2016;54(3):161–72.
65. Johnson TJ, Weaver MD, Borrero S, Davis EM, Myaskovsky L, Zuckerbraun NS, et al. Association of race and ethnicity with management of abdominal pain in the emergency department. Pediatrics. 2013;132(4):e851–8.
66. Zhang L, Losin EAR, Ashar YK, Koban L, Wager TD. Gender biases in estimation of others' pain. J Pain. 2021;22(9):1048–59.
67. Hamberg K, Risberg G, Johansson EE, Westman G. Gender bias in physicians' management of neck pain: a study of the answers in a Swedish national examination. J Womens Health Gend Based Med. 2002;11(7):653–66.
68. Hirsh AT, Hollingshead NA, Matthias MS, Bair MJ, Kroenke K. The influence of patient sex, provider sex, and sexist attitudes on pain treatment decisions. J Pain. 2014;15(5):551–9.
69. Denisco RA, Chandler RK, Compton WM. Addressing the intersecting problems of opioid misuse and chronic pain treatment. Exp Clin Psychopharmacol. 2008;16(5):417–28.
70. Michael GE, Sporer KA, Youngblood GM. Women are less likely than men to receive prehospital analgesia for isolated extremity injuries. Am J Emerg Med. 2007;25(8):901–6.
71. Schafer G, Prkachin KM, Kaseweter KA, Williams AC. Health care providers' judgments in chronic pain: the influence of gender and trustworthiness. Pain. 2016;157(8):1618–25.
72. Wandner LD, Heft MW, Lok BC, Hirsh AT, George SZ, Horgas AL, et al. The impact of patients' gender, race, and age on health care professionals' pain management decisions: an online survey using virtual human technology. Int J Nurs Stud. 2014;51(5):726–33.
73. Safdar B, Heins A, Homel P, Miner J, Neighbor M, DeSandre P, et al. Impact of physician and patient gender on pain management in the emergency department--a multicenter study. Pain Med. 2009;10(2):364–72.
74. Allione A, Pivetta E, Pizzolato E, Lorenzati B, Pomero F, Barutta L, et al. Determinants of inappropriate acute pain management in old people unable to communicate verbally in the emergency department. Turk J Emerg Med. 2017;17(4):160–4.
75. Mion LC, Palmer RM, Anetzberger GJ, Meldon SW. Establishing a case-finding and referral system for at-risk older individuals in the emergency department setting: the SIGNET model. J Am Geriatr Soc. 2001;49(10):1379–86.
76. Herr K, Coyne PJ, Key T, Manworren R, McCaffery M, Merkel S, et al. Pain assessment in the nonverbal patient: position statement with clinical practice recommendations. Pain Manag Nurs. 2006;7(2):44–52.
77. Hadjistavropoulos T, Herr K, Turk DC, Fine PG, Dworkin RH, Helme R, et al. An interdisciplinary expert consensus statement on assessment of pain in older persons. Clin J Pain. 2007;23(1 Suppl):S1–43.
78. Hustey FM, Meldon SW. The prevalence and documentation of impaired mental status in elderly emergency department patients. Ann Emerg Med. 2002;39(3):248–53.
79. Hustey FM, Meldon SW, Smith MD, Lex CK. The effect of mental status screening on the care of elderly emergency department patients. Ann Emerg Med. 2003;41(5):678–84.
80. Quattromani E, Normansell D, Storkan M, Gerdelman G, Krits S, Pennix C, et al. Oligoanalgesia in blunt geriatric trauma. J Emerg Med. 2015;48(6):653–9.
81. McNamara RM, Rousseau E, Sanders AB. Geriatric emergency medicine: a survey of practicing emergency physicians. Ann Emerg Med. 1992;21(7):796–801.
82. Mikelyte R, Abrahamson V, Hill E, Wilson PM. Factors influencing trends in opioid prescribing for older people: a scoping review. Prim Health Care Res Dev. 2020;21:e36.
83. Noble RE. Drug therapy in the elderly. Metabolism. 2003;52(10 Suppl 2):27–30.
84. Lim F, Paguirigan M, Cernivani D. Delivering LGBTQ-sensitive care. Nurs Crit Care. 2018;13(4):14–9.
85. Sabatello M, Burke TB, McDonald KE, Appelbaum PS. Disability, ethics, and health care in the COVID-19 pandemic. Am J Public Health. 2020;110(10):1523–7.
86. Disability impacts all of us. Atlanta: Centers for Disease Control; 2020. Available from: https://www.cdc.gov/ncbddd/disabilityandhealth/infographic-disability-impacts-all.html.
87. Krahn GL, Walker DK, Correa-De-Araujo R. Persons with disabilities as an unrecognized health disparity population. Am J Public Health. 2015;105(Suppl 2):S198–206.
88. Scarry E. The body in pain: the making and unmaking of the world. New York: Oxford Univeristy Press; 1985.
89. Baruch J, Springs S. Opioids and pain in the emergency department: a narrative crisis. Med Humanit. 2018;44(3):213–6.
90. Cohen SP, Baber ZB, Buvanendran A, McLean BC, Chen Y, Hooten WM, et al. Pain management best practices from multispecialty organizations during the COVID-19 pandemic and public health crises. Pain Med. 2020;21(7):1331–46.
91. Manchikanti L, Vanaparthy R, Atluri S, Sachdeva H, Kaye AD, Hirsch JA. COVID-19 and the opioid epidemic: two public health emergencies that intersect with chronic pain. Pain Ther. 2021;10(1):269–86.

92. Ortyl E. Criminal RICO, fighting corruption and fraud in big pharma – United States v. Michael L. Babich. Am J Law Med. 2019;45(1):86–90.
93. Braun E. Big pharma and teh opioid epidemic: from Vicodin to heroin. Mankota: Captsone; 2020.
94. Lajam CM, Cenname J, Hutzler LH, Bosco JA 3rd. Ethics of opioid prescriber regulations: physicians, patients, and pain. J Bone Joint Surg Am. 2019;101(23):e128.
95. McGuire AL, Aulisio MP, Davis FD, Erwin C, Harter TD, Jagsi R, et al. Ethical challenges arising in the COVID-19 pandemic: an overview from the Association of Bioethics Program Directors (ABPD) task force. Am J Bioeth. 2020;20(7):15–27.
96. Brock DW. Children's rights to health care. J Med Philos. 2001;26(2):163–77.
97. Young VB. Effective management of pain and anxiety for the pediatric patient in the emergency department. Crit Care Nurs Clin North Am. 2017;29(2):205–16.
98. Fein JA, Zempsky WT, Cravero JP, Committee on Pediatric Emergency M, Section on A, Pain M, et al. Relief of pain and anxiety in pediatric patients in emergency medical systems. Pediatrics. 2012;130(5):e1391–405.
99. Kleiber C, Jennissen C, McCarthy AM, Ansley T. Evidence-based pediatric pain management in emergency departments of a rural state. J Pain. 2011;12(8):900–10.
100. Drendel AL, Brousseau DC, Gorelick MH. Pain assessment for pediatric patients in the emergency department. Pediatrics. 2006;117(5):1511–8.
101. Birnie KA, Chambers CT, Fernandez CV, Forgeron PA, Latimer MA, McGrath PJ, et al. Hospitalized children continue to report undertreated and preventable pain. Pain Res Manag. 2014;19(4):198–204.
102. Stanford EA, Chambers CT, Craig KD. The role of developmental factors in predicting young children's use of a self-report scale for pain. Pain. 2006;120(1–2):16–23.
103. American Academy of Pediatrics. Committee on Psychosocial Aspects of C, Family H, Task Force on Pain in Infants C, Adolescents. The assessment and management of acute pain in infants, children, and adolescents. Pediatrics. 2001;108(3):793–7.
104. Herr K, Coyne PJ, Ely E, Gelinas C, Manworren RCB. Pain assessment in the patient unable to self-report: clinical practice recommendations in support of the ASPMN 2019 position statement. Pain Manag Nurs. 2019;20(5):404–17.
105. Bromberg R, Goldman RD. Does analgesia mask diagnosis of appendicitis among children? Can Fam Physician. 2007;53(1):39–41.
106. Goyal MK, Chamberlain JM, Webb M, Grundmeier RW, Johnson TJ, Lorch SA, et al. Racial and ethnic disparities in the delayed diagnosis of appendicitis among children. Acad Emerg Med. 2021;28(9):949–56.
107. Gerstman MD, Rolland LR, Tramer MR, Habre W, Elia N. Researchers' choice of pain scales in trials of children undergoing surgery: a cross-sectional analysis of systematically searched randomized controlled trials and survey of authors. Paediatr Anaesth. 2021;31(11):1194–207.
108. Marzona F, Pedicini S, Passone E, Pusiol A, Cogo P. Mandatory pain assessment in a pediatric emergency department: failure or success?: a retrospective study. Clin J Pain. 2019;35(10):826–30.
109. Noble J, Zarling B, Geesey T, Smith E, Farooqi A, Yassir W, et al. Analgesia use in children with acute long bone fractures in the pediatric emergency department. J Emerg Med. 2020;58(3):500–5.
110. Day LM, Huang R, Okada PJ. Management of pain after pediatric trauma. Pediatr Emerg Care. 2020;36(2):e33–e7.
111. Brown JC, Klein EJ, Lewis CW, Johnston BD, Cummings P. Emergency department analgesia for fracture pain. Ann Emerg Med. 2003;42(2):197–205.
112. Alexander J, Manno M. Underuse of analgesia in very young pediatric patients with isolated painful injuries. Ann Emerg Med. 2003;41(5):617–22.
113. Sahyoun C, Cantais A, Gervaix A, Bressan S, Lollgen R, Krauss B, et al. Pediatric procedural sedation and analgesia in the emergency department: surveying the current European practice. Eur J Pediatr. 2021;180(6):1799–813.
114. Johnson TJ, Goyal MK, Lorch SA, Chamberlain JM, Bajaj L, Alessandrini EA, et al. Racial/ethnic differences in pediatric emergency department wait times. Pediatr Emerg Care. 2022;38(2):e929–e35.
115. Bergeron J, Bailey B. Evaluation of pain in the pediatric emergency department and the request of analgesia. Pediatr Emerg Care. 2021;37(7):e356–e9.

Part III

Transitions of Care

Medication Reconciliation

25

Elizabeth A. Cook

Abbreviations

ADE	Adverse drug event
TOC	Transitions of care
CMS	Centers for medicare and medicaid services
JC	Joint commission
IHI	Institute for healthcare improvement
AHRQ	Agency for healthcare research and quality
NPSG	National patient safety goals
HCAHPS	Hospital consumer assessment of health-care providers and systems
HRRP	Hospital readmission reduction program
AMI	Acute myocardial infarction
CABG	Coronary artery bypass graft
COPD	Chronic obstructive pulmonary disease
HF	Heart failure
THA/TKA	Elective primary total hip arthroplasty and/or total knee arthroplasty
TCM	Transitional care management
NPP	Non-physician practitioner
PDMP	Prescription drug monitoring program
DEA	Drug Enforcement Administration
MME	Morphine milligram equivalents
CDC	Centers for disease control and prevention
OTC	Over-the-counter
IR	Immediate release
CR	Controlled release
DR	Delayed release
ER or XR	Extended release
SR	Sustained release
ADR	Adverse drug reaction

E. A. Cook (✉)
Robert J. Dole Veterans Affairs Medical Center, Wichita, KS, USA

Introduction

Medication errors are preventable occurrences that may lead to inappropriate medication use or patient harm. These events can transpire whether a medication is in the control of a healthcare professional or a patient [1]. It is estimated that seven million patients per year in the United States (US) are impacted by preventable medication errors, making this the most common type of medical mistake affecting patient safety [2–4]. While it is possible for medication errors to result in little or no harm to a patient, they may result in adverse drug events (ADE), which are defined as injury or loss of life that results from a missed or inappropriately dosed medication [2, 3]. ADE are estimated to cost the US healthcare system approximately $40 billion in annual spending to treat impacted patients, conduct root-cause analyses, and develop quality improvement processes to prevent recurrent incidents [3, 5]. Medication errors can occur due to a variety of reasons, but more than 40% of all inpatient medication errors, and approximately 20% of all ADE reported overall, are attributed to inadequate medication reconciliation during a transition of care (TOC) [4, 6].

TOC is defined by the Centers for Medicare and Medicaid Services (CMS) as the movement of a patient from one healthcare provider or setting to another as their condition or care needs evolve [7]. This may include patients transitioning from hospital to home; from an intensive care unit to a general medical floor; or from a primary care provider to a pain management specialist. Additional examples of care transitions are depicted in Fig. 25.1 [8–15].

TOC is a vulnerable period for patients due to many factors including confusion that may arise regarding changes to their medications, difficulty following through on care instructions, challenges communicating with ancillary providers, and the expectation of attending follow-up appointments as necessary [16, 17]. If lack of understanding or communication occurs for patients regarding their health status, medications, or care plan, continuity of care may col-

J. P. Reinert et al. (eds.), *Adjunctive Analgesic Strategies for the Bedside Clinician and Beyond*,
https://doi.org/10.1007/978-3-032-21675-5_25

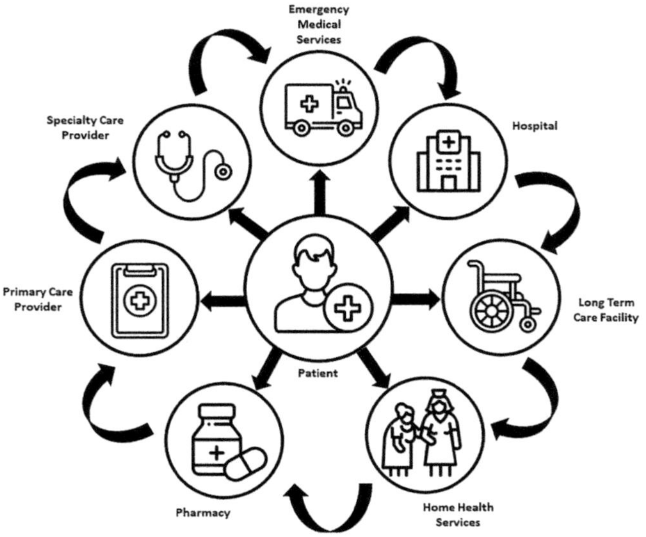

Fig. 25.1 Examples of the patient experience in transitions of care [8–15]

lapse. This dyssynchronous care can result in hospital admission or readmission. Medication reconciliation is an essential component of the communication process at each healthcare transition to ensure that pharmacotherapy changes are relayed to the patient and all members of the patient-centered care team [18, 19].

Medication reconciliation is the process of identifying the most accurate list of all medications that a patient is taking. The healthcare provider doing medication reconciliation compares those medications listed in the medical record to an external list provided by the patient and those obtained from another healthcare facility or provider if necessary [20]. Completing the reconciliation process includes ensuring that changes are appropriately implemented and communicated to others. The intent of conducting a medication reconciliation is to resolve any medication discrepancies, such as omissions, duplications, dosing errors, drug-drug interactions, or contraindications. Furthermore, medication reconciliation allows the medical team to identify opportunities for early intervention to ensure the regimen is feasible and favorable based on patient preferences and to avoid repetition of efforts which helps to conserve medical resources during TOC [21]. Medication reconciliation should be performed at every medical visit, as well as at every care transition, to reduce the likelihood of errors [20].

The risk of medication errors can be compounded in patients with multiple comorbid diseases, or those with complex pharmacotherapeutic regimens, such as those persons with acute or chronic pain conditions. Many analgesic medications are considered high-risk drugs due to their potential for adverse drug events if improperly dosed. Analgesic medications may also be considered high-risk medications in the presence of drug-drug interactions or conflicting health conditions. Persons with pain undergoing a TOC may experience interruptions in their pain management regimen which can result in reduced quality of life; increased risk of adverse events, such as injury or overdose; higher likelihood of hospital readmission; and increased healthcare spending. A comprehensive and reliable medication reconciliation process is crucial to ensure safe and effective pain management at TOC [22].

Standards of Care, Regulatory Bodies, and Reimbursement for Transitions of Care Services

Healthcare systems in the USA spend 15–20 billion dollars annually caring for patients with unplanned hospital readmissions, some of which are a result of potentially preventable ADEs [2, 5]. Use of evidence-based practices that help prevent or reduce ADEs, like medication reconciliation, are important to help minimize unnecessary healthcare expenditures related to readmissions [21, 23–26].

Medication safety organizations such as the Joint Commission (JC), the Agency for Healthcare Research and Quality (AHRQ), and the Institute for Healthcare Improvement (IHI) promote medication reconciliation as an essential practice to [20, 27, 28]. Performance measures related to medication reconciliation during the hospital stay may not only be captured through audits using tools provided by these organizations, but also through the Hospital Consumer Assessment of Healthcare Providers and Systems (HCAHPS) survey and the CMS Core Measures [29–31].

The HCAHPS is a national, standardized survey of patients' perspectives of the care they received during their hospital stay, including doctor and nursing staff communication, staff responsiveness, hospital environment, medication communication, discharge information, care transitions, overall rating of the hospital, and likelihood of recommending the hospital to others. The majority of these domains are directly impacted by ensuring that an accurate medication list is obtained and communicated to patients, their caregivers, and healthcare team, incentivizing a regimented medication reconciliation process for inpatient facilities. Repercussions of receiving low HCAHPS scores can hinder a hospital's reputation among customers and potentially limit distribution of funding from Medicare [29].

The same is true for the CMS Core Measures which are available for both adult and pediatric populations. While medication reconciliation is not an outcome specifically highlighted in the pediatric Core Measures, guidance does emphasize this measure for adult populations as of 2025 [30, 31]. This measure examines the percentage of specified visits where a healthcare worker documents a complete list of a patient's current medications in the medical record. Both

HCAHPS and the CMS Core Measures are examples of the continued shift from fee-for-service to quality-based metrics for reimbursement in the USA. CMS also provides oversight for the Hospital Readmission Reduction Program (HRRP), which is a Medicare value-based program that encourages hospitals to improve care coordination at hospital discharge. HRRP penalizes health systems by reducing payments if patients with chief complaints of acute myocardial infarction (AMI), coronary artery bypass graft (CABG) surgery, chronic obstructive pulmonary disease (COPD), elective primary total hip arthroplasty (THA) and/or total knee arthroplasty (TKA), heart failure (HF), or pneumonia are readmitted within 30-days of hospital discharge [32]. The potential negative financial impact of not adhering to such guidance provides incentive for organizations to develop streamlined medication reconciliation processes.

While penalties exist for not adhering to medication reconciliation best practices during hospital discharge, so do opportunities to increase reimbursement when conducting follow-up with patients transitioning from hospital to home. Transitional Care Management (TCM) services were developed by CMS as an opportunity to increase reimbursement for Medicare patients following hospital discharge. TCM services are composed of two types of visits. The first type of visit is an initial outreach that is conducted within two business days of hospital discharge. This initial contact can be in-person, telephonic, or virtual and can be completed by a physician, a non-physician practitioner (NPP) (physician assistant, nurse practitioner, clinical nurse specialist, certified nurse midwife) or by a licensed clinical staff member under their direction (e.g., registered nurse, pharmacist). Such visits typically include a review of discharge instructions, medication reconciliation, and relevant review of systems so that timely follow-up can be coordinated. A second in-person visit can then be conducted by a physician or non-physician provider within 7–14 days of hospital discharge. Medication reconciliation should also be conducted at this visit, along with a more in-depth workup as dictated by the patients' specific needs and diagnosis. Providers can then bill to receive reimbursement from CMS for these visits provided the patient is designated as moderate or high complexity according to their health conditions, and they are not readmitted within 30 days of their original hospital discharge date [33].

Who Should Conduct a Medication Reconciliation

Ideally, the medication reconciliation process for a given facility should be conducted by an interprofessional team. This includes, but is not limited to medical providers, nurses, medical assistants, pharmacists, and other health disciplines as appropriate. Each team member should be assigned a role suitable for their discipline during the medication reconciliation and TOC processes. Examples of tasks assigned to team members include collecting the medication history, requesting supporting medical documentation from outside sources, critically analyzing the appropriateness of a medication regimen, inputting medication orders, and coordinating discharge prescriptions. Roles should be clearly defined for all parties to safeguard against medication errors by ensuring clear communication among team members and accountability for essential tasks. It is important to note that the process of designating which healthcare professionals should conduct a medication reconciliation is variable depending on the setting of care, available resources, and a healthcare system's own unique standard operating procedures [34–36].

How to Conduct a Medication Reconciliation

All organizations focusing on medication reconciliation endorse utilizing stepwise processes to ensure that the most accurate list is obtained from patients to reduce the likelihood of medication errors leading to poor health outcomes. Suggested formats of reconciling medications per the JC, AHRQ, and IHI are outlined in Table 25.1 [20, 27, 28]. While the phrasing of the medication reconciliation process differs slightly among organizations, the core concepts remain the same. Differences in considerations for medication reconciliation practices in different care settings, such as inpatient versus outpatient arenas, will be highlighted when applicable throughout the chapter.

Verification

The first step of medication reconciliation is collecting a comprehensive medication history from the patient or their caregiver [20, 27, 28]. This not only includes what medications the patient is currently taking but also previous medication trials and adverse reactions [37]. A history of previous allergic or adverse reactions to medications, supplements, additives, food products, or other potential allergens should be collected. Obtaining a complete history of allergies serves multiple purposes including ascertaining whether current medical concerns are possibly a result of the patient's current drug regimen, ruling out use of medications that may be otherwise be indicated as first-line treatments, and preventing adverse events from occurring in the future if agents with cross-reactivity or similar side effect profiles need to be considered. Part of obtaining a complete allergy history is deciphering whether a patient experienced a true immune-mediated allergic reaction versus an adverse drug reaction, defined as a known effect of a drug that is not the

Table 25.1 Steps of reconciling medications as outlined by various US organizations [20, 27, 28]

The Joint Commission	Agency for healthcare research and quality	Institute for healthcare improvement
1. Develop a list of current medications 2. Develop a list of medications to be prescribed 3. Compare the medications on the two lists 4. Make clinical decisions based on the comparison 5. Communicate the new list to appropriate caregivers and to the patient	1. Obtain, document, and verify a patient's current medication list 2. Compare the medication list with medications ordered within the facility 3. Ensure any discrepancies identified are appropriate and intentional based on the patient's care plan 4. Resolve unintended discrepancies with supporting documentation 5. Communicate medication information during transitions of care	1. Verification—Collection of the medication history 2. Clarification—Ensuring that the medications and doses are appropriate 3. Reconciliation—Documentation of changes in the orders

intended therapeutic outcome [38]. An allergy and adverse drug reaction intake should include the name of the causative agent, the timing of the reaction relative to exposure, and sequelae of the event. If possible, the dose of the agent that incited the reaction should be collected if dose-dependent side effects are deemed pertinent. When relevant, healthcare personnel should inquire about a patient's previous history of medication overdose, whether intentional or unintentional, so that appropriateness of their current or future regimens should be considered as well [39].

Next, personnel should obtain a list of medications from the patient or their caregiver. When conducting a medication history, open-ended questions are useful to invite the patient or their caregiver to respond with a free-form answer to elicit additional information. It is often helpful to utilize probing questions in the medication reconciliation interview to identify medications the patient may possibly forget. To trigger patient's memories, personnel completing a medication reconciliation can consider taking a disease-based approach (e.g., "What do you take for your fibromyalgia?"), a symptom-based approach (e.g., "What do you take if you have back pain?"), or a specialist-based approach (e.g., "What medications does your pain management provider prescribe to you?"). Closed-ended questions can be utilized for more targeted intakes, though they can potentially limit opportunities to discover concerns related to health-literacy, adherence, presence or absence of symptoms, or other concerns. Timing of changes to patients' medication regimens may also be relevant, and thus it should be encouraged to inquire about newly initiated or discontinued mediations, as well as when dose adjustments may have occurred [27, 34, 40].

A medication intake should include not only prescription medications, but commonly overlooked items such as herbal products, vitamins, and over-the-counter (OTC) medications [41]. The use of dietary supplements has become increasingly common in the USA, with some estimates citing close to 60% of adults 20 years of age and older utilizing a dietary supplement within the past 30 days [42]. The incidence of dietary and herbal supplement use, and quantity of supplements used, has been shown to increase with age, making older adults more vulnerable to polypharmacy or drug-drug interactions [43]. Approximately 70% of patients do not regularly report the use of herbal products, vitamins, and OTC medications [44]. While not comprehensive, Table 25.2 denotes several commonly used herbal products with the potential for clinically significant drug interactions when used with prescription and OTC analgesic medications [45]. Healthcare personnel should take care to assess total daily doses of commonly used OTC analgesics, such as acetaminophen, when patients are concurrently prescribed, or may be prescribed other acetaminophen containing products (e.g., oxycodone-acetaminophen, hydrocodone-acetaminophen).

Complete medication administration instructions should be obtained, including the name of the product, strength, quantity of medication administered per dose, and route and frequency of administration. When relevant, clinical personnel should inquire if patients are using immediate-release (IR) or modified-release formulations (controlled-release (CR), delayed-release (DR), extended-release (ER or XR), sustained-release (SR) products) as the dosing frequency differs by formulation and should also be evaluated. Clarifying the formulation, especially for modified-release products, ensures that the medications are being appropriately utilized by patients. Furthermore, using the correct dosage form is essential for patients who may need to crush or open products to administer them in cases of dysphagia or administration via feeding tubes [46]. In cases where a liquid product is necessary, it is good clinical practice to document both the concentration and volume of medication administered to prevent errors in dosing.

Clinical staff should probe patients for use of medications with atypical routes of administration or those that would require administration in a medical office, as these may be easily overlooked or forgotten. These may include, but are not limited to, products delivered via the following routes:

- Buccal
- Inhaled
- Intraarticular
- Intracavernosal
- Intramuscular

Table 25.2 Commonly used herbal products and clinically relevant analgesic drug interactions [45]

Analgesic medication class	Herbal products	Potential outcomes
Aspirin Non-steroidal anti-inflammatory drugs (NSAIDs)	Bilberry (*Vaccinium myrtillus*) Garlic (*Allium sativum*) Ginger (*Gingiber officinale*) Ginkgo (*Ginkgo biloba*) Ginseng American (*Panax quinquefolius*) Asian (*Panax ginseng*) Siberian (*Eleutherococcus senticosus*) Meadowsweet (*Filipendula ulmaria*) Turmeric (*Curcuma longa*) Willow (*Salix* sp.)	Decreased platelet aggregation resulting in increased risk of bleeding
	Chamomile (*Matricaria recutita, Chamaemelum mobile*) Fenugreek (*Trigonella foenum-graecum*) Motherworth (*Leonurus cardiaca*)	Anticoagulant effect via coumarin compounds resulting in increased risk of bleeding
Anticonvulsants Antidepressants Antipsychotics Gabapentinoids Ketamine Muscle relaxants Opioids	Kava (*Piper methysticum*) Valerian (*Valeriana officinalis*) Cannabidiol (*Cannabis* sp.) Kratom (*Mitragyna speciosa*)	Central nervous system depression and sedation

- Intranasal
- Intravenous
- Intrathecal
- Intraurethral
- Oral
- Ocular
- Otic
- Rectal
- Subcutaneous
- Sublingual
- Topical.
- Transdermal.
- Vaginal.

Staff should take care to clarify when the last dose of a given medication is administered and when the next dose is intended to be administered to the patient. This ensures that the potential for a lapse in treatment, or overdose, is mitigated, particularly if a patient is being admitted for inpatient care, and timing of medication administration needs to be scheduled in the medication administration record [27, 34, 39]. In particular, patients may forget to mention medications with infrequent dosing regimens, such as fentanyl transdermal patches, which are applied every 72-h. In cases where transdermal patches are utilized for pain management, staff should locate the site of where the patch was applied in addition to noting the time that it was placed and the time it is intended to be removed [39]. An assessment of medication adherence should be conducted as well to determine how often patients may be administering as needed medications and how often they may be forgetting doses of scheduled medications [20, 27, 28, 34, 39]. Additional information regarding identifying and addressing these concerns can be found in Chap. 32.

Clarification

Once a medication history is obtained from the patient or their caregivers, healthcare personnel should seek to clarify any discrepancies identified during the interview. Use of hardcopy or electronic medication lists, smart phone applications, medication bottles, photographs of medication labels, or other modalities provided by the patient or caregiver, may be useful tools to supplement the medication history. However, these may fail to provide an accurate picture of how the patient is actually using the medications at home. Communication from hospitals, providers offices, and pharmacies may also be useful tools to clarify information provided by the patient and can assist with confirming medication adherence through payor and prescription refill histories. In some cases, shared electronic medical records among health systems and health plans may be accessible [47].

State prescription drug monitoring programs (PDMPs) are a resource that healthcare personnel can utilize to improve patient care and safety concerning controlled substances. PDMPs are electronic databases that track prescriptions for controlled substances, which can assist providers with clarifying medication information during medication reconciliation, as well as identifying patients who may be at risk of overdose [48, 49]. PDMPs in several states may also track "drugs of concern" which are defined by the US Department of Justice Drug Enforcement Administration (DEA) as medications that are not formally designated as controlled substances by the Controlled Substances Act, but may have abuse potential. Drugs of concern listed in the PDMP may vary by state and are often identified by state boards of pharmacy [50].

CMS requires qualified PDMPs as having the following characteristics: regulation oversight by the state, records of prescription drug history for controlled substances, requirements for Medicaid providers to check the PDMP prior to prescribing a controlled substance, and integration of information from the PDMP into provider workflow. Additionally, the PDMP must be able to deliver annual reports of the following key metrics: the percentage of providers who check the PDMP, total quantity of prescribed daily morphine milligram equivalents (MME), number and quantity of MME per patient, types of controlled substances prescribed, dates of prescriptions for controlled substances, and prescriptions of controlled substances within specific populations [49]. Ideally, PDMP data should be reviewed prior to dispensing any controlled substance for acute, subacute, or chronic pain. However, the Centers for Disease Control and Prevention (CDC) recommend, at minimum, assessing the PDMP when first initiating controlled substances for acute, subacute, or chronic pain, as well as every 3 months, or more frequently, when continuing a controlled substance [48].

The above sources should not be considered replacements to speaking with the patient or their caregiver, but supplemental information. It is important to interview a patient or their primary care giver directly to gauge the accuracy of, and adherence to, the medication regimen [20, 27, 28, 41]. It should be noted that patients' capacity to recall or communicate their medication regimens may be affected by the acuity of their medical condition if incapacitated or suffering from severe illness that alters their cognitive abilities. In these situations, it may be necessary to verify the patient's medication list upon admission, then again at a later point in the hospital stay when their faculties are no longer impaired. The medical team should clearly document the finalized home medication list in the medical record so that it is accessible by all health professions caring for the patient for future reference [20, 27, 28].

In the clarification phase, a critical review of the patient's verified medication list and the intended treatment plan for the visit should then be performed. It is important for clinical personnel reviewing the patient's allergy and adverse reaction history to interpret whether reactions pose a significant risk should the patient be reexposed to the same agent or one with potential cross-reactivity. Previous adverse drug events related to analgesic medications, such as overdose, sedation, constipation, gastric irritation, etc., should be also catalogued [34, 39]. When applicable, harm reduction strategies should be discussed and provided. These can include dispensing naloxone for treatment of an opioid overdose, provision of a bowel regimen to prevent opioid-induced-constipation, use of acid suppressing medications to prevent gastroduodenal toxicity in those prescribed chronic NSAIDs, among others. Additional information regarding this subject can be found in Chap. 21.

The medical team should document indications for each medication whenever possible to ensure that the drug is a suitable treatment for a given health condition in addition to ensuring all agents have a reason for being prescribed to a patient. A thorough review should be conducted to determine the efficacy and safety of all medications a patient is prescribed and how those best integrate into a proposed care plan at a given visit. Interviews with the patient and their caregivers can assist with determining efficacy and safety of a regimen based on patient satisfaction regarding symptom relief and provide them the opportunity to report possible side effects. When constructing a new medication regimen for a patient, potential drug interactions, contraindications, or precautions to medications should be assessed in relation to patient's home regimen. Those medical conditions without a medication prescribed for treatment should be assessed to determine if nonpharmacologic management is indeed adequate or if additional drug therapy would be beneficial [37].

In addition to confirming that each medication has a specific indication, staff should assess the appropriateness of all aspects of each medication including formulation, route, dose, frequency, and duration of treatment for safety concerns. Clarifying the formulation, especially for modified-release products, helps to ensure that the medications are being appropriately utilized. In situations where patients have dysphagia or require use of feeding tubes, modified-release formulations may be unfavorable due to their alteration of pharmacokinetics if the medication dosage form is damaged in the cutting or crushing process [46, 51]. Destroying the structural integrity of a modified-release product could expedite the onset of action and increase the peak concentration leading to supratherapeutic effects, thus increasing risk of overdose or ADRs. Additionally, destroying the mechanism by which a product is formulated to be modified-release (such as crushing a film-coated tablet) can lead to shortened duration of action potentially resulting in inadequate treatment of pain [51].

The route of medication administration in those patients transitioning to from an outpatient to inpatient setting, and vice versa, can depend on a multitude of factors, such as degree of illness, ability to swallow, scheduled procedures requiring *nil* per os (NPO) status, etc. When assessing a drug regimen for a patient utilizing a feeding tube, it is important to bear in mind that drug absorption also depends on the drug's ability to permeate the intestinal mucosa. In all scenarios where medications must be delivered via a feeding tube, clinical staff should assess whether the location of the feeding tube (e.g., stomach, duodenum, jejunum) will permit proper dissolution and absorption of the medication and whether the formulation may need to be changed. In patients where feeding tubes are utilized as a route to deliver medications, the medical team should consider whether a crushed tablet, opened capsule, powder, or liquid product has the potential to clog tubing [46] or whether continued use of medications with chemical or physical abuse deterrents is warranted [52]. This could become relevant when formulating a hospital discharge regimen in patients requiring long-term use of feeding tubes if a provider mistakenly prescribes a product with such abuse deterrents.

A thorough medication history assessing adherence to opioid medications is essential to ensure that a patients' pain management regimens are appropriately prescribed in an inpatient setting. This includes quantifying the number of missed doses of their scheduled opioid regimen, as well as the number of as-needed doses administered for breakthrough pain [41]. The PDMP can serve as a resource to determine if prescriptions are being refilled in a timely manner based on the quantity dispensed and the fill date [48–50]. Providers should ensure that the total MME is calculated so that the appropriate agent and regimen can be prescribed if an alternative product is necessary per hospital or insurance formulary or based on other patient-specific factors. In patients whose medications must be converted from oral to parenteral route, and vice versa, ordering providers should ensure that medications are converted on an equianalgesic basis [39, 53]. Providers should be cautious when converting between opioid analgesics due to potential differences in cross-tolerance among agents. It is generally recommended to consider reducing the dose of the new opioid analgesic by 25%–50% MME in persons with well-controlled pain, particularly in older adults and persons with renal dysfunction, to reduce the likelihood of overdose. Conversely, in persons whose pain is uncontrolled at the start of transitioning to a new opioid analgesic, it may be reasonable to start at 100% of the MME [53].

Relevant laboratory and diagnostic tests should be obtained to aid in determining if adjustments are necessary to maintain the efficacy and safety of a given regimen from a clinical standpoint including assessment of organ function so that dose and frequency of administration of a medication are appropriately adjusted to permit adequate drug clearance or metabolism. In those patients who are prescribed limited courses of analgesic medications for post-surgical pain, acute pain conditions, and other concerns, the medical team should attempt to define an appropriate duration of use of opioid medications [37, 39].

Reconciliation

After obtaining a medication history and clarifying areas of concern in the patient's regimen, it is important for providers to decisively document changes to the patient's medication regimen in the medical record to reduce risk of discrepancies. Common discrepancies to be aware of include, but are not limited to:

- Dosage form discrepancies
- Dosage discrepancies
- Frequency discrepancies
- Route of administration discrepancies
- Addition of a medication not previously used
- Duplication of therapy
- Omission of a drug previously used
- Substitution from one medication to another targeting the same treatment goals [6, 26, 34, 54]

The justification provided for the changes made to the medication regimen at a given visit should be clearly recorded, for example in progress notes in an outpatient setting or discharge paperwork in the inpatient setting. Changes to a medication regimen should not only align with evidence-based practices, but also take into account a patient's health literacy, socioeconomic status, and personal beliefs to ensure that the regimen aligns with their values and capabilities. It is important to determine if proposed medication changes are feasible based on the regimen complexity and determine if additional assistance is necessary to ensure therapy is delivered as intended. Additionally, the patient's insurance benefits and medication formulary should be reviewed to ensure that preferred treatment options are selected and prior authorization or patient assistance paperwork is completed as necessary prior to discharge. Programs such as bedside medication delivery or clearly defining the patient's preferred pharmacy can also enhance likelihood of them obtaining their medications in a timely manner [18–21, 36]. Methods to evaluate and address the above barriers are highlighted further in Chaps. 30 and 31.

After remedying these concerns, patients should be provided with a finalized medication list at discharge denoting which medications were initiated, discontinued, continued, or had a change in dose. Both written and verbal education should be provided in a manner that is appropriate for the patient and caregivers level of health literacy. In addition to highlighting changes to the medication regimen, the care team should ensure that the patient is aware of potential adverse effects associated with their medications, therapeutic expectations, and nonpharmacologic interventions they can employ if relevant. The patient and their caregiver's ability to appropriately administer their pain regimen, identify signs and symptoms of overdose, utilize a reversal agent for overdose should be assessed, and education regarding disposal of medications when treatment is completed or no longer needed should be discussed [18–21, 27, 36]. In those at high risk for readmission, it is important that their disease state education includes clear instructions as when to seek a higher level of medical care for worsening clinical condition. Closed-loop communication techniques such as the "teach back" method can be useful to assess a patient or caregiver's understanding of instructions. Clinical staff can deploy this technique by asking an individual to explain a concept related to their care in their own words. This allows for the healthcare worker to assess for gaps in recall and comprehension and correct these misunderstandings in real time [40, 55].

At present, there are limited data regarding how frequently patients prescribed analgesics misunderstand their discharge medication instructions. Previous studies have determined, however, that 40% of patients are unable to accurately describe the reason for their hospitalization, 80% have limited understanding of their medication changes, and over 50% are unable to accurately recall follow-up appointment details when transitioning from hospital to home [56, 57]. Thus, the education process at hospital discharge is an essential component to reducing the potential for medication errors, adverse events, and likelihood of hospital readmission.

Patients and their caregivers should be explicitly informed of requirements for follow-up appointments with specialists or their primary care providers post-hospital discharge [21, 27, 28, 36]. Clear documentation and communication of care plans are essential not only to ensure patient and caregiver understanding but also to ensure that continuity of care is maintained between other members of the medical team. Failed handoffs between inpatient and outpatient providers are common. By some estimates, only 12%–34% of hospital discharge summaries are received by outpatient providers for review prior to hospital follow-up appointments, which can potentially limit preparation for those patients with complex medication regimens and pain conditions [58].

Medication reconciliation should be conducted at these follow-up visits to ensure that patients have followed through on their new regimens. Furthermore, these post-discharge appointments should serve to assess the efficacy and safety of those changes made by the inpatient medical team and determine degree of follow-up and additional referrals if necessary [21, 27, 28].

Conclusions

Medication errors and adverse drug reactions are commonly associated with inadequate medication reconciliation practices occurring during TOC [4, 6]. The risk of medication errors during care transitions can be intensified in patients with intricate and high-risk pharmacotherapeutic regimens, such as those persons with acute or chronic pain conditions. Persons with pain undergoing TOC are susceptible to interruptions in their pain management which can result in reduced quality of life and increased risk of adverse events and hospital readmission [22]. Utilizing an interprofessional care team with clearly defined roles and a stepwise process of completing medication reconciliation can increase patient understanding, reduce the likelihood of medication errors, and improve communication among providers as patients transition from one care setting to another [34, 36].

References

1. What is a medication error? Medication error definition. National Coordinating Counsel for Medication Error Reporting and Prevention. https://www.nccmerp.org/about-medication-errors. Accessed 6 Nov 2023.
2. Tariq RA, Vashisht R, Sinha A, et al. Medication dispensing errors and prevention. [Updated 2023 May 2]. In: StatPearls [Internet]. Treasure Island: StatPearls Publishing. p. 2023. https://www.ncbi.nlm.nih.gov/books/NBK519065/.
3. Uhlenhopp DJ, Aguilar O, Dai D, Ghosh A, Shaw M, Mitra C. Hospital-wide medication reconciliation program: error identification, cost-effectiveness, and detecting high-risk individuals on admission. Integr Pharm Res Pract. 2020;9:195–203. https://doi.org/10.2147/IPRP.S269857.
4. Barnsteiner JH. Medication reconciliation: transfer of medication information across settings-keeping it free from error. Am J Nurs. 2005;105(3 Suppl):31–51. https://doi.org/10.1097/00000446-200503001-00007.
5. Lahue BJ, Pyenson B, Iwasaki K, Blumen HE, Forray S, Rothschild JM. National burden of preventable adverse drug events associated with inpatient injectable medications: healthcare and medical professional liability costs. Am Health Drug Benefits. 2012;5(7):1–10. https://pubmed.ncbi.nlm.nih.gov/24991335/
6. Rozich J, Roger R. Medication safety: one organization's approach to the challenge. J Clin Outcomes Manag. 2001;8:27–34.
7. Centers for Medicare and Medicaid Services. Community-Based Care Transitions Program Fact Sheet. https://www.cms.gov/priorities/innovation/files/fact-sheet/cctp-fact-sheet.pdf. Accessed 13 Nov 2023.
8. Icongeek26. Patient. Retrieved from https://www.flaticon.com/free-icon/medical_1512910?term=patient&page=1&position=1&origin=style&related_id=1512910.
9. Freepik. Ambulance. Retrieved from https://www.flaticon.com/free-icon/medical_1512910?term=patient&page=1&position=1&origin=style&related_id=1512910.
10. Joalfa. Hospital. Retrieved from https://www.flaticon.com/free-icon/medical_1512910?term=patient&page=1&position=1&origin=style&related_id=1512910.
11. Madness. Wheelchair. Retrieved from https://www.flaticon.com/free-icon/medical_1512910?term=patient&page=1&position=1&origin=style&related_id=1512910.
12. Nadiinko. Nurse. Retrieved from https://www.flaticon.com/free-icon/medical_1512910?term=patient&page=1&position=1&origin=style&related_id=1512910.
13. Freepik. Medication bottle. Retrieved from https://www.flaticon.com/free-icon/pills_3004423?term=medicine+bottle&page=1&position=14&origin=style&related_id=3004423.
14. Freepik. Clipboard. Retrieved from https://www.flaticon.com/free-icon/pills_3004423?term=medicine+bottle&page=1&position=14&origin=style&related_id=3004423.
15. Srip. Stethoscope. Retrieved from https://www.flaticon.com/free-icon/pills_3004423?term=medicine+bottle&page=1&position=14&origin=style&related_id=3004423.
16. Rattray NA, Sico JJ, Cox LM, Russ AL, Matthias MS, FrankelRM. Crossing the communication chasm: challenges and opportunities in transitions of care from the hospital to the primary care clinic. Jt Comm J Qual Patient Saf. 2017;43(3):127–37. https://doi.org/10.1016/j.jcjq.2016.11.007.

17. Mansukhani RP, Bridgeman MB, Candelario D, Eckert LJ. Exploring transitional care: evidence-based strategies for improving provider communication and reducing readmissions. P T. 2015;40(10):690–4. https://pubmed.ncbi.nlm.nih.gov/26535025/
18. Coleman EA. Falling through the cracks: challenges and opportunities for improving transitional care for persons with continuous complex care needs. J Am Geriatr Soc. 2003 Apr;51(4):549–55. https://doi.org/10.1046/j.15325415.2003.51185.x.
19. Coleman EA, Mahoney E, Parry C. Assessing the quality of preparation for posthospital care from the patient's perspective: the care transitions measure. Med Care. 2005;43(3):246–55. https://doi.org/10.1097/00005650-200503000-00007.
20. Joint Commission. National Patient Safety Goals. https://www.jointcommission.org/-/media/tjc/documents/standards/national-patient-safety-goals/2023/2023-hap-npsg-goals-102122_simple.pdfs. Accessed 9 Nov 2023.
21. Centers for Medicare and Medicaid Services. Improving Care Transitions. https://www.medicaid.gov/medicaid/quality-of-care/quality-improvement-initiatives/improving-care-transitions/index.html. Accessed 13 Nov 2023.
22. IOM (Institute of Medicine). Relieving pain in America: a blueprint for transforming prevention, care, education, and research. Washington, DC: The National Academies Press; 2011. https://doi.org/10.17226/13172.
23. Jencks SF, Williams MV, Coleman EA. Rehospitalizations among patients in the Medicare fee-for-service program [published correction appears in N Engl J Med. 2011 Apr 21;364(16):1582]. N Engl J Med. 2009;360(14):1418–28. https://doi.org/10.1056/NEJMsa0803563.
24. Gillespie U, Alassaad A, Henrohn D, et al. A comprehensive pharmacist intervention to reduce morbidity in patients 80 years or older: a randomized controlled trial. Arch Intern Med. 2009;169:894. https://doi.org/10.1001/archinternmed.2009.71.
25. Schnipper JL, Kirwin JL, Cotugno MC, et al. Role of pharmacist counseling in preventing adverse drug events after hospitalization. Arch Intern Med. 2006;166:565. https://doi.org/10.1001/archinte.166.5.565.
26. Bülow C, Clausen SS, Lundh A, Christensen M. Medication review in hospitalised patients to reduce morbidity and mortality. Cochrane Database Syst Rev. 2023;1:CD008986.
27. Agency for Healthcare Research and Quality. Published April 2023. Accessed November 9, 2023. Medications at Transitions and Clinical Handoffs (MATCH) Toolkit for Medication Reconciliation. https://www.ahrq.gov/sites/default/files/publications/files/match.pdf.
28. Institute for Healthcare Improvement. Prevent adverse drug events by implementing medication reconciliation. Last updated December 2011. http://www.ihi.org/resources/Pages/Tools/HowtoGuidePreventAdverseDrugEvents.aspx.
29. Hospital Consumer Assessment of Healthcare Providers and Systems. HCHAPS Survey. https://hcahpsonline.org/globalassets/hcahps/quality-assurance/2023_survey-instruments_english_mail.pdf. Accessed 16 Nov 2023.
30. Centers for Medicare and Medicaid Services. 2024 core set of adult health care quality measures for Medicaid (Adult Core Set). https://www.medicaid.gov/sites/default/files/2023-08/2024-adult-core-set_0.pdf. Accessed 12 Dec 2023.
31. Centers for Medicare and Medicaid Services. 2024 Mandatory core set of children's health care quality measures for Medicaid and CHIP (Child Core Set). https://www.medicaid.gov/sites/default/files/2023-08/2024-child-core-set_0.pdf. Accessed 12 Dec 2023.
32. Centers for Medicare and Medicaid Services. Hospital Readmission Reduction Program. Published September 10, 2024. Available at https://www.cms.gov/Medicare/Medicare-Fee-for-Service-Payment/AcuteInpatientPPS/Readmissions-Reduction-Program.
33. Centers for Medicare and Medicaid Services. Transitional care management services. Published July 2024. Available at https://www.cms.gov/files/document/mln908628-transitional-care-management-services.pdf.
34. Jarrett T, Cochran J, Baus A. Applying the medications at transitions and clinical handoffs toolkit in a rural primary care clinic: implications for nursing, patients, and caregivers. J Nurs Care Qual. 2020;35(3):233–9. https://doi.org/10.1097/NCQ.0000000000000454.
35. Al-Hashar A, Al-Zakwani I, Eriksson T, Al Za'abi M. Whose responsibility is medication reconciliation: physicians, pharmacists or nurses? A survey in an academic tertiary care hospital. Saudi Pharm J. 2017;25(1):52–8. https://doi.org/10.1016/j.jsps.2015.06.012.
36. Stranges PM, Jackevicius CA, Anderson SL, Bondi DS, et al. Role of clinical pharmacists and pharmacy support personnel in transitions of care. J Am Coll Clin Pharm. 2020;3:532–45. https://doi.org/10.1002/jac5.1215.
37. The patient care process for delivering comprehensive medication management (CMM): optimizing medication use in patient-centered, team-based care settings. CMM in Primary Care Research Team Published July 2018. http://www.accp.com/cmm_care_process. Accessed 12 Dec 2023.
38. Pourpak Z, Fazlollahi MR, Fattahi F. Understanding adverse drug reactions and drug allergies: principles, diagnosis and treatment aspects. Recent Patents Inflamm Allergy Drug Discov. 2008;2(1):24–46. https://doi.org/10.2174/187221308783399289.
39. Island Peer Review Organization – Quality Improvement Network – Quality Improvement Organizations – Centers for Medicare and Medicaid Services iQuality Improvement and Innovation Group. Pain Management Essential Communication Elements for Transitions of Care Guide. https://qi.ipro.org/wp-content/uploads/12SOW-T12-A2-PainMgt-Essentl-Communic-ElementsTool_v1.pdf. Accessed 12 Dec 2023.
40. Perri M. Communication skills for pharmacists. Am J Pharm Educ. 2006;70(1):12.
41. Fitzgerald RJ. Medication errors: the importance of an accurate drug history. Br J Clin Pharmacol. 2009;67(6):671–5. https://doi.org/10.1111/j.1365-2125.2009.03424.x.
42. Gahche J, Bailey R, Burt V, Hughes J, Yetley E, Dwyer J, et al. Dietary supplement use among U.S. Adults has increased since NHANES III (1988–1994), NCHS Data Brief, no 61. Hyattsville: National Center for Health Statistics; 2011.
43. Mishra S, Stierman B, Gahche JJ, Potischman N. Dietary supplement use among adults: United States, 2017–2018, NCHS Data Brief, no 399. Hyattsville: National Center for Health Statistics; 2021. https://doi.org/10.15620/cdc:101131.
44. Johnston BA. Prevention magazine assesses use of dietary supplements. HerbalGram. 2000;48:65–72.
45. Abebe W. Herbal medication: potential for adverse interactions with analgesic drugs. J Clin Pharm Ther. 2002;27(6):391–401. https://doi.org/10.1046/j.1365-2710.2002.00444.x.
46. Grissinger M. Preventing errors when drugs are given via enteral feeding tubes. P T. 2013;38(10):575–6. https://pubmed.ncbi.nlm.nih.gov/24391375/
47. Kini V, Ho PM. Interventions to improve medication adherence: a review. JAMA. 2018;320(23):2461–73. https://doi.org/10.1001/jama.2018.19271.
48. Centers for Disease Control and Prevention. Prescription Drug Monitoring Programs (PDMPs). Overdose prevention. Published May 6, 2024. https://www.cdc.gov/overdose-prevention/hcp/clinical-guidance/prescription-drug-monitoring-programs.html
49. United States Department of Health and Human Services and Centers for Medicare and Medicaid Services. Report to Congress: State Challenges and Best Practices Implementing PDMP Requirements Under Section 5042 of the SUPPORT Act. Published

June 30, 2021. https://www.medicaid.gov/medicaid/data-and-systems/downloads/rtc-5042-state-challenges.pdf.
50. US Department of Justice Drug Enforcement Administration. Drugs of Abuse: A DEA Resource Guide 2024 Edition. Published December 12, 2024. https://www.dea.gov/sites/default/files/2024-12/2024-Drugs-of-Abuse-508.pdf.
51. Gill D, Spain M, Edlund BJ. Crushing or splitting medications: unrecognized hazards. J Gerontol Nurs. 2012;38(1):8–12. https://doi.org/10.3928/00989134-20111213-01.
52. Adler JA, Mallick-Searle T. An overview of abuse-deterrent opioids and recommendations for practical patient care. J Multidiscip Healthc. 2018;11:323–32. https://doi.org/10.2147/JMDH.S166915.
53. Schneider C, Yale SH, Larson M. Principles of pain management. Clin Med Res. 2003;1(4):337–40. https://doi.org/10.3121/cmr.1.4.337.
54. Quélennec B, Beretz L, Paya D, et al. Potential clinical impact of medication discrepancies at hospital admission. Eur J Intern Med. 2013;24(6):530–5. https://doi.org/10.1016/j.ejim.2013.02.007.
55. Schillinger D, Piette J, Grumbach K, et al. Closing the loop: physician communication with diabetic patients who have low health literacy. Arch Intern Med. 2003;163(1):83–90. https://doi.org/10.1001/archinte.163.1.83.
56. Ziaeian B, Araujo KL, Van Ness PH, Horwitz LI. Medication reconciliation accuracy and patient understanding of intended medication changes on hospital discharge. J Gen Intern Med. 2012;27(11):1513–20. https://doi.org/10.1007/s11606-012-2168-4.
57. Horwitz LI, Moriarty JP, Chen C, et al. Quality of discharge practices and patient understanding at an academic medical center. JAMA Intern Med. 2013;173(18):1715–22. https://doi.org/10.1001/jamainternmed.2013.9318.
58. Kripalani S, LeFevre F, Phillips CO, Williams MV, Basaviah P, Baker DW. Deficits in communication and information transfer between hospital-based and primary care physicians: implications for patient safety and continuity of care. JAMA. 2007;297(8):831–41. https://doi.org/10.1001/jama.297.8.831.

Barriers to Patients Receiving Care

26

Troy Lynn Lewis, Faith S. Wellings, Danielle M. Kieck, and Peter Iskander

Introduction

Despite evidence-based recommendations regarding pain management, many patients with pain receive inadequate care [151]. Patient factors such as accessibility, discrimination, health literacy, communication, and financial barriers can contribute to a lack of adequate care, as well as other clinical and health system-related barriers (e.g., reimbursement issues, provider stigmas, and inadequate training).

Socioeconomic and cultural barriers may impede optimal pain assessment and management and, in return, contribute to already existing health disparities. The biopsychosocial pain model can be considered when addressing these disparities [50]. This model includes both disease and illness, involving a complex interaction of biological, psychological, and social factors. Disease is the underlying disruption in the biological structure or body processes, while illness is the subjective experience of the patient and how they live with and respond to symptoms of disease. Addressing the various factors that collectively contribute to health and well-being, while managing the perceptions of both the patient and the healthcare provider, is important in the assessment and achievement of optimal outcomes.

The Centers for Disease Control and Prevention (CDC) recommends that "Clinicians, practices, health systems, and payers should vigilantly attend to health inequities and ensure access to appropriate, affordable, diversified, coordinated, and effective pain management care for all persons" [122].

T. L. Lewis (✉) · F. S. Wellings · D. M. Kieck · P. Iskander
Nesbitt School of Pharmacy, Wilkes University, Wilkes-Barre, PA, USA
e-mail: troy.lewis@wilkes.edu; faith.wellings@wilkes.edu; danielle.kieck@wilkes.edu

Bias, Stigmas, and Stereotypes in Pain Management

Provider biases can influence decisions regarding pain management, affecting expectations about patients and impacting interpersonal interactions, diagnosis, and treatment decisions. The influence of a patient's demographics, including gender, race, and age, among others, can significantly affect the quality and standard of care patients receive [64, 144, 149, 155].

Healthcare providers hold both explicit and implicit biases against several marginalized communities, including, but not limited to, racial and ethnic minorities, individuals with disabilities, and gender and sexual minorities [17]. The American Psychological Association defines implicit bias as "a negative attitude, of which one is not consciously aware, against a specific social group" [9]. It is believed that implicit biases are molded by experiences and established through learned connections between specific attributes and social classifications, such as race or gender. People's perceptions and actions can be impacted by the implicit biases they possess, even if they are unaware of possessing such biases. An explicit bias is one that is consciously endorsed [17, 48, 154]. Refer to Table 26.1 for bias terminology.

When discrimination is embedded into the healthcare system and institutionalized practices, it can cause health inequities by resulting in biased decision-making. Additionally, social and structural determinants of health diminish health outcomes in marginalized patients. In return, biases facilitate, exacerbate, and perpetuate discriminatory practices, creating a feedback loop and vicious cycle powered by confirmation bias that sustains itself (Fig. 26.1) [154]. For example, a clinician who perceives a female patient as sensitive or fabricating her pain may be less inclined to recommend an intensive or evidence-based pain regimen based on the clinician's preconceived notions regarding the pain tolerance of female patients. This clinician believes he/she made the best clinical decision,

J. P. Reinert et al. (eds.), *Adjunctive Analgesic Strategies for the Bedside Clinician and Beyond*,
https://doi.org/10.1007/978-3-032-21675-5_26

Table 26.1 Bias terminology

Implicit bias	"Implicit biases are unconscious mental processes that lead to associations and reactions that are automatic and without intention; actors have no awareness of the associations with a stimulus…Implicit bias goes beyond stereotyping to include favorable or unfavorable evaluations toward groups of people. Although we are not aware these implicit biases exist, they have a significant impact on decision-making" [154]
Explicit bias	"Explicit forms of bias include preferences, beliefs, and attitudes of which people are generally consciously aware, personally endorse, and can identify and communicate." [154]
Confirmation bias	"Confirmation bias is a type of psychological bias in which a decision is made according to the subject's preconceptions, beliefs, or preferences. Such bias results from human errors, including imprecision and misconception. Confirmation bias can also emerge owing to overconfidence, which results in contradictory evidence being ignored or overlooked. In medicine, confirmation bias is one of the main reasons for diagnostic errors and may cause inaccurate diagnosis and improper treatment management" [6]
Stereotype	"A stereotype is a fixed set of attributes associated with a social group" [154]
Stigma	"Stigma is defined as the co-occurrence of labeling, stereotyping, separation, status loss, and discrimination in a context in which power is exercised…because the overall stigma process incorporates several other elements, such as labeling and stereotyping, the stigma concept is broader than discrimination" [57]
Discrimination	"Discrimination, the result of either implicit or explicit biases, is the inequitable treatment and/or impact of general policies, practices, and norms on individuals and communities based on social group membership"[154]

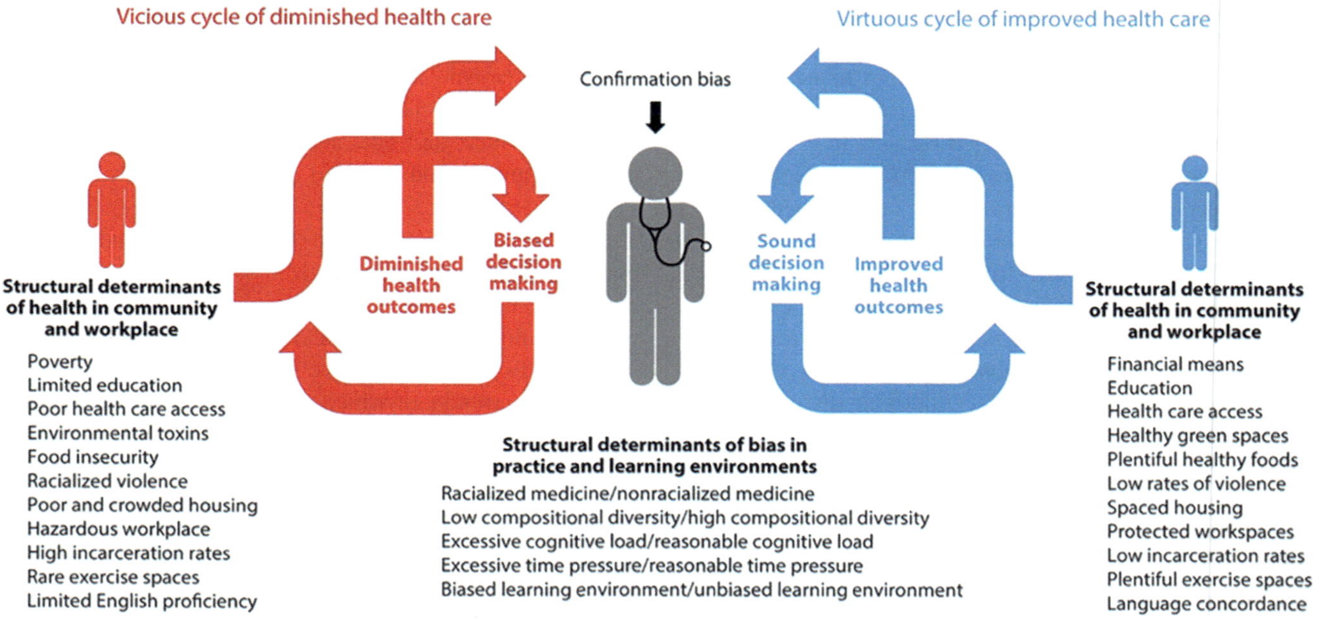

Fig. 26.1 Flow chart illustrating the cycle of healthcare outcomes through the interactions between patient structural determinants and provider implicit bias. On the left, the "Vicious cycle of diminished health care" is shown in red, starting with structural determinants like poverty and limited education, leading to diminished health outcomes and biased decision-making. On the right, the "Virtuous cycle of improved health care" is shown in blue, beginning with positive structural determinants like financial means and education, leading to improved health outcomes and sound decision-making. A central figure represents the influence of confirmation bias on decision-making. (Reproduced from Vela et al. [154])

unaware that his/her perceptions were distorted by implicit biases that, in turn, have an overall effect on patient health outcomes. The clinician's bias is further reinforced as the female patient's pain remains uncontrolled, confirming the provider's biases as true. Moreover, patients can bring their own implicit biases into clinical interactions, which can further complicate communication and hinder the achievement of shared patient-centered clinical goals [17]. Unfortunately, these inequities persist despite many studies identifying implicit biases and stigmas as a potential root cause.

Racial and Ethnic Bias in Pain Management

Decades of research have consistently shown that patients from racial and ethnic minority backgrounds are less likely to receive pain treatment or appropriate management compared to their White counterparts [97]. Studies have shown that patients are less likely to be prescribed pain medication, and when they are, doses are lower and less aggressive and do not follow appropriate management strategies compared to their White counterparts. Additionally, these studies have shown that minority patients are less likely to be prescribed opioids for their pain and are more likely to have their pain underestimated and viewed as having less severe pain [15, 28, 98, 147]. Disparities persist at each level of care (assessment and management); treatment setting (emergency rooms, surgery); and type of pain (acute, chronic, and cancer pain) [55]. These racial and ethnic disparities persist even after statistically adjusting for age, gender, and pain intensity [105].

Prejudices, stigmas, false beliefs, and implicit biases may be driving racial and ethnic disparities in pain management. Physicians' limited awareness of their own cultural beliefs and stereotypes regarding pain and the use of analgesics in patients of ethnic and racial minorities appears to be a major contributing factor to these disparities [105]. Implicit bias from providers has been associated with clinically meaningful differences in pain management compared to Black and White patients, including fewer prescribed pain medications, lower quality of care, and less patient-centered communication [47, 127]. In a study by Hoffman et al., medical trainees' (students and residents) bias was shown to be associated with false beliefs that Black patients have greater pain tolerance, thicker skin, and feel less pain than White patients [66]. Furthermore, the study showed that trainees who endorsed these false beliefs were less likely to prescribe appropriate pain treatments for Black patients as compared with White patients. Failure to address these biases will only perpetuate the inequities of pain assessment and treatment in racial and ethnic minority groups.

Sex and Gender Bias in Pain Management

Sex refers to the biological, genetic, and physiological attributes of an individual, whereas gender refers to the socially constructed norms, roles, relationships, and behavior attributed to women and men, irrespective of biological differences (i.e., anatomy, hormones, etc.) [109, 118]. However, for purposes of this section of the chapter, the multidimensional term "sex/gender" will be utilized to emphasize both the biological and social impacts of pain management. Clinical evidence suggests an underestimation and undertreatment of pain in female patients. Females are less likely to be prescribed analgesics and opioids, referred for specialty care, and wait longer to receive pain treatment [27, 30, 40, 131]. There is a distinction between the definitions of sex and gender, and it is not recommended to use these terms interchangeably.

Sex/gender stereotypes can influence the assessment and treatment of pain in female patients and, in return, result in a lack of equity and access to care [65, 103, 130, 164]. Robinson et al. created the Gender Role Expectations of Pain (GREP) questionnaire. This is a standardized measure developed to assess a subject's perceptions of males and females in relation to their pain sensitivity, pain endurance, and willingness to report pain [124]. Studies using the GREP measurement have found that women are viewed as more willing to report pain, more sensitive to pain, and less able to endure pain than men [34, 158]. Based on a literature review of 77 articles aimed at analyzing sex/gender perceptions and treatment bias of pain in men and women, women were commonly described as sensitive, hysterical, emotional, complaining, fabricating pain, and "all in her head," whereas men were described as stoic, autonomous, in control, and tolerating pain [130]. Other studies provide examples of these stigmas, including that women complain more than men, women are not accurate historians, and women have better pain tolerance and coping skills than men [65]. In instances where both male and female patients report similar pain experiences, female patients tend to be directed toward psychotherapy, while men are prescribed analgesics [16, 65, 130, 164]. These practices can underestimate the female pain experience, as many women express feelings of neglect and minimization by providers [65, 96, 130, 164]. These gender pain stereotypes may represent the underlying gender biases in pain assessment and treatment.

Managing pain in transgender and gender-diverse patients can present unique circumstances and challenges. Strath et al. found that women (whether cisgender or transgender) reported greater chronic pain severity than cisgender men [142]. Adverse childhood experiences, including sexual trauma, in LGBTQ+-identifying patients have been associated with increased chronic pain (Shirsat et al. 2024). In particular, higher rates of chronic pain have been observed in transgender and gender-diverse individuals compared to cisgender participants [167, 168]. In a large cohort study of nearly 100,000 transgender patients, Tabernacki and colleagues found a higher likelihood of chronic pain diagnoses in those receiving gender-affirming hormone therapy with either testosterone or estrogen [168]. However, data from previous studies have shown mixed effects of hormones on pain perception, and additional prospective research is needed.

Lack of trust in the healthcare system, lack of provider education, and bias have created significant disparities in health outcomes for transgender and gender-diverse patients.

The 2011 National Transgender Discrimination Survey found that 28% of respondents had postponed necessary medical care when ill, a third had avoided preventive care, and approximately one in five had been refused care related to their gender identity or expression. The study also found that half of the respondents reported needing to teach their provider about transgender care [54]. Similarly, in the 2015 United States Transgender Survey, 33% of nearly 30,000 participants reported at least one negative experience with a healthcare practitioner in the past year [74].

Specific practices commonly utilized in the transgender and gender-diverse community, including chest binding and genital tucking, can lead to pain. However, these practices can help improve mental health/decrease gender dysphoria. It should not be recommended to avoid these practices, but perhaps suggesting "off days" when patients are at home can be a reasonable suggestion to reduce pain. Clinicians should be sensitive to patient preferences and potential trauma when performing a physical exam or procedure. For example, a clinician can consider if a binder may be left in place rather than automatically instructing the patient to remove all clothing [141].

Age Bias in Pain Management

Negative age stereotypes can contribute to chronic pain in older adults [83]. There is a widely held belief/assumption that the chronic pain of older adults is inevitable and a consequence of aging [33, 89]. A qualitative study by Makris et al. uncovered themes including beliefs about the age-related inevitability of restricting back pain [89]. This study suggests that patient-provider interactions can serve as a deterrent for patients to seek care for their pain.

Negative age stereotypes, age discrimination, and age attribution have been found to act as mediators between negative age stereotypes and chronic pain [83]. A recent cohort study evaluated participants who were pain-free at baseline. Participants who endured negative age stereotypes were 32% more likely to develop chronic pain in the next 7 years than those who had experienced positive age stereotypes [83].

Opioid Use and Substance Use Disorder Stigma

Studies show that patients who are treated with opioid therapy are predisposed to stigmas and discrimination from healthcare providers, family, friends, and society at large [32, 82, 94, 152]. These stigmas can cause patients to feel judged, guilty, and embarrassed, which can worsen mental health. This can lead to an exacerbation of anxiety and depression, ultimately causing further health decline [136].

Patients with substance use disorder (SUD) and chronic pain also face overt stigmas [143]. These stigmas create barriers for comorbid pain treatment, as well as participation in medication-assisted therapy and similar programs for SUD [29, 129]. Studies report significant stigmas associated with naloxone [160], methadone, and buprenorphine treatment [82]. Associated stigmas pose a significant barrier to patients with SUD seeking treatment, with 20.5% not seeking treatment because of negative consequences associated with their work, and around 17% being concerned about negative judgments by friends or community [151].

Patients are not the only ones subjected to stigmas. Healthcare providers who treat acute and chronic pain with opioids can face stigmas from the healthcare system and coworkers that can discourage them from appropriately prescribing opioids [151].

Provider Bias Toward Alternative Treatments

Alternative treatments, also referred to as complementary and integrative health approaches, include meditation, yoga, acupuncture, massage, osteopathic and chiropractic manipulation, naturopathy, and guided imagery/progressive muscle relaxation. Integrative health, by definition, incorporates conventional and complementary health approaches in coordination [151]. Despite being commonly accepted as a valuable component of a multimodal interdisciplinary approach to pain management and being included in guidelines and best practice statements, complementary and integrative health approaches are often underutilized. One reason for this could be secondary to provider bias against the use of complementary and integrated health approaches, potentially due to concerns of a lack of high-quality evidence to clearly support their use. Additionally, a lack of training or knowledge of alternative treatments and cost concerns may play a role.

Mitigation Strategies to Bias, Stigmas, and Stereotypes in Pain Management

Recommendations for addressing the complex challenges surrounding pain management and stigmatized care emphasize the need for targeted and comprehensive education, intentional training, and awareness campaigns at organizational, individual provider, and societal levels (Table 26.2) [25]. General recommendations for culturally and medically appropriate care for transgender and gender-diverse patients are summarized in Table 26.3.

Understanding the influence of race, social determinants, SUD, sex, gender, and age on pain outcomes requires a multilevel approach. Education is paramount in reducing stigma associated with pain and addiction while fostering understanding of underlying disease processes. Medical

Table 26.2 Mitigation Strategies to bias, stigmas, and stereotypes in pain management

Level	Mitigation strategy
Organizational	"Periodically *surveying providers and staff members* to better understand how they perceive the organization's policies and actions related to improving diversity and addressing discrimination" [25]
	"*Administering the implicit association test (IAT)* to assess subconscious feelings, attitudes, and thoughts among providers that may contribute to stereotypes and bias in treatment decisions" [25]
	"*Developing and consistently using a protocol* to investigate reports of discrimination or unfair policies and practices" [25]
	"*Supporting workforce training* that raises awareness about bias and health disparities and teaches strategies that promote health equity" [25]
	"*Leveraging data capabilities* to (a) monitor and compare patient treatment and outcomes by race, gender, and socioeconomic indicators and (b) implement quality improvement initiatives" [25]
	"Devising strategies to *address the burden of high cognitive workload*, which may result in providers defaulting to automatic reasoning and decision-making processes that are vulnerable to bias" [25]
	"*Promoting diversity, empathy, and understanding throughout the organization* via methods such as intergroup and equal-status contact, team building, positive association, and counter-stereotype exposure" [25]
Provider	"*Participating in training* to improve situational awareness and better understand metacognition" [25]
	"Learning and implementing skills such as *perspective-taking, emotional regulation, and partnership-building* to reduce bias and promote empathy, positive feelings, and patient-centered care" [25]
	"Working toward a better *understanding of cultural beliefs, attitudes, and values that affect various patient populations*" [25]
	"Using techniques and methods to *assist in cross-cultural communication, break down health literacy barriers, and improve provider-patient communication*. Examples of such techniques and methods include motivational interviewing" [25]
	"Consciously *making an effort to see each patient as a unique individual* rather than applying stereotypical characteristics, and respecting their personal values, experiences, preferences, and expressed needs" [25]
	"Using clinical pathways, *adhering to established standards of care, and practicing evidence-based medicine*" [25]
	"*Adhering to the ethical principles of autonomy* (patients' right to make decisions about their healthcare), *beneficence* (making decisions and taking actions that will benefit patients), *nonmaleficence* (making decisions and taking actions that will not harm patients), and *justibce* (treating patients fairly and equally according to their situations)" [25]
Societal	"Counter societal attitudes that equate pain with weakness through an awareness campaign that urges early treatment for pain that persists beyond the expected duration for that condition or injury" [151]

Table 26.3 Considerations for providing appropriate care to transgender and gender-diverse patients

Avoid stigmatizing language
Ask pronouns, how they identify, and sex assigned at birth; use current name and pronouns
Assess organ inventory uncoupled from gender when history-taking
Perform trauma-sensitive exams with a chaperone and appropriate pain control procedures
Be aware of bias, undertreatment, possible trauma, anxiety, depression, and substance use
Recognize that more research is needed to inform best practices

Adapted from Strand et al. [141]

school curricula should emphasize not only dispelling myths about biological differences but also fostering structural humility among students [132]. Research efforts should focus on the use of race as an independent variable without considering broader social contexts; this can help ensure that differential opportunities and social vulnerabilities are accounted for [132]. Increasing diversity in medical education admissions and faculty, alongside implementing antiracism and inclusive strategies, is crucial for promoting health equity [132].

Progress has been made toward eliminating barriers to accessing complementary and alternative strategies, leading to increased uptake. More recently, the body of evidence supporting the efficacy of complementary health approaches has increased [135]. Insurance coverage for some interventions, such as acupuncture, has also improved patient access. According to research by Nahin and colleagues, the percentage of respondents from the National Health Interview Survey (NHIS) that reported using at least one complementary health approach increased from 19.2% in 2002 to 36.7% in 2022. Among those using complementary health approaches, the percentage using them for pain management increased from 42.3% in 2002 to 49.2% in 2022 [106].

In summary, a multifaceted approach involving education, organizational strategies, and provider-level interventions is essential for addressing disparities in pain management and promoting health equity in healthcare systems. By implementing these recommendations, healthcare providers can work toward a more just and inclusive healthcare system that delivers high-quality care to all patients.

Therapeutic Alliance and Patient Autonomy

Lack of Trust and Therapeutic Alliance

A trusting relationship between a healthcare provider and patient is critical to providing the highest quality of care and has been shown to predict pain management outcomes [46,

Table 26.4 Example responses for empathetic communication

"Our team is here to help you through this"
"What you just said really helps me understand the situation better"
"Dealing with this has been such a big part of your life and taken so much energy"
"We will work hard to get you the support that you need"
"Help me understand more about…"
"I can see how dealing with this might be (challenging/frustrating/ overwhelming)"
"I'm really impressed by all that you've done to manage your illness"

Excerpted from: National Center for Ethics in Health Care Goals of Care Conversations Skills Training for Clinicians [108]

81]. Correlations have been demonstrated between physician empathy, patient overall trust, trust in the physician's benevolence and competence, and the physician-patient relationship [161]. In particular, physician empathy has a significant positive impact on outcomes in the treatment of chronic pain, including pain scores and quality of life [24]. Barriers to empathic communication include lack of time, not being familiar with the healthcare provider, institutional culture and workload, and medical specialty. Other patient factors, such as the patient's level of clinical dysfunction, personality, self-awareness, level of education, and ability to communicate clearly, can also play a factor [75].

Mitigation Strategies for Lack of Trust and Therapeutic Alliance

Effective Communication

Affirming statements can help engage patients and build trust (Table 26.4). Although rigorously designed studies are relatively few, targeted empathy training has been found efficacious [78, 99, 121, 139]. Numerous tools are available to assess empathy development, including the Jefferson Scale of Physician Empathy (JSPE), the Interpersonal Reactivity Index (IRI), the Hogan Empathy Scale, the Balanced Emotional Empathy Scale (BEES), the Barrett-Lennard Scale, the Accurate Empathy Scale, and the Consultation and Relational Empathy Measure (CARE). Additionally, patient perceptions have been used to evaluate provider empathy [146].

Appropriate language should be utilized in chart documentation to avoid perpetuating bias, as this could affect how future providers treat pain [53]. Not only can implicit and explicit bias affect providers' perceptions and judgment, but negative interpersonal interactions (e.g., providers not listening and not allowing the patient to contribute to decision-making) and unresolved pain have been associated with perceived racial/ethnic discrimination by providers among patients with pain [58] and inequities in patient experience [128], as already discussed.

Shared Decision-Making and Preserving Patient Autonomy

Shared decision-making involves clinicians and patients coming together to discuss the best available practices based on patient values and preferences [43]. Determining the patient's goals and expectations for the management of their pain is an important first step. Asking open-ended questions may improve visit efficiency and allow clinicians to gather valuable details about the patient's past experiences and perceptions about what has been effective in relieving their pain. A recent qualitative review of chronic pain clinic intake forms found that patients often added unprompted information to their intake forms to provide more information [79]. Another study found that qualitative survey respondents would like for their providers to ask how pain affects their lifestyle and inquire about their goals using open-ended questions [14]. It should also be considered that a patient in severe pain may not be able to effectively engage in conversation.

Once goals are set and prioritized, options should be discussed for achieving those goals and weighing the associated risks and benefits. Goal-based decisions should be agreed upon, and a plan to evaluate progress can then be made [44].

According to self-determination theory, autonomy, competence, and relatedness are key in fostering the intrinsic motivation necessary for health behavior change. This theory has been applied to chronic disease, pain management, and medication adherence interventions [80, 112, 126, 159]. Healthcare providers' support of autonomy has been shown to have a significant effect on pain management behavior [80].

Empowered with choice and autonomous motivation, patients can maximize self-management techniques to help achieve individualized goals. Patients should be provided with self-management strategies and encouraged to utilize them. Supported self-management strategies have been shown to improve pain outcomes [39, 117]. Support for self-management can include addressing health literacy and medical obstacles, motivational interviewing, action planning, and problem-solving to address patient concerns; linking patients with peer/community support; and regularly scheduled follow-up (in person, by phone, or by email) with planned time to address self-management needs [31].

Social Determinants of Health

According to Healthy People 2030, "Social determinants of health (SDoH) are the conditions in the environments where people are born, live, learn, work, play, worship, and age that affect a wide range of health, functioning, and quality-of-life outcomes and risks" [63]. Understanding the connection between SDoH and pain management is necessary for addressing the multifaceted needs of individuals living with pain. The five main domains of SDoH—economic stability, education access and quality, healthcare access and quality, neighborhood and built environment, and social and community context—all can have an impact on treatment outcomes, patient satisfaction, and overall well-being [63].

Economic Stability

Chronic pain is an expensive health concern for both patients and the healthcare system. In the United States, approximately 100 million adults experience chronic pain and have expenses for treatment, missed work costs, and lower wages [49]. The financial cost of pain, including healthcare costs and lost productivity, is estimated to be $560 to $635 billion annually. For the most effective pain management, multidisciplinary approaches using non-pharmacological treatments (e.g., physical therapy, acupuncture, or cognitive behavioral therapy) are recommended. Unfortunately, insurance coverage for these non-pharmacological services is variable, and the expenses of seeing multiple providers can become costly for patients [23, 62].

Patients with a lower socioeconomic status are particularly affected by the high cost of pain management. A review of 31 articles found that while opioid prescribing rates were higher among patients with lower socioeconomic status, these patients are less likely to receive other medications commonly used to treat chronic pain [8]. Additionally, lower socioeconomic status has been consistently linked with increased rates of chronic pain [86, 119].

Education Access and Quality

Patient education is a key factor in managing pain. Pain is a complex illness with multiple contributing factors, subjectivity, and various treatment options. Poor understanding of both medical and non-pharmacological treatment strategies, as well as poor knowledge of a patient's own disease state and symptom management, have been identified as barriers to pain management [116]. Studies have found that lack of education and knowledge can lead to increased opioid use, increased reliance on ineffective or harmful self-treatments, and overall worse outcomes [8, 26, 116, 162, 163].

Education on pain management can be complex and, when it does not align with a patient's health literacy, can lead to misunderstanding and confusion. Oosterhaven et al. studied patients' understanding of delivered pain neuroscience education, a form of education commonly provided to patients to explain the neurobiology and neuropsychology of pain, and found patients with low health literacy had difficulties understanding and applying the information explained [115]. It was noted that adjustment of content to health literacy level and the teach-back method were not employed in the education provided to these patients, but they should be considered. More information on assessing pain and health literacy can be found in Chap. 34.

Healthcare Access and Quality

Access to Health Care

Limited access to healthcare can create significant barriers to effective pain management. Geographic distance to pain specialists, transportation concerns, and long wait times for appointments can lead to delays in treatment, undertreatment, and ultimately lower quality of life [36, 145]. This can be particularly concerning for individuals with chronic pain who require long-term care and monitoring. A major factor leading to access issues is the lack of healthcare providers trained in pain management, especially in rural areas [22].

Other vulnerable patient populations with access barriers include those who are incarcerated and those of migrant/refugee populations. Incarcerated patients have reported barriers to receiving health care, including cost, long wait times, lack of resources to research health information, and inadequate pain management [77]. Although the National Commission on Correctional Health Care has put out a statement that incarcerated individuals should receive care following the current guidelines, treatment options, including non-pharmacological management in different facilities, may vary, limiting access to these individuals [111]. In the migrant/refugee population, a systematic review found that a multidisciplinary approach to pain management improves outcomes, similar to other populations [7]. Unfortunately, many of these patients are left uninsured due to either being ineligible for certain federal programs or having difficulty navigating enrollment; without insurance, these patients would be forced to pay out of pocket for their care [3].

Communication Challenges

Effective communication is necessary for providing high-quality healthcare. Communication barriers not only impact understanding, trust, and satisfaction but can also lead to worse health outcomes [2]. Furthermore, the subjective nature of many pain conditions makes understanding the patients' perspective an important factor in providing effective treatment [50]. Communication can be impacted by patients, healthcare providers, and outside factors. According to the Institute for Healthcare Advancement (IHA), common barriers to communication in healthcare include language barriers, cultural and social differences, disabilities and other challenges, low health literacy, complexity of health topics, and lack of time [70].

Language barriers often occur when patients and healthcare personnel speak different native languages [137]. These barriers can result in miscommunication, diminished satisfaction, compromised healthcare quality, and decreased patient safety [2, 37]. In addition to the impact on patients, Limited English Proficiency (LEP) can lead to increased healthcare worker stress and is attributed as one of the largest obstacles for providing timely care [4, 52]. With more than 25 million people in the United States having LEP, this becomes a critical barrier to address [38], especially when dealing with a subjective illness such as pain. A systematic review found that patients with LEP frequently reported lower pain scores, and providers faced challenges interpreting and diagnosing pain in this population, which overall can lead to inadequate pain management [88]. In addition to appropriately assessing and managing the patient's pain, proper communication is necessary for education on safe and appropriate use of any treatments provided. Pain management treatments can be complex, and misunderstanding the indication, directions, or monitoring parameters can lead to medication errors [138].

Communicating using inclusive language and cultural competence is important when working with people from diverse backgrounds. With many stigmas and biases regarding pain management in diverse populations, lack of appropriate communication can lead to mistrust and undertreatment (*see section on stigmas above*). Additionally, recognizing that communication of pain can be largely impacted by a person's cultural, ethnic, and religious background is required for appropriate assessment and management. In some cultures, individuals avoid expressing their pain, while in others, pain is expressed through moaning, crying, or facial expressions [125]. Lor and colleagues observed that patients of the Hmong culture express pain through stories and metaphors and are not as direct about their pain [87]. Religious beliefs have also been shown to impact the expression of pain and coping [107]. Therefore, a lack of understanding of how a patient may respond to pain based on their diverse background can lead to misinterpretation of pain and inadequate treatment.

Individuals with the inability to verbally communicate can have their pain mismanaged and undertreated. Populations at risk are pediatric patients, patients with disabilities (physical or intellectual), and those who are intubated/sedated. While physiologic and behavioral observations have been used to develop several tools for observing pain in nonverbal patients, there is still risk for improper assessment and management of pain [95]. In the pediatric population, studies have found that although physiologic and behavioral observations are helpful, they can result in inaccurate pain scores. Fear or distress could inflate intensity scores, while playing through pain can lead to falsely low scores [73]. In patients with physical or intellectual disabilities impacting verbal communication, there are similar concerns. Lastly, for patients who are intubated/sedated, it has been reported that pain assessments can be forgotten or misused due to organizational challenges, provider attitudes, and lack of knowledge [35, 120].

Pain can be a complex illness to express and assess. Furthermore, once pain is assessed and treatments are initiated, the complexity of regimens can be difficult to understand. Therefore, addressing health literacy barriers becomes increasingly significant (*see* Chap. 34).

Additional communication barriers include a lack of provider time and miscommunication between interprofessional teams. Pain management can be complex and time-consuming, requiring additional appointment time [68]. Healthcare providers need time not only to accurately assess a patient's pain but also to provide appropriate education. In addition to patient communication, appropriate pain management often requires an interdisciplinary approach with referrals and communication with other members of the patient's healthcare team. Although studies have shown an interdisciplinary approach to pain management to be the most effective, in practice, patients frequently report frustration with miscommunication between healthcare providers and can get "stuck in the middle" of opposing views [140].

Neighborhood and Built Environment

The neighborhood and living environment for individuals can impact their health outcomes. Living in impoverished neighborhoods or having low socioeconomic status has been associated with long-term stress that can negatively affect pain response [91]. Unsafe living environments may also lead to increased stress and can impact a patient's physical activity [91], which has been associated with worse pain, decreased physical function, and poorer quality of life [51]. Limited access to green space has also been associated with decreased pain tolerance and worse health outcomes [21, 85].

In addition to living environments, work environments, particularly those with high physical demands, can contribute to the development or exacerbation of chronic pain. Hurwitz and colleagues found that patients with low socioeconomic status are more likely to have occupations associated with higher rates of accidents, leading to pain and disabilities [69]. Furthermore, a systematic review reported that manual jobs and nonformal employment are more associated with disability after back surgery and a decreased chance of returning to work [163].

Social and Community Context

Relationships and community support networks are influential for improving health outcomes and quality of life [67]. Unfortunately, living with chronic pain can lead to withdrawal from social activities, isolation, conflict, and family dysfunction, which in turn can worsen pain outcomes [12, 84]. Patients with a significant disability caused by pain will often need to rely more on their support systems to perform activities of daily living, which can lead to more family dysfunction [84]. Understanding this cyclical connection is important to properly support patients and address pain.

Although relationships and community support networks can improve outcomes when they are positive and encouraging, relationships and other social influences that diminish or invalidate an individual's pain can result in future underrating of pain [18]. Nicola et al. conducted a review and thematic analysis of pain narratives and found that invalidation of pain by self, friends, family, and providers often resulted in emotional distress and threats to individuals' self-image [113]. A pain invalidation scale (Pain-IS) has been developed and can be used as a tool by healthcare providers to identify areas that could be impacting pain management and prompt a discussion with the patient [114].

Mitigation Strategies for SDoH

SDoH Screening and Resources

SDoH can vary greatly, and it is common for patients to have more than one SDoH barrier to overcome when providing care. Identifying SDoH barriers specific to each individual is the first step to overcoming them. There are several reputable SDoH screening tools available; therefore, healthcare workers should work with their team to find one that best fits their and their patient's needs [1, 101]. After screening for SDoH, it is important to provide patients with resources to overcome barriers they may be facing. Connecting patients with social workers can facilitate this process and reduce healthcare inequities for vulnerable patient populations. Healthcare workers can also support change beyond the patient level through advocacy efforts and community partnerships [11]. By overcoming SDoH barriers, this can improve healthcare outcomes and increase the quality of life for patients living with pain [63].

Education

Efforts to address educational barriers must prioritize accessible education and resources, alongside targeted interventions aimed at improving healthcare literacy and patient-provider education among vulnerable populations. Oosterhaven et al. suggest the following:

> Lessons can be learned from the extensive literature on health literacy and patient education: decrease the complexity of the information by using plain language; be specific and limit the information ('Askme3' questions: (1) what their main problem is, (2) what they need to do, and (3) why it is important to them), and make sure that a patient has understood the information given (apply the teach-back method) [115].

Mittinty and colleagues found that participants who observed changes in pain cognition, and self-management after receiving pain education reported lower pain intensity and higher expectations of recovery than those who did not experience a change [100]. In a recent systematic review including 22 randomized controlled trials, mobile health (mHealth) applications used to expand access for patient education, monitoring, and treatment of various chronic pain conditions were shown to reduce pain intensity and improve functional disability and quality of life [102].

Effective Communication

There are many types of communication barriers that can occur when treating pain. To overcome these barriers, it is important that healthcare workers equip themselves with the education and tools necessary for success. To overcome language barriers, language concordance between patient and provider is usually considered ideal but not always possible and, in some cases, results in worse outcomes [37]. When healthcare personnel and patients do not speak the same language, the use of interpreters or translation services like "Google Translate and MediBabble" is encouraged, although it can come with challenges, including accessibility concerns, increased time for service, and the chance of misinterpretation [2, 4]. Other facilitators helping patients with LEP are having specific organizational strategies, bedside tools, and structured assessments for pain [52]. To overcome barriers related to working with patients from different backgrounds and cultures, it is important to use patient-centered language and ensure healthcare personnel are properly trained on cultural competence (Table 26.2). As discussed, pain is a subjective illness that requires the healthcare team to be diligent about frequent, comprehensive assessment of pain, especially for those who are unable to effectively communicate their pain. Building relationships with patients suffering from pain can support bidirectional communication that supports effective assessment and management of pain. Actively listening to patients' concerns, developing a patient-centered plan, remaining nonjudgmental, and being open with communication results in stronger provider-patient relationships [59, 157]. Lastly, healthcare personnel need to diligently communicate information to other members of the team and use support staff for efficiency.

Incorrect Provider Practices and Lack of Evidence-Based Medicine

Inadequate Training and Lack of Credentialing

Inadequate training in pain assessment and management is a challenge affecting members of various healthcare disciplines. It persists across the spectrum of care, from acute inpatient medical and surgical services to outpatient chronic management. Additionally, although many interventional strategies of varying complexity (e.g., trigger point injections, nerve block or ablation, spinal cord stimulation) can be used to help manage chronic pain, more evidence is needed to inform guidelines for the use of these methods, and proper credentialing is needed for clinicians providing these therapies [151].

Barriers to effective pain management in critical care have been extensively evaluated [5, 120]. Numerous barriers were identified; these can include psychological (knowledge) and physical capability, opportunity, motivation, patients' inability to communicate, physicians' prescription of analgesics being independent of pain scores evaluation, and absence of standardized guidelines and protocols for pain evaluation and control. Caregivers may also lack understanding about multimodal analgesia and treating all aspects of what is affecting pain, such as sleep and mood.

Lack of Awareness and Support of Protocols

Lack of awareness of multimodal pain management strategies can lead to poorly controlled acute pain, which is associated with an increased risk of developing chronic pain [134]. This association has been seen across many practice settings, including postsurgical patients and those with medical illnesses.

Multimodal pain management, as part of Enhanced Recovery After Surgery (ERAS) protocols, has become a mainstay of perioperative care worldwide. Barriers to adherence to ERAS protocols include inadequate staff, lack of support/accountability of hospital administration, variability of uptake at different locations, "poor patient-doctor collaboration," poor communication among multidisciplinary team members, and cost [76, 156]. Examples of inconsistent utilization of multimodal pain management strategies in the hospital setting include discharging patients on opioids despite requiring little to no opioids while in the hospital [19] or missed doses of scheduled non-opioids due to patient refusal or nurse non-administration [156].

Mitigation Strategies for Incorrect Provider Practices and Lack of Evidence-Based Medicine

Training and Education for Healthcare Professionals

Educational interventions for both healthcare profession students and continuing education for practicing providers can improve learner perceptions of their knowledge and performance on assessments. There is still room, however, for improvement in the depth and breadth of pain topics, interprofessional education, and application of knowledge to real-world scenarios [13, 60, 61, 90, 133, 150, 153]. Specific recommendations for an interprofessional pain curriculum, as well as curricula for various individual healthcare disciplines, have been made by the International Association for the Study of Pain (IASP). The interprofessional curriculum's broad content categories include the multidimensional nature of pain, pain assessment and measurement, pain management, and clinical conditions (application to various disease states and patient populations). In addition, the IASP has produced a Multidisciplinary Pain Center Development Manual.

Consultation with an interdisciplinary pain medicine team, if available, and specialists for the management of underlying disease states that contribute to pain should be sought to ensure the best patient outcomes [151]. Maintaining frequent and open communication among the primary treatment team or provider and consultants is essential. Unfortunately, in many rural and other underserved areas, pain management specialists and teams are not readily available. Some remedies do exist, however, such as telehealth visits for patients and tele-education to connect primary care doctors in remote areas with specialists in academic medical centers. An example of this is the "Extension for Community Healthcare Outcomes" (ECHO) project, which allows primary care providers to engage in educational activities with experts who also work together with them to comanage patients [148, 165].

Awareness and Support of Protocols

Health system-wide support for interventions and education for both healthcare professionals and patients to improve awareness and share outcomes and successes could improve utilization of appropriate multimodal pain management strategies. More specifically, educational interventions for hospital nurses utilizing a variety of methods (i.e., lecture-based, skills-based, group discussion, role-play, feedback/testing, and ongoing support) have been associated with increased assessment of pain by nurses and, in some studies, improvements in pain scores [42]. Additionally, higher scores on a survey assessing pain knowledge, skills, and attitudes were correlated with higher Hospital Consumer Assessment of Healthcare Providers (HCAHPS) scores [20].

Healthcare System Regulatory and Operational Challenges

When delivering pain management services, it is imperative to acknowledge the substantial impact of healthcare system regulations and resultant barriers. These regulations serve as guiding frameworks that shape the accessibility, quality, and delivery of pain management interventions within healthcare systems. A comprehensive understanding of healthcare system regulations and barriers is essential for healthcare practitioners and policymakers alike, as it informs strategies aimed at optimizing pain management services and improving patient outcomes. Efforts to mitigate these barriers and enhance regulatory frameworks are integral to ensuring equitable access to high-quality pain care for all individuals within the healthcare system.

Regulatory and Insurance Restrictions

Regulatory and insurance restrictions, along with reimbursement issues, present significant challenges to pain management, impacting both healthcare providers and patients. A primary concern is increasing regulations surrounding opioid prescribing in response to the opioid epidemic. Restrictions are in place to limit misuse but can impact access [92]. The American Medical Society (AMA) has put out several statements opposing hard thresholds for opioid prescribing and "high prescriber" lists at pharmacies, as this can limit access to care [123]. The CDC also updated its clinical practice guidelines for prescribing opioids for pain to clarify that the information is a guide and should not be used as a hard limit for developing policies and insurance restrictions for higher-dose opioids [41].

Additionally, insurance reimbursement policies may limit access to certain pain management interventions and therapies. Some insurance plans have restrictions on coverage for non-pharmacological treatments such as physical therapy, acupuncture, or cognitive behavioral therapy, despite evidence supporting their efficacy in managing chronic pain [23, 62]. Patients may encounter barriers to accessing these alternative treatments due to limited insurance coverage, high out-of-pocket costs, or pre-authorization requirements, which restrict their ability to obtain comprehensive care.

Restrictive Healthcare System Policies

Restrictive healthcare system policies intended to stem the opioid epidemic may inadvertently lead to decreased access to appropriate pain management in some cases. For example, it has become common for emergency departments to restrict the use of opioids for pain management. As mentioned previously, bundled payment models may lead to decreased spending on restorative (rehabilitation) services such as physical and occupational therapies [110]. Lastly, formulary limitations in both the inpatient and outpatient settings may lead to a patient being transitioned from a medication that has been effective for them to an alternative based on hospital protocol or insurance coverage.

Laws

Changes to state and federal law have the potential to create barriers to patient access to pain medications. Due to concerns about medication misuse and the opioid epidemic, many states have enacted restrictions on initial opioid day supplies for the treatment of acute pain. Federally, hydrocodone-containing products were reclassified as Schedule II narcotics, which cannot be refilled, and several states have classified gabapentin as a controlled substance or required refill reporting to prescription drug monitoring programs.

Medication Shortages

In recent years, medication shortages have also contributed to limitations in accessing various forms of analgesia. Supplies of both opioid and non-opioid medications have been affected by manufacturing delays, product discontinuations, contamination, shortages of raw materials or ingredients, and legal limits on production. Some examples include injectable ketamine used as monotherapy or for pain cocktails, certain formulations of gabapentin, injectable ketorolac, injectable lidocaine, and topical products [10, 45].

In addition, opioid analgesic availability may be limited in certain neighborhoods, particularly communities of color and low-income areas [56, 104]. The reasons for this disparity have not been fully elucidated, and more recent survey results are conflicting [93].

Mitigating Strategies for Healthcare System Regulatory and Operational Challenges

Advocacy and Research

Healthcare professionals should continue to advocate for decreased restrictions on providing patient care. Several organizations, including the AMA, have put out statements opposing insurance barriers and regulations that impact quality care for patients suffering from pain [123]. Additionally, continued research showing the benefits of non-pharmacological treatments can support increased buy-in and coverage for patients.

Education/Training

As previously discussed, education for both healthcare providers and patients within the system is essential when new policies are put in place. Policies and practices should be regularly reviewed (i.e., medication use evaluations, satisfaction surveys, and evaluation of recent evidence) and updated as needed to ensure goals are being met. Patients should be individually assessed, and treatment regimens should be tailored based on patient-specific factors rather than broadly applying the same process to all situations.

While state and federal laws may be a barrier to prescribing medication in some instances, regulations can also lead to safer medication use and encourage healthcare providers to acquire additional pain management knowledge. Many states now require initial licensure applicants to complete training in pain management and/or require continuing education in pain management topics for licensure renewal.

Addressing Drug Shortages

Although the drug industry landscape is constantly changing, drug shortages have remained a significant concern for many years. Due to the large number of drug shortages and their potential to negatively impact patient care, the U.S. The Food and Drug Administration (FDA) and organizations such as the American Society of Health-System Pharmacists maintain continuously updated drug shortage lists that contain information such as which specific products are unavailable, reasons for the shortage, possible alternatives, and an estimate of the expected duration of the shortage, if known. Shortages are typically managed by placing drugs on allocation and organizational prioritization of use for those who most need them or in situations where there is no acceptable alternative. Substitution with alternate products and compounded versions has led to medication errors and thus should be undertaken with extreme caution and transparency. A Failure Mode and Effects Analysis (FMEA) can be undertaken to proactively assess and mitigate risks associated with switching to alternatives, including, but not limited to, look-alike/sound-alike issues, calculation or administration errors, and toxicity monitoring [71].

Application to Clinical Practice

An interprofessional team is in the best position to overcome the many barriers patients experience when seeking treatment for their pain. It is critical that a well-trained team work effectively together to identify and mitigate barriers to pain management using a variety of strategies to provide holistic, person-first care according to the biopsychosocial model. The IASP's Multidisciplinary Pain Management Clinic Development Manual contains recommendations for necessary staff, desirable team characteristics, and core competencies for interprofessional collaborative practice. These have been published by the Interprofessional Education Collaborative (Table 26.5). Staff should include a physician leader and ideally other provider(s) trained in pain medicine (e.g., additional physicians, nurse practitioners, and physician assistants), nurse(s), clinical psychologist(s), behavioral health specialist(s), physical and occupational therapists, pharmacists, medical social workers, and administrative support. Roles and responsibilities, including clinical and administrative tasks, should be clearly defined.

Table 26.5 Desirable characteristics for pain center personnel and Interprofessional Education Collaborative (IPEC) core competencies for interprofessional collaborative practice

Team characteristics (IASP)	IPEC core competencies
1. Understand the main objectives of the center and act accordingly 2. Commit to working as a member of a multidisciplinary team 3. Understand the contribution of psychosocial issues to chronic pain 4. Show empathy to all patients 5. Possess and use effective communication skills 6. Understand and respect cultural norms in their respective communities 7. Participate in continuing professional development 8. Commit to ethical clinical practice	*Values and ethics:* Work with team members to maintain a climate of shared values, ethical conduct, and mutual respect *Roles and responsibilities:* Use the knowledge of one's own role and team members' expertise to address individual and population health outcomes *Communication:* Communicate in a responsive, responsible, respectful, and compassionate manner with the team members *Teams and teamwork:* Apply values and principles of the science of teamwork to adapt one's own role in a variety of team settings

Excerpted from: International Association for the Study of Pain Multidisciplinary Pain Center Toolkit Advisory Group [72] and Zorek et al. [166]

Key Themes

- Implicit and explicit biases and stigmas can create disparities in access to care for many patients; however, education, organizational strategies, and provider-level intervention can be utilized to help address these disparities.
- Effective communication, shared decision-making, and preserving patient autonomy are key elements to building trust and maintaining therapeutic alliances when managing pain.
- All five main domains of SDoH—economic stability, education access and quality, health care access and qual-

ity, neighborhood and built environment, and social and community context—need to be considered and addressed when caring for patients living with pain.

- Practice gaps related to inadequate healthcare professional training, lack of awareness and/or support for protocols, and the need for more strategic patient education interventions continue to exist. Specialized training and credentialing of providers are needed.
- Healthcare system policies and regulations intended to stem the opioid epidemic and reduce healthcare costs, as well as medication shortages, have impacted access to some forms of analgesia and holistic pain management strategies. Updates to policies and insurance criteria, considering evolving medical literature and current clinical practice guidelines, could benefit millions of patients living with pain.

Conclusion

Pain management is complex, multifaceted, and associated with many barriers to quality care. Although it is impossible to eliminate all barriers, mitigation strategies should be employed to improve the equity and well-being of patients suffering from pain. By collectively addressing these challenges, we can strive toward a healthcare landscape where every individual living with pain receives the comprehensive, compassionate, and evidence-based care they deserve.

References

1. AHRQ. SDOH & practice improvement. Agency for Healthcare Research and Quality; 2023. https://wwwahrqgov/sdoh/practice-improvementhtml Accessed 30 Mar 2024.
2. Al Shamsi H, Almutairi AG, Al Mashrafi S, Al Kalbani T. Implications of language barriers for healthcare: a systematic review. Oman Med J. 2020;35(2):e122. https://doi.org/10.5001/omj.2020.40.
3. Alarcon FJ. The migrant crisis and access to health care. Dela J Public Health. 2022;8(4):20–5. https://doi.org/10.32481/djph.2022.10.006.
4. Ali PA, Watson R. Language barriers and their impact on provision of care to patients with limited English proficiency: nurses' perspectives. J Clin Nurs. 2018;27(5–6):e1152–60. https://doi.org/10.1111/jocn.14204.
5. Alotni M, Guilhermino M, Duff J, Sim J. Barriers to nurse-led pain management for adult patients in intensive care units: an integrative review. Aust Crit Care. 2023;36(5):855–62. https://doi.org/10.1016/j.aucc.2022.09.002.
6. Althubaiti A. Information bias in health research: definition, pitfalls, and adjustment methods. J Multidiscip Healthc. 2016;9:211–7. https://doi.org/10.2147/JMDH.S104807.
7. Altun A, Brown H, Sturgiss L, Russell G. Evaluating chronic pain interventions in recent refugees and immigrant populations: a systematic review. Patient Educ Couns. 2022;105(5):1152–69. https://doi.org/10.1016/j.pec.2021.08.021.
8. Atkins N, Mukhida K. The relationship between patients' income and education and their access to pharmacological chronic pain management: a scoping review. Can J Pain. 2022;6(1):142–70. https://doi.org/10.1080/24740527.2022.2104699.
9. American Psychological Association. Implicit bias. Apaorg; 2022. Published November 2022. https://www.apa.org/topics/implicit-bias
10. American Society of Health-System Pharmacists. Drug shortages. n.d.. https://wwwashporg/drug-shortages. Accessed 30 Mar 2024.
11. Andermann A. CLEAR collaboration. Taking action on the social determinants of health in clinical practice: a framework for health professionals. CMAJ. 2016;188(17–18):E474–83. https://doi.org/10.1503/cmaj.160177.
12. Ashton-James CE, Anderson SR, Mackey SC, Darnall BD. Beyond pain, distress, and disability: the importance of social outcomes in pain management research and practice. Pain. 2022;163(3):e426–31. https://doi.org/10.1097/j.pain.0000000000002404.
13. Barth KS, Guille C, McCauley J, Brady KT. Targeting practitioners: a review of guidelines, training, and policy in pain management. Drug Alcohol Depend. 2017;173(Suppl 1):S22–30. https://doi.org/10.1016/j.drugalcdep.2016.08.641.
14. Becker KL. Tell me your dreams and goals: structuring communication exchanges to improve patient-centered care with chronic pain patients. Appl Nurs Res. 2020;53:151248. https://doi.org/10.1016/j.apnr.2020.151248.
15. Becker WC, Starrels JL, Heo M, Li X, Weiner MG, Turner BJ. Racial differences in primary care opioid risk reduction strategies. Ann Fam Med. 2011;9(3):219–25. https://doi.org/10.1370/afm.1242.
16. Bernardes SF, Costa M, Carvalho H. Engendering pain management practices: the role of physician sex on chronic low-back pain assessment and treatment prescriptions. J Pain. 2013;14(9):931–40. https://doi.org/10.1016/j.jpain.2013.03.004.
17. Blair IV, Steiner JF, Havranek EP. Unconscious (implicit) bias and health disparities: where do we go from here? Perm J. 2011;15(2):71–8. https://doi.org/10.7812/TPP/11.979.
18. Boring BL, Walsh KT, Ng BW, Schlegel RJ, Mathur VA. Experiencing pain invalidation is associated with under-reporting of pain: a social psychological perspective on acute pain communication. J Pain. 2024;25(5):104428. https://doi.org/10.1016/j.jpain.2023.11.011.
19. Brandal D, Keller MS, Lee C, et al. Impact of enhanced recovery after surgery and opioid-free anesthesia on opioid prescriptions at discharge from the hospital: a historical-prospective study. Anesth Analg. 2017;125(5):1784–92. https://doi.org/10.1213/ANE.0000000000002510.
20. Brant JM, Mohr C, Coombs NC, Finn S, Wilmarth E. Nurses' knowledge and attitudes about pain: personal and professional characteristics and patient reported pain satisfaction. Pain Manag Nurs. 2017;18(4):214–23. https://doi.org/10.1016/j.pmn.2017.04.003.
21. Braubach M, Egorov A, Mudu P, Wolf T, Ward Thompson C, Martuzzi M. Effects of urban green space on environmental health, equity and resilience. In: Kabisch N, Korn H, Stadler J, Bonn A, editors. Nature-based solutions to climate change adaptation in urban areas. Theory and practice of urban sustainability transitions. Cham: Springer; 2017. https://doi.org/10.1007/978-3-319-56091-5_11.
22. Breuer B, Pappagallo M, Tai JY, Portenoy RK. U.S. board-certified pain physician practices: uniformity and census data of their locations. J Pain. 2007;8(3):244–50. https://doi.org/10.1016/j.jpain.2006.08.009.
23. Candon M, Nielsen A, Dusek JA. Trends in insurance coverage for acupuncture, 2010–2019. JAMA Netw Open. 2022;5(1):e2142509. https://doi.org/10.1001/jamanetworkopen.2021.42509.

24. Canovas L, Carrascosa AJ, Garcia M, et al. Impact of empathy in the patient-doctor relationship on chronic pain relief and quality of life: a prospective study in Spanish pain clinics. Pain Med. 2018;19:1304–14. https://doi.org/10.1093/pm/pnx160.
25. Cascella LM. Improving health equity and addressing bias in pain management. MedPro Group; n.d.. Accessed from: https://www.medpro.com/bias-pain-management#:~:text=Some%20strategies%20that%20have%20been%20recommended%20at%20the%20provider%20level,can%20affect%20thinking%20and%20reasoning.
26. Charalambous A, Zorpas M, Cloconi C, Kading Y. Healthcare professionals' perceptions on the use of opioid analgesics for the treatment of cancer-related pain in Cyprus: a mixed-method study. SAGE Open Med. 2019;7:2050312119841823. https://doi.org/10.1177/2050312119841823.
27. Chen EH, Shofer FS, Dean AJ, et al. Gender disparity in analgesic treatment of emergency department patients with acute abdominal pain. Acad Emerg Med. 2008;15(5):414–8. https://doi.org/10.1111/j.1553-2712.2008.00100.x.
28. Chen I, Kurz J, Pasanen M, et al. Racial differences in opioid use for chronic nonmalignant pain. J Gen Intern Med. 2005;20(7):593–8. https://doi.org/10.1111/j.1525-1497.2005.0106.x.
29. Chou R, Korthuis PT, Weimer M, et al. Medication-assisted treatment models of care for opioid use disorder in primary care settings [Internet]. Rockville: Agency for Healthcare Research and Quality (US); 2016; (Technical Briefs, No. 28.) findings. Available from: https://www.ncbi.nlm.nih.gov/books/NBK402343/.
30. Clerc Liaudat C, Vaucher P, De Francesco T, et al. Sex/gender bias in the management of chest pain in ambulatory care. Womens Health (Lond). 2018;14:1745506518805641. https://doi.org/10.1177/1745506518805641.
31. Coleman MT, Newton KS. Supporting self-management in patients with chronic illness. Am Fam Physician. 2005;72(8):1503–10.
32. Corrigan PW, Nieweglowski K. Stigma and the public health agenda for the opioid crisis in America. Int J Drug Policy. 2018;59:44–9. https://doi.org/10.1016/j.drugpo.2018.06.015.
33. Davis MM, Bond LA, Howard A, Sarkisian CA. Primary care clinician expectations regarding aging. Gerontologist. 2011;51(6):856–66. https://doi.org/10.1093/geront/gnr017.
34. Defrin R, Shramm L, Eli I. Gender role expectations of pain is associated with pain tolerance limit but not with pain threshold. Pain. 2009;145(1–2):230–6. https://doi.org/10.1016/j.pain.2009.06.028.
35. Deldar K, Froutan R, Ebadi A. Challenges faced by nurses in using pain assessment scale in patients unable to communicate: a qualitative study. BMC Nurs. 2018;17:11. https://doi.org/10.1186/s12912-018-0281-3.
36. Deslauriers S, Roy JS, Bernatsky S, et al. The burden of waiting to access pain clinic services: perceptions and experiences of patients with rheumatic conditions. BMC Health Serv Res. 2021;21(1):160. https://doi.org/10.1186/s12913-021-06114-y.
37. Diamond L, Izquierdo K, Canfield D, Matsoukas K, Gany F. A systematic review of the impact of patient-physician non-English language concordance on quality of care and outcomes. J Gen Intern Med. 2019;34(8):1591–606. https://doi.org/10.1007/s11606-019-04847-5.
38. Dietrich S, Hernandez. Language Use in the United States: 2019. American community Survey Reports. United States Census Bureau; 2022. https://www.census.gov/content/dam/Census/library/publications/2022/acs/acs-50.pdf Accessed 30 March 2024.
39. Dineen-Griffin S, Garcia-Cardenas V, Williams K, Benrimoj SI. Helping patients help themselves: a systematic review of self-management support strategies in primary health care practice. PLoS One. 2019;14(8):e0220116. https://doi.org/10.1371/journal.pone.0220116.
40. Donovan KA, Taliaferro LA, Brock CW, Bazargan S. Sex differences in the adequacy of pain management among patients referred to a multidisciplinary cancer pain clinic. J Pain Symptom Manag. 2007;36(2):167–72. https://doi.org/10.1016/j.jpainsymman.2007.09.013.
41. Dowell D, Ragan K, Jones C, Baldwin G, Chou R. CDC clinical practice guidelines for prescribing opioids for pain – United States, 2022. MMWR Recomm Rep. 2022;77(3):1–95. https://doi.org/10.15585/mmwr.rr7103a1.
42. Drake G, de C Williams AC. Nursing education interventions for managing acute pain in hospital settings: a systematic review of clinical outcomes and teaching methods. Pain Manag Nurs. 2017;18(1):3–15. https://doi.org/10.1016/j.pmn.2016.11.001.
43. Elwyn G, Coulter A, Laitner S, Walker E, Watson P, Thomson R. Implementing shared decision making in the NHS. BMJ. 2010;341:c5146. https://doi.org/10.1136/bmj.c5146.
44. Elwyn G, Vermunt NPCA. Goal-based shared decision-making: developing an integrated model. J Patient Exp. 2020;7(5):688–96. https://doi.org/10.1177/2374373519878604.
45. FDA Drug Shortages Database. U.S. Food and Drug Administration, Silver Spring; n.d.). https://www.accessdata.fda.gov/scripts/drugshortages/ Accessed 30 Mar 2024.
46. Ferreira PH, Ferreira ML, Maher CG, Refshauge KM, Latimer J, Adams RD. The therapeutic alliance between clinicians and patients predicts outcome in chronic low back pain. Phys Ther. 2013;93(4):470–8. https://doi.org/10.2522/ptj.20120137.
47. Fiscella K, Epstein RM, Griggs JJ, Marshall MM, Shields CG. Is physician implicit bias associated with differences in care by patient race for metastatic cancer-related pain? PLoS One. 2021;16(10):e0257794. https://doi.org/10.1371/journal.pone.0257794.
48. FitzGerald C, Hurst S. Implicit bias in healthcare professionals: a systematic review. BMC Med Ethics. 2017;18(1):19. https://doi.org/10.1186/s12910-017-0179-8.
49. Gaskin DJ, Richard P. The economic costs of pain in the United States. In: Institute of Medicine (US) Committee on Advancing Pain Research, Care, and Education. Relieving pain in America: a blueprint for transforming prevention, care, education, and research. Washington, DC: National Academies Press (US); 2011. Appendix C. Available from: https://www.ncbi.nlm.nih.gov/books/NBK92521/.
50. Gatchel RJ, Peng YB, Peters ML, Fuchs PN, Turk DC. The biopsychosocial approach to chronic pain: scientific advances and future directions. Psychol Bull. 2007;133(4):581–624. https://doi.org/10.1037/0033-2909.133.4.581.
51. Geneen LJ, Moore RA, Clarke C, Martin D, Colvin LA, Smith BH. Physical activity and exercise for chronic pain in adults: an overview of Cochrane reviews. Cochrane Database Syst Rev. 2017;4(4):CD011279. https://doi.org/10.1002/14651858.CD011279.pub3.
52. Gerchow L, Burka LR, Miner S, Squires A. Language barriers between nurses and patients: a scoping review. Patient Educ Couns. 2021;104(3):534–53. https://doi.org/10.1016/j.pec.2020.09.017.
53. Goddu AP, O'Conor KJ, Lanzkron S, et al. Do words matter? Stigmatizing language and the transmission of bias in the medical record. J Gen Intern Med. 2018;33(5):685–91. https://doi.org/10.1007/s11606-017-4289-2.
54. Grant JM, Mottet LA, Tanis J, Harrison J, Herman JL, Keisling M. Injustice at every turn: a report of the National Transgender Discrimination Survey. Washington, DC: National Center for Transgender Equality and National Gay and Lesbian Task Force; 2011.
55. Green CR, Anderson KO, Baker TA, et al. The unequal burden of pain: confronting racial and ethnic disparities in pain [published correction appears in Pain Med. 2005 Jan–Feb;6(1):99. Kaloukalani, Donna A [corrected to Kalauokalani,

Donna A]]. Pain Med. 2003;4(3):277–94. https://doi.org/10.1046/j.1526-4637.2003.03034.x.
56. Green CR, Ndao-Brumblay SK, West B, Washington T. Differences in prescription opioid analgesic availability: comparing minority and white pharmacies across Michigan. J Pain. 2005;6(10):689–99. https://doi.org/10.1016/j.jpain.2005.06.002.
57. Hatzenbuehler ML, Phelan JC, Link BG. Stigma as a fundamental cause of population health inequalities. Am J Public Health. 2013;103(5):813–21. https://doi.org/10.2105/AJPH.2012.301069.
58. Hausmann LRM, Jones AL, McInnes SE, Zickmund SL. Identifying healthcare experiences associated with perceptions of racial/ethnic discrimination among veterans with pain: a cross-sectional mixed methods survey. PLoS One. 2020;15(9):e0237650. https://doi.org/10.1371/journal.pone.0237650.
59. Haverfield MC, Giannitrapani K, Timko C, Lorenz K. Patient-centered pain management communication from the patient perspective. J Gen Intern Med. 2018;33(8):1374–80. https://doi.org/10.1007/s11606-018-4490-y.
60. Helms J, Frankart L, Bradner M, Ebersole J, Regan B, Crouch T. Interprofessional active learning for chronic pain: transforming student learning from recall to application. J Med Educat Curri Develop. 2023;10:23821205231221950. https://doi.org/10.1177/23821205231221950.
61. Herr K, Marie BS, Gordon DB, et al. An interprofessional consensus of core competencies for prelicensure education in pain management: curriculum application for nursing. J Nurs Educ. 2015;54(6):317–27. https://doi.org/10.3928/01484834-20150515-02.
62. Heyward J, Jones C, Compton W. Coverage of nonpharmacologic treatments for low Back pain among US public and private insurers. JAMA Netw Open. 2018;1(6). https://jamanetwork.com/journals/jamanetworkopen/fullarticle/2705853.
63. HHS. Healthy people 2030: social determinants of health. U.S. Department of Health and Human Services, Office of Disease Prevention and Health Promotion; 2020. https://odphp.health.gov/healthypeople/priority-areas/social-determinants-health#:~:text=Some%20examples%20of%20SDOH%20include:%20*%20Safe,to%20improve%20the%20conditions%20in%20people's%20environments. Accessed 30 Mar 2024.
64. Hirsh AT, Alqudah AF, Stutts LA, Robinson ME. Virtual human technology: capturing sex, race, and age influences in individual pain decision policies. Pain. 2008;140(1):231–8. https://doi.org/10.1016/j.pain.2008.09.010.
65. Hoffmann DE, Tarzian AJ. The girl who cried pain: a bias against women in the treatment of pain. J Law Med Ethics. 2001;29(1):13–27. https://doi.org/10.1111/j.1748-720x.2001.tb00037.x.
66. Hoffman KM, Trawalter S, Axt JR, Oliver MN. Racial bias in pain assessment and treatment recommendations, and false beliefs about biological differences between blacks and whites. Proc Natl Acad Sci USA. 2016;113(16):4296–301.
67. Holt-Lunstad J, Smith TB, Layton JB. Social relationships and mortality risk: a meta-analytic review. PLoS Med. 2010;7(7):e1000316. https://doi.org/10.1371/journal.pmed.1000316.
68. Hundley HE, Hudson ME, Wasan AD, Emerick TD. Chronic pain clinic efficiency analysis: optimization through use of the Gantt diagram and visit diagnoses. J Pain Res. 2018;12:1–8. https://doi.org/10.2147/JPR.S173345.
69. Hurwitz EL, Randhawa K, Torres P, et al. The global spine care initiative: a systematic review of individual and community-based burden of spinal disorders in rural populations in low- and middle-income communities. Eur Spine J. 2018;27(Suppl 6):802–15. https://doi.org/10.1007/s00586-017-5393-z.
70. IHA. 7 barriers to effective communication in healthcare. IHA Health Literacy Solutions Center; 2023. https://wwwhealthliteracysolutionsorg/blogs/iha-staff1/2023/07/19/7-barriers-to-effective-communication-in-healthcar. Accessed 30 Mar 2024.
71. Institute for Safe Medication Practices. Weathering the storm: managing the drug shortage crisis. ISMP Medication Saf Alert. 2010;15(20):1–4.
72. International Society for the Study of Pain Multidisciplinary Pain Center Toolkit Advisory Group. IASP Multidisciplinary Pain Center Development Manual; 2021. Available at: http://www.iasp--pain.org/MPCManual. Accessed 30 Mar 2024.
73. Ismail A. The challenges of providing effective pain management for children in the pediatric intensive care unit. Pain Manag Nurs. 2016;17(6):372–83. https://doi.org/10.1016/j.pmn.2016.08.005.
74. James SE, Herman JL, Rankin S, Keisling M, Mottet L, Anafi M. The report of the 2015 U.S. transgender survey. Washington, DC: National Center for Transgender Equality; 2016.
75. Jani BD, Blane DN, Mercer SW. The role of empathy in therapy and the physician-patient relationship. Forschende Komplementärmedizin und Klassische Naturheilkunde/Res Complement Class Nat Med. 2012;19(5):252–7. https://doi.org/10.1159/000342998.
76. Kahokehr A, Sammour T, Kamran Zargar-Shoshtari K, Thompson L, Hill AG. Implementation of ERAS and how to overcome barriers. Int J Surg. 2009;7:16–9. https://doi.org/10.1016/j.ijsu.2008.11.004.
77. Kanbergs AN, Durfey SNM. Incarcerated individuals' perspectives on living with serious illness. R I Med J. 2019;102(2):24–7.
78. Kelm Z, Womer J, Walter JK, Feudtner C. Interventions to cultivate physician empathy: a systematic review. BMC Med Educ. 2014;14:219–30. https://doi.org/10.1186/1472-6920-14-219.
79. Kilborn K, Sommer JL, Reynolds K, Roy R, El-Gabalawy R. The need to say more: a qualitative analysis of added free text to chronic pain patient intake packages. Pain Manag Nurs. 2023;24(2):201–8. https://doi.org/10.1016/j.pmn.2022.08.007.
80. Kim R, Kim A. A structural equation model for low Back pain management behavior in patients with spinal disease. Pain Manag Nurs. 2024;26(1):e107–15. https://doi.org/10.1016/j.pmn.2024.10.018.
81. Lakke SE, Meerman S. Does working alliance have an influence on pain and physical functioning in patients with chronic musculoskeletal pain; a systematic review. J Compassionate Health Care. 2016;3(1):1–10.
82. Larance B, Campbell G, Moore T, et al. Concerns and help-seeking among patients using opioids for management of chronic noncancer pain. Pain Med. 2019;20(4):758–69. https://doi.org/10.1093/pm/pny078.
83. Levy BR, Pietrzak RH, Slade MD. Societal impact on older persons' chronic pain: roles of age stereotypes, age attribution, and age discrimination. Soc Sci Med. 2023;323:115772. https://doi.org/10.1016/j.socscimed.2023.115772.
84. Lewandowski AS, Palermo TM, Stinson J, Handley S, Chambers CT. Systematic review of family functioning in families of children and adolescents with chronic pain. J Pain. 2010;11(11):1027–38. https://doi.org/10.1016/j.jpain.2010.04.005.
85. Li H, Zhang X, Bi S, Cao Y, Zhang G. Can residential greenspace exposure improve pain experience? A comparison between physical visit and image viewing. Healthcare (Basel). 2021;9(7):918. https://doi.org/10.3390/healthcare9070918.
86. Liang Y. The mediating effect of allostatic load on the association between life course socioeconomic disadvantage and chronic pain: a prospective finding from the National Survey of Midlife Development in the United States. Front Pain Res (Lausanne). 2023;4:1213750. https://doi.org/10.3389/fpain.2023.1213750.
87. Lor M, Vang X, Rabago D, Brown RL, Backonja M. "It hurts as if…": pain-associated language, visual characterization, and storytelling in Hmong adults. Pain Med. 2020;21(8):1690–702. https://doi.org/10.1093/pm/pnz268.

88. Lor M, Xiong S, Yang NB, Koleck TA. Systematic review of pain research among limited English proficiency patient populations in health care. Pain Manag Nurs. 2023; https://doi.org/10.1016/j.pmn.2023.11.005.
89. Makris UE, Higashi RT, Marks EG, et al. Ageism, negative attitudes, and competing co-morbidities--why older adults may not seek care for restricting back pain: a qualitative study. BMC Geriatr. 2015;15:39. https://doi.org/10.1186/s12877-015-0042-z.
90. Malik Z, Ahn J, Thompson K, Palma A. A systematic review of pain management education in graduate medical education. J Grad Med Educ. 2022;14(2):178–90. https://doi.org/10.4300/JGME-D-21-00672.1.
91. Maly A, Vallerand AH. Neighborhood, socioeconomic, and racial influence on chronic pain. Pain Manag Nurs. 2018;19(1):14–22. https://doi.org/10.1016/j.pmn.2017.11.004.
92. Manchikanti L, Sanapati J, Benyamin RM, Atluri S, Kaye AD, Hirsch JA. Reframing the prevention strategies of the opioid crisis: focusing on prescription opioids, fentanyl, and heroin epidemic. Pain Physician. 2018;21(4):309–26.
93. Mayer JD, Kirlin B, Rehm CD, Loeser JD. Opioid availability in outpatient pharmacies in Washington state. Clin J Pain. 2008;24(2):120–3. https://doi.org/10.1097/AJP.0b013e3181590d4f.
94. McCradden MD, Vasileva D, Orchanian-Cheff A, Buchman DZ. Ambiguous identities of drugs and people: a scoping review of opioid-related stigma. Int J Drug Policy. 2019;74:205–15. https://doi.org/10.1016/j.drugpo.2019.10.005.
95. McGuire DB, Kaiser KS, Haisfield-Wolfe ME, Iyamu F. Pain assessment in noncommunicative adult palliative care patients. Nurs Clin North Am. 2016;51(3):397–431. https://doi.org/10.1016/j.cnur.2016.05.009.
96. McManimen S, McClellan D, Stoothoff J, Gleason K, Jason LA. Dismissing chronic illness: a qualitative analysis of negative health care experiences. Health Care Women Int. 2019;40(3):241–58. https://doi.org/10.1080/07399332.2018.1521811.
97. Meghani SH, Byun E, Gallagher RM. Time to take stock: a meta-analysis and systematic review of analgesic treatment disparities for pain in the United States. Pain Med. 2012;13(2):150–74.
98. Meints SM, Cortes A, Morais CA, Edwards RR. Racial and ethnic differences in the experience and treatment of noncancer pain. Pain Manage. 2019;9(3):317–34. https://doi.org/10.2217/pmt-2018-0030.
99. Miller SR. A curriculum focused on informed empathy improves attitudes toward persons with disabilities. Perspect Med Educ. 2013;2(3):114–25. https://doi.org/10.1007/S40037-013-0046-3.
100. Mittinty MM, Vanlint S, Stocks N, Mittinty MN, Moseley GL. Exploring effect of pain education on chronic pain patients' expectation of recovery and pain intensity. Scand J Pain. 2018;18(2):211–9. https://doi.org/10.1515/sjpain-2018-0023.
101. Moen M, Storr C, German D, Friedmann E, Johantgen M. A review of tools to screen for social determinants of health in the United States: a practice brief. Popul Health Manag. 2020;23(6):422–9. https://doi.org/10.1089/pop.2019.0158.
102. Moreno-Ligero M, Moral-Munoz JA, Salazar A, Failde I. mHealth intervention for improving pain, quality of life, and functional disability in patients with chronic pain: systematic review. JMIR Mhealth Uhealth. 2023;11:e40844. https://doi.org/10.2196/40844.
103. Moretti C, De Luca E, D'Apice C, Artioli G, Sarli L, Bonacaro A. Gender and sex bias in prevention and clinical treatment of women's chronic pain: hypotheses of a curriculum development. Front Med (Lausanne). 2023;10:1189126. Published 2023 Jul 25. https://doi.org/10.3389/fmed.2023.1189126.
104. Morrison RS, Wallenstein S, Natale DK, Senzel RS, Huang LL. "We don't carry that"–failure of pharmacies in predominantly nonwhite neighborhoods to stock opioid analgesics. N Engl J Med. 2000;342(14):1023–6. https://doi.org/10.1056/NEJM200004063421406.
105. Mossey JM. Defining racial and ethnic disparities in pain management (2011). Clin Orthop Relat Res. 2011;469(7):1859–70. https://doi.org/10.1007/s11999-011-1770-9.
106. Nahin RL, Rhee A, Stussman B. Use of complementary health approaches overall and for pain management by US adults. JAMA. 2024;331(7):613–5. https://doi.org/10.1001/jama.2023.26775.
107. Najem C, Mukhtar NB, Ayoubi F, et al. Religious beliefs and attitudes in relation to pain, pain-related beliefs, function, and coping in chronic musculoskeletal pain: a systematic review. Pain Physician. 2021;24(8):E1163–76.
108. National Center for Ethics in Health Care Goals of Care Conversations Skills Training for Clinicians. Empathetic Responses Handout. Updated June 2018. 2018. Retrieved from U.S. Department of Veterans Affairs website: https://www.ethics.va.gov/GoCC.asp. Accessed 29 Mar 2024.
109. National Institutes of Health. Sex & gender. Office of Research on Women's Health; n.d.. orwh.od.nih.gov. Accessed from: https://orwh.od.nih.gov/sex-gender.
110. Navathe AS, Troxel AB, Liao JM, et al. Cost of joint replacement using bundled payment models. JAMA Intern Med. 2017;177(2):214–22. https://doi.org/10.1001/jamainternmed.2016.8263.
111. NCCHC. Management of chronic pain. National Commission on Correctional Health Care; 2023. https://wwwncchcorg/position-statements/management-of-noncancer-chronic-pain-2023/. Accessed 30 Mar 2024.
112. Ng JYY, Ntoumanis N, Thøgersen-Ntoumani C, Deci EL, Ryan RM, Duda JL, Williams GC. Self-determination theory applied to health contexts: a meta-analysis. Perspect Psychol Sci. 2012;7(4):325–40. https://doi.org/10.1177/1745691612447309.
113. Nicola M, Correia H, Ditchburn G, Drummond P. Invalidation of chronic pain: a thematic analysis of pain narratives. Disabil Rehabil. 2021;43(6):861–9. https://doi.org/10.1080/09638288.2019.1636888.
114. Nicola M, Correia H, Ditchburn G, Drummond PD. The pain-invalidation scale: measuring patient perceptions of invalidation toward chronic pain. J Pain. 2022;23(11):1912–22. https://doi.org/10.1016/j.jpain.2022.06.008.
115. Oosterhaven J, Pell CD, Schröder CD, et al. Health literacy and pain neuroscience education in an interdisciplinary pain management programme: a qualitative study of patient perspectives. Pain Rep. 2023;8(6):e1093. Published 2023 Oct 18. https://doi.org/10.1097/PR9.0000000000001093.
116. Orujlu S, Hassankhani H, Rahmani A, Sanaat Z, Dadashzadeh A, Allahbakhshian A. Barriers to cancer pain management from the perspective of patients: a qualitative study. Nurs Open. 2022;9(1):541–9. https://doi.org/10.1002/nop2.1093.
117. Penney LS, Haro E. Qualitative evaluation of an interdisciplinary chronic pain intervention: outcomes and barriers and facilitators to ongoing pain management. J Pain Res. 2019:865–78. https://doi.org/10.2147/JPR.S185652.
118. Pisanu C, Franconi F, Gessa GL, et al. Sex differences in the response to opioids for pain relief: a systematic review and meta-analysis. Pharmacol Res. 2019;148:104447. https://doi.org/10.1016/j.phrs.2019.104447.
119. Prego-Domínguez J, Khazaeipour Z, Mallah N, Takkouche B. Socioeconomic status and occurrence of chronic pain: a meta-analysis. Rheumatology (Oxford). 2021;60(3):1091–105. https://doi.org/10.1093/rheumatology/keaa758.
120. Rababa M, Al-Sabbah S, Hayajneh AA. Nurses' perceived barriers to and facilitators of pain assessment and management in critical care patients: a systematic review. J Pain Res. 2021;14:3475–91. https://doi.org/10.2147/JPR.S332423.

121. Ratka A. Empathy and the development of affective skills. Am J Pharm Educ. 2018;82(10):1140–3. https://doi.org/10.5688/ajpe7192.
122. Rikard SM, Strahan AE, Schmit KM, Guy GP Jr. Chronic pain among adults—United States, 2019–2021. MMWR Morb Mortal Wkly Rep. 2023;72:379–85. https://doi.org/10.15585/mmwr.mm7215a1.
123. Robeznieks A. Get rid of market barriers to appropriate pain management. American Medical Society; 2019. https://wwwama--assnorg/delivering-care/overdose-epidemic/get-rid-market-barriers-appropriate-pain-management. Accessed 30 Mar 2024.
124. Robinson ME, Wise EA. Prior pain experience: influence on the observation of experimental pain in men and women. J Pain. 2004;5(5):264–9. https://doi.org/10.1016/j.jpain.2004.04.003.
125. Rogger R, Bello C, Romero CS, Urman RD, Luedi MM, Filipovic MG. Cultural framing and the impact on acute pain and pain services. Curr Pain Headache Rep. 2023;27(9):429–36. https://doi.org/10.1007/s11916-023-01125-2.
126. Ryan RM, Patrick H, Deci EL, Williams GC. Facilitating health behaviour change and its maintenance: interventions based on self-determination theory. Eur Health Psychol. 2008;10:2–5.
127. Sabin JA, Greenwald AG. The influence of implicit bias on treatment recommendations for 4 common pediatric conditions: pain, urinary tract infection, attention deficit hyperactivity disorder, and asthma. Am J Public Health. 2012;102(5):988–95. https://doi.org/10.2105/AJPH.2011.300621.
128. Salisu M, Blackwell T, Lewis G, et al. Community perceptions of health equity: a qualitative study. J Prim Care Community Health. 2023;14 https://doi.org/10.1177/21501319231211439.
129. Salsitz E, Wiegand T. Pharmacotherapy of opioid addiction: “putting a real face on a false demon”. J Med Toxicol. 2016;12(1):58–63. https://doi.org/10.1007/s13181-015-0517-5.
130. Samulowitz A, Gremyr I, Eriksson E, Hensing G. “Brave men” and “emotional women”: a theory-guided literature review on gender bias in health care and gendered norms towards patients with chronic pain. Pain Res Manag. 2018;2018:6358624. https://doi.org/10.1155/2018/6358624.
131. Schäfer G, Prkachin KM, Kaseweter KA, Williams AC. Health care providers’ judgments in chronic pain: the influence of gender and trustworthiness. Pain. 2016;157(8):1618–25. https://doi.org/10.1097/j.pain.0000000000000536.
132. Schoenthaler A, Williams N. Looking beneath the surface: racial bias in the treatment and management of pain. JAMA Netw Open. 2022;5(6):e2216281. https://doi.org/10.1001/jamanetworkopen.2022.16281.
133. Shipton EE, Bate F, Garrick R, Steketee C, Shipton EA, Visser EJ. Systematic review of pain medicine content, teaching, and assessment in medical school curricula internationally. Pain Ther. 2018;7(2):139–61. https://doi.org/10.1007/s40122-018-0103-z.
134. Sinatra R. Causes and consequences of inadequate management of acute pain. Pain Med. 2010;11(12):1859–71. https://doi.org/10.1111/j.1526-4637.2010.00983.x.
135. Skelly AC, Chou R, Dettori JR, Turner JA, Friedly JL, Rundell SD, Fu R, Brodt ED, Wasson N, Kantner S, Ferguson AJR. Noninvasive nonpharmacological treatment for chronic pain: a systematic review update, Comparative Effectiveness Review No. 227. (Prepared by the Pacific Northwest Evidence-based Practice Center under Contract No. 290-2015-00009-I.) AHRQ Publication No. 20-EHC009. Rockville: Agency for Healthcare Research and Quality; 2020. https://doi.org/10.23970/AHRQEPCCER227.
136. Slade SC, Molloy E, Keating JL. Stigma experienced by people with nonspecific chronic low back pain: a qualitative study. Pain Med. 2009;10(1):143–54. https://doi.org/10.1111/j.1526-4637.2008.00540.x.
137. Slade S, Sergent SR. Language barrier. In: StatPearls. Treasure Island (FL): StatPearls; 2023.
138. Starck PL, Sherwood GD, Adams-McNeill J, Thomas EJ. Identifying and addressing medical errors in pain mismanagement. Jt Comm J Qual Improv. 2001;27(4):191–9. https://doi.org/10.1016/s1070-3241(01)27017-5.
139. Stepien KA, Baernstein A. Educating for empathy: a review. J Gen Intern Med. 2006;21(5):524–30. https://doi.org/10.1111/j.1525-1497.2006.00443.x.
140. Stewart MA. Stuck in the middle: the impact of collaborative interprofessional communication on patient expectations. Should Elbow. 2018;10(1):66–72. https://doi.org/10.1177/1758573217735325.
141. Strand N, Gomez DA, Kacel EL, Morrison EJ, St Amand CM, Vencill JA, Pagan-Rosado R, Lorenzo A, Gonzalez C, Mariano ER, Reece-Nguyen T, Narouze S, Mahdi L, Chadwick AL, Kraus M, Bechtle A, Kling JM. Concepts and approaches in the management of transgender and gender-diverse patients. Mayo Clin Proc. 2024;99(7):1114–26. https://doi.org/10.1016/j.mayocp.2023.12.027.
142. Strath LJ, Sorge RE, Owens MA, Gonzalez CE, Okunbor JI, White DM, Merlin JS, Goodin BR. Sex and gender are not the same: why identity is important for people living with HIV and chronic pain. J Pain Res. 2020;13:829–35. https://doi.org/10.2147/JPR.S248424.
143. Stumbo SP, Yarborough BJ, McCarty D, Weisner C, Green CA. Patient-reported pathways to opioid use disorders and pain-related barriers to treatment engagement. J Subst Abus Treat. 2017;73:47–54. https://doi.org/10.1016/j.jsat.2016.11.003.
144. Stutts LA, Hirsh AT, George SZ, Robinson ME. Investigating patient characteristics on pain assessment using virtual human technology. Eur J Pain. 2010;14(10):1040–5. https://doi.org/10.1016/j.ejpain.2010.04.003.
145. Suntai Z, Won CR, Noh H. Access barrier in rural older adults’ use of pain management and palliative care services: a systematic review. Am J Hosp Palliat Care. 2021;38(5):494–502. https://doi.org/10.1177/1049909120959634.
146. Sulzer SH, Feinstein NW, Wendland CL. Assessing empathy development in medical education: a systematic review. Med Educ. 2016;50(3):300–10. https://doi.org/10.1111/medu.12806.
147. Tamayo-Sarver JH, Hinze SW, Cydulka RK, Baker DW. Racial and ethnic disparities in emergency department analgesic prescription. Am J Public Health. 2003;93(12):2067–73. https://doi.org/10.2105/ajph.93.12.2067.
148. Thies KM, Anderson D, Beals-Reid C. Project ECHO chronic pain: a qualitative analysis of recommendations by expert faculty and the process of knowledge translation. J Contin Educ Health Prof. 2019;39(3):194–200. https://doi.org/10.1097/CEH.0000000000000264.
149. Torres CA, Bartley EJ, Wandner LD, Alqudah AF, Hirsh AT, Robinson ME. The influence of sex, race, and age on pain assessment and treatment decisions using virtual human technology: a cross-national comparison. J Pain Res. 2013;6:577–88. https://doi.org/10.2147/JPR.S46295.
150. Trouvin AP. “Ten-year mixed method evaluation of pre-licensure health professional student self-reported learning in an interfaculty pain curriculum”: a view on pain education. Pain Rep. 2022;7(5):e1031. https://doi.org/10.1097/PR9.0000000000001031.
151. U.S. Department of Health and Human Services. Pain management best practices inter-agency task force. Report: updates, gaps, inconsistencies, and recommendations. Retrieved from U.S. Department of Health and Human; 2019. Services website: https://www.hhs.gov/sites/default/files/pain-mgmt-best-practices-draft-final-report-05062019.pdf

152. Vallerand A, Nowak L. Chronic opioid therapy for nonmalignant pain: the patient's perspective. Part II–Barriers to chronic opioid therapy. Pain Manag Nurs. 2011;11(2):126–31. https://doi.org/10.1016/j.pmn.2009.03.006.
153. Vargovich AM, Schumann ME, Xiang J, Ginsberg AD, Palmer BA, Sperry JA. Difficult conversations: training medical students to assess, educate, and treat the patient with chronic pain. Acad Psychiatry. 2019;43(5):494–8.
154. Vela MB, Erondu AI, Smith NA, Peek ME, Woodruff JN, Chin MH. Eliminating explicit and implicit biases in health care: evidence and research needs. Annu Rev Public Health. 2022;43:477–501. https://doi.org/10.1146/annurev-publhealth-052620-103528.
155. Wandner LD, Stutts LA, Alqudah AF, et al. Virtual human technology: patient demographics and healthcare training factors in pain observation and treatment recommendations. J Pain Res. 2010;3:241–7. https://doi.org/10.2147/JPR.S14708.
156. Wang D, Liu Z, Zhou J, et al. Barriers to implementation of enhanced recovery after surgery (ERAS) by a multidisciplinary team in China: a multicenter qualitative study. BMJ Open. 2022;12:e053687. https://doi.org/10.1136/bmjopen-2021-053687.
157. Wiering B, de Boer D, Krol M, Wieberneit-Tolman H, Delnoij D. Entertaining accurate treatment expectations while suffering from chronic pain: an exploration of treatment expectations and the relationship with patient- provider communication. BMC Health Serv Res. 2018;18(1):706. https://doi.org/10.1186/s12913-018-3497-8.
158. Wesolowicz DM, Clark JF, Boissoneault J, Robinson ME. The roles of gender and profession on gender role expectations of pain in health care professionals. J Pain Res. 2018;11:1121–8. https://doi.org/10.2147/JPR.S162123.
159. Williams GC, Rodin GC, Ryan RM, Grolnick WS, Deci EL. Autonomous regulation and long-term medication adherence in adult outpatients. Health Psychol. 1998;17(3):269–76. https://doi.org/10.1037/0278-6133.17.3.269.
160. Winstanley EL, Clark A, Feinberg J, Wilder CM. Barriers to implementation of opioid overdose prevention programs in Ohio. Subst Abus. 2016;37(1):42–6. https://doi.org/10.1080/08897077.2015.1132294.
161. Wu Q, Jin Z, Wang P. The relationship between the physician-patient relationship, physician empathy, and patient trust. J Gen Intern Med. 2022;37(6):1388–93. https://doi.org/10.1007/s11606-021-07008-9.
162. Yajnik M, Hill JN, Hunter OO, Howard SK, Kim TE, Harrison TK, Mariano ER. Patient education and engagement in postoperative pain management decreases opioid use following knee replacement surgery. Patient Educ Couns. 2019;102(2):383–7. https://doi.org/10.1016/j.pec.2018.09.001.
163. Yap ZL, Summers SJ, Grant AR, Moseley GL, Karran EL. The role of the social determinants of health in outcomes of surgery for low back pain: a systematic review and narrative synthesis. Spine J. 2022;22(5):793–809. https://doi.org/10.1016/j.spinee.2021.11.013.
164. Zhang L, Losin EAR, Ashar YK, Koban L, Wager TD. Gender biases in estimation of others' pain. J Pain. 2021;22(9):1048–59. https://doi.org/10.1016/j.jpain.2021.03.001.
165. Zhou C, Crawford A, Serhal E, Kurdyak P, et al. MHPE. The impact of project ECHO on participant and patient outcomes: a systematic review. Acad Med. 2016;91(10):1439–61. https://doi.org/10.1097/ACM.0000000000001328.
166. Zorek JA, Ragucci K, McKearney S, et al. IPEC Core Competencies for Interprofessional Collaborative Practice: Version 3. 2023. Available at: https://www.ipecollaborative.org/. Accessed 30 Mar 2024.
167. Shirsat N, Finney N, Strutner S, Rinehart J, Higgins KE 3rd, Shah S. Characterizing Chronic Pain and Adverse Childhood Experiences in the Lesbian, Gay, Bisexual, Transgender, or Queer Community. Anesth Analg. 2024;139(4):821-831. https://doi.org/10.1213/ANE.0000000000006922.
168. Tabernacki T, Gilbert D, Rhodes S, et al. The burden of chronic pain in transgender and gender diverse populations: Evidence from a large US clinical database. Eur J Pain. 2025;29(2):e4725. https://doi.org/10.1002/ejp.4725.

27 Assessing Pain Health Literacy

Takova D. Wallace-Gay and Dakota Smith

Introduction

Health literacy (HL) encompasses the ability to seek, comprehend, and apply health-related information to oneself and others. The U.S. Department of Health and Human Services (HHS) categorizes HL into personal and organizational dimensions [1]. Personal health literacy gauges an individual's capacity to utilize health information effectively, while organizational health literacy evaluates how organizations facilitate such information for informed decision-making [2]. This responsibility, evident in the shift from Healthy People 2020 to 2030, extends not only to individuals but also to healthcare professionals [3].

The intricacies of health literacy, from reading to risk assessment, are integral for informed decision-making. Healthcare professionals bear the duty not only to provide information but also to ensure its understanding. In the realm of pain management, a leading cause of medical assistance, more than 50 million U.S. adults experience chronic pain, while nearly 9 out of 10 struggle with everyday health information comprehension [4, 5]. Healthcare professionals play a vital role in bridging this gap by fostering a collaborative approach to initiate and follow appropriate pain management plans. Recognizing the diverse nature of pain, this chapter explores pain, emphasizing the pivotal role of health literacy, and provides strategies for evaluating one's health literacy level [1].

T. D. Wallace-Gay (✉)
School of Medicine, The University of Texas at Tyler, Tyler, TX, USA

Fisch College of Pharmacy, The University of Texas at Tyler, Tyler, TX, USA
e-mail: twallacegay@uttyler.edu

D. Smith
Fisch College of Pharmacy, The University of Texas at Tyler, Tyler, TX, USA
e-mail: dsmith103@patriots.uttyler.edu

Health Literacy: Basics and Assessment

Understanding the fundamental concepts of health literacy is crucial for effective pain management. A lack of health literacy can lead to misunderstandings, nonadherence to treatment strategies, and inadequate pain management [6]. Assessing health literacy levels through various validated tools may allow health professionals to tailor their communication strategies, ensuring that patients receive information in a manner that aligns with their understanding and abilities. Health professionals sometimes assess basic literacy using the patient's highest grade level completed in school; however, this approach is unreliable, as years of education do not consistently reflect an individual's actual literacy or health literacy skills [7]. Valid health literacy tools should be used to more accurately assess health literacy. There are many validated tools available for quick measurement of health literacy in clinical settings. A few common tools are discussed below and listed in Table 27.1. These questionnaires are mostly available in both English and Spanish and may be administered in less than 10 min, making them ideal for both clinical and research settings.

Rapid Estimate of Adult Literacy in Medicine—Short Form (REALM-SF)

The REALM is a widely utilized tool that assesses a patient's ability to pronounce and understand medical terms. It provides healthcare professionals with a quick snapshot of a patient's literacy level, helping them adjust their communication style accordingly. The short-form tool is a 7-item work recognition test that provides assessments ranging from "0—will not be able to read most low-literacy materials" to "7—will be able to read most patient education materials" [8].

J. P. Reinert et al. (eds.), *Adjunctive Analgesic Strategies for the Bedside Clinician and Beyond*,
https://doi.org/10.1007/978-3-032-21675-5_27

Table 27.1 Selected validated health literacy assessment tools

Tool name	Description	Format	Time to complete	Target population
Rapid Estimate of Adult Literacy in Medicine (REALM)	Assesses the ability to pronounce common medical terms	Word recognition test (66 words)	2–3 min	Adults
Test of Functional Health Literacy in Adults (TOFHLA)	Measures reading comprehension and numeracy using healthcare materials (prescription labels, forms, etc.)	Reading passages and numeracy tasks	12–22 min	Adults
Newest Vital Sign (NVS)	Evaluates literacy using a nutrition label and six associated questions	Verbal Q&A based on a nutrition label	3 min	Adults
Short Assessment of Health Literacy—English/Spanish (SAHL-E/S)	Assesses comprehension and word recognition in English or Spanish	Word recognition and comprehension	3–5 min	Adults (English and Spanish speakers)
Health Literacy Questionnaire (HLQ)	Measures multiple dimensions of health literacy, including social support, navigating healthcare, and understanding health info	Self-reported questionnaire (44 items)	10–15 min	Adults
eHealth Literacy Scale (eHEALS)	Measures perceived skills at finding, evaluating, and applying electronic health information	Self-reported questionnaire (8 items)	2–5 min	Adolescents and adults

Test of Functional Health Literacy in Adults (TOFHLA)

The TOFHLA is a functional literacy assessment tool that was designed to assess adult literacy in the health care setting. This tool is especially useful for capturing numeracy and reading comprehension skills [9]. The test was designed using hospital materials and consists of a 50-item reading comprehension test and a 17-item numerical ability test. The comprehension component uses a modified Cloze procedure in which every fifth to seventh word is omitted from a passage, and the test-taker selects from four possible choices. The numeracy portion presents the tester with cue cards or labeled prescription bottles, and they are asked to respond to oral questions related to information on the cards or bottles [9, 10].

Newest Vital Sign (NVS)

The NVS tool assesses health literacy using a nutritional label from an ice cream container. In clinical settings, patients are given the label and then asked a series of six questions. To correctly answer these questions, basic texts must be identified and interpreted, and simple mathematical computations must be performed. Scores ranging from 0 to 1 indicate a high likelihood (50% or more) of having limited health literacy, while scores ranging from 4 to 6 indicate adequate health literacy [11].

Brief Health Literacy Screening Tool (BRIEF)

The BRIEF tool relies on self-reports to evaluate issues related to reading, comprehension, the need for assistance, and confidence, thereby assessing health literacy. After four questions are presented, each of which is assigned a value ranging from one to five points, the assessment categorizes scores into health literacy levels (limited, marginal, or adequate). Administering the BRIEF assessment requires 1–2 min and minimal training [12].

Short Assessment of Health Literacy—Spanish and English (SAHL-S&E)

The SAHL employs word recognition skills, encompassing comprehension and pronunciation of health-related terms, to evaluate health literacy in adults. The assessment involves 18 health-related test terms, each accompanied by two association words: one keyword with a related meaning and one unrelated distractor word. Patients are tasked with selecting the work most akin to the health-related test term. The scoring criteria place individuals into one of two health literacy categories: adequate (15 or more correct answers) or inadequate (fewer than 15 correct answers). Administering the SAHL questionnaire takes 2–3 min, and minimal training is needed [12].

The consequences of limited health literacy may include billions of dollars in health care costs in addition to population health outcomes. When reviewing these consequences, low health literacy may impact health outcomes through mismatched reading abilities and levels of written health information and through a lack of health-related information that may be easily understood [12]. Recognizing and addressing the disparities associated with health literacy is essential for equitable and effective pain management and may be, in part, achieved through careful assessment of health literacy levels.

Pain Management Knowledge

Navigating the complexities of pain management requires a nuanced understanding of health literacy and, specifically, the role of health literacy in comprehending pain, effectively communicating pain management options, deciphering common pain management terminology, and determining the connection between treatment adherence and health literacy levels. Understanding pain goes beyond physical sensations and involves grasping the underlying factors contributing to one's pain experience. Individuals with higher health literacy levels can more effectively interpret and communicate their pain experiences to healthcare professionals, thus fostering more accurate diagnoses and targeted pain management strategies tailored to individual needs. Additionally, individuals with adequate health literacy exhibit less kinesiophobia, which impacts pain intensity and quality of life and may prevent effective treatment [13, 14]. One of the focal points of successful pain management is treatment adherence. Health literacy profoundly influences a patient's ability to understand and follow prescribed pain management plans. Low health literacy may also contribute to opioid misuse among individuals with chronic pain [15]. Other data have demonstrated that higher health literacy does not always translate to patients making appropriate pain management selections, especially for patients with osteoarthritis. However, there was a statistically significant interaction effect between health literacy and the appropriateness of self-management strategies [16]. In the realm of pain management, knowledge is considered empowerment, and health literacy is a tool for unlocking this empowerment for patients.

Barriers to Health Literacy in Pain Management

While recognizing the pivotal role of health literacy in pain management, it is imperative to acknowledge and address barriers that can impede effective communication and understanding. For example, patients may face cultural and linguistic barriers, socioeconomic factors, and limited access to resources. Therefore, it is important to assess and address health literacy and also delve into strategies to identify and overcome accompanying barriers to foster a more inclusive and accessible approach to pain care.

Health care professionals should be cognizant of what may be considered inappropriate or culturally insensitive for some cultures. Health literacy disparities are often intertwined with cultural disparities and should be considered. For example, religion and spirituality significantly influence healthcare decisions, a factor that may be overlooked by healthcare professionals in their evaluation of pain and palliative care. A lack of understanding may negatively affect the clinician-patient relationship, thus posing a substantial barrier to appropriate pain management. In another example, distinct cultural beliefs about the meaning, origin, and role of pain that exist in many cultures may influence how patients interpret and perceive pain. These cultural variations may lead to an over- or underestimation of pain severity, with decreased pain expression mistakenly interpreted by healthcare professionals as an absence of pain [17].

The interplay between health literacy and socioeconomic factors amplifies the challenges faced by certain populations. Limited access to education, economic resources, and healthcare services can compound the difficulty of understanding and managing pain. Data show that individuals with higher health literacy have better health outcomes than do those with lower health literacy [18–20]. Access to information is also a fundamental aspect of health literacy. The level of a patient's health literacy may impact their ability to access, navigate, and benefit from available resources. This might include understanding treatment options, navigating healthcare systems, reading and interpreting educational materials, and communicating with healthcare professionals.

Strategies to Improve Health Literacy in Pain Management

Understanding the role that health literacy plays in effective pain management leads to a discussion on action strategies aimed at enhancing health literacy among patients. By fostering patient-centered communication, utilizing plain language, providing comprehensive health education and resources, and empowering patients to ask questions, healthcare professionals can bridge gaps, ensuring a more informed and engaged patient population. Providing successful treatment to enhance a patient's health literacy involves more than just educating them about their pain and condition. It also encompasses pain management strategies that promote active involvement in healthcare. Factors such as relying solely on physicians, personal motivation, and resistance to accepting their condition can impede the development of literacy [21]. Some strategies to mitigate and address health literacy are described below (Table 27.2).

Table 27.2 Strategies to improve health literacy

Area of improvement	Action items
Patient-centered communication	
Active listening	Encourage health care providers to actively listen to patients, allowing them to express their pain experiences and concerns. Foster trust and open communication by creating a supportive environment where patients feel heard and understood.
Two-way communication	Facilitate a collaborative approach to pain management decisions via bidirectional communication between patients and healthcare professionals. Ensure a personalized and patient-centered care plan by encouraging patients to share their preferences, goals, and expectations.
Cultural competence	Train culturally aware professionals, recognizing and respecting diverse cultural beliefs and practices related to pain. Foster effective and respectful interactions by tailoring communication styles to align with the cultural backgrounds of patients.
Effective use of plain language	
Avoiding jargon	Refrain from using medical jargon and complex technology when discussing pain management. Empower patients to actively participate in their care by utilizing plain language to ensure that information is easily understood.
Use of visual aids	Visual aids, diagrams, and charts can be useful to supplement verbal information thus enhancing comprehension. Visual aids can simplify complex concepts and provide a clear visual representation of pain management strategies.
Health education and resources	
Comprehensive patient education	Include brochures, pamphlets, online resources, and other options to help provide comprehensive educational materials. Ensure accessibility of materials by tailoring the educational materials to varying literacy levels.
Accessible information	Consider diverse linguistic backgrounds. Accommodate different learning preferences by providing various formats, such as audio and video resources.
Empowering patients to ask questions	
Create a supportive environment	Foster an environment where patients feel comfortable asking questions. Discuss the importance of patient participation in the decision-making process.
Encourage questioning	Encourage patients to ask questions about pain, treatment, and potential side effects. Provide opportunities for patients to ask questions, demonstrate understanding, and seek clarification.

[22, 23]

The US Department of Health and Human Services Office of Disease Prevention and Health Promotion developed the National Action Plan to Improve Health Literacy with two main principles in mind. These two principles state that every individual has the entitlement to health information that facilitates informed decision-making and that health services must be provided in a manner that is clear and easily comprehensible and enhances overall health, longevity, and quality of life. The strategies included in this action plan are as follows [24]:

1. Develop and disseminate health and safety information that is accurate, accessible, and actionable.
2. Promote changes in the health care system that improve health information, communication, informed decision-making, and access to health services.
3. Incorporate accurate, standards-based, and developmentally appropriate health and science information and curricula in childcare and education at the university level.
4. Support and expand local efforts to provide adult education, English language instruction, and culturally and linguistically appropriate health information services in the community.
5. Build partnerships, develop guidance, and change policies.
6. Increase basic research and the development, implementation, and evaluation of practices and interventions to improve health literacy.
7. Increase the dissemination and use of evidence-based health literacy practices and interventions.

The Role of Healthcare Professionals

The ability of healthcare professionals to convey information, foster understanding, and promote shared decision-making plays a pivotal role in the overall well-being of individuals experiencing pain. An interdisciplinary team, including physicians, nurses, pharmacists, psychologists, social workers, and physical therapists, would allow for the integration of unique perspectives and varied expertise to help shape the patient's pain experience. Effective collaboration would require the team to develop empathy and active listening skills, tailor communication to the level of the patient, and utilize new tools and strategies, which are all important aspects in the role of the healthcare professional [7, 25].

Empathy lies at the heart of patient-centered care, particularly in the context of pain management. Healthcare professionals must cultivate the ability to understand the feelings of individuals experiencing pain. By acknowledging the emotional and physical aspects of pain, practitioners can build trust and establish a therapeutic alliance with their patients. Empathy and active listening go hand in hand, and the interdisciplinary team should also invest time in understanding the patient's pain experience, qualitatively and quantitatively. This will require paying close attention to nonverbal and verbal cues, validating emotions, and demonstrating concern. Additionally, McNeil et al. introduced the idea of "Health Harmonics," in which the practitioner and the patient bring different levels of nutrition/physical literacy, cognitive literacy, and social literacy and attempt to understand the connection between those during treatment. The idea is to explore the bidirectional transaction between the patient and the practitioner to reduce generalization that has little to no alignment with the patient's frequency on the topic, with no shared meaning [26].

Beyond general understanding and empathy, effective interdisciplinary communication hinges on the ability to convey information in a comprehensible manner. Recognizing and addressing diverse health literacy levels is essential, and healthcare professionals can employ strategies to tailor communication to the specific health literacy levels of the patients. There are a number of tools and strategies that have been outlined below (Table 27.3):

Table 27.3 Strategies and tools to promote health literacy in practice

Area of communication	Strategies	Tools
Verbal communication	Plain language Speak clearly and at a moderate pace Limit content to three key points at a time Confirm patient understanding	Teach-back technique Chunk and check technique
Written communication	Short, simple sentences 5th- to sixth-grade reading level Review educational materials with the patient Bold key words on forms	Use electronic tools to help assess the reading level of written material
Visual aids	Include simple pictures Use videos, models, and photonovelas	Online videos
Patient empowerment	Encourage patient participation Encourage patients to bring a list of questions Provide written or typed medication lists Assess understanding of medications and adherence	AHRQ toolkit

[27]

Future Directions and Conclusion

As we navigate the intricate landscape of health literacy in pain management, it becomes increasingly evident that evolving healthcare policies play a pivotal role in shaping patients' experiences. The recognition of health literacy as a fundamental aspect of effective pain management underscores the need for policymakers to integrate literacy-enhancing strategies into broader healthcare initiatives. A proper start for this need has been outlined in Healthy People 2030, where individuals address personal and organizational health literacy [24]. This calls for healthcare professionals to be proactive in their approach to patient care related to health literacy by championing patient-centered communication, using plain language, and providing patient-focused pain management.

References

1. U.S. Department of Health and Human Services. Pain management best practices Inter-Agency Task Force Report: updates, gaps, inconsistencies, and recommendations. 2019. Retrieved from U. S. Department of Health and Human Services website: https://www.hhs.gov/ash/advisory-committees/pain/reports/index.html.
2. Remarks by vice president Harris at National League of Cities Conference. The White House March 8, 2021. https://www.whitehouse.gov/briefing-room/speeches-remarks/2021/03/08/remarks-by-vice-president-harris-at-national-league-of-cities-conference/. Accessed 12 Nov 2023
3. Health literacy. National Institutes of Health. July 7, 2021. https://www.nih.gov/institutes-nih/nih-office-director/office-communications-public-liaison/clear-communication/health-literacy. Accessed 10 Nov 2023
4. Kutner M, Greenberg E Jin Y, Paulson C. US Department of Education, National Center for Education Statistics, Washington, DC. 2006.
5. Pain. National Institute of Neurological Disorders and Stroke. https://www.ninds.nih.gov/health-information/disorders/pain. Accessed 10 Nov 2023
6. American Academy of Pan Medicine. Health literacy and pain management: a position statement from the American Academy of Pain Medicine. Pain Med. 2019;20(3):429–31. https://doi.org/10.1093/pm/pny200.
7. Institute of Medicine (US) Committee on Health Literacy. Health literacy: a prescription to end confusion. National Academies Press (US); 2004. https://doi.org/10.17226/10883.
8. Agency for Healthcare Research and Quality. Personal health literacy measurement tools. AHRQ. n.d.. https://www.ahrq.gov/health-literacy/research/tools/index.html#rapid
9. Test of functional health literacy in adults: Short Test of Functional Literacy in Adults (STOFHLA). Literacy in Health Care. 1995
10. Parker RM, Baker DW, Williams MV, Nurss JR. The test of functional health literacy in adults: a new instrument for measuring patients' literacy skills. J Gen Intern Med. 1995;10(10):537–41. https://doi.org/10.1007/BF02640361.
11. Weiss BD. The newest vital sign: frequently asked questions. Health Lit Res Pract. 2018;2(3):e125–7. https://doi.org/10.3928/24748307-20180530-02.
12. Fortuna J. Quick and valid tools for measuring health literacy. MEDBRIDGE. 2022. Quick and Valid Tools for Measuring Health Literacy - MedBridge Blog

13. Bittencourt JV, de Souza PAC, Corrêa LA, Volotão AN, Mathieson S, Nogueira LAC. Health literacy, pain-related interference and pain-related distress of patients with musculoskeletal pain. Health Promot Int. 2023;38(4):daab183. https://doi.org/10.1093/heapro/daab183.
14. Malfliet A. Breaking the cycle of misinformation: health literacy's role in managing chronic pain. Pain in Motion. n.d.. http://www.paininmotion.be/blog/detail/breaking-cycle-misinformation-health-literacys-role-managing-chronic-pain
15. Rogers AH, Bakhshaie J, Orr MF, Ditre JW, Zvolensky MJ. Health literacy, opioid misuse, and pain experience among adults with chronic pain. Pain Med. 2020;21(4):670–6. https://doi.org/10.1093/pm/pnz062.
16. Hunter DJ, McLachlan AJ, Carroll PR, Wakefield TAN, Stosic R. Health literacy and appropriateness of self-care and pain management in osteoarthritis: an understanding of the patient's perspective. Arthritis Care Res (Hoboken). 2023 Apr;75(4):848–59. https://doi.org/10.1002/acr.24851.
17. Gilver A, Bhatt H, Maani-Fogelman P. The importance of cultural competence in pain and palliative care. StatPearls Publishing; n.d.. https://www.ncbi.nlm.nih.gov/books/NBK493154/
18. Furuya Y, Kondo N, Yamagata Z, Hashimoto H. Health literacy, socioeconomic status and self-rated health in Japan. Health Promot Int. 2015;30(3):505–13. https://doi.org/10.1093/heapro/dat071.
19. Lastrucci V, Lorini C, Caini S, Florence Health Literacy Research Group, Bonaccorsi G. Health literacy as a mediator of the relationship between socioeconomic status and health: a cross-sectional study in a population-based sample in Florence. PLoS One. 2019;14(12):e0227007. https://doi.org/10.1371/journal.pone.0227007.
20. Nadi T, Poorolajal J, Doosti-Irani A. Socioeconomic status and health literacy as the important predictors of general health in Iran: a structural equation modeling approach. Res Square. 2020; https://doi.org/10.21203/rs.2.22404/v1
21. Edwards M, Wood F, Davies M, Edwards A. The development of health literacy in patients with a long-term health condition: the health literacy pathway model. BMC Public Health. 2012;12:130. https://doi.org/10.1186/1471-2458-12-130.
22. Kountz DS. Strategies for improving low health literacy. Postgrad Med. 2009;121(5):171–7. https://doi.org/10.3810/pgm.2009.09.2065.
23. Hasannejadasl H, Roumen C, Smit Y, Dekker A, Fijten R. Health literacy and eHealth: challenges and strategies. JCO Clin Cancer Inform. 2022;6:e2200005. https://doi.org/10.1200/CCI.22.00005.
24. Healthy People 2023 U.S. Department of Health and Human Services, Office of Disease Prevention and Health Promotion. National action plan to improve health literacy. Washington, DC. 2010.
25. Sørensen K, Van den Broucke S, Fullam J, Doyle G, Pelikan J, Slonska Z, et al. Health literacy and public health: a systematic review and integration of definitions and models. BMC Public Health. 2012;12(1):80. https://doi.org/10.1186/1471-2458-12-80.
26. McNeil A, Arena R. The evolution of health literacy and communication: introducing health harmonics. Prog Cardiovasc Dis. 2017;59(5):463–70. https://doi.org/10.1016/j.pcad.2017.02.003.
27. Hersh L, Salzman B, Snyderman D. Health literacy in primary care practice. Am Fam Physician. 2015;92(2):118–24.

Managing Nonadherence

28

Sarah Aldrich Renner, Marilee Clemons, Brian Tasma, and Derek Gyori

Abbreviations

CMS	Centers for Medicare and Medicaid Services
IAS	Immunoassay Screen
MEMS	Medication event monitoring system
MPR	Medication possession ratio
PDC	Proportion of days covered
PDMP	Prescription drug monitoring program
SMART	Specific, measurable, achievable, realistic, time-bound
THC	Tetrahydrocannabinol

Introduction

Language/Disclaimer: In 2021, the American Medical Association published "Advancing Health Equity: A Guide to Language, Narrative, and Concepts," aiming to promote a deeper understanding of equity-focused, person-first language. Promoting health equity involves ensuring that everyone can attain their highest level of health, regardless of social, economic, or other factors [1]. Language plays a significant role in shaping public perceptions and healthcare practice. Terms such as "nonadherence" and "noncompliance" can be used to describe situations where patients do not follow a medical plan. However, noncompliance generally refers to an intentional refusal to follow a treatment plan, whereas nonadherence recognizes that there may be complex, multifactorial reasons why a patient may not follow a treatment plan [2]. Some may feel that "nonadherence" carries implicit biases and contributes to the stigma that a patient does not follow instructions when the situation may be more complex. It is essential to approach discussions around health and healthcare in a way that is respectful, inclusive, and culturally sensitive [3].

For the context of this chapter, we would like to address the use of the term "nonadherence" in our discussions. It has come to our attention that this word may have unintended connotations and could be perceived as stigmatizing. We want to emphasize that the use of the word "nonadherence" is not meant to discredit any individual or group. Our intention is to communicate medication-taking behaviors in a neutral and inclusive manner.

Introduction Nonadherence can significantly challenge the United States healthcare system, impacting both patient outcomes and healthcare costs. When patients do not take their medications or do not utilize nonpharmacologic therapy as prescribed, it can lead to worsened health conditions, unwanted hospitalizations, and a higher chance of preventable complications [4]. The financial impact of morbidity and mortality associated with medication nonadherence is estimated to cost the United States healthcare system over $500 billion annually [5]. Medication nonadherence in pain management can have negative implications for individual patients and the healthcare team. In general, pain management requires timely and consistent use of medication to reduce pain, improve function, and enhance quality of life. When patients do not appropriately take their pain medications, they can experience inadequate pain relief, poor function, increased healthcare utilization, such as emergency department visits, and strained provider-patient relationships [6].

S. A. Renner (✉) · M. Clemons
General Internal Medicine & Pharmacy Practice, University of Toledo College of Pharmacy and Pharmaceutical Sciences, Toledo, OH, USA
e-mail: sarah.aldrich2@utoledo.edu

B. Tasma
General Internal Medicine & Pharmacy Practice, University of Toledo College of Pharmacy and Pharmaceutical Sciences, Toledo, OH, USA

Department of Internal Medicine, College of Medicine and Life Sciences, The University of Toledo, Toledo, OH, USA

D. Gyori
General Internal Medicine & Pharmacy Practice, University of Toledo College of Pharmacy and Pharmaceutical Sciences, Toledo, OH, USA

VA Ann Arbor Healthcare System, Ann Arbor, MI, USA

J. P. Reinert et al. (eds.), *Adjunctive Analgesic Strategies for the Bedside Clinician and Beyond*,
https://doi.org/10.1007/978-3-032-21675-5_28

A patient-centered approach to addressing medication adherence prioritizes the unique preferences and circumstances of each patient. Rather than relying on a one-size-fits-all model, this strategy tailors interventions to reflect a patient's daily life, which fosters trust and collaboration between the patient and the healthcare team. By recognizing and addressing a patient's personal barriers, such as financial constraints, literacy, or cultural beliefs, clinicians can better support patients in achieving their goals. Literature shows that interventions that include shared decision-making and individualized care are effective at improving adherence and clinical outcomes. Implementing a patient-centered approach in the real world can present challenges. Many adherence strategies developed in clinical trials may not account for the complex nature of life. Time constraints, limited resources, fragmented healthcare systems, and systemic barriers can prevent the consistent application of personalized strategies. Additionally, translating evidence-based models into clinical practice requires training, workflow updates, and sustained commitment from the health care team. Regardless, by trying to understand the individual, healthcare providers can better navigate these challenges and promote healthcare adherence through meaningful and informed solutions [7].

Addressing medication adherence utilizes a patient-centered approach that prioritizes the needs of the individual and the circumstances of the patient to improve their medication-taking behaviors. This approach recognizes that each patient may face various challenges that impact their ability to take their medications as prescribed. Evidence-based strategies provide valuable foundations for adherence interventions; however, it is important to recognize that real-world patient experiences often deviate from what is observed in clinical studies. Literature-based approaches may overlook the details of an individual's life and their challenges. A patient-centered approach focuses on tailoring the medication adherence strategies based on each patient's specific needs. By utilizing a patient-centered approach, the healthcare team can create a collaborative and effective relationship with patients, enhancing the likelihood of positive patient outcomes [7].

Addressing nonadherence in pain management requires a comprehensive approach that includes patient education, regular follow-up visits, and fostering an open channel of communication between the patient and provider. The healthcare team plays a vital role in maintaining an open line of communication, understanding reasons for nonadherence, and working with patients to develop an effective pain management strategy that aligns with the patients' goals [8].

Measures of Nonadherence

To improve medication adherence, the provider must discern if the patient is taking their medication correctly. There are two main methods for assessing adherence: direct measures and indirect measures. Currently, no unanimous agreement exists on the best method or combination to measure adherence [9]. Each measure has its advantages and disadvantages. Combining them can guide treatment decisions but should not replace clinical judgment.

Direct methods utilize objective data to confirm adherence to prescribed opioids. Specifically, toxicology testing is a method of examining blood, urine, saliva, sweat, hair, or feces to identify the presence of drugs. Drugs include prescribed, non-prescribed, recreational, and illicit. Urine is the most common testing medium [10]. However, it may be easier to alter when compared with blood or saliva testing due to not always being able to directly observe sample collection. Toxicology testing includes two main categories: presumptive testing and confirmatory testing. Presumptive testing, also known as immunoassay screening (IAS), is an antibody test used to detect certain drugs or their metabolites [11]. For example, the urine immunoassay screen can be done in minutes and is an easy, widely available, and relatively inexpensive screening method. Presumptive testing is generally considered a qualitative test, as it reports the presence or absence of a drug but will not quantify the result if positive. It can be used to detect natural opioids such as morphine and codeine, benzodiazepines, and illicit/recreational drugs such as amphetamine, cocaine, and tetrahydrocannabinol (THC). However, they may not detect all drugs within a class, such as synthetic/semisynthetic opioids, including oxycodone, hydrocodone, hydromorphone, methadone, fentanyl, and others (see Tables 28.1 and 28.2) [12–15]. Fentanyl and other synthetic opiates are not typically detectable in many immu-

Table 28.1 Frequently screened medications and common false positives

Parent drug	Common false positive agents
Amphetamine	Amantadine, atenolol, bupropion, chlorpromazine, desipramine, fluoxetine, labetalol, methylphenidate, metformin, ofloxacin, phentermine, phenylephrine, promethazine, pseudoephedrine, ranitidine, selegiline, thioridazine, trazodone
Barbiturates	Ibuprofen, naproxen
Benzodiazepines	Efavirenz, oxaprozin, sertraline
Cannabinoids	Dronabinol, ibuprofen, naproxen, proton pump inhibitors (i.e., pantoprazole), sulindac
Cocaine	Coca leaf tea, topical anesthetics containing cocaine
Methadone	Clomipramine, chlorpromazine, diphenhydramine, doxylamine, quetiapine, thioridazine, verapamil
Opiates	Dextromethorphan, diphenhydramine, fluoroquinolone antibiotics (i.e., levofloxacin), poppy seeds, quinine, rifampin
Phencyclidine	Desvenlafaxine, dextromethorphan, diphenhydramine, doxylamine, ibuprofen, imipramine, ketamine, lamotrigine, meperidine, thioridazine, tramadol, venlafaxine
Tricyclic antidepressants	Carbamazepine, cyclobenzaprine, cyproheptadine, diphenhydramine, hydroxyzine, quetiapine

Table 28.2 Frequently screened medications and common false negatives

Parent drug	Common false negative agents
Amphetamine	MDMA (ecstasy)
Benzodiazepines	Alprazolam, clonazepam, lorazepam, triazolam
Opiates	Fentanyl, hydrocodone, hydromorphone, methadone, oxycodone, tramadol

noassay screens [11]. Confirmatory testing often follows to verify the identity of the substance. Generally, providers start with presumptive testing, such as a urine screen, as this tends to be easy, widely available, and cost-effective. Unexpected results from presumptive testing are typically followed by confirmatory testing [11]. Confirmatory testing generally includes chromatography and spectrometry, which is more costly and may have a longer turnaround time [15]. Presumptive and confirmatory testing may also help identify drugs not managed by a healthcare provider, such as illicit substances.

It is recommended to test patients, using presumptive and/or confirmatory testing, before starting opioids and at least every 12 months [10]. Testing can be done more frequently depending on patient risk factors and provider preference. Random testing is preferred over scheduled testing, as it reduces the chance of patients altering their drug use before anticipated tests.

Direct testing may yield unexpected results, such as a false negative, especially in patients who infrequently use opioids. It is also possible that false positives can occur due to cross-reactivity with other drugs [11]. For example, poppy seeds, quinolones, rifampin, verapamil, diphenhydramine, quinine, and naloxone can lead to a false positive for opioids on presumptive testing. Healthcare providers should not stop opioid treatment based on toxicology results alone. Instead, these results should be used along with the overall clinical picture, knowing the limitations of the tests. It is essential to discuss unexpected results with patients in a nonjudgmental manner to better understand the patient and adjust the treatment plan as necessary.

Indirect methods use nonphysical means to assess adherence and are often more straightforward and cost-effective than direct methods. For example, pill counts involve patients bringing in pill bottles and medication organizers during office visits to verify that they contain the appropriate quantity. However, this method can be manipulated if patients bring someone else's pills. Medication event monitoring systems (MEMS) log the time and date a medication container is opened but can overestimate adherence [16]. Prescription drug monitoring programs (PDMPs) allow providers to track controlled substances dispensed in each state. Providers should use PDMPs prior to starting therapy and at a minimum every 3 months; however, reviewing prior to refilling controlled prescriptions is ideal [10]. While PDMPs provide much valuable information to the providers about dispensed controlled substances, they may not include all relevant information and thus should not be used as the sole source of information to assess adherence (Table 28.2).

Questionnaires are another indirect method to measure adherence, though they rely on patient-provided information. Many questionnaires are available, and all include the possibility of recall bias and overestimation of adherence. One example is the Morisky Medication Adherence Scale, a commonly used 4- and 8-point scale used to assess medication adherence in patients with hypertension, diabetes, asthma, and other conditions. Claims data from insurance companies or pharmacies, including the dates of prescriptions filled and days' supply, can demonstrate the time period when medications are dispensed but do not confirm actual administration. Examples of claims data include the proportion of days covered (PDC) and medication possession ratio (MPR). PDC is a percentage calculated using the number of days "covered" in a period divided by the number of days in the period, multiplied by 100. PDC is utilized by insurance companies, Medicare, and studies to measure adherence [17]. A PDC of 80% or greater is considered adherent to therapy. However, these calculations often overestimate adherence and do not demonstrate whether a patient is actually taking a medication. For example, a patient could have 90-day supplies of all medications filled by a mail-order pharmacy, which would show a PDC of 100%, but the patient might never take the medications once they arrive. Therefore, providers are encouraged to consider a holistic approach combining multiple methods to obtain a comprehensive assessment of medication adherence. MPR is a percentage calculated using the sum of dispensed days' supply divided by the number of days in the time period. This is not used as commonly as PDC, as it can overestimate adherence [18].

Dimensions of Nonadherence

The World Health Organization (WHO) suggests five dimensions of nonadherence. The five dimensions of nonadherence are social and economic, health care system-related, condition-related, patient-related, or therapy-related (see Table 28.3) [19, 20]. These relate to and categorize the many reasons patients may experience nonadherence. Adherence is multidimensional, and determining the underlying causes or dimensions of nonadherence can aid in finding an appropriate solution.

The social or economic dimension refers to issues where patients must choose between medical and other priorities. This has not been shown to be an independent predictor of adherence, but these factors can play a role [21]. Examples of nonadherence in this dimension are varied but could be related to low health literacy, medication cost, lack of health

Table 28.3 Nonadherence dimensions and barriers

Dimension of nonadherence	Barriers to adherence
Social and economic	Lack of insurance or inadequate insurance coverage Unemployment High cost of medications, transport or care Poverty or poor socio-economic status Low health literacy, illiteracy, low level of education Lack of social support Lack of stable living conditions, family functioning or environment
Healthcare team or system-related	Lack of care continuity Restricted formularies Poor medication distribution systems or medication recalls Long wait times for care or medications Limited or inadequate health insurance plan reimbursement Poorly developed health services Healthcare team member burnout Lack of knowledge or training for providers on managing chronic conditions or adherence Limited ability to establish community support and patient self-management Short appointment times resulting in limited time for patient education
Condition-related	Lack of symptoms Severity of symptoms or rate of disease progression Level of disability (physical, psychological, social or vocational) Certain conditions resulting in limited motivation such as depression Availability of effective treatments
Therapy-related	Complexity of regimen Frequent changes Actual or perceived side effects Previous treatment failures Timing of therapy effectiveness or beneficial effects Duration of treatment
Patient-related	Forgetfulness or low motivation Inadequate knowledge or skill for managing disease symptoms and treatment Mistrust or frustration with treatment or healthcare providers Visual, hearing or cognitive impairment Perceived risk of disease or need for treatment Perceived risks or effectiveness of treatment Lack of perceived benefits for treatment Psychological stress (anxiety) surrounding treatment or possible adverse effects Low follow-up attendance Stigmatization of disease

insurance, or lack of transportation. Additionally, financial--related factors such as unemployment, unstable living conditions, transportation costs, and poverty can impact adherence.

The healthcare system-related dimension, sometimes called the healthcare team-related dimension, refers to issues navigating and utilizing the healthcare system. This could involve a lack of care continuity, formulary restrictions, long wait times, or poor systems for medication distribution. Additionally, patient-provider relationships can impact adherence positively with good relationships [22] or negatively with care that is not patient-centered, short visits, long follow-up times, or provider burnout. Healthcare teams or systems may have poorly developed services and a lack of knowledge or training for disease or adherence management. Navigating the healthcare system can be a challenge for patients and contribute to nonadherence. In addition, a key area of concern when navigating the healthcare system is during transitions of care, where the movement of patients between settings and providers creates adherence challenges. Chapters 29 and 30 provide more information on these barriers.

The condition-related dimension refers to illness-related demands and challenges faced by patients. The impact is often determined by patient perception. Patients with condition-related nonadherence may be due to a lack of symptoms, symptom severity, disease severity and progression, level of disability related to the condition, or availability of effective treatments [20]. It's important to consider that many treatments for pain may offer improvement of symptoms but may not result in complete relief or resolution. If patients have an expectation of total pain relief and that doesn't happen, they may feel the medication is ineffective and stop taking it. Providers can prevent this from occurring by having clear conversations with patients about expectations of managing their pain vs. eliminating it [8].

The patient-related dimension refers to the resources, knowledge, perceptions, beliefs, and attitudes of the patient. Additionally, a patient's understanding of the perceived risk of disease versus the perceived benefit of treatment can impact adherence to therapy. These beliefs, alongside the patient's expectations for treatment, influence motivation to adhere to prescribed treatment.

The fifth dimension is therapy-related and directly correlates to the treatment regimen. Patients may have difficulty with regimen complexity, frequency of changes, actual side effects, perceived side effects, or treatment duration. Regimen complexity can include frequency of administration, routes of administration, titration or taper instructions, or specific dosing instructions surrounding food or fluids. Additionally, therapy may be impacted by previous treatment experiences or failures. Finally, patients may experience a perceived lack of benefit for certain therapies when symptoms are not impacted, or medications require longer periods of use or titration to demonstrate therapeutic effect [19].

Adherence to pain management can be impacted by all five dimensions of adherence. Research is limited surrounding general adherence to pain management regimens, as most studies focus on misuse and abuse. One systematic review compiled the available literature to determine factors that improve or worsen medication adherence and categorized them into the WHO dimensions of nonadherence. Regarding socio-economic factors, education level was found to negatively impact analgesic adherence in one study, but this was not replicated in two others. Therapeutic relationship challenges, as well as a lack of information, negatively impacted adherence in the healthcare system/team-related dimension. The data surrounding condition-related factors is variable, but pain intensity is commonly associated with changes in adherence. Regimen complexity, including multiple medications and increased dosing frequency, resulted in worsening adherence. Finally, patient-related factors seem to have a significant impact on pain management. Perception of chronic or uncontrollable illness, increased knowledge of medications, and age demonstrated improved adherence. Whereas addiction concerns, tolerance, perceived or actual side effects, and withdrawal were associated with worsening adherence [8].

Strategies to Improve Nonadherence

When it comes to improving patient medication-taking behaviors, there is no one-size-fits-all solution. Every patient and circumstance are different, resulting in the need for a multi-method approach to find a solution. Various strategies can be used to enhance medication adherence (Fig. 28.1) [20].

The SIMPLE strategy [23] is an effective approach to improve medication adherence by simplifying the patient's regimen. It focuses on minimizing complexity and barriers to adherence, making it easier for patients to follow.

- Simplify the regimen: Aim to reduce the number of medications and dosing frequency whenever possible. Utilize combination products, if feasible, to simplify the regimen, making it easier for patients to follow consistently. For example, use once-daily or long-acting formulations when appropriate.
- Impart knowledge: Provide patients with clear and concise information about their medications, including their indications, how to take them, potential side effects, and the importance of taking the medication. For example, tell the patient, "this therapy may reduce your pain by about 50%, not totally eliminate it."
- Modify patient beliefs: Ask patients open-ended questions about the impact of not taking their medications or the reasons why they do not take them. Address any misconceptions or concerns patients may have, clarify misunderstandings, and provide reassurance to alleviate fears.
- Provide communication and trust: Encourage patients to actively participate in discussions about their disease state and medications. Provide emotional support and allow ample time and opportunity for patients to ask questions.

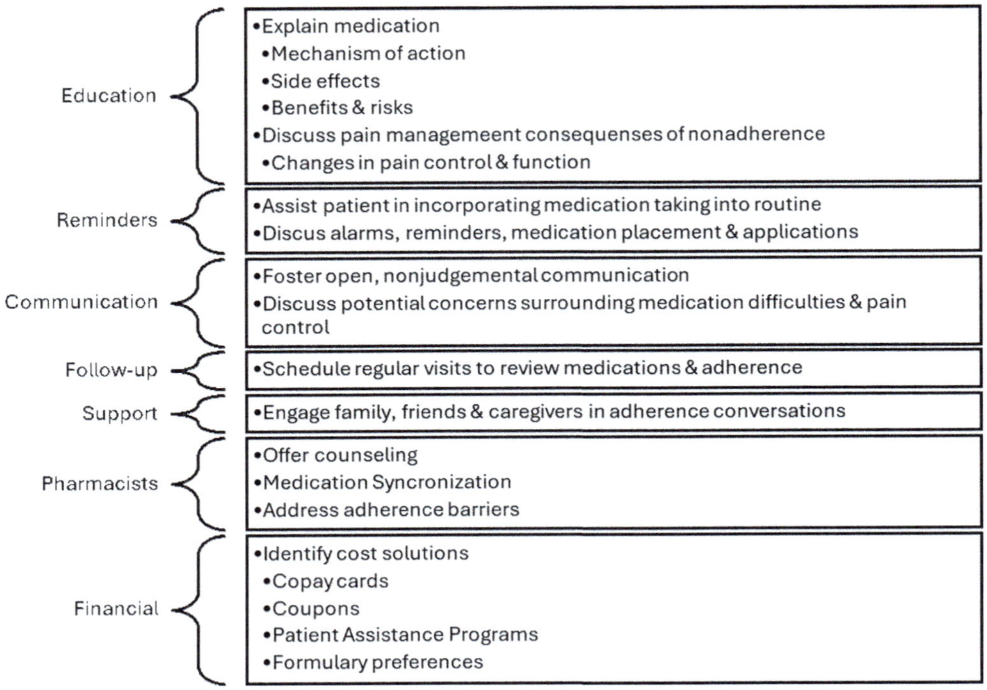

Fig. 28.1 Strategies to improve nonadherence

- Leave the bias: Avoid making assumptions or judgments about patients. Understand that challenges with taking medication can arise from a variety of factors, and it is important to approach each patient with a nonjudgmental attitude.
- Evaluate adherence: Continuously monitor and assess medication adherence. Work with the patient to make needed adjustments. Regular follow-up appointments with the healthcare team are crucial for assessing progress and addressing challenges.

The SIMPLE strategy is an accessible and practical approach to improving medication-taking behaviors. By simplifying medication regimens, providing education, offering tools and support, and involving patients in their care, healthcare professionals can empower patients to manage their health and improve their pain. This approach helps providers set realistic expectations, simplify regimens, and build trust through open communication. By addressing patient beliefs and routinely evaluating adherence, this strategy reinforces a collaborative and effective approach to managing pain and helps patients stay on track with their health.

Adherence to Nonpharmacological Treatment

As with most chronic disease states, nonpharmacological treatments are recommended in addition to pharmacological options for pain management. Nonpharmacologic therapies play a crucial role in.

addressing the complex nature of pain and helping promote self-management [24]. Like medication adherence, following nonpharmacologic recommendations and incorporating them into the A multimodal and multidisciplinary approach to pain management can prevent worsening of health conditions, hospitalization, other complications, and improve health-related quality of life [25]. Numerous nonpharmacological treatments can be used to prevent and treat pain:

- Exercise: walking, running, lifting, cycling, and some aspects of physical therapy.
- Psychological therapies: cognitive behavioral therapy, biofeedback, relaxation techniques.
- Acceptance and commitment therapy.
- Mind-body practices: yoga, tai chi, qigong.
- Mindfulness practice: meditation, mindfulness-based stress reduction.
- Spinal manipulation: chiropractic or osteopathic manipulation.
- Complementary and alternative medicine: acupuncture, massage, art, music.
- Interdisciplinary rehabilitation: functional restoration.
- Physical modalities: traction, ultrasound, transcutaneous electrical nerve stimulation (TENS), low-level laser therapy, superficial heat or cold, bracing for knee, back or neck, electro-muscular therapy, magnets.

As with medication adherence, nonpharmacological treatment relies heavily on direct and indirect measures to assess patients' adherence to treatments. Direct measurements of adherence to nonpharmacologic therapy often come in the form of office visits or therapy sessions with healthcare professionals. For example, adherence to physical therapy can be measured by attending supervised appointments with their physical therapist or physical therapy assistant. In some cases, measuring adherence to nonpharmacological treatments relies solely on attendance (Table 28.4). However, there are instances where unsupervised nonpharmacological therapies may be recommended (i.e., avoiding bed rest, physical therapy exercises at home, yoga twice daily at home, and cold packs twice daily). These unsupervised

Table 28.4 Methods to address nonadherence

Potential reason for nonadherence	Suggested strategies for improvement
Adverse effects	Prescribe alternative medication Switch medication formulation Provide education to address perceived adverse effects
Cost	Investigate insurance formulary Encourage the use of manufacturer coupons Ensure patient is using an in-network pharmacy Utilize pharmacy discount cards Enroll patients in patient assistance programs
Lack of understanding	Educate patient on disease state, lifestyle, and medications Assess and address health literacy Set appropriate expectations with patient on medication effects
Forgetfulness	Set alarms as medication reminders Store medications in a visible place (safe from pets and children) Establish a daily routine to take medications Utilize adherence applications or packaging
Regimen complexity	Deprescribe medications Use medication synchronization programs at the pharmacy Prescribe medication adherence/blister packaging Order 90-day prescriptions for chronic therapy

activities and missing supervised appointments make up the most common form of nonadherence to nonpharmacological treatments [24].

The unsupervised activities recommended by healthcare providers encourage patients to take ownership and promote self-management of their nonpharmacological pain regimen [24]. To ensure patients are completing unsupervised activities, healthcare providers need to be active in conversations with patients to develop a plan, set goals, and discuss realistic expectations [8]. Important concepts to include in developing plans and goals and setting realistic expectations would be to set goals using the SMART goals acronym—Specific, Measurable, Achievable, Relevant, and Time-Based—and utilize motivational interviewing to help patients be an active part in developing their treatment plan by engaging the patients in decisions, showing empathy, and promoting optimism [26, 27]. These techniques can help guide discussion at future appointments and encourage ownership of patient healing and quality of life [24]. In addition to developing a plan and setting patient-centered goals, it is important to ensure that patients set realistic expectations. Often, patients will abandon nonpharmacological therapies due to unexpected difficulty, lack of progress, increased pain initially, lack of motivation or time, and expense [28]. Therefore, it is important to discuss these expectations up front and incorporate them into motivational interviewing and SMART goal setting.

Applications to Clinical Practice + Conclusion

Ensuring adherence is multidimensional and essential for successful pain management. Achieving and maintaining adherence requires a multidisciplinary approach that includes patient education, regular follow-ups, and open communication between the patient and providers. Providers should assess adherence utilizing direct and indirect measures and modify the regimen to achieve optimal pain control. Measuring adherence is complex and requires a multimodal approach. Objective data may indicate a patient has their medication but not identify true adherence, which would necessitate further exploration with the patient. Understanding the root cause of adherence can guide effective interventions. Strategies such as SIMPLE, motivational interviewing, patient-centered conversations, and setting SMART goals can increase adherence across all modalities.

Overall, clinicians and healthcare staff need to take an active role in identifying reasons for nonadherence and addressing barriers. Adherence is different for each patient and requires a patient-centered approach for resolution and prevention.

References

1. American Medical Association. Advancing health equity: a guide to language, narrative, and concepts. Washington, DC. 2021. Available at https://www.ama-assn.org/system/files/ama-aamc-equity-guide.pdf. Accessed 01 Dec 2023.
2. Cooperative of American Physicians. The noncompliant vs. the non-adherent patient. 2016. Available at https://www.capphysicians.com/articles/noncompliant-vs-non-adherent-patient. Accessed 27 May 2025.
3. Johnston Roberts K, Volberding P. Adherence communication: a qualitative analysis of physician-patient dialogue. AIDS. 1999;13(13):1771–8.
4. Chisholm-Burns M, Spivey C. The 'cost' of medication nonadherence: consequences we cannot afford to accept. J Am Pharm Assoc. 2012;52(6):823–6.
5. Klein D. Medication non-adherence: a common and costly problem. PAN Foundation. 2020; Available at https://www.panfoundation.org/app/uploads/2020/05/Issue-Brief-13_Medication-Adherence.pdf. Accessed 01 Dec 2023
6. Morris D, FergusonM. Ask the PharmD: how to improve medication adherence in chronic pain management. Pract Pain Manage. 2021;21(4). Available at https://www.medcentral.com/meds/adherence/how-improve-medication-adherence-chronic-pain-management. Accessed 08 Dec 2023.
7. Brown M, Sinsky CA. Medication adherence: improve patient outcomes and reduce costs. American Medical Association. 2018. Available at https://edhub.ama-assn.org/steps-forward/module/2702595. Accessed 08 Dec 2023.
8. Timmerman L, Stronks D, et al. The relation between patients' beliefs about pain medication, medication adherence, and treatment outcomes in chronic pain patients: a prospective study. Clin J Pain. 2019; https://doi.org/10.1097/AJP.0000000000000760.
9. Lin Y, Liang L, Ding R, et al. Factors associated with nonadherence to lung cancer screening across multiple screening time points. JAMA Netw Open. 2023; https://doi.org/10.1001/jamanetworkopen.2023.15250.
10. Dowell D, Ragan KR, Jones CM, Baldwin GT, Chou R. CDC clinical practice guideline for prescribing opioids for pain—United States. MMWR Recomm Rep. 2022; 71(RR-3), 1–95. Available at https://doi.org/10.15585/mmwr.rr7103a1. Accessed 3 Nov 2023.
11. Raouf M, Bettinger JJ, Fudin J. A practical guide to urine drug monitoring. Fed Pract. 2018;35(4):38–44. PMID: 30766353; PMCID: PMC6368048.
12. Stanbridge J, Adams S, Zotos A. Urine drug screen: a valuable office procedure. Am Fam Physician. 2010;81(5):635–40. Accessed 04 Mar 2025.
13. Brahm N, Yeager L, Fox M, et al. Commonly prescribed medications and potential false-positive urine drug screens. Am J Health Syst Pharm. 2010;67:1344–50. Accessed 04 Mar 2025.
14. Saitman A, Park H, Fitzgerald R. False-positive interferences of common urine drug screen immunoassays: a review. J Anal Toxicol. 2014;38:387–96. Accessed 04 Mar 2025.
15. Moeller K, Lee K, Kissack J. Urine drug screen: practical guideline for clinicians. Mayo Clin Proc. 2008;83(1):66–76. Accessed 04 Mar 2025.
16. van Onzenoort HAW, Verberk WJ, Kessels AGH, Kroon AA, Neef C, van der Kuy P-HM, de Leeuw PW. Assessing medication adherence simultaneously by electronic monitoring and pill count in patients with mild-to-moderate hypertension. Am J Hypertens. 2010;23(2):149–54. https://doi.org/10.1038/ajh.2009.207.
17. Prieto-Merino D, Mulick A, Armstrong C, Hoult H, Fawcett S, Eliasson L, Clifford S. Estimating proportion of days covered (PDC) using real-world online medicine suppliers' datasets. J

Pharm Policy Pract. 2021;14(1):113. https://doi.org/10.1186/s40545-021-00385-w. PMID: 34965882; PMCID: PMC8715592.
18. Pharmacy Times. Do you know the difference between these adherence measures? 2015. Available at https://www.pharmacytimes.com/view/do-you-know-the-difference-between-these-adherence--measures. Accessed 18 June 2025.
19. Sabaté E. Adherence to long-term therapies: evidence for action. Geneva: World Health Organization; 2003.
20. Aldrich Renner S, Clemons M, et al.. Medication adherence: the key to positive patient outcomes. The Ohio Cardiovascular & Diabetes Health Collaborative. 2022. Available at https://www.cardi-oh.org/assets/best-practices/patient-Adherence/Cardi-OH--Medication-Adherence-the-Key-to-Positive-Patient-Outcomes.pdf. Accessed 08 Dec 2023.
21. Alsabbagh W, Lemstra M, Eurich D, et al. Socioeconomic status and nonadherence to antihypertensive drugs: a systemic review and meta-analysis. Value Health. 2014;3(17):288–96.
22. Rose LE, Kim MT, Dennison CR, Hill MN. The contexts of adherence for African Americans with high blood pressure. J Adv Nurse. 2000;32(3):587–94.
23. Atreja A, Bellam N, et al. Strategies to enhance patient adherence: making it simple. MedGenMed. 2005;7(1):4.
24. Hall AM, Kamper SJ, Hernon M, et al. Measurement tools for adherence to non-pharmacologic self-management treatment for chronic musculoskeletal conditions: a systematic review. Arch Phys Med Rehabil. 2015;96:552–62.
25. Turk DC, Wilson HD, Cahana A. Treatment of chronic non-cancer pain. Lancet. 2011;377:2226–35.
26. Werner JJ, Bailey K, Crowe C. Using SMART goals to promote a healthy body weight. 2023. Available at https://www.cardi-OH.org/assets/Capsules/Cardi-OH-Capsule-29-Using-SMaRT-Goals--to-Promote-a-Healthy-Body-Weight.pdf. Accessed 21 Dec 2023.
27. Miller WR, Rollnick S. Motivational interviewing: helping people change. 3rd ed. New York: The Guilford Press; 2013.
28. Silva MA. Predictors of retention in physical therapy: client-, disease-, treatment-related factors (Doctoral dissertation, Marquette University). 2010.

Part IV

Adjunctive Therapies Beyond Medications

29 Physical Therapy and Exercise Science

Andrea L. Miller

Introduction

Pain is complex and based on diverse inputs from socioeconomic status, education, lifestyle, and individual pain perceptions. Pain is a "uniquely individual and subjective experience, among the most controversial and complex" medical issues that providers are currently treating [1]. Chronic pain, defined as pain lasting longer than 3 months, is one of the most common issues for which people seek out medical assistance [1]. Over 100 million Americans suffer from chronic pain, and the cost of helping these individuals is reaching up to a staggering $635 billion per year [1]. Cases of chronic pain could potentially be avoided by early referral to a PT for an acute injury.

Per the CDC, opioid-related deaths reached 645,000 from 1999 through 2021. The first wave of the crisis originated in the 1990s with prescription opioids, evolved to the second wave in 2010 with heroin, and culminated in a third wave in 2013 from synthetic opioids, particularly fentanyl [2]. Prescription opioids were intended for those suffering from acute moderate-to-severe pain post-surgery or injury, or for those diagnosed with cancer. However, they are now being prescribed for chronic pain and noncancer patients, despite a lack of evidence demonstrating efficacy and safety for long-term use in populations for indications like chronic low back pain. Not only are opioids addictive, but they also do not treat the underlying cause of the pain [1]. The most common prescription drug overdoses are from opiates (methadone, oxycodone, and hydrocodone) [3]. As the epidemic continues, we are at a critical crossroads: choose to practice and encourage alternative ways of reducing pain or continue to propagate the epidemic.

A. L. Miller (✉)
Harmony Physical Therapy, Fleetwood, PA, USA

Origins of the Physical Therapist

PTs are movement experts, treating all body systems that facilitate movement, including the musculoskeletal, cardiopulmonary, integumentary, and nervous systems. PT helps to strengthen muscles, bones, heart, lungs, and brain and modulate ascending and descending nociceptive pathways. PTs treat all ages from newborn to end-of-life and focus on improving quality of life through manual techniques, exercises, and various forms of education. PTs skillfully and thoroughly evaluate each patient, identifying key impairments and developing patient-specific rehabilitation plans that improve function, help maintain independence, and reduce pain [13].

In the 2000s, the American Physical Therapy Association (APTA) updated the *Guide to Physical Therapy Practice* and started to focus more on evidence-based treatment, with the goal of PTs practicing as direct patient providers in order to establish standards of practice throughout the profession [4]. With the transition of PT moving to a doctorate-level degree, many PTs are now practicing as short-term direct care providers. PTs treat independently for up to 30 days in most states and refer any patients who are inappropriate for therapy to medical providers [5].

PT and the Cost of Waiting

A systematic review completed by Arnold et al. [6] looked at the outcomes for those who received PT within 30 days for acute low back pain (LBP) versus delayed PT (14–90 days post-injury) (Table 29.1). These authors included randomized control trials (RCTs) along with prospective and retrospective cohort studies, of which 11 met criteria for inclusion.

J. P. Reinert et al. (eds.), *Adjunctive Analgesic Strategies for the Bedside Clinician and Beyond*,
https://doi.org/10.1007/978-3-032-21675-5_29

Table 29.1 Outcome measures and questionnaires

Numeric Pain Rating Scale (NPRS) [25]	Measures pain in adults	0–10 scale; 0 = no pain 10 = worst pain imaginable	High test-retest reliability	Highly correlated with VAS (0.86–0.95)	MCID = reduction by 2 points
Visual Analog Scale (VAS) [26]	Measures intensity/ frequency of pain	0 mm–100 mm scale; 0–4 mm = no pain, 5–44 mm = mild pain, 45–74 mm = moderate pain, and 75–100 mm = severe pain	Test-retest reliability ($r = 0.94$)	Construct validity in patients with rheumatic diseases highly correlated with VAS (rated from 0.71–0.78 ad 0.62–0.91)	MCD = reduction by 11 points
Neck Disability Index (NDI) [27]	Questionnaire regarding functional status secondary to neck pain	Contains 10 items: pain, personal care, lifting, reading, headaches, concentration, work, driving, sleeping, and recreation. Each item has 6 statements in which patient must choose statement closest to their function and are scored 0–5 Scoring: ×/50 then to % 0–4 points (0–8%) = no disability, 5–14 points (10–28%) = mild disability, 25–34 points (50–64%) = severe disability, and 35–50 points (70–100%) = complete disability	Fair-moderate test-retest reliability, although intraclass correlations can change between 0.50 and 0.98	Good construct validity and strong correlations with VAS	MCID = 5 points, or 10%

Northwick Park Pain Questionnaire [28]	Questionnaire that measures pain and disability in those with neck pain	Divided into sections including (1) pain intensity, (2) neck pain and sleeping, (3) pins and needles or numbness in the arms at night, (4) duration of symptoms, (5) carrying, (6) reaching or watching TV, (7) working and/or housework, (8) social activities and (9) driving and (10) aims to compare the current state to the state when the questionnaire was first completed. Each parameter is divided into 5 possible answers with points from 0 to 4 where 0 = no pain and 4 = worst pain; only one answer is selected for each section Neck pain score is the sum of the points scored for the first nine questions; the driving question may or may not be answered If all 9 questions are answered: NPQ percentage = ((neck pain score)/36) ×100% If 8 questions are answered: NPQ percentage = ((neck pain score)/32) ×100% Minimum score is 0, and maximum is 36; the higher the percentage, the greater the disability and pain	High level of internal consistency and sensitivity to change	Construct validity was found to be good and have positive correlation with the NDI and NPRS
McGill Pain Questionnaire (MPQ) [29]	Self-reporting measure of pain assessing both quality and intensity of pain consisting of 3 components including sensory intensity, cognitive evaluation of pain, and emotional impact of pain	Consist of 78 words in which patients choose the words that best describe their pain experience 7 words are selected from the following categories: Dimensions 1–10 (pain descriptors) (3 words) Dimensions 11–15 (affective components of pain) (2 words) Dimension 16: (evaluation of pain), (one word) —Dimensions 17–20 (miscellaneous) (1 word) Scores are tabulated by summing the values associated with each word and range from 0 (no pain) to 78 (severe pain)	Test-retest reliability found to be excellent for both illiterate ($r = 0.95$) and literate ($r = 0.96$)	Good criterion validity, construct validity, and content validity

(continued)

Table 29.1 (continued)

General Health Questionnaire-28 (GHQ-28) [30]	Screening tool for identifying minor psychiatric disorders	Four subscales including somatic symptoms, anxiety and sleepiness, social dysfunction, and severe depression GHQ-28 Maximum score is 84 (28 questions × 3 points) 4 possible answers for each question: not at all, no more than usual, rather more than usual, or much more than usual Scores range from 0 to 3 (first choice =0 and last choice = 3)	Outstanding inter- and intra-rater reliability (Cronbach's 0.9–0.95) and high test-retest reliability (0.79–0.9)		
Fibromyalgia Impact Scale (FIQ) [31]	Measures the components of health that tend to be most affected by FM	First item contains 11 questions related to physical functioning where patients answer 0–3 where 0 = always and 3 = never Items 2 and 3 ask the patient to mark the number of days they felt well along with the number of days they were unable to work due to FM symptoms Items 4–10 are horizontal linear scales marked in 10 increments where the patient rates work difficulty, pain, fatigue, morning tiredness, stiffness, anxiety, and depression	Current assessment indicates the FIQ is sufficient regarding reliability and validity but warrants further testing in clinical situations		

Multidimensional Pain Inventory Subscale [32]	Assesses chronic pain in individuals	Composed of 52 items across 12 subscales and 3 over all domains Domain 1: Assesses pain experience with subscales Perceived interference of pain in various aspects of functioning Perception of support received by others Levels of pain severity Perception of control Perception of affective distress Domain 2: Assesses response of others to the patient's communicated pain with subscales Perceived frequency of punishing responses Perceived frequency of solicitous responses Perceived frequency of distracting responses Domain 3: Assesses the extent to which the patients participate in daily activity with subscales Performance of household chores Performance of outdoor work Performance of activities away from home Performance of social activities Each item rated on 0–6 scale, and the scores for each subscale are calculated by adding the scores for each item in that subscale, divided by the number of items in that subscale to yield a mean score Higher scores indicate greater intensity in that subscale	Excellent test-retest reliability (0.75–0.89)	Adequate internal consistency (Cronbach's alpha of 0.70–0.90) and construct validity

(continued)

Table 29.1 (continued)

Quebec Back Pain Questionnaire (QBPDS) [33]	Condition-specific questionnaire developed to measure the level of functional disability in patients with LBP	Contains 20 daily activities categorized into 6 types of activities, including Bed/rest (items 1–3) sitting/standing (items 4–6) Ambulation (items 709) Movement (items 10–12) Bending/stopping (items 13–16) Handling of large/heavy items (items 17–20) For every activity there are 6 answer categories measured from 0 to 5 where 0 = no effort and 5 = not able Final outcome obtained by summing the scoring of the degree of difficulty in performing the 20 activities with outcome scores ranging from 0 to 100, with higher number meaning higher level of disability	ICC is 0,55 (95% CI = 0,20-0,78) in acute occupational LBP	External construct/ convergent validity: moderate-to-strong correlation between QBPDS and Roland-Morris disability questionnaire: 2 = 0.77–0.81, ODI: 2 = 0.80–0.83	QBPDS highly sensitive to change for the score of the individual domains as for the total score (SRM = 0.80 and effect size = 0.62). Studies found MDC of 19% (955 CI 14–24) in patients with LBP who reported no change during 6 weeks and for patients with chronic LBP, MDC is 15.8.
Orebro Musculoskeletal Pain Questionnaire [34]	Predicts long-term disability and work absenteeism in working adults with acute and chronic MSK pain	Consists of 25 questions, of which 21 are scored on a 0–10 point scale First 4 questions are unscored due to asking demographic information Measures domains including pain site, duration, frequency, coping, stress, depression, and sick leave The total minimum score is 4 and maximum is 210 Lower scores are desirable as higher scores indicate increased disability	Test-retest reliability, 0.90 = ICC with 2–4 days between tests Internal consistency = 0.95 = Cronbach's alpha	Convergent validity: $r = 0.38$ domain score for function as compared to the QBPDS ($p = 0.01$) and $r = 0.47$ domain score for pain compared to the VAS ($p = 0.01$)	MDC: 12 points
Oswestry Disability Index (ODI) [35]	Questionnaire giving a subjective percentage score of level of function (disability) in activities of daily living (ADLs) in those with LBP	Examines the level of disability on 10 ADLs: pain intensity, personal care, lifting, walking, sitting, standing, sleeping, sex (if applicable), social life, and travel Each item consists of 6 statements scored from 0 to 5 where 0 is least disability and 5 is the greatest. Total score is calculated by a percentage where 0% = no disability and 100% = highest level of disability 0–20% = minimal disability 21–40% = moderate disability 41–60% = severe disability 61–80% = crippled 81–100% = patients are bedbound or exaggerating symptoms	Test-retest reliability consistently high across studies (mean ICC value of 0.937 + −0.032) with lowest ICC reported of 0.880) and highest of 0.96	Consistent with validity in many studies	MCID = 5 points or 10%

Roland Morris Disability Questionnaire (RMDQ) [36]	Designed to assess self-related physical disability caused by LBP Recommended for patients with mild-to-moderate disability due to acute, subacute, or chronic LBP	Consists of 24 statements in which the patient is asked to tick the statement if it applies to them on that specific day At the end of the 24 statements, you sum the ticked boxes Scores range from 0 = no disability to 24 = maximum disability Omitted describing various levels of disability	Test-retest reliability for 24-item = ICC from 0.42 to 0.91	Content validity is limited as it only covers physical problems and not physiological or social ones RMDQ correlates well with ODI, NPRS, and QBPDS
Patient Reported Outcomes Measurement Information System (PROMIS) [37]	Person-centered measures that evaluate and monitor physical, mental, and social health in adults aim to improve patient-clinician communication and can also be used to screen for disability Assesses physical health (physical function, fatigue, and pain) and mental health (emotional distress, social health)	10-item patient-reported questionnaire where each question has a 5-point scale (ranging from poor to excellent); the higher the score, the healthier the patient, with a maximum score of 20	Still a new measure needing more studies but has been found to be valid and reliable in conditions including LBP, hip arthroscopy, knee arthroplasty, upper limb issues, and stroke	
Pain Disability Index [38]	Simple and rapid instrument for measuring the impact that pain has on the ability of a person to perform ADLs	Looks at 7 aspects including family and home responsibilities, recreation, social activity, occupation, sexual behavior, self-care, and life-support activity Each aspect is ranked on a 0–10 scale where 0 = no disability and 10 = total disability Scored by summing all 7 parameters; minimal index = 0 and maximal index = 70; the higher the index, the greater the disability due to pain	Modest test-retest reliability	

(continued)

Table 29.1 (continued)

Pain Rehabilitation Expectations Scale (PRES)- Working Alliance Subscale [39]	Clinical tool developed to measure the expectations about rehab treatment outcome for people with LBP	3 subscales, including working alliance, proxy efficacy, and motivation/expectation (total of 49 items) 16 items for working alliance 13 items for proxy efficiency 20 items for motivation/expectations Each item is rated on a 4-point scale where 1 = strongly disagree, 2 = disagree, 3 = agree and 4 = strongly agree, where a higher PRES subscale score indicates a better patient expectation for pain rehab	Cronbach's alpha coefficients are >0.90, which is generally suggested as good internal validity within the subscales, but more studies need to be conducted for more reliability and validity data		
Working Alliance Theory of Chance Inventory (WATOCI) [40]	Evaluates the collaborative relationship between the helper and the client but doesn't encompass all aspects of the relationship such as clinical outcomes	Consists of 36 questions (12 questions short-term form) including 3 domains Task, goal, and bond: 12 questions for each domain Each item scored from 1 to 7 where 1 = minimum (never) and 7 = maximum (always) Minimum total score is 36 to maximum is 252, where higher scores indicate a more positive rating of working alliance	Internal consistency for counseling was found to be excellent with Cronbach alpha = 0.87–0.93; construct validity was found to be excellent with correlation between goal-therapist subscale and task-client subscales was only 0.01 less than the corresponding validity coefficient ($r = 0.76$)		

Seven of these studies discussed specific PT interventions, including patient education, exercises with progressions, modalities, and manual therapy (MT). Authors utilized two of these studies, both retrospective in nature with $n = 785{,}520$, to aggregate data to assess opioid use in those who had early versus delayed PT. A statistically significant reduction in the odds of opioid use (OR = 0.69; 95% CI, 0.53–0.84; $I^2 = 81.1\%$; $n = 2$) was identified with pooled analysis between the two groups ($p < 0.0001$). The same retrospective studies also assessed LBP-related costs between groups, with Childs et al. reporting an average of $1202.29 after 2 years and Fritz et al. an average of $2736.23 less in healthcare costs after 18 months for those choosing early PT intervention for LBP.

A cohort study by Aoyagi et al. [7] posed the question, "Are PT interventions before and after total knee replacement (TKR) associated with lower risk of postoperative long-term use of opioids?" Knee osteoarthritis (OA) is noted as the most common form of OA experienced worldwide. TKR is the method used to reduce the pain and improve quality of life (QOL), with 650,000 surgeries performed in 2008 in the US and projected to be 3.5 million per year by 2030. Postoperatively (post-op), opioids are the most common pain reliever administered, and concern lies with the possibility of becoming a long-term opioid user after exposure. 67,322 individuals over the age of 40 were studied, including both those with prior opioid history, defined as having two or more opioid prescriptions filled 12 months prior to TKR, and those without prior opioid history, defined as having no opioid prescriptions 12 months prior to TKR. The patient was considered to have prehabilitation (prehab) if they saw PT one or more times 90 days prior to TKR and considered to have post-op PT if they had one or more PT sessions within 90 days post-op. This study defined long-term opioid use as 90 days' worth or more, where prescription opioids were filled during assessment periods (12 months after the first 90 days post-op to exclude immediate post-op use). The authors found that 14.3% of participants received prehab. 2.4% without prior opioid history and 35% with prior opioid history had long-term opioid use post-op. However, having any prehab was associated with lower odds of long-term use in both groups: without prior use, adjusted odds ratio (aOR), 0.75 (95% CI, 0.60–0.95); with prior use: (aOR), 0.75 (95% CI, 0.70–0.80). Post-op, 75% of participants received PT within 90 days, and those with prior opioid history lowered their odds of long-term opioid use (aOR, 0.75 (95% CI, 0.70–0.79)), whereas no statistically significant difference was discovered for the cohort with no prior opioid use (aOR, 0.89 (95% CI, 0.75–1.04)). A statistically significant difference was found for the prior opioid use group regarding the number of sessions of PT they received post-op, with 6 to 12 sessions (aOR, 0.82 (95% CI, 0.75–0.90)) and 13 or more sessions (aOR, 0.71 (95% CI, 0.65–0.77)) showing lower odds of long-term opioid use versus only 1–5 sessions. No statistically significant difference was found for the no prior opioid use group regarding the number of PT sessions; however, if care was started after 31 days post-op in this cohort, they were more likely to have long-term opioid use (aOR, 1.45 (95% CI, 1.19–1.77)).

Horn and Fritz [8] conducted a retrospective cohort study looking at the timing of PT consultation for those with cervical spine pain and how it impacted healthcare use and expense. Cervical pain has been estimated to be the third largest condition that contributes to health care costs in the US and is estimated at $87.6 billion per year. They looked at 308 patients located in Utah with a new onset of neck pain, defined as having no recorded incident of neck pain 90 days prior to initial contact with a healthcare provider, a majority of whom were women and an average age of 48. They categorized PT timing into early PT (consult within 14 days), delayed PT (between 15 and 90 days), and late PT (between 91 and 364 days) and monitored the use of injections, imaging, opioids, and costs between the groups over 1 year. Of the 308 eligible patients, 160 (52%) consulted PT within 14 days, and 98 (61%) of the 160 patients sought PT through direct access (DA). 74 patients (24%) had delayed PT, and 74 patients (24%) had late PT. No statistically significant difference between groups was found regarding comorbid depression, anxiety, fibromyalgia, or obesity; however, groups differed in prevalence of LBP ($p = 0.01$) (81.1% late PT group), chronic/generalized pain ($p < 0.0001$) (47.3% late PT group), substance abuse ($p = 0.01$) (23.0% late PT group), and tobacco use ($p = 0.05$) (24.3% late PT group). The authors found that 193 patients (62.7%) were prescribed prescription opioids within the one-year follow-up. Of these 193 patients, 61 (82.4%) were in the late PT group, 44 (59.5%) were in the delayed PT group, and 88 (55%) were in the early PT group. After adjusting for covariates, late PT was associated with increased odds of being prescribed opioids as compared to early PT after a one-year follow-up (aOR = 2.79, 95% CI, 1.35–5.79). Adjusted healthcare cost for early PT was $1853 (95% CI $1172–$2536), delayed PT was \$2917 (95% CI \$1969–\$3866), and late PT was associated with the highest one-year cost at \$4026 (95% CI \$2377–\$5674, $p < 0.001$). The one-year healthcare cost comparing late versus early PT demonstrated a statistically significant difference, with late PT costing \$2172 more (95% CI \$557–\$3786, $p < 0.01$) than the early PT group.

While the quality of research available is inconsistent, the three studies imply that early PT could have a positive impact on healthcare costs and potential exposure to opioids. Early PT could potentially reduce unnecessary opioid prescribing and reduce long-term healthcare costs in a variety of settings and patient groups.

Analgesic Effects of Specific PT Modalities

Therapeutic Exercise

Therapeutic exercise (TE) "involves movement prescribed to correct impairments, restore muscular and skeletal function and/or maintain a state of well-being…can theoretically involve all joints..and the main benefits of exercise involve long-term adaptation include the effects upon the musculoskeletal, metabolic, cardiovascular, and respiratory systems" [9]. TE is expertly prescribed after a PT performs an initial evaluation, which includes a thorough patient history, physical examination, special testing to rule in or out specific diagnoses, evaluation of information gathered, and finally, the formation of a diagnosis and prognosis. Goal-setting is also an essential part of the evaluation, helping to determine the best TE for the patient going forward. TE has a wide variety of benefits, with some of the most noted being QOL, health, general function, and reducing pain.

The three main categories of TE are endurance, resistance, and flexibility training. In simple terms, endurance training focuses on the use of large muscle groups to achieve a greater VO2max, which is the gold standard for cardiovascular fitness. VO2max "reflects the ability of a person to imbibe, transport, and use oxygen, which defines that person's functional aerobic capacity," and the focus for TE endurance training is usually between a person's 50–60% calculated VO2max [9]. Resistance training focuses on improving a patient's strength and utilizes the principles of three forms, including isometrics, isotonics, and isokinetics. Isometric means that there is a consistent muscle contraction with no change in muscle length. Isotonic is defined as a consistent load through a dynamic movement. Isokinetic is defined as a consistent velocity but with a variable load. Flexibility training improves range of motion in one or various joints by using slow and controlled exercises, including static stretching (stretch position held for prolonged time), dynamic stretching (target muscles are stretched by being repetitively utilized in activity-specific movement), and proprioceptive neuromuscular facilitation (PNF) ("alternating contraction and relaxation of agonist/antagonist muscles at specific joints..") [9].

Bertozzi et al. [10] performed a systematic review and meta-analysis of RCTs on the effect of TE on pain and disability for those suffering from chronic cervical spine pain (CNSNP), defined as pain lasting longer than 3 months. CNSNP, without any specific underlying cause, is one of the most common MSK disorders, a close second behind LBP, with a prevalence in the work population of 30–50%, and has been reported to contribute to substantial healthcare costs. Disability, in this study, was assessed as a primary outcome measure if it measured the impact of chronic neck pain on everyday life, not just on work or leisure. Researchers utilized only RCTs that had a control group and comparison group, with comparison groups including (1) placebo, (2) non-exercise or comparator (e.g., advice for self-care), and (3) standard practice (e.g., wait list or usual care, with no further explanation given). Trials were excluded if participants had diagnoses including radiculopathy, myelopathy, fracture, infection, dystonia, tumor, inflammatory disease, osteoporosis, whiplash-associated disorders, myofascial neck pain, trauma-associated neck pain, degenerative changes, or fibromyalgia. TE was the only intervention considered in this study, and the authors excluded studies focusing on the use of patient education, MT, traction, modalities, cognitive behavioral therapy (CBT), and multidisciplinary rehabilitation. Nine RCTs fit criteria for Bertozzi's systematic review and meta-analysis regarding TE, where TE interventions varied accross the studies but included: strength training for the upper extremities, neck musculature and postural muscles (posterior and anterior chain) and included the use of dumbbells, machines and Thera-Band tubing and used isometrics, isotonics and isokinetics. The Upper Body Ergometer (UBE/cycling) was utilized for endurance training; stretching (dynamic and static) and postural retraining were other included TE interventions. Interventions ranged from being performed two times per week to daily and spanned 2 weeks to 52 weeks. Outcomes assessed included pain using the Numeric Pain Scale (NPRS) (0–10) and Visual Analog Scale (VAS) (0–100) and disability using the Neck Disability Index (NDI) (1–00), Northwick Park Neck Pain Questionnaire, and Disability Index (0–80), and outcomes were assessed at short-term (0–1 month), intermediate-term (1–6 months), and long-term (>6 months) as available by study. The overall effect size of TE on pain was medium and significant ($g = 0.53$, with a range from −0.86 to −0.20) at short-term and medium and significant at intermediate-term ($g = -0.45$, with a range from −0.82 to −0.07). Unfortunately, no significant findings were associated with TE and disability at any range, and only one of the included RCTs had a follow-up beyond 6 months, which was also found to have no significant findings. However, TE is still suggested as an effective way to reduce chronic neck pain.

An RTC completed in 2017 by Dehghani et al. [11] sought to assess the effectiveness of Pilates and McKenzie training versus a control group for general health and pain relief in men aged 40–55 with chronic LBP, defined as pain lasting longer than 3 months without any pathological symptom. Exclusion criteria included spinal tumors, fractures, inflammatory diseases, previous spinal surgery, nerve root compromise, spondylolysis or spondylolisthesis, spinal stenosis, neurological disorders, systemic diseases, cardiovascular diseases, and receiving other therapies. The examiner who assessed outcome measures was blinded to group assignment, with outcome measures given 24 h prior to training, including the McGill Pain Questionnaire (MPQ) and General Health Questionnaire −28 (GHQ-28). The MPQ is a self-reported measure that assesses the quality and intensity of the pain by using 78 words put into four dimensions: pain descriptors (subject chooses 3 words), affective components of pain (subject chooses 2 words), evaluation of pain (subject chooses one word), and miscellaneous (subject chooses one word). Scores range from 0 (no pain) to severe (78) and are calculated by summing the numerical value of the seven chosen words. Thirty-six subjects were separated into three groups: Pilates, McKenzie, and control. The Pilates group participated in 1-hour sessions, 3 times a week for 6 weeks. The McKenzie group exercised for 1 hour a day for 20 days with six exercises used, including four lumbar-extension-based exercises performed in prone and sitting and two lumbar-flexion-based exercises performed in supine and sitting, ten times for each exercise. The control group did not participate in any exercise. All groups completed the MPQ and GHQ-28 after treatment for analysis. Researchers found a statistically significant reduction in pain index pretest and posttest for the Pilates and McKenzie groups: Pilates ($P < 0.0001$), McKenzie ($P < 0.006$), whereas the control group demonstrated a statistically significant increase in pain pre-to-post test ($P < 0.009$). General health was also found to be statistically significant pre-to-post test in the McKenzie group ($P < 0.0001$).

The effect of TE on fibromyalgia was investigated by Sosa-Reina et al. [12] via a systematic review and meta-analysis of RCTs. Fibromyalgia is characterized by widespread pain and is estimated to globally impact 2.7% of the population, with a majority being female (3:1 ratio). In this study, TE included aerobic activity, coordination and balance, gait training, posture and body mechanics retraining, flexibility, relaxation, and muscle strengthening. RCTs were included if they contained TE or compared TE with a control group or group receiving standard care. They assessed outcome measures, including pain via VAS, the Fibromyalgia Impact Scale (FIQ), and the Multidimensional Pain Inventory subscale. Depression, global well-being, and health-related QOL were also measured. Standard mean differences (SMDs) were calculated from the means, and SMDs for each intervention were reported as 95% CIs. Hedge's (adjusted) g was utilized secondary to small sample sizes (<40 participants) in each group. Combined effects were assessed using a random effects model; Cohen's g was used to evaluate the magnitude of the effect sizes calculated by the SMD, with $g > 0.2–0.4$ indicating a small effect size, $g > 0.4–0.8$ a medium effect size, and $g > 0.8$ a large effect size. Overall effects were assessed using Z statistics, with $p < 0.05$ indicating a statistically significant difference. Fourteen RCTs met criteria and included 715 participants, with 700 being women, and the average age was 42 years old. Data analysis revealed that there was strong evidence per intention-to-treat (ITT) that exercise reduces pain (−1.11 (95% CI)—1.52, −0.71), overall effect $p < 0.001$. Data analysis revealed that aerobic exercise was found to produce a large reduction in pain (−1.05 (95% CI) -1.78, −0.33; overall effect $p < 0.001$), muscle strengthening decreases pain (−1.39 (95% CI) -2.16, −0.62; overall effect $p < 0.001$), and a combination of exercise produces a large decrease in pain (−0.51 (95% CI) −0.99, −0.44; overall effect $p < 0.05$). Synthesized data suggests that completing aerobic exercise for 30–60 minutes at an intensity of 50–80% heart rate max 2–3 times per week for 4–6 months and muscle-strengthening exercises (1–3 sets of 8–11 repetitions with a load of 45% 1 repetition maximum) is the most effective in reducing pain severity.

The above studies include a wide array of TE interventions and chronicity of symptoms among the body systems. It is vital to note that the conclusion for most studies is that TE in almost any shape or form has a positive impact on general health and pain. PTs often tell patients that "motion is lotion" and that the more you move, the better you are going to feel. The patient/therapist relationship helps ensure that the exercise program is tailored to individual needs. Considerations must include patient access to exercise equipment, time available to exercise, their highest motivating factors, and their beliefs about exercise.

Manual Therapy

MT is defined by the APTA as "the synergistic application of movement-oriented strategies integrating exercise and manually applied mobilization and manipulation procedures" [13]. MT techniques can include, but are not limited to, manual resistance, manual stretching/range of motion, manual traction, joint mobilization, myofascial release, strain counterstrain, positional release, muscle energy technique (MET), neural tissue tension techniques, instrument-assisted soft tissue mobilization (IASTM), cupping, and trigger point therapy.

Santos et al. [14] completed a systematic review with meta-analysis looking at the effectiveness of MET for the treatment of nonspecific LBP on pain and disability in the short term (8 weeks). MET is a technique practiced for over 50 years that is targeted to the lumbopelvic region and has the patient complete a controlled, voluntary muscle contraction with the hopes that it can help with strength, stretching, pain relief, and improved joint mobility around that muscle contraction. They included 19 RCTs in their review, in which 822 total patients aged 18–55 with subacute or chronic nonspecific LBP received MET versus other therapies or exercises or MET versus sham interventions, including but not limited to cranial sacral therapy, Mulligan neural tissue mobilization, hot/cold packs to the lower back, the McKenzie extension exercise program, dynamic stabilization exercises, core stability exercises, the strain-counter strain technique, back care education, and stretching for the lower limbs. Pain evaluation was performed via the VAS, NPRS, MPQ, Quebec Back Pain Questionnaire, Orebro Musculoskeletal Pain Questionnaire, and pain provocation test. Functional disability was evaluated through the Oswestry Disability Index (ODI), the modified Oswestry Disability Index (mODI), and the Roland Morris Disability Questionnaire (RMDQ). Mean differences between groups in the post-intervention and 95% CIs were calculated to quantify the effect of results. For meta-analysis for studies using the same pain scales, results were presented as mean differences (MD) and 95% CIs. Disability was calculated using SMDs and 95% CIs. A small effect size was defined as MD < 10% or SMD < 0.4; moderate included MD between 10% and 20% or SMD between 0.41 and 0.7; big included MD > 20% or SMD > 0.7. Values referring to treatment effect were considered statistically significant if $P < 0.05$. A meta-analysis of MET versus other therapies for pain and disability found a significant difference in favor of MET for pain intensity (MD = -0.67 (95% CI, −1.16 to −0/17), $P = 0.008$, $N = 416$, studies = 13, $I^2 = 87\%$) for chronic LBP. A significant difference was also observed when comparing MET to the control group for pain intensity for chronic LBP (MD = −1.88 (95% CI, −3.23 to 0.54), $P = 0.006$, $N = 237$, studies = 5, $I^2 = 97\%$); however, no significant effect was found for disability in patients with chronic or subacute LBP in both the MET versus other therapies and MET versus control groups.

A systematic review completed by Namnaqani et al. [15] assessed the effectiveness of the McKenzie method versus manual therapy on pain and disability for the treatment of chronic LBP (>12-week history of pain in this study). The McKenzie method, in the simplest of terms, is finding if your patient has a spinal extension or flexion-based preference and prescribing exercises based on their preference with hopes of reducing their LBP. They compared McKenzie treatment versus other interventions that included, but are not limited to chiropractic manipulation, postural correction exercises, treadmill training, manual mobilization, MT, advice "to be active only," and manual trigger point release (MTPR). Five studies were included in this review and they explored pain levels between groups at 3 months, 6 months, and 12 months post-intervention. Both genders were included, with an average age of 41, and most were employed. Participants were excluded if they had underlying pathologies, including spinal stenosis, scoliosis, radiculopathy, or pregnancy; were less than 6 months postoperative; had severe metabolic or cardiovascular disease; or presented with red flag items. Regarding pain, the authors looked at the NPRS, VAS, Symptoms Bothersomeness Scale, and the MPQ. The ODI and RMDQ were assessed for disability. I^2 statistics and Chi^2 tests were used to assess statistical heterogeneity between trials; meta-analysis was not performed secondary to large variability in methodologies between studies. Pain and disability were equal across groups at baseline; however, immediately posttreatment, two studies found that the McKenzie group had a significant decrease in pain ($p = 0.01$, $p = 0.001$, respectively) along with significant improvement in RMDQ ($p = 0.03$). These studies included McKenzie versus manual mobilization/therapy, individual exercises, and advice to stay active. At 3 months, all groups had a significant reduction in pain. 6 months post-intervention, two studies observed a statistically significant reduction in disability for the McKenzie group ($p < 0.028$; $p < 0.05$, respectively), whereas the other groups received manual therapy and advice to stay active. At 12 months, they found no significant difference between groups regarding pain, but the McKenzie group improved disability scores as compared to the manual therapy group ($p = 0.05$, $p = 0.028$, $p = 0.030$, respectively).

Munoz-Gomez et al. [16] completed an RCT that explored the effect of MT on women with pelvic pain lasting more than 1 year secondary to endometriosis. Forty-one women with an average age of 36 were split into two groups. One received manual therapy (MTG): a combination of eight soft tissue and articular techniques at the cervical spine, thoracic spine, lumbar spine, sacroiliac joint, abdomen, broad ligament, pelvic diaphragm, sphenoid, and fourth ventricle. The other received a placebo intervention (PG): light contact at the same points and for the same amounts of time as the MT group over the course of 8 weeks, including one 30-minute session every 15 days. Patients were excluded if they were pregnant, had rheumatic or degenerative neurological disease, had another cause of pelvic pain, had pelvic surgery in the past year, or had PT in the previous 3 months. The authors assessed pain via VAS before intervention (T0), immediately after intervention (T1), 1 month after intervention (T2), and 6 months post-intervention (T3). Cohen's d was utilized for the effect size of continuous variables, rated as small

(0.20–0.50), medium (0.50–0.80), or large (>0.80). The study found that there was a significant reduction in pain for the MTG at T1 ($P < 0.001$; $d = 1.00$), T2 ($p < 0.001$; $d = 0.89$), and T3 ($p < 0.001$; $d = 2.28$). The MTG also significantly reduced their pain scores as compared to the PG at T1 ($p = 0.03$; $d = 0.71$) and T3 ($p < 0.01$; $d = 1.81$). They found no significant difference for the PG at follow-up regarding pain ($p > 0.05$).

The above studies cover a plethora of MT interventions along with common diagnoses that are large contributors to pain worldwide. Although it is almost impossible to cover all aspects of MT and diagnoses in the scope of this chapter, these studies provide guidance and suggest that various forms and dosages of MT can have a positive impact on pain and disability in both the long and short term, especially when compared to non-intervention groups.

Patient Education and Pain Neuroscience Education

Traditional patient education regarding pain tends to focus on directly correlating tissue damage to pain, utilizing anatomical, biomechanical, and pathoanatomical models. However, there has been compounding evidence that tissue damage does not necessarily correlate to pain, especially regarding persistent pain (PNE 101) [17]. Furthermore, practice is moving away from the traditional model of pain education, as research demonstrates how different types of education can impact long-term patient outcomes regarding pain. Traditional education techniques can increase pain, catastrophizing, and fear avoidance behaviors, driving a shift toward pain neuroscience education (PNE) (PNE 101). PNE is a way of educating a patient by explaining the biological and physiological aspects of pain and how this impacts their pain experience. It is ideally applied one-on-one with the provider for 30 min, 1–2 times a week for 4–6 weeks, and uses metaphors, books, examples, and pictures. The focus of this education, beyond reducing pain and fear avoidance, is to also reduce healthcare-seeking behaviors and assist the patient in more independently managing their symptoms.

Ibrahim et al. [18] studied the effectiveness of patient education (PE) plus motor control exercise (MCE) versus each treatment separately on those suffering from chronic LBP. Inclusion criteria included both genders from ages 18 to 70 and nonspecific LBP with or without leg pain for more than 12 weeks. Patients were excluded if they had a history of spine surgery, spine or lumbar deformities, serious spinal pathologies (i.e., infection, metastasis, fracture, or cauda equina syndrome), severe chronic cardiovascular and pulmonary disease, poor hearing or vision, previous PT in the past 3 months (including exercise and/or education), a body mass index (BMI) >35 kg/cm^2, or pregnancy. A total of 120 participants were included, with 60% being male, an average age of 46 years old, and over 66% having no formal education. Three groups were established, including (group 1) PE only: PE followed by stretching and aerobic exercise; (group 2) MCE only: received stretching followed by MCE and aerobic exercise (consisting of non-supervised continuous overground walking or bicycling for a minimum of 30 minutes, 5 times per week); and (group 3) MCE plus PE: PE was followed by stretching, then MCE and aerobic exercise. PE was completed once a week for 8 weeks for a total of eight sessions. Each session was 60–80 minutes and held face-to-face with the lead author. Each session covered a different topic, where the topics and goals of PE were to gain a better understanding of what LBP is and its causes; to educate about the spine and its function; to understand the truths about LBP and dispel myths; to understand what causes pain and current beliefs/understanding of pain; to encourage return to normal activities and to remain active despite pain; to promote better active coping strategies; to promote positive self-management strategies; and to improve healthy posture habits with ergonomic education. Stretching and MCE were completed twice a week for a total of 16 sessions. Three different booklets were distributed to the groups. Group 3 received a booklet including information about the PE program, along with picture models of stretching and MCE. Group 1 received the same booklet as group 3, with the exception of the MCE program, and group 2 obtained a booklet that contained only stretching and the MCE program. Researchers primarily assessed intensity of pain via the NPRS and disability via the ODI, and secondary outcomes included QOL, global perceived recovery, fear avoidance beliefs, catastrophizing, and pain medication use. They assessed these outcomes immediately after intervention and 8 weeks post-intervention. Statistical analysis utilized an alpha level of 0.05. Data were summarized using mean (SD) for continuous variables and percentage for discrete variables. ANOVA was utilized for continuous variables, whereas Fisher's exact test was used for cell counts <5, and the Chi^2 test was used for cell counts>5. ITT was the main focus of this study, and it used linear mixed-effects models (LMMs) to assess the effects on primary and secondary outcome measures. The treatment effect was summarized as the adjusted between-group difference and associated 95% CI at 8 and 20 weeks, as compared to baseline. A Bonferroni adjustment with an alpha of 0.017 was applied for NPRS and ODI. All groups had similar pain intensity at baseline. Findings indicated that the PE plus MCE group showed a significant treatment effect versus PE alone regarding pain intensity by an additional −1.15 (95% CI, −2.04 to −0.25) points 8 weeks after intervention and −1.25 (95% CI, −2.14 to −0.35) points 20 weeks after intervention. Mean disability levels (0–100 scale) were also found to be similar between groups at baseline. Interventions indicated that the PE plus MCE and MCE alone groups demonstrated a significant treatment effect with reduced disability by −5.04% (95% CI, −9.57 to −0.52) and 5.68% (95% CI, 1.15 to 10.2) points, respectively, at 8 weeks post-intervention and −5.96% (CI, −9.84 to −2.07) and 6.57% (95% CI, 2.69 to 10.4) points, respectively, 20 weeks post-intervention.

A Cochrane Review was completed by Engers et al. [19], who assessed individual patient education and how it impacted patients aged 16 or older with nonspecific subacute, acute, or chronic LBP. Patients were excluded if their LBP was caused by infection, neoplasm, metastasis, osteoporosis, RA, fracture, or radiculopathy. Pain was defined as being localized below the lower ribs but above the inferior gluteal fold. For this study, PE included having a discussion with a professional, taking a special class, obtaining a take-home booklet, or watching videos specific to PNE. The authors wanted to assess pain via the VAS and Symptom Bothersomeness Scale; function via the RDQ and ODI; and return-to-work in the short-term (<6 months post-intervention) and long-term (>6 months post-intervention). RCTs were included if they assessed (1) individual PE versus no intervention, (2) individual PE versus non-education intervention, or (3) individual PE versus another type of individual PE. Data analysis was conducted separately for acute versus subacute LBP versus chronic LBP and short-term versus long-term outcomes. "The effect size was considered relevant when at least one of these criteria was met: (1) there was a group difference of more than 10 mm on a VAS scale for pain (100 mm); (2) there was a group difference of more than two points on the RMDQ; or (3) there was a group difference of more than 10% on any of the other primary outcomes." Clinical homogeneity was evaluated by looking at the difference between RCTs with regard to the study population, intervention types, and the outcomes and measurement instruments. Meta-analysis was not performed secondary to many trials failing to provide sufficient data; therefore, authors summarized results using a rating system consisting of five levels of scientific evidence, including (1) strong evidence—consistent findings with multiple high-quality RCTs, (2) moderate evidence—consistent findings with multiple low-quality RCTs and/or one high-quality RCT, (3) limited evidence—1 low-quality RCT, (4) conflicting evidence—inconsistent findings among trials, and (5) no evidence—no RCTs. Consistency was defined as 75% or more RCTs having similar results and was considered effective when the difference between intervention and reference treatment was statistically significant and clinically significant on at least one primary outcome measure in favor of education. Researchers utilized 24 studies for review, 14 of which were rated as high-quality. They concluded that there is strong evidence for the use of individualized PE for approximately 2.5 hours of oral education for those with subacute LBP in the short and long term in getting these patients back to work, reducing long-term pain, and demonstrating global improvements. For those with chronic LBP, the effect of PE is less clear, and these patients may benefit from more intense interventions, although their definition of "more intense interventions" was not made clear in the conclusion.

A systematic review completed by Lepri et al. [20] looked at the effectiveness of PNE in those >18 years old with chronic MSK pain and central sensitization (CS) with a focus on how PNE affects pain, disability, and psychosocial factors. Primary chronic MSK pain is considered the "chronic pain experienced in muscles, bones, joints, or tendons that (1) is characterized by significant emotional distress (such as anxiety, anger, frustration, or depressed mood) or functional disability (interference in daily life activities and reduced participation in social roles), and (2) cannot be attributed directly to a known disease or damage process." Authors included participants suffering from fibromyalgia (FM), chronic fatigue syndrome (CFS), LBP, and chronic spinal pain (CSP). Included in this study were RCTs with patients over the age of 18 with chronic MSK pain (> 3 months) secondary to CS. CS criteria were screened using various questionnaires and outcome measures, including Central Sensitization Inventory (CSI) >40 and Quantitative Sensory Testing (QST) positive scores or any other criteria, including FM, CFS, psychosocial, or maladaptive pain beliefs. Patients were excluded if they were under age 18 or had acute, subacute, or recurrent LBP secondary to pathologies such as pulmonary, cardiac, neurological, oncological, visceral, cognitive, or psychiatric or had surgical intervention on the back less than a year prior. RCT interventions included PNE in any format with or without other interventions and compared PNE to other education, waiting lists, placebo interventions, and active (exercise) versus passive (MT) interventions, and outcome measures were required to assess either pain, disability, or psychosocial factors. Secondary to high heterogeneity, no meta-analysis was able to be conducted. Instead, a qualitative synthesis in a narrative and tabular format was written. Both between-group and within-group differences were reported for each outcome, and when possible, CIs, SDs, effect size, statistical significance (p), MCID, and punctual estimates were reported. Fifteen RCTs were included in this study, and the findings were subdivided by diagnosis. The authors concluded that PNE was effective in reducing pain, disability, and psychosocial factors in those diagnosed with FM and chronic LBP. PNE was most effective when combined with other therapeutic approaches and when given in a one-on-one session in which written reinforcement materials were given.

Sleep Management

Sleep hygiene is one of the most underrated facets of PT's care and a piece of the puzzle often missing when treating patients dealing with pain, especially chronic pain.

As movement experts, one of the first questions regarding sleep is typically "how are you sleeping and what position are you mostly in?" Many times, PTs are able to educate the patient on more appropriate sleeping positions to offload painful structures or advise on using more pillows around their body for the same purpose.

Timing and consistency of sleep are other crucial parts of sleep hygiene [21]. A consistent sleep schedule is key, even on the weekends; therefore, going to sleep and waking up at the same time every day is fundamentally important, as is getting enough sleep every night. The sleep target depends on the age of the patient in question. Newborns can sleep up to 17 hours a day, while adults should get at least 7–8 hours of quality sleep per night. Sleep is when the body does its healing, and thus it is important to figure it out early on in treatment.

It is also important to find out what the patient's nighttime routine is to identify modifications needed to facilitate a good night's sleep. Room temperature, light, noise, electronic stimulation, and caffeine or alcohol intake can adversely affect sleep.

In 2019, de la Vega et al. [22] conducted a study looking at the benefit of an interdisciplinary treatment plan utilizing psychologists, PTs, and occupational therapists (OTs) on quality sleep and fatigue for those suffering from chronic pain. Sleep quality and pain have been hypothesized to affect each other in a bidirectional way. Poor sleep is also associated with fatigue, which could lead to reduced QOL, increased disability, and increased depressive symptoms, which is why the authors wanted to evaluate the role of a change in sleep quality on these factors. They included 125 adults who had a mean age of 54 years; 76% were women, had a pain duration average of almost 10.5 years, and had an average baseline pain of 6.35/10 on the VAS, and 20% of patients were suffering from either chronic LBP or cervical pain. Participants were included if they had a history of chronic pain and could commit to a 4-week program and were excluded if they were found to be unable to handle the physicality of a 4-week program, were cognitively impaired, or had active suicidal thoughts. Participants attended a 4-week program in which treatment was 3-hour sessions, 3 days per week, and was offered in a group setting. These sessions included education on pain, setting realistic goals, relaxation techniques, coping strategies, and how to pace their activities. Two sessions were specifically for sleep, including sleep hygiene (i.e., sleep/wake cycle, reducing daytime napping), the role of the circadian rhythm, and sleep drive. Another session discussed sleep positioning for better pain management, including the use of supportive bolsters and pillows. Measurements for depressive symptoms, pain-related disability, sleep disturbance, and pain intensity were all taken during the first week of treatment and then after the 4 weeks of treatment using the Patient-Reported Outcomes Measurement Information System (PROMIS) with subscales looking at fatigue severity, sleep disturbance, pain intensity, and depressive symptoms. The Pain Disability Index, or PDI, was also used in this study. For data analysis, the authors used numbers and percentages for categorical variables, means and SDs for continuous variables, and Cohen's d to determine effect size. SD changes of 0.5 or higher were deemed clinically meaningful. Authors also conducted three linear multiple regressions, one for each of the criterion variables: posttreatment variables of (1) average pain intensity, (2) depressive symptoms, and (3) disability. Results indicated statistically significant pre-to-posttreatment effects for all outcome variables, with small (Cohen's $d < 0.2$) to moderate (Cohen's $d > 0.2$) effect sizes. Regarding pain intensity, this study found that a change in sleep and fatigue independently made a statistically significant impact on predicting a change in pain intensity (I^2 = a^^, 0.24 and 0.25, $P < 0.01$); the more that sleep and fatigue decreased during treatment, the more the pain intensity also decreased. Authors also found that a change in pain was able to predict a change in disability ($I^2 = 0.27$, $P < 0.01$). Lastly, they also found that a change in fatigue made an independent contribution to a change in depression ($I^2 = 0.16$, $P < 0.05$). Their most significant finding was that the quality of sleep has the biggest impact on pain intensity, suggesting that sleep should potentially have a bigger role in treatment programs when dealing with chronic pain.

Therapeutic Alliance

Therapeutic alliance (TA) is establishing a collaborative and respectful relationship between the PT and the patient by establishing collaborative treatment and goals that are meaningful for the patient. In order to establish TA, active listening is key, along with finding what will motivate the patient while being respectful and empathetic about what matters most to them.

Kinney et al. [23] completed a systematic review that looked at the impact of TA on those suffering from chronic MSK pain. Their aim was to focus on the value of TA in a PT setting with chronic MSK pain with three main objectives: (1) assess the impact of TA and PT; (2) identify elements that influence the strength of TA between the PT and their patient; and (3) determine a working definition of TA in the PT profession. Studies were selected if they included

(1) adults with pain lasting >3 months, (2) interventions assessing TA, (3) any pain management PT interventions, (4) RCTs, cohort trials, observational trials, case series, and mixed model studies, and (5) outcome measures associated with pain and TA. Studies were excluded if participants were younger than 18, had cancer, or had no treatment by a PT. 7 total studies met the inclusion criteria, with three studies looking specifically at the effect of TA on chronic MSK pain management. One study looked at the relationship between the VAS and the Working Alliance subscale of the Pain Rehabilitation Expectations Scale (PRES), which demonstrated a 0.23 cm impact on pain intensity for every 1-point increase in TA ($\beta = -0.23$, $p = 0.002$). Another study found a 0.044 cm improvement in pain measured by the VAS for every 1-point increase in the Working Alliance Theory of Change Inventory (WATOCI) ($\beta = -0.044$, 95% CI = −0.070–0.017, $p = 0.001$). The third study found a statistically significant improvement in pain measured by the NPRS for groups with enhanced TA ($p < 0.01$). Overall, they found that there was a positive correlation between a strong TA and pain outcomes, and this may be even more beneficial when combined with traditional PT interventions such as MT and TE. Positive influences for TA included trust, open communication, positive support from the PT, the patient feeling that the PT had their best interest in mind, patient values and barriers being identified, the PT working with the whole person, individualized and flexible treatment plans, and the ability to work through challenges that may have been presented during the plan. Negative influences for TA included hostility and expressions of anger.

A qualitative study on TA and PT expectations before and after PT intervention was performed by Unsgaard-Tondel & Soderstrom [24]. They found that pre-PT, most patients expected the focus to be on exercises and their diagnoses. However, after PT, they found that patients were pleasantly surprised at how PT was able to personalize their experience and help with self-managing pain. They were able to do this by actively listening to the patient, educating them, and empowering them. Patients found this to be one of the most meaningful aspects of their care, and hence, the writers conclude that TA can have a very strong correlation to patient outcomes and should be a focus when treating them.

Applications for Clinical Practice

There is still a long road ahead of us in order to get the opioid crisis under control, and it is going to take the collaboration of healthcare professionals to bring it to fruition. PT should be considered as a first line of defense when it comes to both acute and chronic MSK disorders. Although the quality of research varied for each section of this chapter, the research still suggests that early referral to PT for highly prevalent conditions such as LBP could reduce the long-term odds of using opioids and reduce the overall cost of healthcare. PT has a unique approach secondary to the various modalities that can be used, including but not limited to manual therapy, therapeutic exercise, PNE, and sleep hygiene. These strategies allow the PT to help the patient in various aspects that can be tailored in ways that other interventions or medications may not be able to. TA is another aspect that could be considered an asset, where most patients get to spend multiple times a week with their PT, allowing for a more well-rounded and meaningful intervention for the patient. Overall, research seems to suggest that PT, in collaboration with other healthcare providers and/or non-opioid modalities, could lead to better outcomes regarding pain, disability, and function and should be considered as a highly important part of fighting the opioid crisis.

References

1. APTA white paper. 2021. Retrieved 2023, from https://www.apta.org/contentassets/b9421650038941469c75d06a0a191069/beyond-opioids-white-paper.pdf.
2. Centers for Disease Control and Prevention. Understanding the opioid overdose epidemic. Centers for Disease Control and Prevention; 2023. https://www.cdc.gov/opioids/basics/epidemic.html
3. Centers for Disease Control and Prevention. Prescription opioids. Centers for Disease Control and Prevention; 2017. https://www.cdc.gov/opioids/basics/prescribed.html
4. Moffat M. The history of physical therapy practice in the United States. J Phys Ther Educ. 2003;17(3):15–25. https://doi.org/10.1097/00001416-200310000-00003.
5. Ramanayake RPJC, Basnayake BMTK. Evaluation of red flags minimizes missing serious diseases in primary care. J Family Med Prim Care. 2018; https://www.ncbi.nlm.nih.gov/pmc/articles/PMC6060920/
6. Arnold E, La Barrie J, DaSilva L, Patti M, Goode A, Clewley D. The effect of timing of physical therapy for acute low back pain on health services utilization: a systematic review. Arch Phys Med Rehabil. 2019;100(7):1324–38. https://doi.org/10.1016/j.apmr.2018.11.025.
7. Aoyagi K, Neon T, Peloquin C, Dubreuil M, Marinko L, Camarinos J, Felson DT, Kumar D. Association of physical therapy interventions with long-term opioid use after total knee replacement. JAMA Netw Open. 2021; https://doi.org/10.1001/jamanetworkopen.2021.31271.
8. Horn ME, Fritz JM. Timing of physical therapy consultation on 1-year healthcare utilization and costs in patients seeking care for neck pain: a retrospective cohort. BMC Health Serv Res. 2018;18(1) https://doi.org/10.1186/s12913-018-3699-0.
9. Bielecki JE, Tadi P. Therapeutic exercise. National Library of Medicine; 2023. https://www.ncbi.nlm.nih.gov/books/NBK555914/
10. Bertozzi L, Gardenghi I, Turoni F, Villafañe JH, Capra F, Guccione AA, Pillastrini P. Effect of therapeutic exercise on pain and disability in the management of chronic nonspecific neck pain: systematic review and meta-analysis of randomized trials. Phys Ther. 2013;93(8):1026–36. https://doi.org/10.2522/ptj.20120412.
11. Dehghani A, Hasanpour-Dehkordi A, Solati K. A comparison of the effects of pilates and Mckenzie training on pain and general health in men with chronic low back pain: A randomized trial. Indian J Palliat Care. 2017;23(1):36. https://doi.org/10.4103/0973-1075.197945.
12. Sosa-Reina MD, Nunez-Nagy S, Gallego-Izquierdo T, Pecos-Martín D, Monserrat J, Álvarez-Mon M. Effectiveness of therapeutic exercise in fibromyalgia syndrome: a systematic review

and meta-analysis of randomized clinical trials. Biomed Res Int. 2017;2017:1–14. https://doi.org/10.1155/2017/2356346.
13. APTA Guidelines to Clinical Practice. APTA: American Physical Therapy Association. (2023). https://guide.apta.org/search
14. Santos GK, Gonçalves de Oliveira R, Campos de Oliveira L, Ferreira C. de Oliveira C, Andraus RA, Ngomo S, Fusco A, Cortis C, da Silva RA. Effectiveness of muscle energy technique in patients with nonspecific low back pain: a systematic review with meta-analysis. Eur J Phys Rehabil Med. 2022;58(6) https://doi.org/10.23736/s1973-9087.22.07424-x.
15. Abrahim Namnaqani F, Salah Mashabi A, Mohhammed Yaseen K, Abdullah Alshehri M. The effectiveness of McKenzie method compared to manual therapy for treating chronic low back pain: a systematic reviewF. J Musculoskelet Nueronal Interact. 2019;19(42) https://www.ncbi.nlm.nih.gov/pmc/articles/PMC6944795/
16. Muñoz-Gómez E, Alcaraz-Martínez AM, Mollà-Casanova S, Sempere-Rubio N, Aguilar-Rodríguez M, Serra-Añó P, Inglés M. Effectiveness of a manual therapy protocol in women with pelvic pain due to endometriosis: a randomized clinical trial. J Clin Med. 2023;12(9):3310. https://doi.org/10.3390/jcm12093310.
17. PNE 101 - EIM post-professional education; n.d.. https://evidenceinmotion.com/wp-content/uploads/2020/02/PNE101.pdf
18. Ibrahim AA, Akindele MO, Ganiyu SO. Effectiveness of patient education plus motor control exercise versus patient education alone versus motor control exercise alone for rural community-dwelling adults with chronic low back pain: a randomised clinical trial. BMC Musculoskelet Disord. 2023;24(1):142. https://doi.org/10.1186/s12891-022-06108-9.
19. Engers AJ, Jellema P, Wensing M, van der Windt DA, Grol R, van Tulder MW. Individual patient education for low back pain. Cochrane Database Syst Rev. 2008; https://doi.org/10.1002/14651858.cd004057.pub3.
20. Lepri B, Romani D, Storari L, Barbari V. Effectiveness of pain neuroscience education in patients with chronic musculoskeletal pain and central sensitization: a systematic review. Int J Environ Res Public Health. 2023;20(5):4098. https://doi.org/10.3390/ijerph20054098.
21. Sleep Education. Healthy sleep habits. American Academy of Sleep Medicine; 2023. https://sleepeducation.org/healthy-sleep/healthy-sleep-habits/
22. De la Vega R, Racine M, Castarlenas E, Solde E, Roy R, Jensen MP, Miro J, Cane D. The role of sleep quality and fatigue on the benefits of an interdisciplinary treatment for adults with chronic pain. Pain Pract. 2019;19(4):354–62. https://doi.org/10.1111/papr.12746.
23. Kinney M, Seider J, Floyd Beaty A, Coughlin K, Dyal M, Clewley D. The impact of therapeutic alliance in physical therapy for chronic musculoskeletal pain: a systematic review of the literature. Physiother Theory Pract. 2020;36(8):886–98. https://doi.org/10.1080/09593985.2018.1516015.
24. Unsgaard-Tondel M, Soderstrom S. Therapeutic alliance: patients' expectations before and experiences after physical therapy for low back pain- a qualitative study with 6-month follow-up. Phys Ther Rehab J. 2021;101(11):1–9. https://doi.org/10.1093/ptj/pzab187.
25. Numeric pain rating scale. Physiopedia; n.d.. https://www.physio-pedia.com/Numeric_Pain_Rating_Scale
26. Visual analogue scale. Physiopedia; n.d.. https://www.physio-pedia.com/Visual_Analogue_Scale
27. Neck disability index. Physiopedia; n.d.. https://www.physio-pedia.com/Neck_Disability_Index?utm_source=physiopedia&utm_medium=search&utm_campaign=ongoing_internal
28. The Northwick Park Questionnaire. Physiopedia; n.d.. https://www.physio-pedia.com/The_Northwick_Park_Questionnaire?utm_source=physiopedia&utm_medium=search&utm_campaign=ongoing_internal
29. McGill Pain Questionnaire. Physiopedia; n.d.. https://www.physio-pedia.com/McGill_Pain_Questionnaire?utm_source=physiopedia&utm_medium=search&utm_campaign=ongoing_internal
30. 28-Item general health questionnaire. Physiopedia; n.d.. https://www.physio-pedia.com/28-Item_General_Health_Questionnaire?utm_source=physiopedia&utm_medium=search&utm_campaign=ongoing_internal
31. Fibromyalgia impact questionnaire (FIQ). Physiopedia; n.d.. https://www.physio-pedia.com/Fibromyalgia_Impact_Questionnaire_(FIQ)?utm_source=physiopedia&utm_medium=search&utm_campaign=ongoing_internal.
32. West Haven-yale multidimensional pain inventory. Shirley Ryan AbilityLab; n.d.. https://www.sralab.org/rehabilitation-measures/west-haven-yale-multidimensional-pain-inventory
33. Quebec back pain disability scale. Physiopedia; n.d.. https://www.physio-pedia.com/Quebec_Back_Pain_Disability_Scale?utm_source=physiopedia&utm_medium=search&utm_campaign=ongoing_internal
34. Orebro Musculoskeletal pain questionnaire (OMPQ). APTA; n.d.. https://www.apta.org/patient-care/evidence-based-practice-resources/test-measures/orebro-musculoskeletal-pain-questionnaire-ompq
35. Oswestry disability index. Physiopedia; n.d.. https://www.physio-pedia.com/Oswestry_Disability_Index?utm_source=physiopedia&utm_medium=search&utm_campaign=ongoing_internal
36. Roland-Morris disability questionnaire. Physiopedia. n.d.. https://www.physio-pedia.com/Roland%E2%80%90Morris_Disability_Questionnaire?utm_source=physiopedia&utm_medium=search&utm_campaign=ongoing_internal
37. Patient-reported Outcomes Measurement Information System Global Health (promis GH-10). Physiopedia; n.d.. https://www.physio-pedia.com/Patient-Reported_Outcomes_Measurement_Information_System_Global_Health_(PROMIS_GH-10)?utm_source=physiopedia&utm_medium=search&utm_campaign=ongoing_internal.
38. The pain disability index (PDI); n.d.. https://cme.dmu.edu/sites/default/files/The Pain Disability Index (PDI).pdf.
39. Cheing GLY, Lai AKM, Vong SKS, Chan FH. Factorial structure of the pain rehabilitation expectations scale: a preliminary study. Int J Rehabil Res. 2010;33(1):88–94. https://doi.org/10.1097/mrr.0b013e32832e9884.
40. Working Alliance Inventory. Shirley Ryan AbilityLab; n.d.. https://www.sralab.org/rehabilitation-measures/working-alliance-inventory

Art Therapy

30

Giustino Varrassi, Alberto Corriero, Giacomo Farì, Christopher Gharibo, Alena Javurkova, Matteo Luigi Giuseppe Leoni, Filomena Puntillo, and Jaroslava Raudenska

Introduction

Pain is a universal human experience, deeply personal and profoundly complex [1]. While it can serve as a biological warning system indicating injury or illness, chronic pain often becomes a source of suffering that transcends physical sensations [2]. Millions globally endure persistent pain that resists conventional medical explanations or fails to respond to pharmacological treatments [3]. In such cases, pain extends beyond the physical, impacting psychological, emotional, and social domains [4].

Traditional pain management has centered on pharmacological, interventional, and surgical approaches. While these methods have provided relief to many, they frequently fall short when faced with the multifaceted nature of chronic pain [2, 5]. Patients often cycle through treatments offering only temporary benefits or encounter adverse effects that intensify their distress [6]. This has spurred interest in integrative therapies that address the broader human experience of pain.

Art therapy has emerged as a promising integrative approach, gaining recognition for its role in pain management [7, 8]. Situated at the crossroads of psychology, creativity, and healing, it offers a unique way for individuals to process and transform their pain. Unlike talk therapies that depend on verbal articulation, art therapy accesses the nonverbal, symbolic, and sensory dimensions of the mind [9]. This is crucial for those who struggle to express the complexities of their condition.

The power of art therapy lies not in artistic talent but in the act of creation itself [9]. Through painting, drawing, or sculpting, patients shift focus from suffering to meaning-making. This process has been linked to reduced anxiety, alleviation of depressive symptoms, and modulation of pain perception [7]. Additionally, it nurtures a sense of autonomy, accomplishment, and identity, qualities often eroded by chronic illness [10].

A growing body of research underscores the tangible benefits of art therapy in pain settings [7, 11]. These include psychological gains and physiological effects such as reduced cortisol levels, improved sleep, and lower heart rate. Increasingly, art therapy is being integrated into pain clinics, hospitals, cancer centers, and mental health facilities as part of holistic care plans that treat the whole person [12]. Nevertheless, art therapy remains underutilized and frequently misunderstood [13]. Medical professionals may lack familiarity with its methods, and patients may see it as irrelevant or feel intimidated by notions of artistic ability [14]. Bridging these gaps in understanding and accessibility is essential for broader implementation.

This chapter explores art therapy's role in pain management from a biopsychosocial perspective. It reviews the limitations of conventional treatments and examines the theoretical and clinical foundations of art therapy. Drawing on empirical evidence and case studies, it illustrates how art-

G. Varrassi (✉)
Fondazione Paolo Procacci, Rome, Italy

A. Corriero · F. Puntillo
Department of Interdisciplinary Medicine, ICU Section, University of Bari Aldo Moro, Bari, Italy

G. Farì
Department of Experimental Medicine, University of Salento, Lecce, Italy

C. Gharibo
Department of Pain Management, NYU Langone Health, New York, NY, USA

A. Javurkova
Department of Clinical Psychology, University Hospital Kralovske Vinohrady and 3rd Faculty of Medicine, Prague, Czech Republic

M. L. G. Leoni
Department of Medical and Surgical Sciences and Translational Medicine, Sapienza University of Rome, Rome, Italy

J. Raudenska
Department of Nursing, 2nd Faculty of Medicine, Charles University, Prague, Czech Republic

J. P. Reinert et al. (eds.), *Adjunctive Analgesic Strategies for the Bedside Clinician and Beyond*,
https://doi.org/10.1007/978-3-032-21675-5_30

making can foster relief, resilience, and transformation, reframing pain not as an endpoint but as a potential gateway to creative empowerment.

Understanding Pain

Pain, though often regarded as a simple physical sensation, is in reality a multifaceted and deeply subjective experience. It arises from a complex interplay of biological, psychological, and social factors, challenging purely physiological explanations [15]. To appreciate the value of art therapy in pain management, one must first understand the nature of pain itself.

Acute vs. Chronic Pain

Pain is commonly classified as either acute or chronic. Acute pain typically has a sudden onset and is associated with a specific injury or illness—such as a broken bone, a surgical procedure, or an infection [16]. It serves a vital protective role, prompting rest and recovery, and usually resolves as the underlying issue heals. Chronic pain, in contrast, persists beyond the expected healing time—generally over 3–6 months. It often lacks a clear cause and may result from changes in the nervous system that heighten or misfire pain signals [17]. This form of pain is not simply a symptom but often evolves into a condition itself, frequently accompanied by depression, anxiety, or post-traumatic stress [18]. It resists straightforward biomedical solutions and affects all areas of life, from sleep and work to mood and relationships [19].

The Biopsychosocial Model of Pain

Historically, pain was understood through a narrow biomedical lens that emphasized physical injury or disease. Yet this view faltered when patients reported ongoing pain despite normal imaging or recovery. The biopsychosocial model, introduced in 1977, now underpins modern pain medicine [20]. This model, illustrated in Fig. 30.1, recognizes that pain is shaped not only by biological factors (such as nerve function, inflammation, and genetics) but also by psychological elements (mood, trauma, and beliefs) and social conditions (relationships, culture, and healthcare access).

Art therapy aligns well with this model, as it offers a platform to explore and influence the emotional and cognitive dimensions of pain [13]. Through creative expression, individuals can address unresolved trauma, shift maladaptive beliefs, and cultivate resilience, each of which can directly modify their pain experience [21].

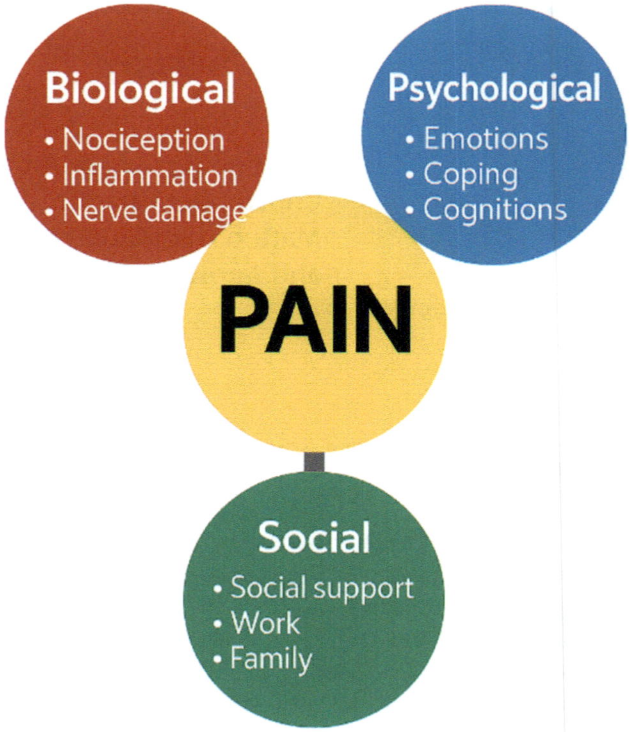

Fig. 30.1 Biopsychosocial model for pain [AI-generated image]

Psychological and Emotional Impacts of Pain

The emotional toll of chronic pain is profound [22]. Conditions like depression and anxiety often emerge alongside persistent pain, compounding the distress in a self-reinforcing cycle. Pain can erode one's identity and purpose, leading individuals to feel isolated, disbelieved, or invisible [21, 23]. These emotional burdens further amplify pain perception. Moreover, chronic pain can trigger central sensitization, a state where the nervous system becomes hypersensitive and poorly regulates discomfort [24].

While conventional pain treatments focus on physical symptoms, they often neglect the psychological landscape. Art therapy offers a nonverbal and symbolic avenue for exploring suffering, helping patients regain a sense of coherence, self-worth, and emotional control [25].

Pain and Communication: When Words Fail

A major challenge in pain care is its invisibility. Unlike external injuries, pain is internal and subjective, often leading to skepticism from clinicians or family members [20]. Language alone frequently fails to convey the nuance, depth, and persistence of the experience [26, 27].

Art therapy provides an alternative language. Metaphor, color, and image can express what words cannot. A visual representation may effectively communicate sensations like burning, stabbing, or tightness. In this way, art functions both diagnostically and therapeutically, offering clinicians insight and enabling patients to externalize and reframe their pain [7, 28].

Cultural Perspectives on Pain

Culture heavily influences how pain is perceived, expressed, and managed. Some societies valorize stoicism, while others encourage vocal expression of suffering. Cultural beliefs also shape how patients are treated by healthcare professionals [29].

Art therapy can be adapted to fit these cultural frameworks. It can incorporate indigenous symbols, culturally relevant stories, or traditional art forms, thereby making it more relatable and effective. A poignant example is the Southern Italian myth of the "*taranta,*" a folkloric belief linking the bite of a tarantula to agonizing pain and agitation, cured only by music and dance. This story, rooted in the region of Salento (Italy), reflects a symbolic cultural representation of pain as seen in Fig. 30.2.

In this way, art therapy's adaptability across cultures makes it a respectful, inclusive, and meaningful intervention for diverse populations [30].

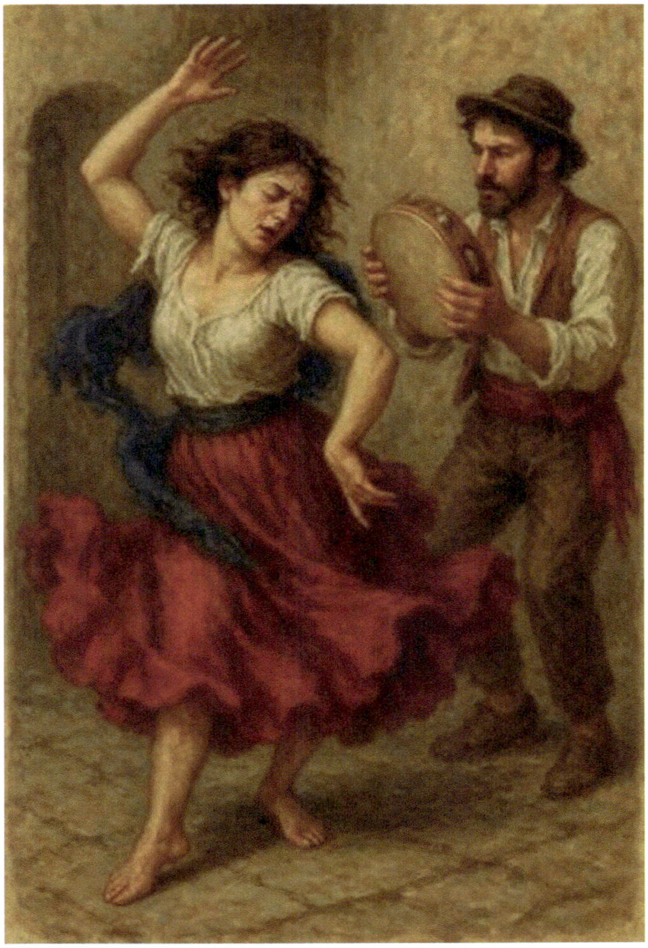

Fig. 30.2 The "taranta" dance [AI-generated image]

The Foundations of Art Therapy

Art therapy is a structured, evidence-informed practice integrating psychology and creative expression [7]. It supports emotional regulation, insight, and personal growth, offering those with chronic pain not just symptom relief but a path to reclaim identity and well-being amid suffering [31].

Definition and Scope

The American Art Therapy Association (AATA) provides a broad definition, which reflects the versatility of art therapy across a wide range of populations, settings, and conditions [32]. In the context of pain management, art therapy can serve many functions: helping individuals process trauma related to injury or illness, manage the emotional burden of persistent discomfort, increase adherence to treatment, and regain a sense of agency and autonomy. Art therapy is not dependent on a person's artistic talent or training. The focus lies not on producing a technically "good" piece of art, but on the therapeutic process, the exploration, creation, reflection, and meaning-making that occur through engagement with visual media [33]. The art itself becomes a language through which inner experiences can be seen, heard, understood, and treated.

Historical Evolution

The origins of art therapy can be traced back to early twentieth-century movements in psychiatry, psychoanalysis, and education [34]. As interest in the therapeutic potential of unconscious processes and symbolic expression expanded, key figures such as Margaret Naumburg and Edith Kramer emerged as foundational pioneers in the development of art therapy as a legitimate psychotherapeutic practice. Margaret Naumburg, often hailed as the "mother of art therapy" in the United States, believed that spontaneous artistic expression served as a symbolic language of the unconscious. Through free drawing or painting, she argued, individuals could reveal repressed thoughts and emotions, thereby gaining psychological insight and facilitating healing. In contrast, a couple of decades later, Edith Kramer emphasized the intrinsic value of the creative process itself. She proposed that art-making could support ego development and emotional integration even without verbal analysis. Kramer's approach, known as "art-as-therapy," underscored the healing power of the act of creation and helped differentiate art therapy from purely interpretive models. Together, their contributions laid the groundwork for the diverse methodologies used in contemporary art therapy [35]. From its early psychoanalytic roots, art therapy has evolved to incorporate a variety of psychological theories and models, including cognitive behavioral therapy (CBT), trauma-informed care, mindfulness, and neurobiological research [36, 37]. This pluralistic foundation makes it adaptable and integrative, qualities particularly valuable in complex cases like chronic pain.

Core Principles and Theoretical Frameworks

While art therapy encompasses diverse methods and styles, several unifying principles distinguish it from recreational art or creative hobbies. The understanding that the creative process itself is therapeutic is central, fostering states of flow that promote emotional regulation and reduce distress through sensory engagement with color, texture, and movement [38]. Art also serves as a nonverbal language, providing a critical outlet for individuals—particularly those living with pain—who struggle to articulate complex emotions or experiences [39]. Through this medium, pain, trauma, and grief may be symbolically expressed when words are insufficient.

Importantly, the artwork functions as a reflective tool, externalizing internal states in a tangible form [40]. This perspective enables individuals to process their pain with greater insight and agency. The therapeutic relationship between the patient and the art therapist is equally central, establishing a safe, empathetic space where trust and emotional exploration can occur [41]. Finally, the use of symbolism and metaphor enhances healing by transforming abstract pain experiences into visual forms—such as storms, cages, or dark spaces—that can be explored, reinterpreted, and gradually transformed through therapy [42]. Together, these principles underpin art therapy's unique role in fostering psychological resilience and emotional healing in pain management.

The Role of the Art Therapist

An art therapist is a trained mental health professional with specialized education in both psychology and the visual arts. Certification typically involves a master's degree, supervised clinical experience, and ongoing professional development. Art therapists work in a variety of settings, including hospitals, rehabilitation centers, mental health clinics, schools, and private practices. In pain management settings, art therapists work collaboratively with interdisciplinary teams—comprising physicians, psychologists, nurses, physiotherapists, and social workers—to support patient care. They guide meaningful use of art materials, encourage emotional expression, foster coping and resilience, and assess therapeutic progress by observing changes through patients' creative processes [43]. Importantly, art therapists are trained to witness and contain strong emotional reactions that may arise during art-making, especially when dealing with trauma or body-related distress [36]. This makes art therapy a safe space for deep and often transformative work.

Differences Between Art Therapy and Other Creative Activities

While many individuals engage in creative activities like painting or journaling for relaxation, art therapy is distinct in its therapeutic intent and structure and provides interesting results also in stress indicators [44]. It is guided by specific goals tailored to each individual, with a trained art therapist facilitating the process to help safely explore emotions and foster insight. Art therapy is integrated into broader treatment plans, supporting psychological, medical, or rehabilitative outcomes. Crucially, the emphasis is on the process rather than the final product, aiming not for aesthetic success but for emotional expression, regulation, and healing.

This distinction is important in medical settings where patients might initially be hesitant, believing they "aren't artistic." With guidance and support, these same individuals often discover that the power of art therapy lies in self-expression, not skill.

Mechanisms of Art Therapy in Pain Relief

To understand how art therapy alleviates pain, one must look beyond the physical body and into the cognitive, emotional, and neurological dimensions of the pain experience. Unlike interventions aimed solely at physical symptoms, art therapy engages the whole person, addressing not just what hurts but *how* it hurts, *why* it hurts, and *what the pain means* [8]. The mechanisms through which art therapy influences pain are diverse and interconnected, offering multiple pathways to relief and healing.

Distraction and Attentional Shift

When someone is in pain, especially chronic pain, their attention is often consumed by the sensation, amplifying its intensity. Art therapy offers an attentional shift, a means of engaging the mind in focused, meaningful activity that draws attention away from pain [45]. Creating art can induce a flow state, characterized by deep immersion, a loss of self-consciousness, and an altered perception of time [38]. During flow, pain signals may still exist, but the brain's attentional resources are redirected, reducing the perception of pain. This is more than distraction; it is constructive absorption in an activity that fosters agency and mastery. Moreover, art-making often engages multiple sensory systems—visual, tactile, and kinesthetic—which can override or dampen the internal signals of pain [46]. Manipulating clay, painting with broad strokes, or choosing colors for a collage activates the brain in novel ways, temporarily disrupting habitual pain pathways.

Emotional Expression and Catharsis

Chronic pain is frequently intertwined with unprocessed emotions such as grief, anger, fear, guilt, or shame. These emotional burdens often intensify the pain experience and may even be stored somatically, particularly in cases where pain is linked to trauma. Art therapy provides a safe, nonverbal outlet for these emotions, enabling catharsis, the release and expression of pent-up feelings [47]. Through metaphor, symbolism, and visual language, individuals can express what may be too overwhelming or complex to articulate [42]. A person who cannot say "I am scared of being disabled" might instead draw a shattered bridge or a darkening sky. In doing so, they begin the work of externalizing and processing emotional pain, which can reduce psychological stress and, in turn, alleviate physical symptoms. Art therapy also helps individuals name and reframe their emotions [48]. Through therapeutic reflection, the artwork becomes a mirror, allowing people to explore their feelings from a different perspective and consider alternative narratives that promote healing.

Neurobiological and Physiological Effects

The benefits of art therapy extend beyond psychological relief, exerting measurable neurological and physiological effects. Engaging in creative processes influences brain chemistry and structure in ways that modulate pain perception and promote healing [46]. Activation of reward pathways through art-making stimulates dopamine release, counteracting the disruptions commonly observed in chronic pain patients, such as anhedonia and depression [49, 50]. This restores positive reinforcement mechanisms and enhances emotional well-being.

Simultaneously, art therapy contributes to stress reduction, as evidenced by lowered cortisol levels, reduced heart rate, and decreased blood pressure [44]. By attenuating sympathetic nervous system arousal, it mitigates the physiological amplification of pain responses. Moreover, art therapy facilitates neural plasticity, fostering the formation of new, adaptive neural connections while reducing sensitization in chronic pain pathways [31, 51]. This adaptive rewiring enhances self-regulation and promotes resilience.

Additionally, art therapy promotes the integration of left and right brain functions, which is essential for processing the often nonverbal nature of pain. While language-based therapies may inadequately address right hemisphere-mediated experiences, art therapy engages both hemispheres—combining visual, emotional, and intuitive elements with cognitive reflection and interpretation [52, 53]. This hemispheric integration supports a more cohesive and comprehensive processing of the pain experience, reinforcing art therapy's role as a valuable component in multidisciplinary pain management.

Enhancing Agency and Control

One of the most psychologically damaging aspects of chronic pain is the loss of control [54]. Medical interventions often place the patient in a passive role, with doctors prescribing treatments or procedures that the patient undergoes. Art therapy, in contrast, places the individual in an active, creative, and empowered role [55]. The act of choosing materials, deciding what to create, and shaping an artistic image restores a sense of personal agency. Even when the pain cannot be eliminated, the individual can take control of how they express and relate to it. This shift from helplessness to empowerment can have profound implications for mood, motivation, and self-efficacy. Additionally, through ongoing creative work, individuals may track their progress over time. Artwork becomes a visual record of emotional states, insights, and changes. This evidence of growth and adaptation reinforces hope and resilience.

Facilitating Insight and Meaning-Making

Pain disrupts life stories [56]. People often describe chronic pain as something that "steals their life," "changes who they are," or "breaks their sense of meaning." Art therapy offers a way to reconstruct meaning, to reinterpret suffering in a way that honors the struggle while also opening space for transformation [57]. Creating images of pain, strength, memory, and hope allows individuals to explore their personal narratives. For some, this might involve confronting loss or trauma; for others, it might mean imagining a future self that copes with pain in new ways. These symbolic acts help people move from a fragmented sense of self to a more integrated identity that includes, but is not defined by, their pain. In this way, art therapy facilitates what Viktor Frankl called "meaning-making," the ability to find purpose or significance even in suffering [58]. This existential dimension of healing is often overlooked in medical settings but is central to long-term well-being. Figure 30.3 illustrates the multifac-

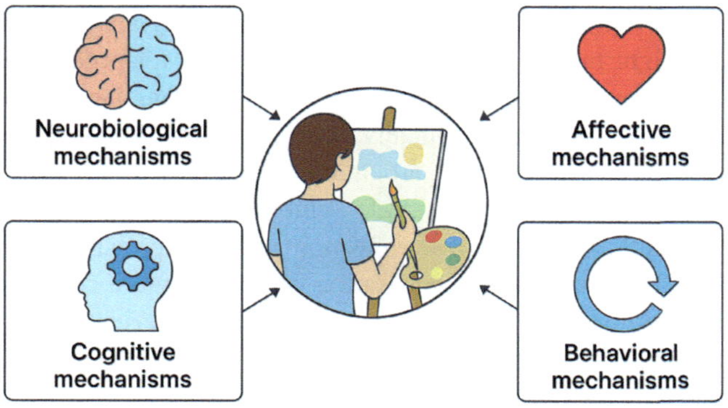

Fig. 30.3 Mechanisms of art therapy in pain relief. The diagram shows the key pathways through which art therapy may alleviate pain, including neurobiological, affective, cognitive, and behavioral mechanisms, each interacting to support holistic pain management

eted mechanisms through which art therapy contributes to pain relief, encompassing neurobiological, affective, cognitive, and behavioral domains.

Evidence-Based Research

In recent decades, a growing body of research has explored the therapeutic potential of art therapy, including its application in pain management. While the subjective and complex nature of pain presents unique challenges for empirical measurement, a range of quantitative, qualitative, and mixed-methods studies have demonstrated the benefits of art therapy in reducing pain intensity, improving mood, enhancing quality of life, and promoting emotional resilience [7]. This section examines key findings from clinical trials, meta-analyses, and case studies, highlighting how art therapy has become an evidence-informed component of holistic care for individuals living with pain.

Overview of the Research Landscape

Art therapy research spans diverse fields such as psychology, medicine, neuroscience, nursing, and public health [59–62]. Despite varying methodologies, studies consistently highlight its beneficial outcomes. These include reductions in perceived pain intensity, anxiety, depression, and stress levels. Art therapy also improves coping skills, self-efficacy, and emotional communication, while fostering a greater sense of agency and well-being. These effects are particularly well-documented in oncology, palliative care, rehabilitation, and chronic illness contexts, where pain is often complex and persistent [63, 64]. The interdisciplinary nature of this research underscores the broad applicability and therapeutic potential of art-based interventions across healthcare settings.

Clinical Studies in Pain Management

Art therapy has demonstrated significant value across a range of pain contexts, including cancer-related, chronic, and acute pain conditions. In cancer pain, patients often experience complex physical, emotional, and spiritual suffering. Art therapy offers a complementary means of addressing these multidimensional challenges. Monti et al. [65] showed in a randomized controlled trial that women with cancer participating in an eight-week mindfulness-based art therapy (MBAT) program reported marked reductions in psychological distress and improved quality of life versus controls. Subsequent studies confirmed similar benefits across diverse cancer populations [66]. Likewise, Lin et al. [67] found that terminal cancer patients engaged in art appreciation and painting within hospice care experienced enhanced emotional relaxation and physical comfort, benefits also documented in pediatric palliative settings [63]. Qualitative research further highlights art therapy's capacity to help patients express fears, grief, and physical suffering, contributing to improved emotional regulation and pain perception [68–70].

In chronic pain conditions such as fibromyalgia, arthritis, migraines, and neuropathic pain, art therapy has emerged as an effective adjunct. A study has demonstrated that creative engagement reduces stress and depression, enhancing coping among patients with chronic musculoskeletal pain [71]. Mindfulness-based art therapy has shown benefits in reducing depression and stress and enhancing happiness in migraine sufferers [72]. Clinical trials in fibromyalgia also report reductions in pain intensity, improvements in quality of life, and positive effects on body image [73, 74].

In acute and postsurgical pain, art therapy interventions have proven beneficial, particularly in pediatric care. A scoping review demonstrated that art-based activities reduce pain, anxiety, stress, and fear during treatment [75]. In adults, a randomized trial in burn units showed mandala coloring reduced pain and anxiety during dressing changes [76]. Similarly, in postpartum care, art-based interventions alleviate depression and anxiety while improving maternal-infant bonding, as supported by a recent meta-analysis [77]. Collectively, these findings affirm art therapy's versatility as an evidence-informed, non-pharmacological tool for managing diverse pain experiences across clinical settings.

Neuroimaging and Psychophysiological Research

Advancements in neuroimaging and physiological monitoring have provided objective evidence supporting the efficacy of art therapy in pain management. Functional MRI studies indicate that engaging in creative activities activates brain regions associated with pleasure and emotional processing, such as the anterior cingulate cortex and somatosensory cortex, while reducing activity in areas linked to pain perception [78]. Electroencephalogram (EEG) research has demonstrated that art-making can increase alpha wave activity, which is associated with relaxation and decreased cortical arousal, correlating with reduced pain perception [79]. Furthermore, studies measuring salivary cortisol levels, a biomarker for stress, have found significant reductions following art therapy sessions, particularly in individuals experiencing pain-related anxiety and tension [44]. These findings suggest that art therapy not only alters subjective experiences but also induces measurable changes in brain function and physiological stress responses, offering a multifaceted approach to pain mitigation.

Limitations and Challenges in Research

Despite encouraging findings, research on art therapy in pain management faces notable limitations. A major concern is the heterogeneity of methodologies across studies, including variations in intervention duration, art modality, sample size, and assessment tools, which makes direct comparisons and meta-analyses difficult. Additionally, many investigations rely on small sample sizes, often from pilot studies, limiting the generalizability of outcomes.

The nature of art therapy also makes it challenging to implement double-blind designs, increasing the risk of bias. Furthermore, most outcome measures are subjective, relying on self-reported pain and emotional states, which can be influenced by expectations and placebo effects. These methodological constraints underscore the need for more robust, longitudinal research designs with larger, more diverse populations and the inclusion of objective biomarkers. Multidisciplinary approaches integrating neuroimaging, physiological monitoring, and standardized outcome metrics may offer a clearer understanding of art therapy's efficacy and mechanisms in the context of pain and psychological distress.

Patient Perspectives and Qualitative Insights

While quantitative data provides measurable outcomes, qualitative research reveals the profound personal impact of art therapy on individuals experiencing pain. Patient interviews and narrative analyses consistently highlight themes of nonverbal expression, autonomy, and emotional renewal. Participants often describe art-making as a means to communicate pain without words, offering relief from the constant role of "patient" and restoring a sense of self. Statements such as "It made me feel like a person again, not just someone in pain" and "I saw myself differently. Stronger" illustrates art therapy's role in identity reconstruction and empowerment. Beyond symptom relief, these insights emphasize its contribution to emotional expression and social reconnection.

Applications Across Different Populations

Art therapy is inherently adaptable, making it suitable for a wide variety of individuals experiencing pain. Whether the source of pain is physical, psychological, or a combination of both, art therapy can be modified to fit the developmental, cultural, medical, and emotional needs of different populations. In this section, we examine how art therapy is used effectively among children, adults, the elderly, trauma survivors, individuals with disabilities, and those in palliative or hospice care.

Pediatric Populations

Children and adolescents experience pain differently from adults [80]. Their limited cognitive and emotional vocabulary can make it difficult to articulate where or how much something hurts. Art therapy offers a nonverbal language through which children can communicate discomfort, fear, and anxiety [63]. Art therapy plays a pivotal role in pediatric care by addressing both emotional and physical challenges faced by children [81, 82]. In hospital settings, it serves as a valuable tool to alleviate anxiety and fear associated with medical procedures, providing children with a sense of control and emotional resilience. For those managing chronic illnesses like juvenile arthritis, sickle cell anemia, or cancer, art therapy offers a medium to externalize pain, foster hope, and enhance coping mechanisms. Additionally, incorporating creative activities such as drawing and storytelling aids in pain education, enabling children to identify, label, and express their discomfort, which in turn improves emotional regulation and treatment adherence. Art therapists employ developmentally appropriate materials—like markers, clay, and paint—to engage children in a therapeutic process that encourages both creativity and communication, ultimately supporting their overall well-being.

Adolescents and Young Adults

Adolescence is a pivotal period marked by identity formation, heightened sensitivity to peer perception, and a quest for autonomy. Experiencing pain, whether physical, chronic, or emotional, can significantly disrupt this developmental trajectory. Art therapy offers adolescents a constructive outlet to navigate these challenges [82]. For instance, a study by Huang et al. [83] demonstrated that group art therapy sessions enhanced self-concept and peer relationships among adolescents, mitigating feelings of social isolation and fostering a sense of belonging. Additionally, Mittal et al. [84] found that art therapy interventions positively impacted adolescents' mental health, aiding in emotional expression and reducing psychological distress. Moreover, recent research highlighted that art therapy facilitated emotional competence and identity resolution in adolescents facing stressors related to self-exploration and peer pressure [85]. These findings underscore the efficacy of art therapy in addressing the multifaceted challenges adolescents face, promoting emotional well-being, and aiding in the development of a cohesive self-identity.

Adults with Chronic Pain

Adults in treatment for chronic pain often grapple with more than just physical discomfort; they face identity challenges, financial stress, shifts in family roles, and emotional fatigue. Art therapy may result in both a coping mechanism and a reconstructive tool, facilitating long-term adaptation. Narrative art therapy encourages individuals to explore and reframe their personal pain stories, fostering resilience and growth. Such narrative approaches have been shown to restore self-awareness and hope in chronic pain sufferers [86]. Body mapping, where patients illustrate their bodies to depict areas of pain or emotion, enhances body awareness and communication with healthcare providers. Recent studies highlight its effectiveness in capturing the complexity of chronic pain and facilitating personalized care [87]. Engaging in mandala art therapy, involving repetitive, soothing artistic processes like coloring, has been associated with stress reduction, decreased anxiety, and improved emotional well-being. A systematic review suggests that mandala art may improve negative symptoms and relieve pain [88].

Collectively, these art therapy interventions not only alleviate symptoms but also help adults reclaim a sense of productivity and creativity, especially when chronic pain has disrupted their work, hobbies, or identity.

Elderly and Geriatric Populations

Older adults often face chronic pain from conditions like arthritis, neuropathy, or degenerative diseases, compounded by cognitive decline, social isolation, and physical limitations. Art therapy offers multifaceted benefits in managing these challenges.

Reminiscence and life review: Engaging in art therapy allows older adults to reflect on life experiences, fostering a sense of meaning and distracting from pain. A randomized controlled study demonstrated that life review therapy significantly improved the quality of life in the elderly [89].

Fine motor engagement: Simple creative tasks can maintain or improve dexterity and reduce stiffness in arthritic joints. A very recent publication has shown that activities like Zentangle drawing improve fine motor skills and reduce anxiety in older adults [90].

Cognitive stimulation: For those with dementia, visual and tactile art-making stimulates memory and communication. A scoping review by Galassi et al. [91] highlighted the value of creative arts therapies in promoting healthy aging and cognitive function.

Combating isolation: Group art therapy sessions encourage connection, enhancing mood and reducing the psychological burden of pain. A randomized controlled study showed that clay-based group art therapy decreased loneliness and hopelessness in older adults living alone [92].

To accommodate mobility and vision limitations, adaptations such as using larger tools, bright colors, or seated group formats are often implemented, ensuring accessibility and effectiveness of art therapy interventions for older adults.

Trauma Survivors and PTSD-Related Pain

For individuals with a history of trauma, pain often manifests both physically and psychophysically and presents different challenges for both diagnosis and therapy [93]. Trauma survivors frequently experience somatic symptoms, including chronic pain without a clear medical cause. Art therapy offers a trauma-informed approach to address these complexities [94]. Creating sensory-safe environments in art therapy allows patients to engage in the creative process without fear of judgment or triggering stimuli, fostering a sense of safety and control. Symbolic expression through art enables survivors to process traumatic experiences indirectly, using metaphors that can feel safer than direct confrontation. Empowering patients with choices over materials and pacing restores autonomy often compromised by trauma. Trauma-focused art therapy techniques, such as collage, mask-making, and visual storytelling, assist survivors in re-authoring their experiences and managing the physical manifestations of trauma. The cited meta-analysis demonstrated that creative arts therapy significantly reduces PTSD symptoms, highlighting its efficacy in trauma treatment [94].

Individuals with Physical Disabilities

Individuals with physical disabilities often contend with chronic pain, societal stigma, and emotional challenges [95]. Art therapy offers tailored interventions to address these multifaceted issues.

Adaptive materials and tools: Art therapists customize tools, such as adaptive brushes, textured surfaces, or digital platforms, to accommodate various physical abilities, ensuring meaningful participation [96]. This approach fosters inclusivity and empowers patients to engage in creative expression despite physical limitations.

Self-representation: Through art, patients explore and express their identities, perceptions, and aspirations [97]. This process can lead to increased self-acceptance and empowerment, as individuals depict how they perceive themselves and how they wish to be seen by others.

Pain coping strategies: Visualizing pain and constructing personal symbols through art can enhance insight and coping capacity [42]. Engaging in creative processes provides a nonverbal outlet for expressing discomfort and developing personalized strategies for pain management.

By focusing on creative potential rather than limitations, art therapy helps individuals with physical disabilities transition from narratives of loss to ones of capability and strength.

Palliative Care and End-of-Life Contexts

In palliative and hospice care, where pain is often persistent and not fully resolvable, art therapy serves as a source of comfort, meaning, and emotional closure.

Legacy work: Patients engage in creating memory books, letters, or symbolic objects to leave behind, reinforcing purpose and reducing existential pain [98]. Such legacy-making interventions have been found to improve quality of life and foster adaptive coping mechanisms in pediatric palliative-care settings.

Spiritual expression: Art therapy provides a medium to explore questions of faith, the afterlife, and identity beyond the physical self [99]. This creative process aids in managing chronic pain, regulating emotions, strengthening family connections, and creating meaningful legacies for those in palliative care.

Emotional release: Through art-making, patients can process grief, fear, and regret [100]. Caregivers and family members may also use art therapy to prepare for loss, facilitating emotional expression and coping.

Nonverbal support: When verbal communication becomes challenging due to cognitive decline or emotional overwhelm, art offers an alternative means of expression [101]. Art therapy enables patients to process complex emotions, including grief, fear, and acceptance, which might otherwise be difficult to articulate verbally.

In these settings, art therapists prioritize the comfort and individual needs of patients, ensuring the process is soothing, affirming, and tailored to each person's capabilities and preferences.

Implementation and Practical Considerations

Pain is complex, not only a physical sensation but also a psychological, emotional, social, and spiritual experience. As such, its effective management often requires a multidisciplinary approach, drawing on the strengths of various therapeutic modalities and healthcare professionals. Within this integrative framework, art therapy has emerged as a vital complementary intervention, bridging biomedical treatment with holistic care. In this section, we explore how art therapy fits into interdisciplinary pain management teams, the benefits of collaborative care, and the practical considerations for implementing art therapy in clinical settings.

The Multidisciplinary Pain Management Model

A multidisciplinary pain management team typically includes a range of healthcare professionals working in concert to deliver comprehensive, individualized care (Fig. 30.4). These teams may involve physicians (such as pain specialists, neurologists, or oncologists), alongside nurses, physical and occupational therapists, psychologists, psychotherapists, pharmacists, and social workers. Additionally, complementary therapists (like acupuncturists and massage therapists) and creative arts therapists, including art therapists, contribute to the holistic approach. Together, they implement the biopsychosocial model of pain, which recognizes that pain is influenced not only by physical factors but also by emotional and social dimensions [20]. Within this framework, art therapy plays a unique and vital role. It enhances patient communication, particularly when verbal expression is limited, supports emotional processing, encourages behavioral engagement, and fosters resilience and coping skills [102]. In both inpatient and outpatient settings, art therapists offer nonverbal, experiential modalities that complement traditional medical and psychological interventions [55]. Their presence enriches the care team, ensuring that treatment is not only effective but also empathetic and responsive to the full spectrum of the patient's lived experience.

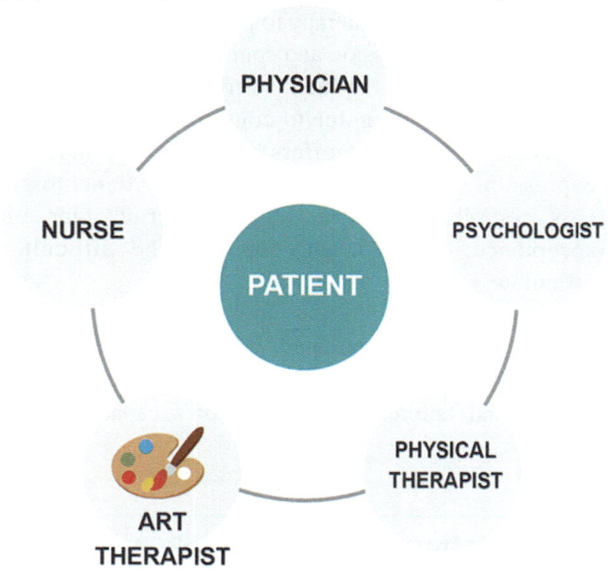

Fig. 30.4 Art therapy in multidisciplinary pain care. A circular team model showing the collaborative integration of the art therapist alongside physicians, psychologists, nurses, and physical therapists in delivering comprehensive care centered around the patient

Complementarity with Other Disciplines

Art therapy integrates seamlessly with various healthcare disciplines, offering unique benefits that enhance patient care across multiple domains.

Medical providers: Art therapy provides clinicians with deeper insights into patients' experiences of illness and treatment [28]. Techniques like body mapping and pain drawings enable patients to visually express subjective symptoms, aiding in more accurate diagnoses and tailored care plans.

Psychological therapies: When combined with approaches such as Cognitive Behavioral Therapy (CBT) and Dialectical Behavior Therapy (DBT), art therapy enhances emotional awareness and expression [25]. It is particularly beneficial for individuals who face challenges with verbal communication due to trauma, age, or cultural factors.

Physical and occupational therapies: Engaging in art-making activities supports both fine and gross motor skills, aligning with movement and coordination goals [103]. Collaborative efforts between art and occupational therapists can develop adaptive strategies, ensuring continued creative engagement despite physical limitations.

Social work and case management: Art therapy facilitates life review, identity exploration, and future planning, complementing the advocacy and support roles of social workers [104]. It can uncover underlying social and emotional needs, leading to more effective referrals and resource allocation.

Incorporating art therapy into multidisciplinary teams enriches the holistic care approach, addressing the physical, emotional, and social aspects of patient health.

Case Integration Example

Patient: Laura, age 65, with chronic lower back pain.

Team: Pain specialist, psychologist, physiotherapist, and art therapist.

Integrated Plan:

- *Physician*: Managed medications and injections.
- *Psychologist*: Addressed mood disorders and catastrophizing thoughts.
- *Physiotherapist*: Facilitated movement and flexibility.
- *Art Therapist*: Worked with Laura to express her fears about dependency, loss of mobility, and identity shifts through visual journaling and sculpture.

Result: Laura became more compliant with her exercise plan after exploring her resistance artistically. Her mood improved, and her perceived pain levels decreased over 8 weeks.

Benefits of Integrative Collaboration

Integrating art therapy into multidisciplinary healthcare teams enhances patient-centered care by offering nonverbal avenues for expression, particularly beneficial for individuals facing communication challenges due to trauma, age, or cultural barriers [55, 100]. Art therapy facilitates emotional processing, fosters empowerment, and supports continuity of care by aligning with therapeutic goals across disciplines. In both inpatient and outpatient settings, art therapists contribute to holistic treatment plans, addressing the physical, emotional, and social dimensions of health.

Challenges and Solutions in Integration

Integrating art therapy into multidisciplinary healthcare teams presents several challenges, including limited awareness among medical professionals, funding constraints, and siloed care models [105]. Medical staff may lack familiarity with art therapy's scope and referral processes, while budget limitations can hinder the inclusion of creative therapies in clinical programs. Additionally, isolated departmental operations can impede collaborative efforts. To address these issues, cross-disciplinary education through in-service and collaborative rounds can enhance understanding of art therapy's benefits. Art therapists contributing to interdisciplinary documentation and research can increase visibility and legitimacy within healthcare settings. Involving art therapists in shared treatment planning ensures alignment with team goals, fostering therapeutic synergy. Recent studies underscore the importance of integrating art therapy into healthcare systems. A narrative review highlights the growing support for art therapy in developed nations, emphasizing its role in improving mental health outcomes through nonverbal, creative expression, particularly for individuals who struggle with conventional therapies [106]. Furthermore, research indicates that art therapy facilitates emotional expression and self-discovery, contributing to overall well-being. By addressing these challenges through education, documentation, and collaborative planning, art therapy can be more effectively integrated into multidisciplinary teams, enhancing patient care and outcomes.

Guidelines for Effective Collaboration

For successful integration of art therapy into multidisciplinary teams, the following guidelines are recommended:

- *Clear role definition*: Establish the specific functions and scope of art therapy within the team.
- *Mutual respect*: Encourage open dialogue and shared decision-making among all disciplines.
- *Regular communication*: Hold consistent interdisciplinary meetings where patient progress and challenges are discussed holistically.
- *Referral pathways*: Create simple and clear procedures for making art therapy referrals.
- *Ethical coordination*: Ensure consent, confidentiality, and cultural competence are maintained across all providers.

Art Therapy in Integrative Pain Clinics

In many countries, integrative pain clinics are beginning to include creative arts therapy departments [107]. These clinics serve as models for how art therapy can be fully embedded into patient care. In such settings, patients may receive art therapy as part of a standard treatment plan alongside medication, counseling, and physical rehabilitation. They may participate in individual or group-based sessions, depending on the patient's needs. Outcomes are tracked collaboratively, with art therapists contributing visual documentation and progress notes. These models exemplify how art therapy not only complements but also enriches pain treatment, resulting in more humanized, comprehensive, and effective care.

Vision for the Future

As the healthcare field increasingly acknowledges the limitations of current approaches to pain management, there is growing momentum to integrate art therapy into multidisciplinary care models [71]. This integration aims to promote clinical research and individualized treatment plans that highlight the efficacy and safety of art therapy, educate medical students and clinicians on the value of expressive therapies, incorporate art therapy into national pain management guidelines, and include it in insurance reimbursement models [108]. Art therapy's role in pain management is expanding, offering non-pharmacological interventions that address the emotional and psychological aspects of chronic pain. By facilitating emotional expression and enhancing coping strategies, art therapy complements traditional medical treatments and contributes to holistic patient care.

Challenges and Ethical Considerations

While the implementation of art therapy in pain management shows tremendous promise, it is not without challenges. From logistical barriers to ethical complexities, art therapists must navigate a range of issues that can impact the effectiveness, accessibility, and safety of their work. This section explores some of the most pressing challenges in clinical practice and the ethical frameworks needed to maintain professional integrity and patient well-being.

Emotional Risk and Re-traumatization

A core strength of art therapy—its capacity to access unconscious emotions—also presents risks, particularly for individuals with unresolved trauma or comorbid psychological conditions. Simple creative tasks may evoke deeply buried feelings related to pain, loss, or abuse, especially in vulnerable populations such as veterans or survivors of violence [109]. To prevent harm, therapists must be trained to identify signs of distress, apply grounding and regulation techniques, and provide referrals when necessary [25, 110]. Sessions should include emotional "cool-down" periods and ensure appropriate follow-up care, especially following intense expressive work.

Scope of Practice and Professional Boundaries

A clear distinction must be upheld between art therapy and recreational art activities [111]. While both use creative materials, only trained art therapists are equipped to guide psychological healing through art [112]. Misunderstanding this boundary can underestimate the emotional depth and potential risks involved. Furthermore, therapists must maintain professional boundaries regarding physical touch, dual relationships, and emotional involvement. Regular supervision and ongoing education are essential to managing complex therapeutic dynamics, preventing over-identification, and mitigating compassion fatigue or burnout.

Informed Consent and Autonomy

Patients must be fully informed about the nature, goals, and potential emotional impact of art therapy prior to treatment. Informed consent—covering session structure, expected outcomes, risks of emotional distress, and policies on artwork storage and sharing—must be documented and periodically revisited as treatment evolves. Equally, respecting patient autonomy is an ethical cornerstone of art therapy, ensuring individuals retain control over their creative process [113]. Patients must be free to choose materials, set personal goals, and determine the pace and direction of therapy. They also maintain authority over what they create, including whether to discuss their art, how it is interpreted, and whether it is displayed or shared. This respect fosters trust and empowerment, critical for individuals whose pain may have eroded their sense of control.

Confidentiality and Privacy of Artwork

In art therapy, the confidentiality and respectful handling of patient-created artwork are paramount. Such artwork often encapsulates deeply personal thoughts, emotions, and experiences, warranting the same level of confidentiality as verbal disclosures. Unauthorized display or photography of these creations without explicit consent constitutes a breach of ethical standards. The American Art Therapy Association (AATA) emphasizes that patient artwork is considered protected information and, in many settings, forms part of the clinical record [114]. Patients have the right to access their artwork during therapy and upon its conclusion, in alignment with therapeutic objectives and benefits. Art therapists are responsible for ensuring that any exhibition of patient artwork is conducted with informed consent, safeguarding against exploitation or misrepresentation. Proper storage of physical artwork involves secure, labeled systems that maintain confidentiality and allow patient access upon request. Clear policies should outline the disposition of artwork post-therapy, ensuring patients are informed about the handling of their creations. The advent of digital platforms introduces additional considerations. Art therapists must navigate data privacy concerns, ensuring compliance with regulations such as the Health Insurance Portability and Accountability Act (HIPAA) in the U.S. and the General Data Protection Regulation (GDPR) in the European Union. This includes secure digital storage, obtaining informed consent for online sharing, and implementing measures to protect patient confidentiality in digital communications. Adhering to these ethical and legal standards is essential in fostering a safe and respectful therapeutic environment, upholding the integrity of the art therapy process, and protecting patient well-being.

Cultural, Religious, and Social Sensitivities

Art therapy necessitates the practice of cultural humility, recognizing and respecting the diverse cultural backgrounds of patients. This involves an awareness of cultural nuances such as color symbolism, where, for instance, white may signify mourning in certain Eastern cultures, and understanding artistic taboos or religious restrictions, like prohibitions against depicting the human form [115]. Additionally, therapists must be attuned to varying communication styles, storytelling traditions, and differences in pain expression and coping mechanisms across cultures. To foster an inclusive therapeutic environment, practitioners should employ open-ended questions, utilize interpreters when necessary, and encourage patients to share culturally significant references or materials. Such practices are emphasized in the literature on multicultural approaches in art therapy, which advocates for the integration of diverse perspectives and the adaptation of materials and techniques to suit individual cultural contexts. Moreover, social determinants significantly influence access to art therapy services. Individuals from marginalized communities often encounter barriers, including economic constraints, transportation challenges, lack of insurance coverage, and experiences of discrimination within healthcare systems [116]. Addressing these issues requires systemic changes, such as advocating for inclusive policies, offering sliding-scale services, and developing outreach programs tailored to underserved populations. Research highlights the impact of social and economic discrimination on healthcare access, underscoring the need for interventions that consider these determinants to ensure equitable care.

Legal and Institutional Compliance

Art therapists operating within hospital or clinical settings are required to adhere to institutional protocols, including infection control measures and patient safety guidelines. They must also engage in comprehensive documentation within electronic health records (EHRs), participate in interdisciplinary team meetings and case conferences, and comply with billing and coding procedures when applicable. Documentation should be concise and medically pertinent and avoid speculative interpretations of artwork. For instance, noting that a "patient used red paint to express anger" is appropriate, whereas stating "patient is angry at mother" without explicit patient disclosure is not. The American Art Therapy Association emphasizes the importance of maintaining accurate and confidential records, ensuring that patient artwork is treated as protected information and stored securely [114]. In situations where patient artwork reveals indications of suicidal ideation, abuse, neglect, or threats to others, art therapists are mandated reporters and must follow legal requirements. This includes disclosing confidential information when mandated by law in civil, criminal, or disciplinary actions arising from art therapy services [114]. Policies regarding such disclosures should be clearly communicated to patients during the informed consent process. Furthermore, therapists must ensure that any use of patient artwork, such as for educational or promotional purposes, is conducted with explicit written consent, maintaining the confidentiality and integrity of the therapeutic relationship [117]. By adhering to these protocols and ethical guidelines, art therapists contribute to a safe and effective therapeutic environment, upholding both institutional standards and the well-being of their patients.

Therapist Self-Care and Burnout Prevention

Art therapists working with chronic pain patients often encounter complex emotional landscapes, which can lead to emotional exhaustion or vicarious trauma. Symptoms such as emotional numbing, increased irritability, withdrawal, decreased job satisfaction, and compassion fatigue are common indicators of burnout in this context. To mitigate these risks, art therapists should prioritize self-care strategies [118]. Engaging in regular supervision or peer consultation provides a platform for processing challenging cases and receiving support. Personal art-making serves as a reflective practice, aiding in emotional processing and maintaining creative engagement. Continuing education and professional development ensure therapists remain informed about best practices and emerging research. Additionally, maintaining bounded work schedules and managing caseloads effectively are crucial for sustaining well-being. Organizational support plays a vital role in therapist resilience. Providing mental health days, implementing wellness programs, and fostering a supportive workplace culture can significantly reduce burnout rates. Research indicates that art therapy-based interventions are effective in addressing burnout and psychosocial distress among healthcare workers, emphasizing the importance of both individual and systemic approaches to therapist self-care [119].

Ethical Use of Technology and Virtual Art Therapy

The expansion of virtual art therapy during the COVID-19 pandemic has enhanced accessibility but also introduced ethical and practical challenges [120, 121]. Key concerns include ensuring patient privacy, adapting therapeutic materials for home use, and addressing digital equity issues, such as patients lacking devices or reliable internet access. Therapists are advised to use secure, HIPAA-compliant video platforms and to provide patients with accessible materials, like digital drawing applications or common household art supplies. Maintaining therapeutic presence online requires deliberate strategies. Therapists should employ clear verbal communication to compensate for the reduced ability to read nonverbal cues and be mindful of potential technical issues that may disrupt sessions. Encouraging patients to establish a private, focused space for therapy can enhance engagement. Regular check-ins regarding the patient's experience with the virtual format are essential to ensure the effectiveness of the therapeutic process. These adaptations are crucial for delivering effective and ethical virtual art therapy, ensuring that patients receive the support they need despite the challenges posed by remote sessions.

The Future of Art Therapy in Pain Management

As the field of pain management evolves, so too must the integration of complementary therapies like art therapy. While significant progress has been made in recognizing its value, the path ahead demands rigorous research, broader implementation, and ongoing innovation. This section examines the key frontiers in art therapy for pain care, what we know, what we need to learn, and how we can expand access and impact.

Expanding the Evidence Base

Despite growing interest in art therapy for chronic pain management, large-scale, controlled studies remain limited. To fully integrate art therapy into conventional medical frameworks, several research priorities must be addressed.

Randomized Controlled Trials (RCTs): There is a need for more RCTs comparing art therapy to standard care or other complementary therapies. Specific populations, such as stomatology surgical patients, should be studied in targeted trials [122]. A recent review highlights the scarcity of such studies, emphasizing the need for rigorous research designs to establish efficacy [7].

Longitudinal studies: Investigating the long-term effects of art therapy on chronic pain can help assess the sustainability of benefits. Pain flare-up management and relapse prevention can be studied over time. Longitudinal research can provide insights into the enduring impact of art therapy interventions [81, 123].

Standardized measures: The use of validated tools for pain intensity (e.g., Visual Analog Scale), pain interference (e.g., Brief Pain Inventory), and quality of life (e.g., SF-36) will allow for more comparable results. The inclusion of neurophysiological biomarkers (e.g., cortisol levels, fMRI) can provide biological correlates of improvement. Standardization is crucial for comparing outcomes across studies [124].

Cost-benefit analyses: Demonstrating that art therapy reduces hospital stays, emergency visits, or medication use may support funding and integration into healthcare systems. Evidence suggests that arts interventions can be cost-effective, reducing healthcare utilization and improving patient outcomes [125].

Addressing these research priorities will enhance the evidence base for art therapy in chronic pain management, facilitating its integration into standard care practices.

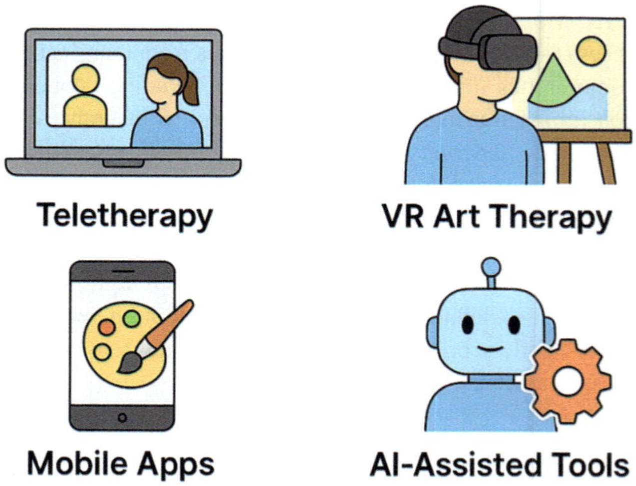

Fig. 30.5 Digital innovations in art therapy. Emerging technologies such as teletherapy platforms, virtual reality (VR) art sessions, mobile applications, and AI-assisted tools are transforming access and delivery of art therapy in pain management, enabling remote, personalized, and engaging therapeutic experiences

Innovations in Practice and Technology

The integration of digital technologies into art therapy has significantly expanded its reach and potential, particularly in pain management (Fig. 30.5).

Digital and virtual art therapy: The COVID-19 pandemic accelerated the adoption of telehealth art therapy, providing essential access to remote and underserved populations. Innovations such as shared digital canvases, virtual reality (VR) painting, and interactive tools have enhanced pain distraction and self-expression. Research indicates that VR applications can effectively reduce pain intensity and improve psychological outcomes in chronic pain management, also in cancer patients [126].

Mobile health applications: Mobile apps guiding individuals through art-based pain management techniques, like coloring for anxiety or pain journaling prompts, serve as valuable adjunctive tools. The incorporation of wearable devices to monitor physiological changes during creative activities, such as heart rate and stress indicators, is an emerging area of interest, even if it still has some ethical problems [127].

Artificial intelligence and image analysis: Artificial intelligence (AI) holds promise in analyzing artwork for emotional content, identifying trends over time, and detecting indicators of distress. Such technologies could provide clinicians with new insights, supporting, but not replacing, the human interpretation central to art therapy. Also in this area, the ethical aspects should be considered [128].

These advancements underscore the evolving landscape of art therapy, highlighting the importance of continued research and ethical considerations in integrating technology into therapeutic practices.

Expanding Access and Inclusion

To establish art therapy as a widely accessible component of pain management, several systemic barriers must be addressed:

Insurance coverage and policy: Advocacy is essential to include art therapy services under national health plans and private insurance. Demonstrating clinical effectiveness and cost savings can influence policy decisions. Currently, in the USA, insurance coverage for art therapy varies, with some private plans offering partial reimbursement, while others do not recognize art therapy services at all [129]. In most of the other countries, the topic is not even considered.

Workforce development: There is a shortage of trained, credentialed art therapists in most of the countries. Investments in training programs, continuing education, and cultural competency are essential. The limited number of accredited graduate programs and supervised clinical training opportunities contributes to this shortage [130].

Community-based programming: Integrating art therapy into schools, community centers, and correctional facilities can address pain in vulnerable populations often excluded from clinical services. Collaborations with nonprofits and public health departments can expand reach. For instance, arts-based programs have been shown to help at-risk and justice-involved youths cope with trauma and develop resilience [131].

Cultural and linguistic adaptation: Art therapy methods should be adapted to be culturally sensitive and linguistically accessible. Research into indigenous and traditional art forms can broaden the therapeutic toolbox. Incorporating culturally significant art practices in therapy can enhance engagement and effectiveness [30].

Addressing these barriers through policy advocacy, educational investment, community engagement, and cultural adaptation is crucial for the integration of art therapy into comprehensive pain care strategies.

Ethical Considerations in Research

As is the hope of everyone, art therapy increasingly integrates into scientific research, but adherence to ethical principles is paramount to ensure the safety and dignity of participants. To obtain it, there are cornerstones not to forget.

Consent and confidentiality: Artworks produced in therapy are deeply personal and must be treated with the same confidentiality as verbal disclosures. Informed consent is essential, especially when artwork is used for research or educational purposes. The American Art Therapy Association emphasizes obtaining written consent before reproducing or exhibiting patient artwork, ensuring patients' rights and privacy are protected [114].

Interpretation sensitivity: Art therapists must approach the analysis of symbolic artwork with care, avoiding reductive or pathologizing interpretations. Recognizing the subjective nature of art, therapists should refrain from making assumptions about a patient's emotional state based solely on their creations. Ethical guidelines advocate for interpretations grounded in patient discussions and context [132].

Trauma-informed practices: Given that many individuals seeking art therapy have trauma histories, it's crucial to prioritize safety, consent, and autonomy throughout the therapeutic process. Therapists should be trained to recognize signs of distress and employ trauma-informed approaches that empower patients and prevent re-traumatization [132].

By upholding these ethical standards, art therapy can continue to be a respectful and effective modality within both clinical and research settings.

Vision for the Future

Art therapy is poised to become a standardized, evidence-based component of comprehensive pain management, integrated across hospitals, rehabilitation centers, palliative care, and community wellness programs. Emerging developments support this trajectory.

Certified clinical guidelines: Initiatives like the Creative Forces Clinical Research Agenda are laying the groundwork for standardized protocols that incorporate art therapy into pain management strategies, particularly for military-connected populations [133].

AI-assisted tools: Innovations such as TherAIssist demonstrate how artificial intelligence can aid therapists in tracking patient themes and progress, enhancing the personalization and effectiveness of art therapy interventions [134].

Global art therapy networks: Scientific and professional organizations like the American Art Therapy Association (AATA) and the International Expressive Arts Therapy Association (IEATA) facilitate the sharing of culturally relevant interventions and outcome data, promoting global collaboration and standardization in the field.

Policy recognition: There is a growing acknowledgment of the role of creative therapies in public health frameworks, with calls for their inclusion in healthcare policies to address chronic pain and mental health challenges [125, 135].

As societies confront increasing rates of chronic pain, mental distress, and reliance on medication, the integration of non-pharmacological interventions like art therapy becomes essential. Recognizing art therapy not as an alternative but as a vital component of holistic pain management can lead to more effective and compassionate care.

Conclusion

Art therapy offers a transformative, evidence-informed approach to the management of pain, addressing critical emotional, existential, and psychosocial dimensions often marginalized within conventional biomedical models. Pain is not merely a physiological event but a complex, dynamic experience shaped by neurobiological, psychological, and environmental interactions. Art therapy, grounded in both scientific knowledge and creative practice, aligns with the biopsychosocial model by fostering nonverbal, symbolic expression, enhancing emotional processing, and empowering patients to take an active role in their care.

Through mechanisms such as distraction, emotional release, modulation of stress responses, neuroplastic adaptation, and activation of brain networks linked to reward and meaning, art therapy can significantly influence pain perception. Clinical trials and neuroimaging studies increasingly document its capacity to reduce pain intensity, elevate mood, and improve functional outcomes and quality of life. Its flexibility and accessibility make it especially valuable across diverse clinical populations, including children, individuals with cognitive or language barriers, and patients in palliative care, where conventional verbal or pharmacologic interventions may be limited.

Ethical practice remains foundational, requiring strict attention to informed consent, confidentiality, and trauma-informed care. As with any therapeutic modality, it is essential to respect patient autonomy and to contextualize imagery within a safe, supportive therapeutic relationship. For art therapy to achieve broader implementation within multidisciplinary pain management, current systemic challenges, including funding constraints, limited insurance coverage, and shortages of trained professionals, must be actively addressed through targeted advocacy, expanded training programs, and the development of clinical guidelines.

In an era of escalating chronic pain prevalence and concerns regarding overmedication, art therapy represents a timely and compassionate complement to established treatments. As digital technologies and artificial intelligence begin to shape new avenues for delivery and assessment, it remains crucial to preserve the central role of human connection in the therapeutic process. With continued research, interdisciplinary collaboration, and a strong commitment to equitable access, art therapy is poised to become an integral component of comprehensive, modern pain care.

Acknowledgments The authors are grateful to *Fondazione Paolo Procacci* for the support during the publishing process.

References

1. Rogger R, Bello C, Romero CS, Urman RD, Luedi MM, Filipovic MG. Cultural framing and the impact on acute pain and pain services. Curr Pain Headache Rep. 2023;27(9):429–36. https://doi.org/10.1007/s11916-023-01125-2.
2. Aaron RV, Ravyts SG, Carnahan ND, Bhattiprolu K, Harte N, McCaulley CC, Vitalicia L, Rogers AB, Wegener ST, Dudeney J. Prevalence of depression and anxiety among adults with chronic pain: A systematic review and meta-analysis. JAMA Netw Open. 2025;8(3):e250268. https://doi.org/10.1001/jamanetworkopen.2025.0268.
3. Camilloni A, Nati G, Maggiolini P, Romanelli A, Carbone G, Giannarelli D, Terrenato I, De Marinis MG, Rossi A, D'Angelo D, Ferrara R, Iacorossi L, Paladini A, Varrassi G, Tarsitani G, Latina R. Chronic non-cancer pain in primary care: an Italian cross-sectional study. Signa Vitae. 2021;7(2):54–62. https://doi.org/10.22514/sv.2020.16.0111.
4. Meints SM, Edwards RR. Evaluating psychosocial contributions to chronic pain outcomes. Prog Neuro-Psychopharmacol Biol Psychiatry. 2018;87(Pt B):168–82. https://doi.org/10.1016/j.pnpbp.2018.01.017.
5. Moncada MAA, Tamayo MAN, Encinas MAN, Leoni MLG, Varrassi G. Immuno-Inflammatory Mechanisms in the Chronification of Pain. Pain Ther. 2026 Mar 7. doi: 10.1007/s40122-026-00818-x.
6. Bae J, Lim YH, Hong SJ, Jeong JH, Choi HR, Park SK, Kim JE, Kim JH. Perceptions of treatment, accompanying symptoms, and other problems in patients with chronic pain: a multicenter cross-sectional study in Korea. Korean J Pain. 2025;38(1):69–78. https://doi.org/10.3344/kjp.24314.
7. Raudenská J, Šteinerová V, Vodičková Š, Raudenský M, Fulková M, Urits I, Viswanath O, Varrassi G, Javůrková A. Arts therapy and its implications in chronic pain management: a narrative review. Pain Ther. 2023;12(6):1309–37. https://doi.org/10.1007/s40122-023-00542-w.
8. Joschko R, Klatte C, Grabowska WA, Roll S, Berghöfer A, Willich SN. Active visual art therapy and health outcomes: A systematic review and meta-analysis. JAMA Netw Open. 2024;7(9):e2428709. https://doi.org/10.1001/jamanetworkopen.2024.28709.
9. Corriero A, Giglio M, Soloperto R, Varrassi G, Puntillo F. Harnessing the healing power of creativity: exploring the role of art in healthcare through art, dance, and music therapy. Adv Health Res. 2024:1. https://doi.org/10.4081/ahr.2024.17.
10. Shojaei F, Shojaei F, Osorio Torres J, Shih PC. Insights from art therapists on using AI-generated art in art therapy: mixed methods study. JMIR Form Res. 2024;8:e63038. https://doi.org/10.2196/63038.
11. Thompson K, Milligan J, Murphy A, Tabasam G, Johnson MI. 'Unmasking pain' through creativity: a phenomenological study of person-centred pain exploration for people living with chronic pain. PLoS One. 2024;19(10):e0312014. https://doi.org/10.1371/journal.pone.0312014.
12. Sajnani N, Fietje N. The Jameel Arts & Health Lab in collaboration with the WHO-lancet global series on the health benefits of the arts. Lancet. 2023;402(10414):1732–4. https://doi.org/10.1016/S0140-6736(23)01959-1.
13. Hadjipanayi C, Banakou D, Michael-Grigoriou D. Art as therapy in virtual reality: a scoping review. Front Virtual Real. 2023;4 https://doi.org/10.3389/frvir.2023.1065863.
14. Millard E, Medlicott E, Cardona J, Priebe S, Carr C. Preferences for group arts therapies: a cross-sectional survey of mental health patients and the general population. BMJ Open. 2021;11(8):e051173. https://doi.org/10.1136/bmjopen-2021-051173.
15. Kovačević I, Pavić J, Filipović B, Ozimec Vulinec Š, Ilić B, Petek D. Integrated approach to chronic pain-the role of psychosocial factors and multidisciplinary treatment: a narrative review. Int J Environ Res Public Health. 2024;21(9):1135. https://doi.org/10.3390/ijerph21091135.
16. Zuqui-Ramírez MA, Belalcazar-López VM, Urenda-Quezada A, González-Rebatu Y, González A, Sander-Padilla JG, Lugo-Sánchez LA, Rodríguez-Vázquez IC, Rios-Brito KF, Arguedas-Núñez MM, Canales-Vázquez E, González-Canudas J. Multimodal analgesia approach in acute low Back pain management: a phase III study of a novel analgesic combination of etoricoxib/tramadol. Pain Ther. 2024;13(6):1511–28. https://doi.org/10.1007/s40122-024-00653-y.
17. Riddle DL, Dumenci L. The measurement of "high-impact chronic pain": limitations and alternative methods. Eur J Pain. 2025;29(1):e4710. https://doi.org/10.1002/ejp.4710.
18. Gasperi M, Afari N, Goldberg J, Suri P, Panizzon MS. Pain and trauma: the role of criterion A trauma and stressful life events in the pain and PTSD relationship. J Pain. 2021;22(11):1506–17. https://doi.org/10.1016/j.jpain.2021.04.015.
19. Aboushaar N, Serrano N. The mutually reinforcing dynamics between pain and stress: mechanisms, impacts and management strategies. Front Pain Res (Lausanne). 2024;5:1445280. https://doi.org/10.3389/fpain.2024.1445280.
20. Engel GL. The need for a new medical model: a challenge for biomedicine. Science. 1977;196(4286):129–36. https://doi.org/10.1126/science.847460.
21. Wang J, Zhang B, Yahaya R, Abdullah AB. Colors of the mind: a meta-analysis of creative arts therapy as an approach for post-traumatic stress disorder intervention. BMC Psychol. 2025;13(1):32. https://doi.org/10.1186/s40359-025-02361-4.
22. De La Rosa JS, Brady BR, Ibrahim MM, Herder KE, Wallace JS, Padilla AR, Vanderah TW. Co-occurrence of chronic pain and anxiety/depression symptoms in U.S. adults: prevalence, functional impacts, and opportunities. Pain. 2024;165(3):666–73. https://doi.org/10.1097/j.pain.0000000000003056.
23. Danilov A, Danilov A, Badaeva A, Kosareva A, Popovskaya K, Novikov V. State-of-the-art personalized therapy approaches for chronic non-specific low back pain: understanding the mechanisms and drivers. Pain Ther. 2025;14(2):479–96. https://doi.org/10.1007/s40122-025-00706-w.
24. Inoue S, Hashizume H, Murata S, Oka H, Kozaki T, Minakata K, Taiji R, Teraguchi M, Iwasaki H, Tsutsui S, Takami M, Mure K, Nakagawa Y, Miyai N, Yamada H. Association between central sensitization and multisite pain in the general population: a cross-sectional analysis of the Wakayama Health Promotion Study. J Orthop Sci. 2025;S0949-2658(25):00039. https://doi.org/10.1016/j.jos.2025.02.001.
25. Czamanski-Cohen J, Weihs KL. The role of emotion processing in art therapy (REPAT) intervention protocol. Front Psychol. 2023;14:1208901. https://doi.org/10.3389/fpsyg.2023.1208901.
26. Wakefield EO, Belamkar V, Sandoval A, Puhl RM, Edelheit B, Zempsky WT, Rodrigues HA, Litt MD. Does diagnostic certainty matter?: pain-related stigma in adolescents with juvenile idiopathic arthritis. J Pediatr Psychol. 2023;48(4):341–51. https://doi.org/10.1093/jpepsy/jsac092.
27. Anselmo A, Pagano M, Corallo F, Cappadona I, Cardile D, Russo F, Laudisio A, Papalia GF, Quartarone A, Calabrò RS. Psychosocial assessment as a key component in an integrated, personalized care pathway: a protocol for a low back pain randomized controlled trial. Pain Ther. 2025;14(3):1155–68. https://doi.org/10.1007/s40122-025-00741-7.

28. Harasymchuk SJ, Howard AF, Noga H, Kelly MT, Yong PJ. The use of arts-based research in chronic pain: A scoping review. Can J Pain. 2024;8(1):2352876. https://doi.org/10.1080/24740527.2024.2352876.
29. Lavin R, Park J. A characterization of pain in racially and ethnically diverse older adults: a review of the literature. J Appl Gerontol. 2014;33(3):258–90. https://doi.org/10.1177/0733464812459372.
30. Arslanbek A, Malhotra B, Kaimal G. Indigenous and traditional arts in art therapy: value, meaning, and clinical implications. Arts Psychother. 2022;77:101879. https://doi.org/10.1016/j.aip.2021.101879.
31. Barnett KS, Vasiu F. How the arts heal: a review of the neural mechanisms behind the therapeutic effects of creative arts on mental and physical health. Front Behav Neurosci. 2024;18:1422361. https://doi.org/10.3389/fnbeh.2024.1422361.
32. https://arttherapy.org/what-is-art-therapy/.
33. Hu J, Zhang J, Hu L, Yu H, Xu J. Art therapy: A complementary treatment for mental disorders. Front Psychol. 2021;12:686005. https://doi.org/10.3389/fpsyg.2021.686005.
34. Bieber I, Herkimer JK. Art in psychotherapy. Am J Psychiatry. 1948;104(10):627–31. https://doi.org/10.1176/ajp.104.10.627.
35. Junge MB. History of art therapy. The Wiley handbook of art therapy. 2015:7–16.
36. Woollett N, Bandeira M, Hatcher A. Trauma-informed art and play therapy: pilot study outcomes for children and mothers in domestic violence shelters in the United States and South Africa. Child Abuse Negl. 2020;107:104564. https://doi.org/10.1016/j.chiabu.2020.104564.
37. Bokoch R, Hass-Cohen N, Espinoza A, O'Reilly T, Levi E. A scoping review of integrated arts therapies and neuroscience research. Front Psychol. 2025;16:1569609. https://doi.org/10.3389/fpsyg.2025.1569609.
38. Chilton G. Art therapy and flow: A review of the literature and applications. Art Ther. 2013;30(2):64–70. https://doi.org/10.1080/07421656.2013.787211.
39. Shukla A, Choudhari SG, Gaidhane AM, Quazi SZ. Role of art therapy in the promotion of mental health: A critical review. Cureus. 2022;14(8):e28026. https://doi.org/10.7759/cureus.28026.
40. Campbell M, Decker KP, Kruk K, Deaver SP. Art therapy and cognitive processing therapy for combat-related PTSD: a randomized controlled trial. Art Ther (Alex). 2016;33(4):169–77. https://doi.org/10.1080/07421656.2016.1226643.
41. Gazit I, Snir S, Regev D, Bat OM. Relationships between the therapeutic alliance and reactions to artistic experience with art materials in an art therapy simulation. Front Psychol. 2021;12:560957. https://doi.org/10.3389/fpsyg.2021.560957.
42. Kirkham JA, Smith JA, Havsteen-Franklin D. Painting pain: an interpretative phenomenological analysis of representations of living with chronic pain. Health Psychol. 2015;34(4):398–406. https://doi.org/10.1037/hea0000139.
43. Johnson MI, Chazot P, Cole F, Cruickshank R, Fuller D, Keyse C, Singh B, Strickson AJ, Tabasam G, Tregidden E, Thompson K, Woodall J. Pain through the perspective of art and creativity: insights from the unmasking pain project. Front Pain Res (Lausanne). 2023;4:1179116. https://doi.org/10.3389/fpain.2023.1179116.
44. Kaimal G, Ray K, Muniz J. Reduction of cortisol levels and participants' responses following art making. Art Ther (Alex). 2016;33(2):74–80. https://doi.org/10.1080/07421656.2016.1166832.
45. Shella TA. Art therapy improves mood, and reduces pain and anxiety when offered at bedside during acute hospital treatment. Arts Psychother. 2018;57:59–64. https://doi.org/10.1016/j.aip.2017.10.003.
46. Crawford C, Lee C, Bingham J, Active Self-Care Therapies for Pain (PACT) Working Group. Sensory art therapies for the self-management of chronic pain symptoms. Pain Med. 2014;15(Suppl 1):S66–75. https://doi.org/10.1111/pme.12409.
47. Weiskittle RE, Gramling SE. The therapeutic effectiveness of using visual art modalities with the bereaved: a systematic review. Psychol Res Behav Manag. 2018;11:9–24. https://doi.org/10.2147/PRBM.S131993.
48. Haeyen S, Van Hooren S, Hutschemaekers G. Perceived effects of art therapy in the treatment of personality disorders, cluster B/C: a qualitative study. Arts Psychother. 2015;45:1. https://doi.org/10.1016/j.aip.2015.04.005.
49. Kaimal G, Ayaz H, Herres J, Dieterich-Hartwell R, Makwana B, Kaiser DH, Nasser JA. Functional near-infrared spectroscopy assessment of reward perception based on visual self-expression: coloring, doodling, and free drawing. Arts Psychother. 2017;55:85–92. https://doi.org/10.1016/j.aip.2017.05.004.
50. Badaeva A, Danilov A, Kosareva A, Lepshina M, Novikov V, Vorobyeva Y, Danilov A. Neuronutritional approach to fibromyalgia management: a narrative review. Pain Ther. 2024;13(5):1047–61. https://doi.org/10.1007/s40122-024-00641-2.
51. He Y, Wang J, Zhao P, Wang R, Li M. Correlations of the central sensitization inventory, conditioned pain modulation, cognitions and psychological factors in individuals with chronic neck pain: a cross-sectional study. Pain Ther. 2024;13(4):843–56. https://doi.org/10.1007/s40122-024-00601-w.
52. Joseph R. The right cerebral hemisphere: emotion, music, visual-spatial skills, body-image, dreams, and awareness. J Clin Psychol. 1988;44(5):630–73. https://doi.org/10.1002/1097-4679(198809)44:5<630::aid-jclp2270440502>3.0.co;2-v.
53. Strang CE. Art therapy and neuroscience: evidence, limits, and myths. Front Psychol. 2024;15:1484481. https://doi.org/10.3389/fpsyg.2024.1484481.
54. Gerdle B, Dragioti E, Rivano Fischer M, Ringqvist Å. Pain intensity and psychological distress show different associations with interference and lack of life control: A clinical registry-based cohort study of >40,000 chronic pain patients from SQRP. Front Pain Res (Lausanne). 2023;4:1093002. https://doi.org/10.3389/fpain.2023.1093002.
55. Martinelli V, Lumer ELL, Fusar Poli L, Chiappedi M, Politi P. Active visual art therapy in the general hospital: facts and challenges from an ethical perspective. Int J Environ Res Public Health. 2025;22(2):316. https://doi.org/10.3390/ijerph22020316.
56. Nimbley E, Caes L, Noel M, Jordan A. Distress and resilience narratives within pain memories of adolescents and young adults with complex regional pain syndrome: A multi-method study. J Pain. 2023;24(7):1275–87. https://doi.org/10.1016/j.jpain.2023.02.025.
57. Laranjeira C, Querido A. An in-depth introduction to arts-based spiritual healthcare: creatively seeking and expressing purpose and meaning. Front Psychol. 2023;14:1132584. https://doi.org/10.3389/fpsyg.2023.1132584.
58. Frankl VE. Search for meaning. Milwaukee: Mount Mary College; 1984.
59. Zhou S, Yu M, Zhou Z, Wang L, Liu W, Dai Q. The effects of art therapy on quality of life and psychosomatic symptoms in adults with cancer: a systematic review and meta-analysis. BMC Complement Med Ther. 2023;23(1):434. https://doi.org/10.1186/s12906-023-04258-4.
60. Emblad SYM, Mukaetova-Ladinska EB. Creative art therapy as a non-pharmacological intervention for dementia: a systematic review. J Alzheimers Dis Rep. 2021;5(1):353–64. https://doi.org/10.3233/ADR-201002.
61. Jenabi E, Bashirian S, Ayubi E, Rafiee M, Bashirian M. The effect of the art therapy interventions on depression symptoms among older adults: a meta-analysis of controlled clinical tri-

als. J Geriatr Psychiatry Neurol. 2023;36(3):185–92. https://doi.org/10.1177/08919887221130264.

62. Liu S, Huang X, Liu Y, Yue J, Li Y, Chen L. A scoping review of the use of creative activities in stroke rehabilitation. Clin Rehabil. 2024;38(4):497–509. https://doi.org/10.1177/02692155241227049.
63. Motlagh EG, Bakhshi M, Davoudi N, Ghasemi A, Moonaghi HK. The physical and psychological outcomes of art therapy in pediatric palliative care: a systematic review. J Res Med Sci. 2023;28:13. https://doi.org/10.4103/jrms.jrms_268_22.
64. Fan YC, Hsiao FH, Hsieh CC. The effectiveness of compassion-based interventions among cancer patients: a systematic review and meta-analysis. Palliat Support Care. 2023;21(3):534–46. https://doi.org/10.1017/S1478951522001316.
65. Monti DA, Peterson C, Kunkel EJ, Hauck WW, Pequignot E, Rhodes L, Brainard GC. A randomized, controlled trial of mindfulness-based art therapy (MBAT) for women with cancer. Psychooncology. 2006;15(5):363–73. https://doi.org/10.1002/pon.988.
66. Bafghi ZR, Ahmadi A, Mirzaee F, Ghazanfarpour M. The effect of mindfulness-based art therapy (MBAT) on the body image of women with polycystic ovary syndrome (PCOS): a randomized controlled trial. BMC Psychiatry. 2024;24(1):611. https://doi.org/10.1186/s12888-024-06057-8.
67. Lin MH, Moh SL, Kuo YC, Wu PY, Lin CL, Tsai MH, Chen TJ, Hwang SJ. Art therapy for terminal cancer patients in a hospice palliative care unit in Taiwan. Palliat Support Care. 2012;10(1):51–7. https://doi.org/10.1017/S1478951511000587.
68. Bar-Sela G, Atid L, Danos S, Gabay N, Epelbaum R. Art therapy improved depression and influenced fatigue levels in cancer patients on chemotherapy. Psychooncology. 2007;16(11):980–4. https://doi.org/10.1002/pon.1175.
69. Thyme Egberg K, Sundin EC, Wiberg B, Oster I, Aström S, Lindh J. Individual brief art therapy can be helpful for women with breast cancer: a randomized controlled clinical study. Palliat Support Care. 2009;7(1):87–95. https://doi.org/10.1017/S147895150900011X.
70. Forzoni S, Perez M, Martignetti A, Crispino S. Art therapy with cancer patients during chemotherapy sessions: an analysis of the patients' perception of helpfulness. Palliat Support Care. 2010;8(1):41–8. https://doi.org/10.1017/S1478951509990691.
71. Stuckey HL, Nobel J. The connection between art, healing, and public health: a review of current literature. Am J Public Health. 2010;100(2):254–63. https://doi.org/10.2105/AJPH.2008.156497.
72. Demir V, Eryürek S, Savaş E. The effect of mindfulness-based art therapy on psychological symptoms and happiness levels in patients with migraine: a pilot study. Curr Psychol. 2024;43(19):17664–72. https://doi.org/10.1007/s12144-024-05634-0.
73. Baptista AS, Jones A, Cardoso FP, Schaffir B, Coelho ER, Orlandi A, Natour J. THU0341 assessment of art therapy program for women with fibromyalgia: randomized, controlled, blinded study. Ann Rheum Dis. 2012;71:271. https://doi.org/10.1136/annrheumdis-2012-eular.2306.
74. Rüütel E, Kruus K, Ivanova A, Laas K. Structured short-term group art therapy in patients with fibromyalgia. a pilot study. Reabilitacijos mokslai: slauga, kineziterapija, ergoterapija. 2018;1(18) https://doi.org/10.33607/rmske.v1i18.753.
75. Giordano F, Messina R, Riefolo A, Rutigliano C, Perillo T, Grassi M, Santoro N, Signorelli F. Music therapy in children affected by brain tumors. World J Pediatr Surg. 2021;4(3):e000307. https://doi.org/10.1136/wjps-2021-000307.
76. Sadeqi H, Rahzani K, Hekmatpou D, Rakei IS. The effect of adult coloring (zhang pattern) on pain and anxiety associated with dressing changes in burn patients: a randomized controlled trial. Scars, Burns & Healing. 2024;10:20595131231218062. https://doi.org/10.1177/20595131231218062.
77. Qian J, Sun S, Wang M, Sun X, Yu X. Art-based interventions for women's mental health in pregnancy and postpartum: a meta-analysis of randomised controlled trials. Front Psych. 2023;14:1112951. https://doi.org/10.3389/fpsyt.2023.1112951.
78. Sun G, McCartin M, Liu W, Zhang Q, Kenefati G, Chen ZS, Wang J. Temporal pain processing in the primary somatosensory cortex and anterior cingulate cortex. Mol Brain. 2023;16(1):3. https://doi.org/10.1186/s13041-022-00991-y.
79. Pénzes I, Engelbert R, Heidendael D, Oti K, Jongen EM, van Hooren S. The influence of art material and instruction during art making on brain activity: a quantitative electroencephalogram study. Arts Psychother. 2023;83:102024. https://doi.org/10.1016/j.aip.2023.102024.
80. Tong H, Maloney TC, Payne MF, King CD, Ting TV, Kashikar-Zuck S, Coghill RC, López-Solà M. Processing of pain by the developing brain: evidence of differences between adolescent and adult females. Pain. 2022;163(9):1777–89. https://doi.org/10.1097/j.pain.0000000000002571.
81. Olaizola S, Lalloo C, Vickers V, Kelenc L, Tariq S, Brown SC, Stinson JN. Art therapy for paediatric pain: a scoping review. Children (Basel). 2024;11(6):619. https://doi.org/10.3390/children11060619.
82. Zhou S, Li H, Yang Y, Qi Y, Liu W, Mo L, Wong CL. Effects of art therapy on psychological outcomes among children and adolescents with cancer: a systematic review and meta-analysis. BMC Complement Med Ther. 2025;25(1):149. https://doi.org/10.1186/s12906-025-04866-2.
83. Huang CY, Su H, Cheng SM, Tan CS. The effects of group art therapy on adolescents' self-concept and peer relationship: a mixed-method study. New Dir Child Adolesc Dev. 2021;2021(179):75–92. https://doi.org/10.1002/cad.20435.
84. Mittal S, Mahapatra M, Ansari SA. Effect of art therapy on adolescents' mental health. Российский психологический журнал. 2022;19(4):71–9. https://doi.org/10.21702/rpj.2022.4.4.
85. Kelemen LJ, Shamri-Zeevi L. Art therapy open studio and teen identity development: helping adolescents recover from mental health conditions. Children (Basel). 2022;9(7):1029. https://doi.org/10.3390/children9071029.
86. Georgiadis E, Johnson MI. Incorporating personal narratives in positive psychology interventions to manage chronic pain. Front Pain Res (Lausanne). 2023;4:1253310. https://doi.org/10.3389/fpain.2023.1253310.
87. https://cjni.net/journal/?p=14007.
88. Zhang MQ, Liu X, Huang Y. Does mandala art improve psychological Well-being in patients? A systematic review. J Integr Complement Med. 2024;30(1):25–36. https://doi.org/10.1089/jicm.2022.0780.
89. Casini I, Ladisa V, Clemente L, Delussi M, Rostanzo E, Peparini S, Aloisi AM, de Tommaso M. A personalized Mediterranean diet improves pain and quality of life in patients with fibromyalgia. Pain Ther. 2024;13(3):609–20. https://doi.org/10.1007/s40122-024-00598-2.
90. McCord A, McKenny S, Horstmanshof L. Effects of Zentangle on older adults' anxiety, happiness, and dexterity. Act Adapt Aging. 2025;49(1):88–115. https://doi.org/10.1080/01924788.2024.2317026.
91. Galassi F, Merizzi A, D'Amen B, Santini S. Creativity and art therapies to promote healthy aging: a scoping review. Front Psychol. 2022;13:906191. https://doi.org/10.3389/fpsyg.2022.906191.
92. Aydın M, Kutlu FY. The effect of group art therapy on loneliness and hopelessness levels of older adults living alone: a randomized controlled study. Florence Nightingale J Nurs. 2021;29(3):271–84. https://doi.org/10.5152/FNJN.2021.20224.
93. Hansen M, Vaegter HB, Ravn SL, Andersen TE. Validation of the Danish PTSD checklist for DSM-5 in trauma-exposed chronic pain patients using the clinician-administered PTSD scale for

DSM-5. Eur J Psychotraumatol. 2023;14(1):2179801. https://doi.org/10.1080/20008066.
94. Schouten KA, de Niet GJ, Knipscheer JW, Kleber RJ, Hutschemaekers GJ. The effectiveness of art therapy in the treatment of traumatized adults: a systematic review on art therapy and trauma. Trauma Violence Abuse. 2015;16(2):220–8. https://doi.org/10.1177/1524838014555032.
95. Perugino F, De Angelis V, Pompili M, Martelletti P. Stigma and chronic pain. Pain Ther. 2022;11(4):1085–94. https://doi.org/10.1007/s40122-022-00418-5.
96. Coleman MB, Cramer ES, Park Y, Bell SM. Art educators' use of adaptations, assistive technology, and special education supports for students with physical, visual, severe and multiple disabilities. J Dev Phys Disabil. 2015;27:637–60. https://doi.org/10.1007/s10882-015-9440-6.
97. El-Tallawy SN, Pergolizzi JV, Vasiliu-Feltes I, Ahmed RS, LeQuang JK, Alzahrani T, Varrassi G, Awaleh FI, Alsubaie AT, Nagiub MS. Innovative applications of telemedicine and other digital health solutions in pain management: A literature review. Pain Ther. 2024;13(4):791–812. https://doi.org/10.1007/s40122-024-00620-7.
98. Deng C, Zheng R, Hong J, Guo Q. Legacy-making interventions in pediatric palliative care: a mixed methods systematic review. Asia Pac J Oncol Nurs. 2025;28:100694. https://doi.org/10.1016/j.apjon.2025.100694.
99. Webb AJ. The therapeutic power of art: exploring the mechanisms behind art therapy's efficacy. Authorea Preprints. 2023; https://doi.org/10.22541/au.169531401.17663927/v1.
100. Nelson K, Lukawiecki J, Waitschies K, Jackson E, Zivot C. Exploring the impacts of an art and narrative therapy program on participants' grief and bereavement experiences. Omega (Westport). 2024;90(2):726–45. https://doi.org/10.1177/00302228221111726.
101. Zhuo X, Yan Y, Lin R, Lin S, Zheng X, Shao T, Zhang H, Chen L, Li H. Effects of an art-based intervention in older adults with dementia: a randomized controlled trial. Sci Rep. 2025;15(1):10406. https://doi.org/10.1038/s41598-025-95051-5. Erratum in: Sci Rep 2025 May 1;15(1):15303. https://doi.org/10.1038/s41598-025-99769-0.
102. Angheluta AM, Lee BK. Art therapy for chronic pain: applications and future directions. Can J Couns Psychother. 2011;45(2) Available from: https://cjc-rcc.ucalgary.ca/article/view/59289.
103. Chan MWM, Lo SHS, Sit JWH, Choi KC, Tao A. Effects of visual arts-based interventions on physical and psychosocial outcomes of people with stroke: A systematic review and meta-analysis. Int J Nurs Stud Adv. 2023;5:100126. https://doi.org/10.1016/j.ijnsa.2023.100126.
104. Ravid-Horesh RH. "A temporary guest": the use of art therapy in life review with an elderly woman. Arts Psychother. 2004;31(5):303–19. https://doi.org/10.1016/j.aip.2004.07.001.
105. MacRitchie J, Short AE, Dion S, Chow JS. Foundations for change management in integrating the arts into healthcare: an empirical study. Approaches: an interdisciplinary. J Music Ther. 2024;16(2):354. https://doi.org/10.56883/aijmt.2024.62.
106. Hiang KS, Fong C, Tripathi S. Art therapy in mental health treatment: a narrative review of efficacy and application in developed countries. Psychology. 2025;16(2):202–13. https://doi.org/10.4236/psych.2025.162012.
107. Youngwerth J, Coats H, Jones A, Wibben A, Somes E, Felton S, Anderson A, Flarity K, Elliot K, Kutner J. Therapeutic effects: the integration of creative arts therapy in palliative care. OBM Integr Complement Med. 2020;5(1):1–9. https://doi.org/10.21926/obm.icm.2001004.
108. Guo L, Reddy KP, Van Iseghem T, Pierce WN. Enhancing data practices for whole health: strategies for a transformative future. Learn Health Syst. 2024;8(Suppl 1):e10426. https://doi.org/10.1002/lrh2.10426.
109. Heijman J, Wouters H, Schouten KA, Haeyen S. Effectiveness of trauma-focused art therapy (TFAT) for psychological trauma: study protocol of a multiple-baseline single-case experimental design. BMJ Open. 2024;14(1):e081917. https://doi.org/10.1136/bmjopen-2023-081917.
110. Bosgraaf L, Spreen M, Pattiselanno K, van Hooren S. Affect regulating art therapy for children and adolescents experiencing psychosocial problems. Int J Art Therapy. 2024;29(2):88–96. https://doi.org/10.1080/17454832.2023.2208198.
111. Pamelia E. Therapeutic art-making and art therapy: Similarities and differences and a resulting framework. Available at: https://scholarworks.indianapolis.iu.edu/server/api/core/bitstreams/2a6cfeaf-d61a-4c18-bbd5-ae4bd80f5e37/content
112. Rubin JA. The art of art therapy: what every art therapist needs to know. Routledge; 2011. Available at: https://www.taylorfrancis.com/books/mono/10.4324/9780203893845/art-art-therapy-judith-rubin
113. Green AR. Ethical considerations in art therapy. Can Art Therapy Assoc J. 2012;25(2):16–21. https://doi.org/10.1080/08322473.2012.11415567.
114. American Art Therapy Association: Ethical principles for art therapists. Available at: https://arttherapy.org/wp-content/uploads/2017/06/Ethical-Principles-for-Art-Therapists.pdf?utm_source=chatgpt.com
115. Bodlovic A, Jackson L. A cultural humility approach to art therapy multicultural pedagogy: barriers to compassion. Int J Divers Educ. 2018;19(1):1. https://doi.org/10.18848/2327-0020/CGP/v19i01/1-9.
116. Garcia J, Crosby RA. Social determinants of discrimination and access to health care among transgender women in Oregon. Transgend Health. 2020;5(4):225–33. https://doi.org/10.1089/trgh.2019.0090.
117. Art Therapy Credential Board: Code governing Standards of Practice, Eligibility for and Regulation of Credentials, and Disciplinary Procedures. Available at: https://atcb.org/ethics-appeals-lp/code-of-ethics-conduct-and-disciplinary-procedures/
118. Chung EV. Self Care for therapists: pillars to protect your mental health. Available at: https://www.blueprint.ai/blog/self-care-for-therapists-pillars-to-protect-your-mental-health?utm_source=chatgpt.com
119. Tjasink M, Keiller E, Stephens M, Carr CE, Priebe S. Art therapy-based interventions to address burnout and psychosocial distress in healthcare workers-a systematic review. BMC Health Serv Res. 2023;23(1):1059. https://doi.org/10.1186/s12913-023-09958-8.
120. Zubala A, Kennell N, Hackett S. Art therapy in the digital world: an integrative review of current practice and future directions. Front Psychol. 2021;12:595536. https://doi.org/10.3389/fpsyg.2021.600070.
121. Walters JA. Online art therapy: experiences of art therapists during the COVID-19 pandemic. In: Virtual art therapy. Routledge; 2022. p. 26–35. Available at: https://www.taylorfrancis.com/chapters/edit/10.4324/9781003149538-4/online-art-therapy-jessica-walters.
122. Giordano F, Giglio M, Sorrentino I, Dell'Olio F, Lorusso P, Massaro M, Tempesta A, Limongelli L, Selicato L, Favia G, Varrassi G, Puntillo F. Effect of preoperative music therapy versus intravenous midazolam on anxiety, sedation and stress in stomatology surgery: A randomized controlled study. J Clin Med. 2023;12(9):3215. https://doi.org/10.3390/jcm12093215.
123. Fenner P, Crane T, Byrne L, Scottney F, Boatman T, Schofield MJ. The impact of group art therapy in post-acute cancer care: A longitudinal qualitative study. Arts Psychother. 2024;87:102122. https://doi.org/10.1016/j.aip.2024.102122.

124. Williamson PR, Altman DG, Blazeby JM, Clarke M, Devane D, Gargon E, Tugwell P. Developing core outcome sets for clinical trials: issues to consider. Trials. 2012;13:132. https://doi.org/10.1186/1745-6215-13-132.
125. Crealey G, McQuade L, O'Sullivan R, O'Neill C. Arts and creativity interventions for improving health and wellbeing in older adults: a systematic literature review of economic evaluation studies. BMC Public Health. 2023;23(1):2496. https://doi.org/10.1186/s12889-023-17369-x.
126. Shafiei SB, Shadpour S, Pangburn B, Bentley-McLachlan M, de Leon-Casasola O. Pain classification using functional near infrared spectroscopy and assessment of virtual reality effects in cancer pain management. Sci Rep. 2025;15(1):8954. https://doi.org/10.1038/s41598-025-93678-y.
127. Pergolizzi JV Jr, LeQuang JAK, El-Tallawy SN, Varrassi G. What clinicians should tell patients about wearable devices and data privacy: a narrative review. Cureus. 2025;17(3):e81167. https://doi.org/10.7759/cureus.81167.
128. Cascella M, Shariff MN, Viswanath O, Leoni MLG, Varrassi G. Ethical considerations in the use of artificial intelligence in pain medicine. Curr Pain Headache Rep. 2025;29(1):10. https://doi.org/10.1007/s11916-024-01330-7.
129. Ou, Jiayu, "Art Therapy Business Plan" 2024. MA Projects 198. Available at: https://digitalcommons.sia.edu/stu_proj/198
130. Torpey E. Art therapist, Career Outlook, U.S. Bureau of Labor Statistics, April 2015. Available at: https://www.bls.gov/careeroutlook/2015/youre-a-what/art-therapist.htm?utm_source=chatgpt.com
131. Arts-based programs and arts therapies for at-risk, justice-involved, and traumatized youths. Available at: https://ojjdp.ojp.gov/model-programs-guide/literature-reviews/arts-based-programs-and-arts-therapies-risk-justice-involved-and-traumatized?utm_source=chatgpt.com
132. Rudolph K. Ethical considerations in trauma-informed care. Psychiatr Clin North Am. 2021;44(4):521–35. https://doi.org/10.1016/j.psc.2021.07.001.
133. Clinical Research Priorities for Creative Arts Therapies Addressing Service Members and Veterans with TBI and Associated Psychological Health Conditions. Available at: https://www.creativeforcesnrc.arts.gov/wp-content/uploads/2024/10/State-of-the-Science-Report-July-2024.pdf?utm_source=chatgpt.com.
134. Liu D, Bai J, Zhang Z, Zhang Y, Zhang Z, Zhao J, An P. TherAIssist: assisting art therapy homework and client-practitioner collaboration through human-AI interaction. arXiv preprint arXiv:2502.12443. 2025. https://doi.org/10.48550/arXiv.2502.12443.
135. Keaten J. Stressed? Sick? Swsiss town lets doctors prescribe free museum visits as art therapy for patients. Available at: https://apnews.com/article/museum-art-therapy-neuchatel-switzerland-55bcf5c4830261e35a3b8704671418f8.

Music Therapy

31

Rachel T. Lazim

Keywords and Definitions

- *Music therapy*: The clinical and evidence-based use of music interventions to accomplish individualized goals within a therapeutic relationship by a credentialed professional who has completed an accredited music therapy program.
- *Music medicine* (also called passive or receptive music therapy): Music offered by medical personnel for symptom management. Depending on the study, music was either curated for a desired tempo or theme or chosen by the patient.

Introduction

Since ancient times, music has played an important role in human societies across the world. In preliterate societies, the medicine man or shaman incorporated music and dance into healing rituals; for example, Native American healing songs utilized differing rhythms and lengths depending on the illness being treated [1]. Music was used to appeal to the gods, causing illness in ancient Babylon (1850 BC), and was considered "physic for the soul in Egypt" (1500 BC) [1]. Similarly, the Hebrew Old Testament describes how the shepherd boy (and eventual King) David played the harp to calm the "evil spirit" tormenting then-King Saul (1100 BC) [1]. When the Greeks conquered Egypt, scholars borrowed many of the Egyptian ideas about medicine and developed them further. Pythagoras explored the relationship between music and the universe, postulating that the physics of music paralleled that of the natural world and could be used for healing [1]. Aristotle recognized the connection between music and emotional states, and Asclepiades (124 BC) used ideas from both Pythagoras and Aristotle to advocate for the treatment of mental illness using modal scales [1]. The Algerian physician Caelius Aurelianus (fifth century AD) had a more nuanced view of music, on the one hand recommending it to treat nerve pain but cautioning against "indiscriminate" use that could "cause madness" [1]. In Islamic culture, mystics in what are now Iran, Azerbaijan, and Turkey developed "spiritual music" for "soul care," a practice continued in the modern-day Sufi sect [2]. Traditional Chinese medicine views music as the "best reflection" of Shen (spirit) and thus integral for healing [3]. In fact, the Chinese character for "herbal medicine" is built on the character for "music" [3]. The scientific basis for music as therapy is much more recent, having developed over the past 100 years in conjunction with the modernization of medicine and psychology [1]. Many scientific research papers informing the adjunctive use of music for analgesia have been published in the past 20 years. Given the short- and long-term potential adverse effects associated with analgesic medications, music is an attractive adjunctive therapy with negligible risk of harm.

The current definition of music therapy was postulated in 2007 and makes the distinction between music therapy (MT), which is the use of music interventions by a licensed music therapist as part of a therapeutic relationship with a patient, and music medicine (MM) , where patients are given prerecorded music to listen to as an intervention in a healthcare setting [2]. Studying music as a therapeutic intervention for pain is challenging in part because assessment of pain is subjective and because finding a suitable placebo for music in randomized controlled trials is difficult. The scope of potential musical interventions is broad; in some studies, patients select music or are given the choice of preselected options; in others, the authors choose music. Modern music therapists use many of the same whole-body techniques used by ancient healers, involving patients not only in passive listening but also in creating music using rhythmic instruments, singing, or vocalizing, often incorporating therapeutic movement.

R. T. Lazim (✉)
South College School of Pharmacy, Knoxville, TN, USA
e-mail: rlazim@south.edu

J. P. Reinert et al. (eds.), *Adjunctive Analgesic Strategies for the Bedside Clinician and Beyond*,
https://doi.org/10.1007/978-3-032-21675-5_31

Music's Influence on Pain and the Brain

Multiple areas of the brain are involved in sensing and processing pain, including the primary and secondary somatosensory cortices, insular cortex, anterior cingulate cortex, prefrontal cortex, thalamus, and amygdala [5]. Depending on the type of pain (acute, chronic, inflammatory, or neuropathic), different neurochemical pathways are involved (endorphins, oxytocin, dopamine, and serotonin) and could be potential therapeutic targets [6]. The "mechanism-of-action" for music in analgesia is similarly multifaceted and involves nociceptive modulation, emotion, cognition, neurotransmitters, and external factors (context) [7].

Music influences pain perception via the descending pain-modulating system (DPMS) [8], activating brain areas associated with reward and emotional arousal [8, 9] and suppressing the sympathetic nervous response [10]. The impact of context on music-associated analgesia has not been the focus of much study, except for the observation that familiarity with, or patient self-selection of, music being played has a greater positive impact on suppressing pain response [8]. On a cognitive level, music is effective at distracting patients from the painful stimulus, offering a soothing alternative focus [10] and providing an "aesthetic experience" that can provide comfort and peace [4]. Music also induces physiologic changes in humans, including reducing blood pressure, heart rate, and muscle tension [4, 11].

Neuroimaging studies of subjects exposed to pleasurable music have demonstrated that the brain releases dopamine (reward system) and endogenous opiates (antinociception and pleasure) in response to music [9] which has been validated in trials of healthy human subjects [10].

Evidence for use Music-based interventions have been studied in many different clinical settings for procedural, acute, and chronic pain across the globe. The predominant music intervention is music medicine (patients listening to music), but in recent years, more studies have been designed with music therapist-led interventions. Differentiating between the interventions requires observation of the study methods; some studies referring to "music therapy" are passive or receptive in nature and do not involve music therapists; thus, they are actually "music medicine." Use of validated pain scales (Visual analog scale (VAS), numerical rating scale (NRS)) before and after musical intervention is standard to assess the analgesic effect of music. An SMD of 0.2 typically represents a small effect, 0.5 a moderate effect, and 0.8 a large effect [8]. Finally, some studies measure mg of analgesic used with or without musical intervention to collect more objective data.

Acute and Procedural Pain

Nilsson and colleagues (2005) conducted a randomized, controlled trial looking at the effects of MM on stress reduction and pain in adult Swedish patients undergoing outpatient hernia repair. Over a 4-month period, 75 patients who were scheduled for morning surgery with the same surgeon and the same anesthesia regimen were enrolled. The patients were randomized by computer into one of three treatment groups: intraoperative music only, postoperative music only, or no music, with 25 patients in each group. The principal investigator did all music interventions and outcome assessments. All patients wore noise-canceling headphones during surgery and smaller headphones during their time in the postanesthesia care unit (PACU), and all had either a fake CD player or a real one with them, so the nurses and staff caring for the patients were blinded to their treatment. All patients receiving the music intervention listened to the same music, a new age synthesizer. Pain was assessed 30 minutes prior to surgery and 1 hour after PACU admission using the numerical rating scale (NRS), and the mg of morphine required in PACU for pain control was recorded for each patient. Patient-reported pain at 1 hour post-op as well as mg of morphine used in PACU were statistically significantly different ($p < 0.05$ and $p < 0.01$, respectively) from the control for patients in the postoperative music group [12]. The intraoperative group also had a statistically significant decrease in pain scores compared to control patients ($p < 0.05$), but the mg of morphine administered on demand was the same as that of control patients [12].

A 2013 meta-analysis by the Cochrane Heart Group sought to explore the efficacy of music in reducing stress and anxiety in adult patients with coronary artery disease with a randomized or quasi-randomized trial design. The effect of music on pain was studied as a subgroup. 8 studies from 1999 to 2012 met criteria for inclusion and described the effect of music on pain in patients with CHD. The trials were divided into those with one music intervention ($n = 5$) and those with two or more music intervention sessions ($n = 3$). The effect of music on patient-reported pain, though lower than the control, was not statistically significant in the one intervention group (SMD −0.55 (−0.8–0.07)) with significant heterogeneity between studies [4]. The effect of music on patient-reported pain in the trials with two or more music interventions was small but statistically significant (SMD −0.27 (−0.55–0.00)) [4]. The type of musical intervention (MM vs MT) was not described.

Mondanaro and colleagues (2017) conducted a randomized study looking at the impact of a music therapy session on pain in adult patients in the US recovering from spinal fusion surgery. Intervention patients had one 30-minute session with a music therapist in the 72 hours after surgery. The music therapy sessions were conducted by two licensed music therapists and included warm-up, patient-selected live music, improvisation, singing, and/or drumming, and breathwork or visualization. Pain scales for both groups were recorded using the VAS before and after the 72-hour study period. Patients who were randomized to the control group were given the opportunity to have a music therapy session after the study period. Mean VAS pain scores in the control group increased from baseline after the study period from 5.2 to 5.87, while the MT group had a decrease in mean VAS from 6.2 pre-intervention to 5.09 ($p = 0.01$) [13].

A 2018 French study by Jacq and colleagues studied the influence of MM on pain experienced by adult mechanically ventilated patients during bathing. Sixty consecutive mechanically ventilated patients with Richmond Agitation-Sedation Scores (RASS) between −3 (moderately sedated) and +4 (combative) were included in the study. The first 30 patients were the control group, and the second 30 patients were the experimental group. The experimental group listened to Mozart through headphones, starting with the beginning of the bath and continuing for 30 minutes after. Nurses not involved in the care of the patient assessed pain using the behavioral pain scale (BPS) before the bath, multiple times during the bath, at the end of the bath, and then 30, 60, and 120 minutes after the end of the bath. All patients had a mean BPS of three at baseline. The proportion of time patients spent with BPS over 5 ($p < 0.001$) and at their maximal pain level ($p = 0.005$) was lower for intervention patients compared to control [14]. Both groups returned to their baseline pain level within 2 hours after bathing.

Bashiri and colleagues conducted a randomized, controlled trial of MM in Turkish patients undergoing endoscopy/colonoscopy published in 2018. The study involved four treatment groups, which were chosen at random by drawing lots. Patients were asked to select their favorite type of music prior to the procedure, then all patients were given headphones to wear; those in the music groups heard their favorite type of music. The treatment differed by group as follows: Group 1 ($n = 25$, light sedation with 2 mg midazolam only), Group 2 ($n = 33$, light sedation with 2 mg midazolam and MM), Group 3 ($n = 55$, deep sedation by an anesthesiologist), and Group 4 ($n = 41$, deep sedation with MM). Pain scores assessed by NRS were obtained before and after the procedure for all patients. For the deep sedation groups (3 and 4), the mg of sedation/anesthesia drugs used were compared between Group 3 (no music) and Group 4 (MM). In the light sedation groups (1 and 2), Group 1 had a statistically significant increase in pain at the end of the procedure compared to the beginning ($p < 0.05$) [15]. In the deep sedation groups, patients in Group 3 had a statistically significant increase in pain from beginning to end of procedure ($p < 0.05$) and used more mg per case of propofol, midazolam, and ketamine than did Group 4 (MM plus deep sedation group), with $p = 0.0001$ for each drug [15].

A meta-analysis of the effects of music on pain in postoperative patients was published by Kuhlmann et al. in 2018. The authors included 46 full-text RCTs with adult subjects studying the effects of music interventions on surgery requiring anesthesia, where pain scales were reported (most used VAS). Subgroup analysis evaluated the effect of music selection (patient selected from list vs music chosen by investigator vs patient provided), timing of the music intervention (preoperative vs perioperative vs postoperative), number of musical interventions, and type of anesthesia provided. Overall, in the 46 trials focused on musical intervention for pain reduction, there was a statistically significant decrease in post-intervention pain scores compared to pre-intervention SMD –0.50 (−0.66, −0.34) $p < 0.001$. With respect to music selection, music chosen by the patient from the provided list (SMD –0.55 (−0.81, −0.28)) and chosen by the investigator (SMD –0.47 (−0.67, −0.6)) both showed statistically significant reduction in pain ($p < 0.001$), but music provided by patients did not (SMD –0.26 (−0.56, 0.04) $p = 0.09$) [19]. Preoperative and perioperative music intervention did not statistically reduce pain, but postoperative music reduced pain SMD –0.53 (−0.79, −0.28) $p < 0.001$ [19]. Both single music interventions and multiple music interventions reduced pain scores SMD –0.47 (−0.65, −0.29) and –0.62 (−0.93, −0.30), both $p < 0.001$ [16]. Finally, music interventions had significant impact on pain scores for both general anesthesia SMD –0.55 (−0.72, −0.39) $p < 0.001$ and to a lesser extent for regional anesthesia SMD –0.41 (−0.80,−0.03) $p = 0.04$ [16]. The type of musical intervention was not described by the authors.

Mandel et al. published a 2019 study describing patient perception of pain before and after MT sessions offered in a US ED setting. Over a period of 3 years, nurses could refer patients in the ED for music therapist services during their ED stay. Patients 18 years or older who were in the ED for pain-related services and could speak or read English or Spanish were eligible for inclusion ($n = 1102$). The therapist worked with the patient in their private ED room using live instruments (guitar, keyboard, and percussion) or recorded music on a digital tablet, depending on patient preference. Before and after the therapy session, the therapist asked patients to assess their level of pain using a verbal analog scale. The MT offered services in a procedural setting for 155 of the patients and in non-procedural situations for 947. Overall, patients who received MT services during their ED visit reported a small but statistically significant decrease in pain (3.99 presession to 3.22 post-session, $p < 0.001$) [17]. The impact of MT on analgesia was more pronounced when the session was used for "procedural support" or to decrease the pain associated with a specific procedure (venipuncture, suturing, or setting a bone). When compared to MT sessions for non-procedural pain (decrease of 0.68 in VAS between pre- and post-session), patients reported a decrease of 2.46 in VAS for procedural pain ($p < 0.001$) [17].

Lin and colleagues conducted a 2019 meta-analysis looking specifically at the effects of music therapy on pain after orthopedic surgery in adult patients. The authors included RCTs of adult patients where MT or MM was used as an intervention, pain scores were reported, and patients did not have mental illness. Nine studies met the inclusion criteria. The primary study outcome was the effect of the intervention on pain; subgroup analyses included the effect of MT on pain, the effect of MM on pain, the difference in mg of analgesic required with or without music, and the effect of patient selection of music on pain. Both MM ($n = 5$) and MT studies ($n = 3$) showed small but statistically significant impact on pain; SMD –0.41 (−0.75, −0.07) for MM and –0.31 (−0.57, −0.04) for MT. [18] Looking at the studies with MM ($n = 3$) and MT ($n = 2$) where patients chose their own music, the effect on pain was slightly greater for both: MM $p = 0.002$ and MT $p = 0$ 02 [18]. Dai and colleagues (2020) conducted a retrospective analysis looking that the effect of MM on pain in adult postoperative coronary artery bypass graft (CABG) patients in China. Patients ($n = 30$ per group) were randomized to either receive music of their choice for 30 minutes, quiet rest for 30 minutes, or normal care for 30 minutes at 8 pm after transfer to the general medical floor. Pain was measured using the NRS before and after the intervention, and all patients were given headphones to wear. Mean post-intervention pain scores for patients in the MM group were lower (4.2) compared with the rest group (7.2) and normal care group (7.4), $p < 0.13$, despite all groups having a pre-intervention NRS score of 7 [19]. In their 2020 meta-analysis, Santivanez-Acosta et al. sought to describe the role of music therapy interventions during labor. Their analysis included 12 randomized controlled trials published between 2003 and 2018, where the primary outcome of pain was measured with VAS. The authors do not describe whether the music interventions were MT or MM in nature. Although the studies evaluated demonstrated the efficacy of music interventions on reducing pain in the various stages of labor, the quality of evidence was low for all but active labor. The three trials of music for pain in active labor were rated moderate quality. No adverse or unfavorable outcomes related to the music intervention were reported [20].

Dong et al. (2023) conducted a randomized controlled trial looking at MM for pain in 86 adult Chinese patients following cardiac valve replacement. All patients had a 30-minute rest period on three separate occasions during their hospitalization: 2 hours post-extubation, after transfer to the general medical floor, and one day prior to discharge, and were provided headphones to wear during the rest period. The MM intervention group ($n = 43$) had 15 minutes of pre-selected music at the end of each rest session, and the control group did not. Vital signs and pain assessment using the VAS were recorded before and after each of the rest/music sessions. Both groups had improvement in pain scores when comparing pre- and post-rest sessions; and the reduction in pain scores between the control and MM groups was statistically significant at each endpoint ($p < 0.03$, $p < 0.001$, and $p < 0.001$, respectively) [21].

Chronic Pain and Cancer Pain

Bradt et al. conducted an RCT comparing MM to MT interventions for the treatment of pain in adult cancer patients in the US, published in 2014. Patients were eligible if currently receiving treatment for cancer, were over 18 years of age, proficient in English, had no cognitive or hearing impairment, and had no psychotic disorder. Thirty-one patients received two MM sessions and two MT sessions in a 2-week timeframe. The order of the interventions (MM then MT or vice versa) was randomized, and patients self-reported pain using NRS. Both MM (pre 3.8, post 2.7, $p = 0.0001$) and MT (pre: 3.6, post 2.7, $p < 0.0004$) sessions were effective at reducing patient-reported pain, and there was no statistical difference between treatment groups [10]. Patients participated in interviews about their experiences at the end of the study period and expressed a preference for music therapy over music medicine interventions [10].

Garza-Villareal and colleagues performed a meta-analysis in 2017 reviewing the effects of music-induced analgesia on chronic pain conditions. RCTs reporting any type of music intervention for adults with chronic pain through 2016 were reviewed for inclusion in the study. Chronic pain was defined as pain persisting or recurring for at least 12 weeks. The primary outcome was reduction in self-reported pain using a validated pain scale (VAS, NRS, McGill Pain Questionnaire, or West Haven-Yale Multidisciplinary Pain Inventory). Subgroup analyses included the selection of music (familiar vs unfamiliar and researcher vs patient selected). Music interventions showed a statistically significant decrease in patient-reported chronic pain SMD –0.5 (−0.72, −0.48) [8]. There was no difference between familiar or unfamiliar music, but patient-selected music had a greater analgesic effect (5 trials, SMD –81 (−1.02, −0.59)) [8] compared to researcher-selected (9 RCTs, SMD –0.51 (−0.65, −0.36)) [8]. The authors reported high heterogeneity but low risk of bias for the analysis.

Low et al. sought to determine the effect of a 12-week vocal MT program for chronic pain patients in a study published in the US in 2020. Participants in the vocal MT intervention group ($n = 22$) were compared to controls ($n = 21$). Participants had to be English-speaking adults 18 or older with at least a 3-month history of chronic pain and a pain impact score of 27 or higher (moderate impact). Patients with hearing deficiency, progressive medical or neurological disorder, psychiatric or cognitive disorder, concurrent drug or alcohol addiction, or currently receiving other MT services were excluded. During the study period, MT intervention patients participated in weekly 90-minute group vocal MT sessions at the study center. The control patients participated in standard therapy available at the same center (medication, physical therapy, yoga, and fitness classes). Pain outcomes were assessed using Patient-Reported Outcomes Measurement Information System (PROMIS) short forms for pain interference (SF-6b), pain intensity (SF-3a), and pain-related self-efficacy (SF-6). Only 33 patients in the intervention group successfully completed all 12 sessions, resulting in a 23% attrition rate [9]. The patients who completed the study reported a large effect on pain-related self-efficacy 5.10 (1.52, 8.68) and smaller, non-statistically significant effects on pain intensity −3.85 (−8.19, 0.49) and pain interference −2.01 (−5.17, 1.15) [7]. Pain-related self-efficacy is an important factor in chronic pain management, as it reflects the subject's ability to function physically, participate in physical activities, increase performance satisfaction, enhance health and work status, and decrease pain intensity [9].

Lin et al. (2021) evaluated the effect of MM on chronic pain for patients after mechanical valve replacement. Adult patients undergoing cardiac valve replacement between January 2017 and September 2018 were offered enrollment in the study and randomized into music or control groups (43 in each group). There were no statistically significant differences between the groups. Both groups chose a quiet room in their house and rested for 30 minutes between 8 and 10 pm for 6 months following their valve replacement. The music group listened to music (patient selected from a list provided by researchers) during the daily rest period. Pain was assessed using VAS in both groups at their 6-month follow-up appointment and was similar between both groups [22].

In 2022, the Cochrane Collaboration published an updated intervention review of music interventions for improving physical outcomes in people with cancer. RCTs or quasi-randomized controlled trials with music as an intervention for improving physical outcomes in adults and children with cancer were reviewed. Studies of biopsies for cancer diagnosis were excluded. Twelve studies ($n = 632$) were included, and the pooled analysis showed a moderate mean effect on pain perception of SMD −0.67 (−1.07, −0.26), $p = 0.001$, with very low certainty of evidence [21]. A subgroup analysis demonstrated that both MT (SMD −0.47 (−0.86, −0.07) $p = 0.02$) and MM (SMD −0.81 (−1.38, −0.24) $p = 0.005$) had a moderate effect on pain [23]. The MT interventions had a consistent effect on pain, whereas the MM study benefits varied widely [23]. Both patient-selected and researcher-selected music led to lower pain scores [23].

Applications for Clinical Practice

In 2016, Lee published a comprehensive meta-analysis of randomized controlled trials published between 1995 and 2014 focused on the effects of music on pain. Studies with two or more therapeutic approaches (i.e., music plus another therapy), nontraditional comparator groups, or uncommon interventions (MM with live music, for example) were excluded to minimize heterogeneity. The author identified 97 studies that met the inclusion criteria and sought to answer the following specific research questions:

(a) *Effectiveness of music at reducing pain versus standard care in various patient populations*: Music interventions decreased pain by a mean of 1.3 units (95% CI −1.44, −0.82, $P < 0.00001$) in the 76 studies using 0–10 pain scales (VAS, NRS), but the results were highly variable. For the 15 studies using other types of scales, the SMD was −0.39 (95% CI −0.68, −0.09) $p = 0.01$, with high heterogeneity of results [24].

(b) *Effectiveness of music at reducing analgesic use compared to standard care*. Seven studies ($n = 382$) detailed the mg of anesthetic (propofol, isoflurane, sevoflurane) used and showed a statistically significant moderate reduction with music intervention, SMD of −0.56 (95% CI −0.88, −0.25) $p = 0.0005$. Twelve studies ($n = 1761$) described the use of opiates (morphine, fentanyl, tramadol) with or without musical intervention and with a small but homogenous and statistically significant reduction in the music intervention groups SDM −0.24 (95% CI −0.34, −0.14) $p < 0.00001$. Three studies ($n = 258$) showed a moderately significant effect on a decrease in non-opiate analgesia in patients with music intervention, SMD −0.54 (95% CI −0.78, −0.29) $p < 0.0001$ with no heterogeneity. The seven studies reporting the effect of music intervention on sedative use found no significant difference with music intervention [24].

(c) *Differentiating between the efficacy of MM and MT vs standard care*. Pain intensity: Using 0–10 point scales, MT interventions (9 trials, $n = 505$) showed a reduction of −1.5 (95% CI −2.09, −0.91, $p < 0.0001$) with moderate heterogeneity, and MM (67 studies, 5925 participants) showed a reduction of −1.08 (95% CI −1.42, −0.75) with high heterogeneity. The differences between the MT and MM effects were not statistically significant. Few MT studies included information about drug dosing in conjunction with interventions, but 21 MM studies detailing opiate mg administered showed a small but statistically significant reduction, SDM −0.25 (95% CI −0.35, −0.14) $p < 0.00001$ [24].

(d) *Effect of MM and MT on different subtypes of pain*. MT had a statistically significant but variable effect on acute/postoperative pain (MD –1.53 (95% CI –3.03, –0.03)) $p = 0.05$ and a moderate and more consistent effect on chronic/cancer pain (MD –1.42 (95% CI. MM –1.99, –0.84)) $p < 0.00001$. MM produced statistically significant but heterogeneous reductions in pain for both acute/procedural (MD –1.09 (95% CI –1.44, –0.74)) $p < 0.00001$ and chronic/cancer pain (MD –0.92 (95% CI –1.41, –0.43)) $p < 0.001$ [24].

The author concluded that both types of musical interventions (MM and MT) benefit patients by reducing pain intensity and decreasing analgesic use [24]. MT appears more effective than MM at reducing self-reported pain intensity, while MM demonstrated a reduction in analgesic use and MT did not [24]. Children seem to benefit more from musical interventions than adults, but outcomes were also more heterogeneous than those reported in adults [24].

Musical interventions with (MT) and without (MM) a music therapist have been studied extensively over the past two decades in a variety of clinical settings for acute, procedural, chronic, and cancer pain. Compared to trials using medications, music therapy studies are more difficult to standardize and conduct with consistent methodology, which introduces a large amount of variability in interpretation. Large meta-analyses support a mild to moderate effect of musical intervention on analgesia. Treatment of pain is complex and subjective, and available pharmacotherapy, while effective, carries the risk of adverse effects and, in the case of opiates, physical and/or psychological dependence. In contrast, studies on musical interventions document no adverse effects. While it is possible that certain types of music may produce adverse outcomes in certain individuals, this has not been described in the current body of evidence.

Music medicine (or listening to music as an intervention in a healthcare setting) is inexpensive, easy to administer, and safe. The optimal genre of music for analgesic effect remains unclear, but it is conceivable that individual preferences impact the efficacy of the analgesic effect of listening to music. Providing relaxing music to patients is likely an effective adjunct to medication-induced analgesia in multiple types of care settings. Further research is needed to determine the optimal timing of music intervention, the most beneficial type of music, and the optimal number of interventions.

Other areas that need further exploration are the potential impact that medications that alter neurotransmitter levels might have on the efficacy of music therapy and whether specific types of music therapy are more effective for specific types of pain (acute vs chronic, neuropathic vs inflammatory, etc.). In a 2019 placebo-controlled trial, Ferreri et al. demonstrated that subjects who received a dopamine blocking agent (risperidone) prior to music exposure experienced decreased pleasure, whereas those who received a dopamine agonist (levodopa) had an increase in hedonistic response, and subjects with a placebo (lactose) had no change in response, so it is conceivable that drugs that modulate dopamine may impact the "reward" a person experiences from music intervention [10]. Studies with stimulants (cocaine and amphetamine) and hallucinogens (LSD) show augmentation of effects of music on mood and creativity so perhaps medications that modulate serotonin or norepinephrine pathways could be used to augment the analgesic effects of music [10]. More research is needed.

Music therapy interventions for pain are an area for ongoing active research. Music therapy is effective for a range of clinical diagnoses and is likely most effective when the therapist is able to conduct ongoing therapeutic sessions and establish a strong bond with the patient. The human pain response is complex and involves cognitive, contextual, and emotional areas of the brain. Licensed music therapists are uniquely qualified to administer musical interventions in the way most likely to benefit patients and adjust to their unique needs. The larger effect of MT on chronic or cancer pain described in the Lee meta-analysis may affirm this supposition [24].

Key Themes

- Music therapy
- Music medicine
- Visual analog scale (VAS)
- Numerical rating scale (NRS)
- Analgesia
- Pain relief

Conclusions

Music has been a key modality in healing since ancient times, but its effect on pain has only been quantified in modern times and is still not completely understood. Musical interventions, whether music medicine or music therapy, can decrease pain associated with acute or chronic conditions and potentially reduce the amount of analgesic medications required with minimal or no harm.

References

1. Thaut M. Music as therapy in early history. Prog Brain Res. 2015;217:143–57.
2. Isgandarova N. Music in Islamic spiritual care: a review of classical sources. Relig Stud Theol. 2015;34(1):101–14.

3. Zhang H, Han L. Five phases music therapy (FPMT) in Chinese medicine: fundamentals and application. Open Access Library J. 2017;4(12):1–11.
4. Bradt J, Dileo C, Potvin N. Music for stress and anxiety reduction in coronary heart disease patients. Cochrane Database Syst Rev. 2013;12:1–87.
5. Ong W, Stohler C, Herr D. Role of the prefrontal cortex in pain processing. Mol Neurobiol. 2018;56:1137–66.
6. Arnold C, Bagg M, Harvey A. The psychophysiology of music-based interventions and the experience of pain. Front Psychol. 2024;15:1361857.
7. Lunde S, Vuust P, et al. Music-induced analgesia: how does music relieve pain? Pain. 2019;160(5):989–93.
8. Garza-villareal E, Pando V, et al. Music-induced analgesia in chronic pain conditions: a systematic review and meta-analysis. Pain Physician. 2017;20:597–610.
9. Low M, Lacson C, et al. Vocal music therapy for chronic pain: a mixed methods feasibility study. J Altern Compl Med. 2020;26(2):113–22.
10. Bradt J, Potvin N, et al. The impact of music therapy vs music medicine on psychological outcomes and pain in cancer patients: a mixed methods study. Support Care Cancer. 2015;23:1261–71.
11. Speranza L, Pulcrano S, et al. Music affects functional brain connectivity and is effective in the treatment of neurological disorders. Rev Neurosci. 2022;33(7):789–801.
12. Nilsson U, Unosson M, Rawal N. Stress reduction and analgesia in patients exposed to calming music postoperatively: a randomized controlled trial. Eur J Anesth. 2005;22:96–102.
13. Mondanaro J, et al. Music therapy increases comfort and reduces pain in patients recovering from spine surgery. Am J Orthop. 2017:E13–21.
14. Jacq G, et al. Music for pain relief during bed bathing of mechanically ventilated patients: a pilot study. PLoS One. 2018;13(11):1–17.
15. Bashiri M, et al. Evaluation of pain and patient satisfaction by music therapy in patients with endoscopy/colonoscopy. Turkish J Gastroenterol. 2018;29(5):574–9.
16. Kuhlman A, et al. Meta-analysis evaluating music interventions for anxiety and pain in surgery. BJS. 2018;105:773–83.
17. Mandel S, et al. Patient satisfaction and benefits of music therapy services to manage stress and pain in the hospital emergency department. J Music Ther. 2019;56(2):149–73.
18. Lin C, et al. Effect of music therapy on pain after orthopedic surgery-a systematic review and meta-analysis. Pain Pract. 2019;20(4):422–36.
19. Dai W, et al. The effect of music therapy on pain, anxiety, and depression after coronary artery bypass grafting. J Cardiothoracic Surg. 2020;15(81):1–5.
20. Santivanez-Acosta R, et al. Music therapy in pain and anxiety management in labor: a systematic review and meta-analysis. Medicina. 2020;56(526):1–11.
21. Dong Y, et al. Music therapy for pain and anxiety in patients after cardiac valve replacement: a randomized controlled trial. BMC Cardiovasc Disord. 2023;23:32.
22. Lin Z, et al. Effect of music therapy on the chronic pain and mid-term quality of life of patients after mechanical valve replacement. Ann Thorac Cardiovasc Surg. 2020;26:196–201.
23. Bradt J, et al. Music interventions for improving physiological and psychological outcomes for people with cancer. Cochrane Database Syst Rev. 2021;10:1–224.
24. Lee J. The effects of music on pain: a meta-analysis. J Music Ther. 2016;53(4):430–77.

Psychotherapy Approaches and Behavioral Modification Strategies

32

Estíbaliz Royuela-Colomer, Jaime Navarrete, Juan P. Sanabria-Mazo, Randy Neblett, and Juan V. Luciano

Keywords and Definitions

- *Acceptance and Commitment Therapy (ACT)*: A form of cognitive behavioral therapy that promotes acceptance of negative internal experiences and commitment to actions guided by personal values, with the main goal of enhancing psychological flexibility.
- *Behavioral activation (BA)*: A behavioral intervention aimed at increasing engagement in rewarding and meaningful activities to reduce avoidance, improve mood, and decrease disability related to pain or depression.
- *Biofeedback*: A therapeutic technique in which biological signals are measured and fed back to the patient and clinician to enhance awareness and promote voluntary control of physiological processes, thereby strengthening self-regulation skills for managing symptoms such as pain.
- *Biopsychosocial model*: A framework that explains health and illness as the result of interactions among biological, psychological, and social factors, widely applied to the understanding and treatment of chronic pain.
- *Chronic pain (CP)*: Pain that lasts for three or more months and is normally associated with distress and disability.
- *Cognitive behavioral therapy (CBT)*: A structured, evidence-based treatment approach that combines cognitive and behavioral techniques to modify dysfunctional thoughts, negative beliefs, and maladaptive behaviors related to pain and disability.
- *Emotion regulation skills-focused (ERSF)*: Interventions that focus on teaching and strengthening emotional regulation skills to improve distress tolerance and decrease the intensity of suffering associated with chronic pain.
- Fibromyalgia (FMS): A chronic pain syndrome characterized by widespread musculoskeletal pain, typically co-occurring with fatigue, sleep disturbance, cognitive difficulties, distress, and heightened pain sensitivity.
- *Kinesiophobia / pain-related fear avoidance*: An excessive and irrational fear of movement or physical activity, often due to the belief that it may cause (re)injury or exacerbate pain, contributing to avoidance behaviors and disability.
- *Low back pain (LBP)*: Pain localized in the lumbar region, one of the most common forms of musculoskeletal pain and a leading cause of disability worldwide.
- *Mindfulness-based interventions (MBI)*: Interventions that foster mindfulness skills to increase present-moment awareness, emotional regulation, and acceptance, applied in the management of pain and stress.
- *Mindfulness-based stress reduction (MBSR)*: A standardized 8-week program developed by Dr. Jon Kabat-Zinn in the 1980s, incorporating mindfulness and meditation

E. Royuela-Colomer
Department of Clinical & Health Psychology, Autonomous University of Barcelona (UAB), Bellaterra, Spain

Centre for Biomedical Research in Epidemiology and Public Health (CIBERESP), Madrid, Spain

J. Navarrete
Centre for Biomedical Research in Epidemiology and Public Health (CIBERESP), Madrid, Spain

Teaching, Research & Innovation Unit, Parc Sanitari Sant Joan de Déu (PSSJD), Sant Boi De Llobregat, Spain, Madrid, Spain

J. P. Sanabria-Mazo
Unit for the Study and Treatment of Pain-ALGOS, Department of Psychology, Universitat Rovira i Virgili, Tarragona, Spain

Institut d'Investigació Sanitària Pere Virgili, Universitat Rovira i Virgili, Tarragona, Spain

R. Neblett
PRIDE Research Foundation, Dallas, TX, USA

J. V. Luciano (✉)
Department of Clinical & Health Psychology, Autonomous University of Barcelona (UAB), Bellaterra, Spain

Centre for Biomedical Research in Epidemiology and Public Health (CIBERESP), Madrid, Spain

Teaching, Research & Innovation Unit, Parc Sanitari Sant Joan de Déu (PSSJD), Sant Boi De Llobregat, Spain, Madrid, Spain
e-mail: JuanVicente.Luciano@uab.cat

J. P. Reinert et al. (eds.), *Adjunctive Analgesic Strategies for the Bedside Clinician and Beyond*,
https://doi.org/10.1007/978-3-032-21675-5_32

practices to reduce stress, anxiety, depression, and chronic pain symptoms.

- *Multicomponent treatment*: Treatment packages that combine different therapeutic ingredients (e.g., psychological, physical, pharmacological, and educational) to address the complex and multidimensional nature of chronic pain.
- *Multidisciplinary treatment*: A treatment approach where professionals from different disciplines (e.g., physicians, health psychologists, physical therapists, nurses, and occupational therapists) work in parallel, each addressing pain from their own specialty. Coordination is limited, and treatments are usually delivered separately.
- *Interdisciplinary treatment*: An integrated model of care in which professionals from different disciplines collaborate closely, share information, and develop a coordinated treatment plan with common goals. The patient is considered an active member of the team, and interventions are delivered in a harmonized manner rather than separately.
- *Musculoskeletal pain (MSK)*: Pain affecting muscles, bones, joints, tendons, and ligaments, frequently related to overuse, injuries, and chronic conditions.
- *Pain catastrophizing*: A cognitive style involving exaggerated negative expectations about pain, including feelings of helplessness, rumination, and magnification of symptoms, which are associated with poor outcomes in pain management.
- *Pain neuroscience education (PNE)*: Evidence-based instruction in modern pain biology reframes pain as a protective, context-dependent "alarm" mechanism of the nervous system rather than a direct measure of tissue damage.

Introduction

Chronic pain (CP) is defined as pain in one or more parts of the body that persists for at least three months and is associated with psychological distress and/or functional disability [1]. Beyond its clinical consequences, CP involves a considerable economic impact in terms of direct costs (e.g., healthcare use) and indirect costs (e.g., work absenteeism) [2]. According to recent studies, the lifetime prevalence of CP in the adult population is estimated to range between 13% and 34% [3, 4], and includes a variety of conditions, such as general musculoskeletal pain, low back pain, fibromyalgia, and rheumatoid arthritis, among others.

Pharmacological approaches, particularly opioids, remain the most common treatment for CP; however, growing evidence indicates that medication alone is insufficient for long-term effectiveness and overlooks the psychological and social dimensions of pain and their bidirectional interactions [5–7]. In recent years, the biopsychosocial model of CP has gained considerable attention, as it acknowledges the dynamic interplay among biological, psychological, and social factors in the development, maintenance, and exacerbation of CP. Although CP has diverse origins and causes, evidence indicates a considerable overlap in its underlying mechanisms, as well as in the psychological processes and comorbidities observed across different pain conditions [5]. Moreover, CP is frequently accompanied by substantial psychological distress—including anxiety, anger, frustration, and depressed mood [1]—underscoring the central role of psychological therapies in its management. Given its high prevalence and profound personal and societal impact, developing and implementing effective psychological strategies for both treatment and prevention is essential for mitigating the adverse consequences of CP.

This chapter provides a brief overview of psychological approaches and behavioral modification strategies for managing CP. We begin by examining the psychological factors commonly associated with CP, including comorbidities, as well as risk, precipitant, and protective factors, together with approaches to their assessment. We then describe evidence-based interventions alongside emerging and other psychological approaches. Key process variables shared across different therapeutic models are also discussed. Finally, we address barriers to treatment and variations in delivery modalities and conclude with clinical recommendations for specialists working with patients suffering from CP.

Psychological Factors in Chronic Pain

Regardless of its etiology, people with CP frequently report symptoms of psychopathology. Several studies have demonstrated an association between CP and psychological variables, providing consistent evidence for this relationship [8, 9]. One meta-analysis, including 110 studies, found that people with CP reported significantly higher levels of depression, anxiety, somatization, anger, and hostility, as well as lower levels of self-efficacy, self-esteem, and overall emotional functioning compared to people without pain [8]. Interestingly, evidence suggests that pain-related psychological factors are often similar across different pain conditions [9]. It is also common to see CP patients with comorbid psychiatric disorders, including major depressive disorder, generalized anxiety disorder, substance use disorders, and post-traumatic stress disorder [8, 10–14].

While some studies indicate a unidirectional link from pain to psychological consequences, others highlight a bidirectional relationship, where pain and psychological factors can mutually influence each other. For instance, in a prospective cohort study, Bondesson and colleagues [15] reported comparable incidence rate ratios for the development of mental illness following CP and for the onset of CP following mental illness. Moreover, evidence suggests that longitudinal changes in pain are closely associated with changes in mental health, indicating that effective pain management may alleviate psychological symptoms, while improvements in psychological conditions can, in turn, contribute to pain relief [16]. In line with this, the HUNT Pain Study [17], which followed a random sample from the general population over 4 years, concluded that depression and pain catastrophizing were predictors of the future development of CP.

Thus, these findings align with the biopsychosocial model of pain, emphasizing the importance of integrating psychosocial factors alongside biological factors in the management of CP. In the following section, we describe key psychological variables closely related to CP that can influence prevention, development, persistence, and treatment.

Psychological Distress

Psychological distress—encompassing symptoms of depression, anxiety, and stress—is an evident part of the experience of CP [3, 5]. It may manifest as depressive symptoms (e.g., dysphoria, anhedonia, low energy, feelings of worthlessness, loss of interest), anxiety symptoms (e.g., excessive worry, rumination, tension, fear), and stress-related manifestations (e.g., irritability, difficulty relaxing, sleep disturbance).

While CP can contribute to the onset of psychological distress, evidence also supports a bidirectional relationship whereby psychological distress exacerbates both the experience and impact of pain [15, 16]. According to Lerman and colleagues [18], psychological distress can negatively influence pain, coping strategies, treatment adherence, and overall functional outcomes. Similarly, higher levels of depression and anxiety have been associated with greater pain intensity and increased pain-related disability [19].

Given this complex interplay between pain and psychological distress, it is essential to assess the latter as part of a comprehensive evaluation in individuals with CP. Early identification and management of psychological distress can inform personalized treatment planning, improve engagement with interventions, and enhance prognosis. Standardized tools such as the Depression Anxiety Stress Scales (DASS) [20], the Hospital Anxiety and Depression Scale (HADS) [21], and the Patient Health Questionnaire (PHQ) [22] are commonly used to assess levels of psychological distress in CP.

Sleep Disturbance

Sleep disturbance is highly prevalent among individuals with CP, with a pooled prevalence of approximately 75% [23]. Common problems include insomnia, fragmented sleep, poor sleep quality, waking unrefreshed, excessive daytime sleepiness, and sleep-related breathing disorders. Poor sleep functions both as a risk factor and a maintaining factor for CP, with evidence supporting a bidirectional relationship between sleep and pain [17]. Specifically, sleep disturbance is associated with greater pain severity, while pain contributes to further sleep disruption and increased psychological distress [14]. Similarly, a review by Husak and Bair [24] indicated that people with CP and comorbid sleep disturbance tend to experience more severe and persistent pain, greater disability, reduced physical activity, and higher levels of depression, anxiety, pain catastrophizing, and suicidal ideation.

Given this strong interaction between sleep, pain, and psychological symptoms, it is essential to assess sleep quality and, when appropriate, treat sleep disturbance as part of a comprehensive CP management plan. Commonly used instruments for evaluating sleep include the Pittsburgh Sleep Quality Index (PSQI) [25] and the Insomnia Severity Index (ISI) [26].

Pain Catastrophizing

Pain catastrophizing, a term coined by Sullivan and collaborators 30 years ago [27], is a maladaptive coping strategy characterized by persistent negative thinking about pain, including rumination, feelings of helplessness, and the tendency to perceive pain as threatening, overwhelming, and unmanageable [28–30]. Typical cognitions include beliefs that pain is intolerable and will never improve, worrying constantly about its persistence, perceiving it as overwhelming, or even thinking that life is not worth living. Evidence suggests that pain catastrophizing contributes to pain-related suffering and predicts both the development and maintenance of CP and disability [16, 17, 29].

Pain catastrophizing is a key variable in evaluating the effectiveness of interventions for CP. It is often included as an outcome in randomized controlled trials (RCTs), and several meta-analyses have shown that psychological interventions such as cognitive behavioral therapy (CBT), behavioral activation (BA), and pain neuroscience education (PNE) effectively reduce pain catastrophizing [31, 32]. Beyond its role as an outcome, pain catastrophizing is also considered a process variable that reflects underlying psychological mechanisms influencing treatment response [33]. Supporting this perspective, a meta-analysis found that pain catastrophizing predicted both pain intensity and disability and mediated the effectiveness of treatment outcomes [34].

The Communal Coping Model (CCM) conceptualizes pain catastrophizing not only as a cognitive coping strategy but also as an interpersonal coping response that leads to assistance or empathetic responses from significant others. Evidence from daily diary studies with couples shows that catastrophizing is linked to changes in spouse perceptions and responses, highlighting its role in shaping the interpersonal dynamics of pain [35]. In addition, Haythornthwaite and colleagues [29] have proposed a developmental model of pain catastrophizing, suggesting that it emerges during childhood and adolescence and that early prevention strategies may serve as protective factors against the later development of CP. Accordingly, the adequate assessment of pain catastrophizing is important. The gold standard measure to assess pain catastrophizing is the Pain Catastrophizing Scale (PCS) [27].

Fear Avoidance and Kinesiophobia

Pain-related fear-avoidance beliefs and behaviors are believed to be an essential feature in the development of chronic musculoskeletal pain from acute pain for a substantial number of patients [36]. The fear avoidance model suggests two primary responses to pain-related fear: confrontation and avoidance [36]. Confrontation, defined as the gradual continuation of activity despite pain, tends to reduce fear over time. In contrast, avoidance can lead to a vicious cycle of increased disability, heightened pain perception, and sustained or exacerbated fear, with significant physical and psychological consequences.

The term "kinesiophobia," or fear of movement, has been used to describe pain-related fear-avoidance behaviors [8]. Kinesiophobia is characterized by the avoidance of movement and physical activity due to a perceived vulnerability to pain or injury [37]. It is associated with greater pain intensity, higher disability, increased functional limitation, and reduced quality of life [38, 39]. Moreover, longitudinal evidence suggests that elevated levels of kinesiophobia predict the progression of disability, increased pain severity, and persistent impairments in quality of life over time [40].

Psychological interventions such as CBT, BA, and PNE have demonstrated effectiveness in reducing fear-avoidance beliefs and behaviors in individuals with CP [31, 32, 38, 41, 42]. These findings suggest that one of the mechanisms through which CP interventions exert their effects may be by targeting and reducing fear of movement [43]. Therefore, assessing kinesiophobia should be an integral part of the initial evaluation in people with CP. The most widely used instrument for this purpose is the Tampa Scale for Kinesiophobia in its different forms (TKS) [37].

Stigma

Stigma refers to attitudes and behaviors that devalue or discredit individuals or groups perceived as deviating from societal norms, typically involving exclusion and shame [44]. Stigma is frequently reported by individuals living with CP, partly because pain is invisible to others, and in many cases lacks a clear biomedical explanation [45, 46]. Contemporary frameworks distinguish between enacted and internalized stigma [47, 48]. The former (also named social stigma) reflects negative judgments and discriminatory behaviors expressed by others, for example, toward individuals with health conditions, whereas the latter (self-stigma) emerges when those affected internalize such negative attitudes and direct them toward themselves [47].

Growing evidence in CP populations shows that stigma contributes to heightened psychological distress, feelings of loneliness, reduced social support, and poorer quality of life [45, 49–51]. Internalized stigma has been linked to elevated depression, anxiety, and pain catastrophizing, alongside diminished self-esteem [48, 50–52]. The 24-item Stigma Scale for Chronic Illnesses (SSCI) [48] is a self-report measure commonly used to assess both enacted and internalized stigma in individuals with chronic illness in research and clinical practice [53].

Self-Efficacy of Pain

Bandura [54] in 1977 defined self-efficacy as the belief in one's capacity to successfully perform the actions required to produce desired outcomes. Within the context of CP, self-efficacy refers to an individual's confidence in engaging in such actions despite the presence of pain [55]. For example, individuals with higher pain self-efficacy can enjoy activities, manage household chores, pursue personal goals, maintain employment, socialize with friends and family, and sustain a normal lifestyle, even while experiencing pain. However, people with CP often report low self-efficacy in managing their symptoms [56].

Self-efficacy has been associated with prognosis in CP. A meta-analysis by Martinez-Calderon and colleagues [57] found that higher levels of self-efficacy are associated with better physical functioning, greater participation in physical activity, improved health and work status, higher satisfaction with performance, stronger efficacy beliefs, and lower levels of pain intensity, disability, disease activity, depressive symptoms, fatigue, tender points on the body, and presenteeism. Conversely, lower self-efficacy has been associated with worse clinical outcomes, including higher pain intensity, greater disability, and poorer psychological functioning [56].

Self-efficacy has also been identified as a key psychological mechanism in treatment responsiveness. A meta-analysis found that increases in self-efficacy mediated the effects of CBT on disability outcomes [43]. Similarly, Hayes and colleagues [58] identified self-efficacy as one of the core process variables through which psychological interventions for CP exert their therapeutic effects. For all these reasons, it is essential to assess self-efficacy, most commonly with the Pain Self-Efficacy Questionnaire (PSEQ) [55].

Mindfulness, Pain Acceptance, and Psychological Flexibility

Emerging evidence suggests that "third-wave" psychological variables, such as mindfulness, pain acceptance, and psychological flexibility, can act as protective factors in the development and exacerbation of CP and can also contribute to its treatment [59]. Dispositional mindfulness has been defined as "the awareness that emerges through paying attention on purpose, in the present moment, and nonjudgmentally to the experience moment by moment" ([60], p. 145). It emphasizes an accepting and nonreactive attitude toward pain, encouraging individuals to acknowledge their symptoms without allowing them to dominate or restrict daily life. In this way, mindfulness can facilitate improved coping and reduced emotional reactivity in CP. Indeed, a meta-analysis by Tomlinson and colleagues [61] found that dispositional mindfulness is associated with adaptive cognitive strategies, including lower levels of rumination and pain catastrophizing. However, two separate systematic reviews found only limited evidence that mindfulness-based stress reduction was effective for improving pain intensity and disability in patients with low back pain [62, 63].

Psychological flexibility involves "the ability to contact the present moment more fully as a conscious human being and to change or persist in behavior when doing so serves valued ends" ([64], p. 7). Thus, pain-related psychological flexibility is the ability to experience pain without letting it dominate one's thoughts, emotions, or behavior or to interfere with engagement in meaningful activities [65]. Psychological flexibility is at the core of Acceptance and Commitment Therapy (ACT), which seeks to lessen the impact of pain and associated restrictive experiences in daily life by enhancing psychological flexibility processes, such as pain acceptance and mindfulness [65, 66]. A related construct is pain acceptance, which refers to the willingness to experience pain without attempting to control or avoid it [67].

Gold-standard self-report measures for assessing these protective factors in CP populations are the Multidimensional Psychological Flexibility Inventory (MPFI) [68], the Psy-Flex [69], the Psychological Inflexibility in Pain Scale (PIPS)[70], the Chronic Pain Acceptance Questionnaire (CPAQ) [71], and the Five Facets of Mindfulness Questionnaire (FFMQ) [72].

Other Clinical, Biological, Social, and Contextual Factors

In addition to the psychological factors discussed above, several other variables are important to consider in the psychological management of CP. The biopsychosocial model of health and disease, involving interactions among biological, psychological, and social factors, was proposed by Engel in 1977 [73]. More recently, spirituality has been recommended as a fourth component of the model [74]. The proposed "biopsychosociospiritual model" proposes that spiritual beliefs, practices, and experiences may contribute uniquely to patients' coping processes, quality of life, and health outcomes, thereby offering a more comprehensive approach to the assessment and management of health conditions in general and CP in particular (see [75]).

As detailed by Miaskowski and co-authors [76] and by Gatchel and colleagues [77], multiple biological factors can influence pain and its management, including sex, age, comorbidities, fatigue, and sleep disturbance. Lifestyle and health behaviors are also relevant, such as smoking, substance use, body mass index, physical activity, nutrition, and exposure to sunlight/vitamin D. Equally influential are social factors, including race/ethnicity, culture, socioeconomic status, social support, and social isolation. Other highly relevant contributors include a history of violent injury, interpersonal violence, and abuse [73, 74]. As noted by Miller and colleagues [78], clinical variables must also be considered, particularly those directly related to pain, such as its type, location, severity, interference, and management. Additional variables include genetic predispositions, multimorbidity, mortality, history of surgical or medical interventions, body weight, and sleep disorders.

Notwithstanding, a detailed analysis of all these factors is beyond the scope of this chapter. However, clinicians are strongly encouraged to conduct an individualized assessment, as such factors can significantly influence the psychological management of CP, either facilitating or complicating the course of treatment. Readers interested in a more comprehensive examination of these variables are referred to the biopsychosocial model of CP for older adults by Miaskowski and co-authors [76] and the review on the epidemiology of pain and associated factors by Mills and colleagues [79].

Summary

To sum up, when planning treatment for CP, it is essential to conduct an individualized evaluation that considers all relevant biopsychosocial factors and comorbid conditions influencing the multidimensional experience of pain. Attention to these variables can help explain why some individuals develop CP while others do not and why people with similar pain conditions often experience different trajectories of pain severity and disability. Moreover, biopsychosocial factors play a key role in the psychological management of CP and can strongly influence treatment efficacy. Importantly, some of these variables, such as pain catastrophizing or psychological flexibility, also operate as mechanisms of change in psychological therapies. Table 32.1 summarizes the main biopsychosocial factors associated with CP, along with commonly used assessment tools.

Evidence-Based Cognitive Behavioral and Related Therapies for Chronic Pain

Psychological therapies for CP aim to reduce disability and psychological distress while improving overall quality of life. Seven types of interventions, with strong empirical evidence and contextualized in cognitive and behavioral paradigms, will be highlighted: Behavioral Activation (BA), Cognitive Behavioral Therapy (CBT), Acceptance and Commitment Therapy (ACT), mindfulness-based interventions (MBIs), Emotion Regulation Skills-Focused (ERSF) therapies, biofeedback, and pain neuroscience education (PNE).

Table 32.1 Assessment of biopsychosocial factors associated with chronic pain (CP) and its management

Factors	Description	Assessment tools
Biological and social	Biological and social aspects, such as age, sex, ethnicity and cultural background, socioeconomic background, employment status and occupational factors, social support, stigma, isolation, violent injury, interpersonal violence, abuse, and life-threatening events	Clinical interview
Lifestyle and behavior	Factors such as, smoking, drugs, alcohol, physical activity, nutrition, sunshine and vitamin D can influence the development and maintenance of CP, as well as treatment effectiveness	Clinical interview
Clinical	Clinical variables such as multimorbidity, history of surgical or medical interventions, body weight, and sleep disorders	Clinical interview
Pain	Type of pain, location, interference, and intensity	Clinical interview The Brief Pain Inventory (BPI) [153] Visual analog scale or the numerical rating scale Pain drawing
Sleep disorders	Sleep problems, such as insomnia, fragmented sleep, poor sleep quality, excessive daytime sleepiness, and sleep-related breathing disorders, are common in CP	Pittsburgh Sleep Quality Index (PSQI) [25] Insomnia Severity Index (ISI) [26]
Psychological		
Mental health comorbidities	CP frequently co-occurs with other psychological and psychiatric conditions, including major depressive disorder, generalized anxiety disorder, substance use disorders, and post-traumatic stress disorder	Diagnosis of comorbidities typically relies on clinical interviews complemented by standardized assessment tools (e.g., DSM-5 [154], ICD-11 [155])
Pain catastrophizing	Persistent negative thinking about pain, including rumination, feelings of helplessness, and a tendency to perceive pain as threatening, overwhelming, and unmanageable	Pain catastrophizing scale (PCS) [27]
Fear avoidance/ Kinesiophobia	Kinesiophobia is a maladaptive pain-related fear characterized by the avoidance of movement and physical activity due to a perceived vulnerability to pain or injury	Tampa scale for Kinesiophobia (TKS) [156]
Self-efficacy of pain	The belief in one's capacity to successfully perform the actions required to produce desired outcomes, and confidence to engage in such actions despite the presence of pain	Pain Self-Efficacy Questionnaire (PSEQ) [55]
Emotional distress	Emotional distress includes symptoms of depression, anxiety, and stress, such as dysphoria, anhedonia, feelings of worthlessness, loss of interest, tension, and fear, as well as stress-related manifestations, including irritability and difficulty relaxing	Depression anxiety stress scales (DASS) [20] Hospital Anxiety and Depression Scale (HADS) [21] Patient Health Questionnaire (PHQ) [22]
Mindfulness	Dispositional mindfulness emphasizes an accepting and nonreactive attitude toward pain, encouraging individuals to acknowledge their symptoms without allowing them to dominate or restrict daily life	Mindfulness attention awareness scale (MAAS) [157] Five Facet of Mindfulness Questionnaire (FFMQ) [72]
Pain acceptance	Pain acceptance refers to the willingness to experience pain without attempting to control or avoid it, while continuing to engage in meaningful activities despite pain	Chronic Pain Acceptance Questionnaire (CPAQ) [71]
Psychological flexibility	Psychological flexibility is the ability to experience pain without letting it dominate one's thoughts, emotions, or behavior, and maintaining engagement in meaningful activities	Psychological Inflexibility in Pain Scale (PIPS) [70]

According to several meta-analyses, CBT remains the most widely studied and methodologically robust intervention, consistently showing positive outcomes [32, 80]. CBT is also the most recommended therapy according to national and international clinical guidelines [81, 82]. ACT has also shown strong evidence and is recommended by the NICE guideline for CP management [82, 83]. The following section describes common therapeutic modalities in more detail. Table 32.2 provides a summary of the main psychological therapies for CP.

Cognitive Behavioral Therapy (CBT)

CBT was originally developed for the treatment of depression and is now one of the most extensively studied psychological therapies for CP. It aims to modify maladaptive thoughts and behaviors related to pain, teach coping strategies to reduce distress and disability, and improve self-management [84]. CBT for pain includes cognitive restructuring, Socratic dialogue, identification of cognitive biases, and relaxation training strategies.

Table 32.2 Overview of psychological therapies in chronic pain management

Therapy	Description	Evidence of effectiveness	References
Cognitive Behavioral Therapy (CBT)	CBT aims to modify maladaptive thoughts and beliefs related to pain and to teach coping strategies to reduce distress, disability, and improve self-management. CBT for pain includes cognitive restructuring, behavioral activation, and relaxation training strategies	High (multiple meta-analyses) Recommended by most clinical guides as the primary option	[32, 80, 158]
Acceptance and Commitment Therapy (ACT)	ACT promotes psychological flexibility by fostering acceptance of pain and commitment to valued activities, rather than attempting to control or eliminate pain	Moderate-high Recommended by clinical guides	[159, 160]
Behavioral Activation (BA)	BA is a structured approach that increases engagement in meaningful and rewarding activities to reduce avoidance and withdrawal, improving mood and functioning despite pain	Moderate-high	[94, 96]
Mindfulness-Based Interventions (MBIs)	MBIs teach nonjudgmental awareness of present-moment experiences through meditation practices, aiming to reduce stress, pain, and improve well-being. Normally, MBIs are delivered in group or online formats	Moderate Recommended as a complementary therapy in several clinical guides	[100, 161]
Biofeedback	Biofeedback training teaches skills for self-regulating psychophysiological processes and managing symptoms such as muscle tension, emotional distress, and pain	Moderate-high	[108, 111, 107] https://www.va.gov/WHOLEHEALTHLIBRARY/tools/biofeedback.asp
Pain Neuroscience Education (PNE)	This educational modality teaches patients about the biological mechanisms and biopsychosocial nature of chronic pain to help reduce maladaptive pain beliefs, encourage adaptive pain management strategies, and improve function with activities of daily living	Moderate when combined with multimodality treatments, including exercise	[116–118]
Emotion Regulation Skill Focused Interventions (ERSF)	ERSF enhance adaptive emotion regulation strategies to decrease emotional distress and improve coping with chronic pain	Emerging	[124]
Positive Psychology (PP)	PP focuses on enhancing strengths, positive emotions, and resilience through interventions such as gratitude, optimism, and meaning-making, aiming to improve well-being despite chronic pain	Emerging	[129–131]
Compassion Focused Therapy (CFT)	CFT cultivates self-compassion and reduces self-criticism to alleviate suffering and enhance emotional resilience in chronic pain patients	Emerging	[162, 163]
Dialectical Behavior Therapy (DBT)	DBT integrates CBT and mindfulness with emphasis on emotion regulation, distress tolerance, and interpersonal effectiveness, supporting better coping with chronic pain and comorbid emotional dysregulation	Emerging	[99, 164, 165]
Functional Analytic Psychotherapy (FAP)	FAP uses the therapeutic relationship as a context to shape adaptive behaviors, reinforcing in-session improvements in interpersonal and emotional functioning that generalize to pain management	Emerging	[166, 167]
Metacognitive Therapy (MCT)	MCT targets unhelpful metacognitive beliefs and worry/rumination cycles, aiming to reduce maladaptive cognitive processes that exacerbate pain-related distress	Emerging	[168, 169]

CBT is currently the only psychological approach with sufficiently robust evidence to be recommended as the first-line psychological treatment for CP [80]. CBT focuses on problem-solving and promoting an active role for the patient through the recognition, examination, and restructuring of maladaptive thoughts. The main goals of CBT in pain management are to reduce pain-related distress and improve physical functioning.

Multiple meta-analyses have shown CBT to be effective in reducing pain and disability as well as improving quality of life and pain-related distress [80, 85]. In addition, it has been found to improve secondary outcomes such as self-efficacy, psychological distress, and return-to-work rates [86]. Despite being a widely used and standardized therapy, there is considerable variation in its delivery. According to a review of reviews, there is no universally accepted protocol for CBT in CP, and further research is needed to determine the most effective duration, delivery mode (e.g., online, group-based), and intensity [85]. Evidence also suggests that CBT achieves the best results when integrated with other active treatments, such as exercise or physiotherapy, or within multidisciplinary interventions [85, 87].

Several factors may influence the effectiveness of CBT. A review of predictors of treatment outcomes for CBT in CP identified baseline sociodemographic, physical, and emotional variables as important determinants of success [88]. The most reported predictors were higher baseline anxiety and depression levels, as well as negative cognitions about pain and coping strategies.

Acceptance and Commitment Therapy (ACT)

ACT is a psychological therapy that integrates cognitive, behavioral, and mindfulness-based approaches, with the primary aim of increasing psychological flexibility to live a value-driven life [89]. It is structured around six core processes: acceptance, self-as-context, cognitive defusion, present-moment awareness, values clarification, and committed action, which represent its proposed mechanisms of action [90]. In the context of CP, ACT encourages people to engage in behaviors consistent with their personal values despite the persistence of pain and discomfort, particularly when previous efforts to control or reduce pain have been ineffective.

A meta-analysis including 25 RCTs reported improvements in key outcomes such as pain interference, disability, depression, and quality of life, alongside consistent associations between increased psychological flexibility and positive treatment outcomes [91]. Similarly, a meta-analysis of 21 studies found significant effects on pain severity, pain-related functioning, anxiety, depression, and quality of life [92, 93]. This latter study also suggested that longer session duration and extended treatment length were associated with larger effects, although the overall methodological quality of the included studies was heterogeneous.

Furthermore, an umbrella review encompassing 84 systematic reviews concluded that, at posttreatment, ACT can reduce depression and anxiety symptoms, psychological inflexibility, and pain catastrophizing, while improving mindfulness and pain acceptance [83]. Some of the results were maintained at 3–6 months after treatment; however, not all studies included a follow-up period, limiting the certainty of long-term effects.

Behavioral Activation (BA)

BA was originally developed as a treatment for depression and has been adapted for the management of CP [94, 95]. It is based on the principle that scheduling and engaging in pleasurable or meaningful activities can improve mood. In the context of CP, BA focuses on identifying and promoting activities that are personally reinforcing and consistent with the individual's values and goals. The aim of BA is to help people overcome fear and avoidance behaviors and enhance their motivation to remain physically active. Evidence indicates that progressively increasing participation in previously avoided activities can break the negative cycle linking pain, fear, avoidance, and low mood [39].

A recent meta-analysis concluded that BA has the potential to reduce pain, possibly through its impact on depressive symptoms [96]. However, most of the included studies were rated as having a high risk of bias, indicating overall low study quality and warranting caution in interpreting the findings.

Mindfulness and Acceptance-Based Interventions (MBIs)

MBIs cover different therapeutic approaches, including mindfulness-based stress reduction (MBSR) [97], Mindfulness-Based Cognitive Therapy (MBCT) [98], ACT [89], and Dialectical Behavioral Therapy (DBT)[99]; as well as psychological interventions that integrate meditation practices and compassion- and acceptance-based strategies. They are based on teaching strategies to cultivate present-moment awareness and a nonjudgmental attitude toward thoughts, emotions, and bodily sensations. In the context of CP, it means shifting the attention away from pain and pain-related thoughts or ruminations and instead cultivating an open, accepting observation of current experiences and feelings.

Scientific interest in MBIs has grown in recent years. A meta-analysis of 30 RCTs on mindfulness meditation for CP reported small but significant improvements in pain symptoms, reductions in depressive symptoms, and improvements in quality of life [62, 100]. However, the authors suggested interpreting these findings with caution due to the heterogeneity of the included studies, small sample sizes, and the low methodological quality of some trials. Similar concerns were raised in a recent study on MBIs for low back pain [101], which found that MBIs may help reduce pain intensity but emphasized that the evidence is limited and inconsistent, with potential problems related to high variability in study designs, small samples, risk of bias, and lack of studies assessing long-term effects.

A systematic review comparing group-based MBIs with CBT found no significant differences in treatment benefits between the two approaches, with both demonstrating superiority over control conditions. Specifically, both MBSR and CBT showed clinically meaningful improvements in physical functioning, pain intensity, and depression relative to control groups [102]. In addition, an umbrella review of 19 systematic reviews on MBIs for chronic musculoskeletal pain reported mixed findings, though some evidence suggests potential benefits for pain, quality of life, and depression [103]. The authors concluded that MBIs were comparable to CBT and superior to no treatment. However, they highlighted substantial heterogeneity across studies in the definition of MBIs, as well as in session length, number, frequency, and overall treatment duration, which might affect the results.

More recently, a meta-analysis exploring the mechanisms of action reported that mindfulness practices promote pain acceptance and modify pain control beliefs, which are key process variables for pain outcomes [104]. Furthermore, long-term mindfulness practice was associated with increased pain thresholds and reduced pain unpleasantness, potentially mediated by higher activation in brain regions involved in attentional control.

Biofeedback

Biofeedback is a procedure in which biological information is measured and "fed back" to a patient and clinician [105]. The use of biofeedback as a clinical tool has a long history, going back to the 1960s [106]. It can be performed as a single modality or in conjunction with cognitive behavioral therapy or physical therapy [107]. Modern biofeedback assessment and training is most often done with computer equipment, using visual feedback on a computer graph, sometimes with the addition of auditory feedback through computer speakers [105]. Multiple biofeedback modalities can be used in CP treatment/rehabilitation, including biomechanical measures (force and pressure); neuromuscular measures (surface electromyography); autonomic nervous system measures (hand temperature, skin conductance, and heart rate); and central nervous system measures (electroencephalography) [106].

The primary goals of biofeedback training are to learn increased awareness and control over biological processes and self-regulation skills for managing symptoms such as pain [105]. A recent systematic review of 25 published studies determined that biofeedback training can produce significant reductions in pain intensity and enhancements in quality of life across a variety of different clinical populations, including those with low back pain, headaches, fibromyalgia, and pelvic pain [108]. A separate systematic review and meta-analysis of 21 studies focused on chronic low back pain concluded that biofeedback can lead to improvements in pain intensity, depression, muscle tension, disability, and cognitive coping [107]. Mental health professionals may be especially drawn to the potential reductions in stress, anxiety, and pain that can be achieved with heart rate variability biofeedback training, which is usually done in conjunction with paced breathing [109–112].

Pain Neuroscience Education (PNE)

Pain-related fear-avoidance and catastrophizing are tied to the belief that pain means harm, it is always a sign of tissue damage, and increased pain indicates that the damage is getting worse [113]. However, modern science has shown that pain can occur without any sign of tissue damage; this is especially true of CP [114]. PNE uses contemporary pain science to teach patients about the biopsychosocial nature of their CP experience, encourage reconceptualization of pain as less threatening, reduce maladaptive beliefs, facilitate the acquisition of adaptive pain coping strategies, and improve symptom management and function [115]. When combined with exercise and multimodality treatments, systematic reviews have consistently found PNE to be effective in improving pain intensity, pain catastrophizing, fear-avoidance beliefs, and disability with a variety of CP disorders [116–119]. However, PNE as a stand-alone treatment approach has demonstrated limited effectiveness for these outcome variables [42, 120].

Emotion Regulation Skills-Focused (ERSF) Interventions

In recent years, researchers and clinicians have shown growing interest in the association between emotion regulation and CP. To explain the high comorbidity and co-occurrence between CP and emotional disorders, several theoretical models have been proposed. For example, the shared vulnerability model proposes that these conditions arise from shared psychological and biological vulnerabilities, common triggers, and maintaining physiological, cognitive, and behavioral factors [121]. Similarly, transdiagnostic models of CP suggest that CP and emotional problems share some psychological processes, such as catastrophizing, worry, rumination, emotional suppression, and avoidance behaviors [122]. In line with this, a systematic review reported that psychological factors, including emotionality, anxiety, and negative mood, mediate the association between emotion regulation and pain [123]. These authors also suggest that difficulties in emotion regulation represent a risk factor for the development and maintenance of CP, highlighting the importance of addressing emotion regulation in CP interventions.

ERSF interventions aim to teach people emotion regulation skills and strategies, such as increasing awareness, understanding, and acceptance of emotions; identifying emotional triggers; and developing adaptive ways to express emotions [124]. Examples of ERSF interventions are the Emotional Awareness and Expression Therapy and the Transdiagnostic Emotion-Focused Exposure treatment [125, 126]. Findings from a systematic review indicate that ERSF interventions reduce pain intensity and are at least as effective as CBT [124]. While further research is needed, these results represent an important step toward incorporating emotion regulation into the psychological management of CP.

Emerging and Other Therapies

In addition to the aforementioned psychological approaches summarized above, there are other psychological therapies that, although they have received comparatively less research attention, are worth briefly discussing. Within the family of cognitive and behavioral psychological therapies, there are several options beyond ACT and MBIs that can also be applied to CP management.

The term "third-wave" therapies includes a variety of approaches that focus on processes such as acceptance, mindfulness, cognitive defusion, dialectics, values clarification, spirituality, and interpersonal relationships. According to several authors [127, 128], the most frequently cited third-wave therapies include ACT, DBT, MBCT, MBSR, Functional Analytic Psychotherapy (FAP), and BA. Other approaches include mindfulness training, metacognitive therapy, schema therapy, mode deactivation therapy, integrative behavioral couple therapy, compassionate mind training, the cognitive behavioral analysis system of psychotherapy, mindfulness-based training groups, positive psychotherapy, the Unified Protocol, and compassion focused therapy.

Although ACT has received the greatest attention within "third-wave" approaches for CP, other modalities also seem promising. For example, several meta-analyses support the efficacy of positive psychology interventions (PPIs) in individuals with CP [129–131]. PPIs aim to enhance positive personal attributes—such as happiness, quality of life, and overall well-being—by focusing on concepts including pleasure, engagement, and meaning. Evidence from these studies suggests that PPIs can improve psychological well-being, emotional functioning, hope, pain self-efficacy, pain intensity, happiness, and life satisfaction. However, the authors caution that the results should be interpreted carefully due to methodological limitations, including the low quality of some studies, limited evidence on long-term efficacy, and scarce findings on effects related to physical functioning.

Beyond third-wave approaches, other therapeutic modalities have been explored for CP, including virtual reality-based therapies, artificial intelligence-assisted interventions, and supportive psychotherapy (for more information, see [5, 7, 80]). Finally, there is growing interest in integrative approaches (also known as multidisciplinary or multicomponent treatments) that combine elements from different therapeutic traditions, involve multidisciplinary teams, and incorporate diverse perspectives. Evidence suggests that multicomponent interventions may provide greater benefits in treating CP than single interventions alone [132]. Such approaches may offer new opportunities to address the multifaceted nature of CP. Indeed, clinical guidelines recommend integrating different therapeutic approaches, including psychological and physical components.

Delivery Formats and Implementation

The format of delivery is also a relevant factor to consider when administering psychological therapies. For example, if the treatment is delivered in a group format, where group cohesion itself can act as a therapeutic mechanism, it can facilitate adherence and enhance treatment outcomes [133]. The delivery format—whether in-person, online, or even outdoors—can also influence effectiveness [134]. Indeed, online therapies have expanded notably in recent years, especially following the COVID-19 pandemic. We dedicated the next section to internet-based therapeutic approaches. We also discuss barriers and contextual factors that may influence the implementation of psychological therapies for individuals with pain.

Digital Therapeutics

The evidence-based psychological therapies described above are most often provided in person, either individually or in groups. Nevertheless, adults with chronic health conditions frequently face challenges in accessing these traditional face-to-face services. Barriers include the scarcity of free public health programs, the inability of such services to fully address the needs of people with long-term illnesses, geographical distance or scheduling conflicts, physical limitations imposed by the illness itself, and limited availability of trained therapists with accredited experience [135, 136]. To overcome these obstacles, psychological treatments have been adapted into digital formats to make therapeutic support more accessible. In fact, an increasing amount of research points to the cost-effectiveness and positive health outcomes of digital interventions [137]. Within the field of digital health, four main modalities can be distinguished: Internet-Based Interventions (IBIs), smartphone applications, Virtual Reality (VR), and Augmented Reality (AR).

Internet-Based Interventions (IBIs) are therapeutic programs delivered through computers or mobile devices, often organized into modules or lessons such as internet-based CBT. These can be guided with therapist support or unguided and are commonly used to treat depression and anxiety, promote healthy behaviors, and prevent mental health problems. For example, Sanabria-Mazo and colleagues [138] tested a synchronous videoconference group format of ACT and BATD in individuals with chronic low back pain and comorbid depression. Both interventions were delivered remotely in real time, with structured sessions led by a therapist in groups, and compared to treatment as usual. Results were positive, thus highlighting how IBIs can replicate the structure of traditional CBT-based approaches while overcoming barriers to access.

Smartphone applications extend therapeutic access via mobile devices such as smartphones and tablets. They often incorporate ecological momentary assessment/intervention, enabling real-time adaptive support. Apps are increasingly applied for prevention, diagnosis, relapse prevention, and as complements or substitutes for face-to-face therapy for CP. A clear example is Stanza®, a smartphone-based, self-guided digital ACT program developed for fibromyalgia management. It offers 41 structured ACT lessons, mindfulness practices, and daily skills training. The United States phase 3 multicenter RCT [139] showed that a 12-week course of Stanza®, structured into daily self-guided lessons including acceptance, mindfulness, and values-based behavior change exercises, produced significantly higher rates of patient-reported improvement compared to an active control with symptom tracking and pain management education [139].

Lastly, Virtual Reality (VR) and Augmented Reality (AR) are immersive technologies increasingly used in CP management. VR employs head-mounted displays or motion systems to create 3D environments for distraction, gamified rehabilitation, or exposure therapy, with evidence showing significant improvements in pain, functioning, and quality of life [140]. AR, by contrast, overlays digital elements on the real world through smartphones, tablets, or headsets, supporting rehabilitation, exposure, and self-management tasks. A review of 46 studies found that 78% of RCTs using AR, VR, or mixed reality improved pain outcomes, mainly in the short term [141].

Barriers and Limitations of Psychological Treatments for CP

Although current evidence and clinical guidelines support a shift from a predominantly pharmacological model to a more comprehensive biopsychosocial approach [76], multiple barriers continue to limit access to psychological therapies. For example, Driscoll and colleagues [7] described patient, treatment provider, and system/organizational barriers. Regarding the patient perspective, there is often limited recognition of the benefits of psychological interventions for some individuals with CP, and patients tend to favor pharmacological treatments, which are perceived as requiring less time and active involvement. Moreover, there is also some stigma associated with attending psychological therapies, which can negatively affect help-seeking attitudes [142]. To address this stigma, it is essential to educate patients about the rationale and expected outcomes of psychological therapies, and in required cases, combining psychotherapy with medication may also enhance engagement and effectiveness [143].

Similarly, treatment providers (especially when they are nonmental health professionals) may lack understanding of the rationale behind psychological treatments, question their efficacy, or fail to recommend them to patients. These provider beliefs can negatively influence patients' expectations and willingness to engage in therapy. As Wampold [144] highlights in his book *Great Psychotherapy Debate*, common factors in psychological treatment, such as the therapist's beliefs and the patient's expectations, play a crucial role in treatment outcomes. Therefore, training healthcare providers in evidence-based psychological approaches and fostering their confidence in delivering these interventions are critical steps. Allowing flexibility in the choice of psychological strategies—based on clinicians' competencies—alongside adequate training could also improve treatment delivery.

Finally, system and organizational barriers, such as a lack of insurance coverage or therapist scarcity, can impede access to psychological care in CP. These challenges might be improved by providing cost-effective treatment formats, such as virtual or group-based interventions, particularly for people with lower clinical risk.

Intervention Provider

Another key aspect concerns the provider: while interventions may be delivered by physicians, nurses, physiotherapists, or psychologists, some evidence suggests that psychological therapies are more effective when administered by a trained mental health professional [145]. As discussed in the previous section, multicomponent interventions, delivered by different professionals, have also shown promise in the management of CP. These interventions require careful coordination, ideally with each professional focusing on their area of expertise, typically including physiotherapists, physicians, nurses, and psychologists or other licensed mental health professionals.

Process and Common Factors

In recent years, there has been progress in evaluating the effectiveness of psychological therapies for CP. According to McCracken [146], most approaches have relied on standardized, protocol-driven interventions applied uniformly to all patients, without adequately accounting for the individual characteristics of each person. This has led to calls for a shift toward more personalized treatment models, such as process-based therapies [147].

Some researchers suggest that different psychological therapies, and specifically those for CP, tend to yield similar outcomes, suggesting that what truly matters may be less about the specific theoretical model underpinning an intervention and more about the common factors and mechanisms of change involved [102, 144]. From this perspective, several researchers have proposed a paradigm shift—focusing more on identifying and targeting the processes that drive change and on tailoring interventions to individual characteristics and needs toward personalized treatment [147–149].

Proposed mechanisms of change in CP interventions include improvements in emotional regulation, psychological flexibility, acceptance, behavioral exposure, and cognitive restructuring [7, 88, 148, 150]. In addition, several common factors have been identified across different therapeutic approaches, such as the therapeutic working alliance, group climate or cohesion (in the context of group-based therapies), and therapist competence or quality [151].

Although CBT remains the most extensively studied and evidence-supported psychological strategy for managing CP, findings from both pain and broader mental health research suggest that psychological therapies in general can be effective. This effectiveness may stem from a combination of shared therapeutic elements and specific change processes, each contributing in different ways depending on the intervention. In sum, it appears that while various psychological therapies may operate through distinct underlying mechanisms, they also share certain common factors that contribute to their efficacy.

Recommendations for Clinicians

Psychological aspects play a crucial role in the management of CP, and clinicians should therefore adopt a biopsychosocial or even a biopsychosociospiritual approach that incorporates psychological therapies for CP management. As we have discussed above, the therapeutic approaches that have received considerable empirical support in the treatment of CP are BA, CBT, MBIs, ACT, and ERST. Specifically, CBT and ACT are the recommended treatments by several national and international clinical guidelines [81, 82]. Also, MBIs, meditation, psychoeducation, emotional support, or emotion regulation strategies are recommended by clinical, national, and international guidelines as complementary approaches. In addition, there are also other alternative approaches that may also be beneficial and deserve further empirical exploration.

Multimodal or multicomponent interventions that integrate biological, psychological, and social perspectives are strongly recommended. Evidence suggests that integrated approaches—particularly those that address co-occurring mental health conditions such as depression and anxiety—tend to be more effective than treatments focusing on pain symptoms alone. These approaches integrate several therapeutic components, such as psychological therapy, supervised physical exercise, pain neuroscience education, and pharmacological treatment. Moreover, multicomponent interventions are often delivered within a multidisciplinary or interdisciplinary framework, involving the coordination of various professionals such as psychologists, physiotherapists, and physicians, among others.

Moreover, group therapy formats can be particularly useful—not only for their clinical benefits but also for the added value of social support and shared experience among participants. Also, online and eHealth-based interventions have shown promising results in improving access, adherence, and scalability, especially for those facing mobility or geographical barriers.

Despite differences across therapeutic models, many share common process variables, such as acceptance, psychological flexibility, and overcoming fear-avoidance of activities of daily living. Targeting these transdiagnostic processes may enhance outcomes by increasing protective factors and reducing risk factors, regardless of the specific therapeutic orientation. Thus, clinicians are encouraged to focus on these core mechanisms.

Recent evidence highlights the importance of moving toward personalized and process-based approaches in the assessment and treatment of CP [147]. Given the complexity and heterogeneity of CP experiences and individual profiles, clinicians are encouraged to tailor interventions to the specific needs, individual characteristics, and contextual factors of each patient. In that sense, moving toward a transdiagnostic and process-based approach is recommended.

It is also important to recognize that individuals with the same CP diagnosis may respond very differently to the same treatment approach. This variability may be caused by differences in the underlying mechanisms of pain, individual differences in psychological functioning or belief systems, or the presence of comorbid conditions. Therefore, treatment should not be based only on the pain diagnosis but must consider the patient's full context—biological, psychological, and social—to move from a "one-size-fits-all" approach to personalized psychotherapy.

Clinicians must also be aware that individuals with CP often have long histories of consultations with various health professionals, frequently accompanied by frustration, invalidation, and stigma. Importantly, some individuals may hold stigma toward psychological interventions themselves. Therefore, the therapeutic approach should emphasize nonjudgmental attitudes, active listening, and a comprehensive understanding of the patient's experience. The primary goal of treatment should not focus exclusively on reducing pain intensity but rather on improving overall functioning and quality of life.

Meeting patients "where they are"—both emotionally and contextually—can help build a strong therapeutic alliance, which is a key predictor of treatment adherence and long-term outcomes. Ultimately, the aim is to provide integrative, patient-centered care that acknowledges the complexity of CP and its frequent overlap with mental health conditions in a bidirectional relationship.

Finally, a recommendation is the implementation of early intervention strategies, even before pain becomes chronic. Identifying individuals at risk of developing CP through the assessment of personal, psychological, and contextual risk factors may help prevent the progression to chronicity and reduce health care costs [152]. This proactive approach supports a shift from reactive treatment to preventive care.

In summary, current research supports a paradigm shift toward personalized, process-based, and context-sensitive care in the clinical management of CP. This approach emphasizes flexibility, integration, and empathy as essential components for effective and sustainable treatment outcomes.

Conclusions

CP can be complex and difficult to treat. From a biopsychosociospiritual model perspective, CP is associated with several factors and characteristics that can be addressed successfully with psychological treatments, including pain catastrophizing, kinesiophobia, psychological distress, and maladaptive attitudes and beliefs. Evidence suggests that most psychological treatments for CP show small to moderate effects (with differences depending on treatment) for improving pain intensity, disability, kinesiophobia, catastrophizing, psychological distress, self-efficacy, quality of life, and healthcare costs associated with CP. The strongest evidence was found for CBT, ACT, and MBI. It is essential, however, that clinicians evaluate each case individually to explore the patient's unique characteristics and adapt treatment accordingly.

References

1. Nicholas M, Vlaeyen JWS, Rief W, et al. The IASP classification of chronic pain for ICD-11: chronic primary pain. Pain. 2019;160(1):28–37. https://doi.org/10.1097/j.pain.0000000000001390.
2. Stubhaug A, Hansen JL, Hallberg S, Gustavsson A, Eggen AE, Nielsen CS. The costs of chronic pain—long-term estimates. Eur J Pain. 2024;28(6):960–77. https://doi.org/10.1002/ejp.2234.
3. Rometsch C, Martin A, Junne F, Cosci F. Chronic pain in European adult populations: a systematic review of prevalence and associated clinical features. Pain. 2025;166(4):719–31. https://doi.org/10.1097/j.pain.0000000000003406.
4. Yong RJ, Mullins PM, Bhattacharyya N. Prevalence of chronic pain among adults in the United States. Pain. 2022;163(2):e328–32. https://doi.org/10.1097/j.pain.0000000000002291.
5. Cohen SP, Vase L, Hooten WM. Chronic pain: an update on burden, best practices, and new advances. Lancet. 2021;397(10289):2082–97. https://doi.org/10.1016/S0140-6736(21)00393-7.
6. Welsch P, Petzke F, Klose P, Häuser W. Opioids for chronic osteoarthritis pain: an updated systematic review and meta-analysis of efficacy, tolerability and safety in randomized placebo-controlled studies of at least 4 weeks double-blind duration. Eur J Pain. 2020;24(4):685–703. https://doi.org/10.1002/ejp.1522.
7. Driscoll MA, Edwards RR, Becker WC, Kaptchuk TJ, Kerns RD. Psychological interventions for the treatment of chronic pain in adults. Psychol Sci Public Interest. 2021;22(2):52–95. https://doi.org/10.1177/15291006211008157.
8. Burke ALJ, Mathias JL, Denson LA. Psychological functioning of people living with chronic pain: a meta-analytic review. Br J Clin Psychol. 2015;54(3):345–60. https://doi.org/10.1111/bjc.12078.
9. Fillingim R, Ohrbach R, Greenspan J, et al. Associations of psychologic factors with multiple chronic overlapping pain conditions. J Oral Facial Pain Headache. 2020;34:s85–s100. https://doi.org/10.11607/ofph.2584.
10. Csupak B, Sommer JL, Jacobsohn E, El-Gabalawy R. A population-based examination of the co-occurrence and functional correlates of chronic pain and generalized anxiety disorder. J Anxiety Disord. 2018;56:74–80. https://doi.org/10.1016/j.janxdis.2018.04.005.
11. Edwards KA, Buonora MJ, Merlin JS, Liebschutz JM. Recent advances in the treatment of chronic pain and substance use disorders. Curr Opin Psychol. 2025;62:101977. https://doi.org/10.1016/j.copsyc.2024.101977.
12. Johnston KJA, Huckins LM. Chronic pain and psychiatric conditions. Complex Psychiatry. 2023;9(1–4):24–43. https://doi.org/10.1159/000527041.
13. Sharp TJ, Harvey AG. Chronic pain and posttraumatic stress disorder: mutual maintenance? Clin Psychol Rev. 2001;21(6):857–77. https://doi.org/10.1016/S0272-7358(00)00071-4.

14. Ohayon MM, Schatzberg AF. Chronic pain and major depressive disorder in the general population. J Psychiatr Res. 2010;44(7):454–61. https://doi.org/10.1016/j.jpsychires.2009.10.013.
15. Bondesson E, Larrosa Pardo F, Stigmar K, et al. Comorbidity between pain and mental illness—evidence of a bidirectional relationship. Eur J Pain. 2018;22(7):1304–11. https://doi.org/10.1002/ejp.1218.
16. Angst F, Benz T, Lehmann S, et al. Extended overview of the longitudinal pain-depression association: a comparison of six cohorts treated for specific chronic pain conditions. J Affect Disord. 2020;273:508–16. https://doi.org/10.1016/j.jad.2020.05.044.
17. Landmark T, Dale O, Romundstad P, Woodhouse A, Kaasa S, Borchgrevink PC. Development and course of chronic pain over 4 years in the general population: the HUNT pain study. Eur J Pain. 2018;22(9):1606–16. https://doi.org/10.1002/ejp.1243.
18. Lerman SF, Rudich Z, Brill S, Shalev H, Shahar G. Longitudinal associations between depression, anxiety, pain, and pain-related disability in chronic pain patients. Psychosom Med. 2015;77(3):333–41. https://doi.org/10.1097/PSY.0000000000000158.
19. Michaelides A, Zis P. Depression, anxiety and acute pain: links and management challenges. Postgrad Med. 2019;131(7):438–44. https://doi.org/10.1080/00325481.2019.1663705.
20. Lovibond SH, Lovibond PF. Manual for the depression anxiety stress scales. 2nd ed. Psychology Foundation; 1995.
21. Stern AF. The hospital anxiety and depression scale. Occup Med (Chic Ill). 2014;64(5):393–4. https://doi.org/10.1093/occmed/kqu024.
22. Spitzer RL. Validation and utility of a self-report version of PRIME-MD: the PHQ primary care study. Primary care evaluation of mental disorders. Patient health questionnaire. JAMA. 1999;282(18):1737. https://doi.org/10.1001/jama.282.18.1737.
23. Sun Y, Laksono I, Selvanathan J, et al. Prevalence of sleep disturbances in patients with chronic non-cancer pain: a systematic review and meta-analysis. Sleep Med Rev. 2021;57:101467. https://doi.org/10.1016/j.smrv.2021.101467.
24. Husak AJ, Bair MJ. Chronic pain and sleep disturbances: a pragmatic review of their relationships, comorbidities, and treatments. Pain Med. 2020;21(6):1142–52. https://doi.org/10.1093/pm/pnz343.
25. Buysse DJ, Reynolds CF, Monk TH, Berman SR, Kupfer DJ. The Pittsburgh sleep quality index: a new instrument for psychiatric practice and research. Psychiatry Res. 1989;28(2):193–213. https://doi.org/10.1016/0165-1781(89)90047-4.
26. Bastien C. Validation of the insomnia severity index as an outcome measure for insomnia research. Sleep Med. 2001;2(4):297–307. https://doi.org/10.1016/S1389-9457(00)00065-4.
27. Sullivan MJL, Bishop SR, Pivik J. The pain catastrophizing scale: development and validation. Psychol Assess. 1995;7(4):524–32. https://doi.org/10.1037/1040-3590.7.4.524.
28. Flink IL, Boersma K, Linton SJ. Pain catastrophizing as repetitive negative thinking: a development of the conceptualization. Cogn Behav Ther. 2013;42(3):215–23. https://doi.org/10.1080/16506073.2013.769621.
29. Haythornthwaite JA, Campbell CM, Edwards RR. When thinking about pain contributes to suffering: the example of pain catastrophizing. Pain. 2024;165(11S):S68–75. https://doi.org/10.1097/j.pain.0000000000003372.
30. Neblett R. Pain catastrophizing: an historical perspective. J Appl Biobehav Res. 2017;22(1) https://doi.org/10.1111/jabr.12086.
31. Cuenca-Martínez F, López-Bueno L, Suso-Martí L, et al. Implementation of online behavior modification techniques in the management of chronic musculoskeletal pain: a systematic review and meta-analysis. J Clin Med. 2022;11(7):1806. https://doi.org/10.3390/jcm11071806.
32. Niknejad B, Bolier R, Henderson CR, et al. Association between psychological interventions and chronic pain outcomes in older adults. JAMA Intern Med. 2018;178(6):830. https://doi.org/10.1001/jamainternmed.2018.0756.
33. Gilliam WP, Schumann ME, Cunningham JL, et al. Pain catastrophizing as a treatment process variable in cognitive behavioural therapy for adults with chronic pain. Eur J Pain. 2021;25(2):339–47. https://doi.org/10.1002/ejp.1671.
34. Wertli MM, Burgstaller JM, Weiser S, Steurer J, Kofmehl R, Held U. Influence of catastrophizing on treatment outcome in patients with nonspecific low back pain. Spine (Phila Pa 1976). 2014;39(3):263–73. https://doi.org/10.1097/BRS.0000000000000110.
35. Burns JW, Gerhart JI, Post KM, et al. The communal coping model of pain catastrophizing in daily life: a within-couples daily diary study. J Pain. 2015;16(11):1163–75. https://doi.org/10.1016/j.jpain.2015.08.005.
36. Vlaeyen JWS, Linton SJ. Fear-avoidance and its consequences in chronic musculoskeletal pain: a state of the art. Pain. 2000;85(3):317–32. https://doi.org/10.1016/S0304-3959(99)00242-0.
37. Kori S, Miller RP, Todd DD. Kinesiophobia: a new view of chronic pain behavior. Pain Manag. 1990;3:35–43.
38. Bordeleau M, Vincenot M, Lefevre S, et al. Treatments for kinesiophobia in people with chronic pain: a scoping review. Front Behav Neurosci. 2022;16 https://doi.org/10.3389/fnbeh.2022.933483.
39. Lozano-Meca J, Gacto-Sánchez M, Montilla-Herrador J. Association of kinesiophobia with pain, disability and functional limitation in adults with knee osteoarthritis: a systematic review and meta-analysis. Geriatr Nurs (Minneap). 2024;60:481–90. https://doi.org/10.1016/j.gerinurse.2024.10.013.
40. Luque-Suarez A, Martinez-Calderon J, Falla D. Role of kinesiophobia on pain, disability and quality of life in people suffering from chronic musculoskeletal pain: a systematic review. Br J Sports Med. 2019;53(9):554–9. https://doi.org/10.1136/bjsports-2017-098673.
41. Louw A, Zimney K, Puentedura EJ, Diener I. The efficacy of pain neuroscience education on musculoskeletal pain: a systematic review of the literature. Physiother Theory Pract. 2016;32(5):332–55. https://doi.org/10.1080/09593985.2016.1194646.
42. Watson JA, Ryan CG, Cooper L, et al. Pain neuroscience education for adults with chronic musculoskeletal pain: a mixed-methods systematic review and meta-analysis. J Pain. 2019;20(10):1140.e1–1140.e22. https://doi.org/10.1016/j.jpain.2019.02.011.
43. Murillo C, Vo TT, Vansteelandt S, et al. How do psychologically based interventions for chronic musculoskeletal pain work? A systematic review and meta-analysis of specific moderators and mediators of treatment. Clin Psychol Rev. 2022;94:102160. https://doi.org/10.1016/j.cpr.2022.102160.
44. De Ruddere L, Craig KD. Understanding stigma and chronic pain: a-state-of-the-art review. Pain. 2016;157(8):1607–10. https://doi.org/10.1097/j.pain.0000000000000512.
45. Hickling LM, Allani S, Cella M, Scott W. A systematic review with meta-analyses of the association between stigma and chronic pain outcomes. Pain. 2024;165(8):1689–701. https://doi.org/10.1097/j.pain.0000000000003243.
46. Perugino F, De Angelis V, Pompili M, Martelletti P. Stigma and chronic pain. Pain Ther. 2022;11(4):1085–94. https://doi.org/10.1007/s40122-022-00418-5.
47. Molina Y, Choi SW, Cella D, Rao D. The stigma scale for chronic illnesses 8-item version (SSCI-8): development, validation and use across neurological conditions. Int J Behav Med. 2013;20(3):450–60. https://doi.org/10.1007/s12529-012-9243-4.
48. Rao D, Choi SW, Victorson D, et al. Measuring stigma across neurological conditions: the development of the stigma scale for

chronic illness (SSCI). Qual Life Res. 2009;18(5):585–95. https://doi.org/10.1007/s11136-009-9475-1.
49. Bean DJ, Dryland A, Rashid U, Tuck NL. The determinants and effects of chronic pain stigma: a mixed methods study and the development of a model. J Pain. 2022;23(10):1749–64. https://doi.org/10.1016/j.jpain.2022.05.006.
50. Lavefjord A, Sundström FTA, Buhrman M, McCracken LM. The role of stigma in health and functioning in chronic pain: not just catastrophizing. Eur J Pain. 2024;28(4):620–32. https://doi.org/10.1002/ejp.2207.
51. Scott W, Yu L, Patel S, McCracken LM. Measuring stigma in chronic pain: preliminary investigation of instrument psychometrics, correlates, and magnitude of change in a prospective cohort attending interdisciplinary treatment. J Pain. 2019;20(10):1164–75. https://doi.org/10.1016/j.jpain.2019.03.011.
52. Waugh OC, Byrne DG, Nicholas MK. Internalized stigma in people living with chronic pain. J Pain. 2014;15(5):550.e1–550.e10. https://doi.org/10.1016/j.jpain.2014.02.001.
53. Sanabria-Mazo JP, Navarrete J, Serrat M, et al. Assessment of stigma in Spanish people with chronic pain using the 8-item stigma scale for chronic illnesses (SSCI-8). J Pain. 2025;37:105538. https://doi.org/10.1016/j.jpain.2025.105538.
54. Bandura A. Social learning theory. Prentice-Hall International; 1977.
55. Nicholas MK. The pain self-efficacy questionnaire: taking pain into account. Eur J Pain. 2007;11(2):153–63. https://doi.org/10.1016/j.ejpain.2005.12.008.
56. Hayward R, Stynes S. Self-efficacy as a prognostic factor and treatment moderator in chronic musculoskeletal pain patients attending pain management programmes: a systematic review. Musculoskeletal Care. 2021;19(3):278–92. https://doi.org/10.1002/msc.1533.
57. Martinez-Calderon J, Zamora-Campos C, Navarro-Ledesma S, Luque-Suarez A. The role of self-efficacy on the prognosis of chronic musculoskeletal pain: a systematic review. J Pain. 2018;19(1):10–34. https://doi.org/10.1016/j.jpain.2017.08.008.
58. Hayes SC, Ciarrochi J, Hofmann SG, Chin F, Sahdra B. Evolving an idionomic approach to processes of change: towards a unified personalized science of human improvement. Behav Res Ther. 2022;156:104155. https://doi.org/10.1016/j.brat.2022.104155.
59. Miller RM, Kaiser RS. Psychological characteristics of chronic pain: a review of current evidence and assessment tools to enhance treatment. Curr Pain Headache Rep. 2018;22(3):22. https://doi.org/10.1007/s11916-018-0663-y.
60. Kabat-Zinn J. Mindfulness-based interventions in context: past, present, and future. Clin Psychol Sci Pract. 2003;10(2):144–56. https://doi.org/10.1093/clipsy/bpg016.
61. Tomlinson ER, Yousaf O, Vittersø AD, Jones L. Dispositional mindfulness and psychological health: a systematic review. Mindfulness (N Y). 2018;9(1):23–43. https://doi.org/10.1007/s12671-017-0762-6.
62. Cramer H, Haller H, Lauche R, Dobos G. Mindfulness-based stress reduction for low back pain. A systematic review. BMC Complement Altern Med. 2012;12(1):162. https://doi.org/10.1186/1472-6882-12-162.
63. Anheyer D, Haller H, Barth J, Lauche R, Dobos G, Cramer H. Mindfulness-based stress reduction for treating low back pain. Ann Intern Med. 2017;166(11):799–807. https://doi.org/10.7326/M16-1997.
64. Hayes SC, Luoma JB, Bond FW, Masuda A, Lillis J. Acceptance and commitment therapy: model, processes and outcomes. Behav Res Ther. 2006;44(1):1–25. https://doi.org/10.1016/j.brat.2005.06.006.
65. Feliu Soler A, Montesinos F, Gutiérrez-Martínez O, Scott W, McCracken L, Luciano J. Current status of acceptance and commitment therapy for chronic pain: a narrative review. J Pain Res. 2018;11:2145–59. https://doi.org/10.2147/JPR.S144631.
66. Baranoff J, Hanrahan SJ, Kapur D, Connor JP. Acceptance as a process variable in relation to catastrophizing in multidisciplinary pain treatment. Eur J Pain. 2013;17(1):101–10. https://doi.org/10.1002/j.1532-2149.2012.00165.x.
67. McCracken LM, Vowles KE. Acceptance of chronic pain. Curr Pain Headache Rep. 2006;10(2):90–4. https://doi.org/10.1007/s11916-006-0018-y.
68. Rolffs JL, Rogge RD, Wilson KG. Disentangling components of flexibility via the Hexaflex model: development and validation of the multidimensional psychological flexibility inventory (MPFI). Assessment. 2018;25(4):458–82. https://doi.org/10.1177/1073191116645905.
69. Gloster AT, Block VJ, Klotsche J, et al. Psy-flex: a contextually sensitive measure of psychological flexibility. J Contextual Behav Sci. 2021;22:13–23. https://doi.org/10.1016/j.jcbs.2021.09.001.
70. Wicksell RK, Lekander M, Sorjonen K, Olsson GL. The psychological inflexibility in pain scale (PIPS) – statistical properties and model fit of an instrument to assess change processes in pain related disability. Eur J Pain. 2010;14(7):771.e1–771.e14. https://doi.org/10.1016/j.ejpain.2009.11.015.
71. McCracken LM, Vowles KE, Eccleston C. Acceptance of chronic pain: component analysis and a revised assessment method. Pain. 2004;107(1):159–66. https://doi.org/10.1016/j.pain.2003.10.012.
72. Baer RA, Smith GT, Lykins E, et al. Construct validity of the five facet mindfulness questionnaire in meditating and nonmeditating samples. Assessment. 2008;15(3):329–42. https://doi.org/10.1177/1073191107313003.
73. Engel GL. The need for a new medical model: a challenge for biomedicine. Science. 1977;196(4286):129–36. https://doi.org/10.1126/science.847460.
74. Siddall PJ, Lovell M, MacLeod R. Spirituality: what is its role in pain medicine? Pain Med. 2015;16(1):51–60. https://doi.org/10.1111/pme.12511.
75. Katerndahl D, Oyiriaru D. Assessing the Biopsychosociospiritual model in primary care: development of the Biopsychosociospiritual inventory (BioPSSI). Int J Psychiatry Med. 2007;37(4):393–414. https://doi.org/10.2190/PM.37.4.d.
76. Miaskowski C, Blyth F, Nicosia F, et al. A biopsychosocial model of chronic pain for older adults. Pain Med. 2020;21(9):1793–805. https://doi.org/10.1093/pm/pnz329.
77. Gatchel RJ, Peng YB, Peters ML, Fuchs PN, Turk DC. The biopsychosocial approach to chronic pain: scientific advances and future directions. Psychol Bull. 2007;133(4):581–624. https://doi.org/10.1037/0033-2909.133.4.581.
78. Miller ET, Abu-Alhaija DM. Cultural influences on pain perception and management. Pain Manag Nurs. 2019;20(3):183–4. https://doi.org/10.1016/j.pmn.2019.04.006.
79. Mills SEE, Nicolson KP, Smith BH. Chronic pain: a review of its epidemiology and associated factors in population-based studies. Br J Anaesth. 2019;123(2):e273–83. https://doi.org/10.1016/j.bja.2019.03.023.
80. de Williams ACC, Fisher E, Hearn L, Eccleston C. Psychological therapies for the management of chronic pain (excluding headache) in adults. Cochrane Database Syst Rev. 2020;2021(11) https://doi.org/10.1002/14651858.CD007407.pub4.
81. Chou R, Fanciullo GJ, Fine PG, et al. Clinical guidelines for the use of chronic opioid therapy in chronic noncancer pain. J Pain. 2009;10(2):113–130.e22. https://doi.org/10.1016/j.jpain.2008.10.008.
82. National Institute for Health and Care Excellence (NICE). Chronic pain (primary and secondary) in over 16s: assessment of

all chronic pain and management of chronic primary pain, NICE Guideline No. NG193. NICE; 2021. https://www.nice.org.uk/guidance/ng193. Accessed 26 Sept 2025.
83. Martinez-Calderon J, García-Muñoz C, Rufo-Barbero C, Matias-Soto J, Cano-García FJ. Acceptance and commitment therapy for chronic pain: an overview of systematic reviews with meta-analysis of randomized clinical trials. J Pain. 2024;25(3):595–617. https://doi.org/10.1016/j.jpain.2023.09.013.
84. Beck AT. Cognitive therapy: nature and relation to behavior therapy. Behav Ther. 1970;1(2):184–200. https://doi.org/10.1016/S0005-7894(70)80030-2.
85. Leung T, Low MK, Yao PC, Pinho-Gomes AC. The effect of cognitive behavioural therapy on pain and disability in chronic non-specific low back pain: an overview of systematic reviews. PLoS One. 2025;20(6):e0325122. https://doi.org/10.1371/journal.pone.0325122.
86. Yang J, Lo WLA, Zheng F, Cheng X, Yu Q, Wang C. Evaluation of cognitive behavioral therapy on improving pain, fear avoidance, and self-efficacy in patients with chronic low back pain: a systematic review and meta-analysis. Pain Res Manag. 2022;2022:1–15. https://doi.org/10.1155/2022/4276175.
87. Tran TH, Pham VM. Effects of cognitive behavioral therapy combined with physical therapy on improving outcomes in chronic low back pain. J Phys Ther Sci. 2025;37(6):2025-003. https://doi.org/10.1589/jpts.37.291.
88. Forden G, Ronaghan S, Williams P, Fish S, Ford C. Predictors of treatment outcome in cognitive behavioural therapy for chronic pain: a systematic review. Disabil Rehabil. 2024;46(21):4877–88. https://doi.org/10.1080/09638288.2023.2283113.
89. Hayes S. Acceptance and commitment therapy, relational frame theory, and the third wave of behavioral and cognitive therapies. Behav Ther. 2004;35(4):639–65.
90. Dindo L, Van Liew JR, Arch JJ. Acceptance and commitment therapy: a transdiagnostic behavioral intervention for mental health and medical conditions. Neurotherapeutics. 2017;14(3):546–53. https://doi.org/10.1007/s13311-017-0521-3.
91. McCracken LM, Yu L, Vowles KE. New generation psychological treatments in chronic pain. BMJ. 2022:e057212. https://doi.org/10.1136/bmj-2021-057212.
92. Veehof MM, Oskam MJ, Schreurs KMG, Bohlmeijer ET. Acceptance-based interventions for the treatment of chronic pain: a systematic review and meta-analysis. Pain. 2011;152(3):533–42. https://doi.org/10.1016/j.pain.2010.11.002.
93. Ma TW, Yuen ASK, Yang Z. The efficacy of acceptance and commitment therapy for chronic pain. Clin J Pain. 2023;39(3):147–57. https://doi.org/10.1097/AJP.0000000000001096.
94. Kim EH, Crouch TB, Olatunji BO. Adaptation of behavioral activation in the treatment of chronic pain. Psychother. 2017;54(3):237–44. https://doi.org/10.1037/pst0000112.
95. Turner JS, Leach DJ. Behavioural activation therapy: philosophy, concepts, and techniques. Behav Chang. 2012;29(2):77–96. https://doi.org/10.1017/bec.2012.3.
96. Walsh S, Moseley GL, Gray RJ, et al. Use of behavioural activation to manage pain: a systematic scoping review. BMJ Open. 2022;12(6):e056404. https://doi.org/10.1136/bmjopen-2021-056404.
97. Kabat-Zinn J. An outpatient program in behavioral medicine for chronic pain patients based on the practice of mindfulness meditation: theoretical considerations and preliminary results. Gen Hosp Psychiatry. 1982;4(1):33–47. https://doi.org/10.1016/0163-8343(82)90026-3.
98. Segal ZV, Williams JMG, Teasdale JD. Mindfulness-based cognitive therapy for depression: a new approach to preventing relapse. Guilford Press; 2002.
99. Linehan M. Cognitive-behavioral treatment of borderline personality disorder. Guilford Press; 1993.
100. Hilton L, Hempel S, Ewing BA, et al. Mindfulness meditation for chronic pain: systematic review and meta-analysis. Ann Behav Med. 2017;51(2):199–213. https://doi.org/10.1007/s12160-016-9844-2.
101. Paschali M, Lazaridou A, Sadora J, et al. Mindfulness-based interventions for chronic low back pain. Clin J Pain. 2024;40(2):105–13. https://doi.org/10.1097/AJP.0000000000001173.
102. Khoo EL, Small R, Cheng W, et al. Comparative evaluation of group-based mindfulness-based stress reduction and cognitive behavioural therapy for the treatment and management of chronic pain: a systematic review and network meta-analysis. Evid Based Ment Health. 2019;22(1):26–35. https://doi.org/10.1136/ebmental-2018-300062.
103. Cardle P, Kumar S, Leach M, McEvoy M, Veziari Y. Mindfulness and chronic musculoskeletal pain: an umbrella review. J Multidiscip Healthc. 2023;16:515–33. https://doi.org/10.2147/JMDH.S392375.
104. Ploesser M, Martin D. Mechanism of action of mindfulness-based interventions for pain relief—a systematic review. J Integr Complement Med. 2024;30(12):1162–78. https://doi.org/10.1089/jicm.2023.0328.
105. Neblett R. Surface electromyographic (SEMG) biofeedback for chronic low back pain. Healthcare. 2016;4(2):27. https://doi.org/10.3390/healthcare4020027.
106. Giggins OM, Persson U, Caulfield B. Biofeedback in rehabilitation. J Neuroeng Rehabil. 2013;10(1):60. https://doi.org/10.1186/1743-0003-10-60.
107. Sielski R, Rief W, Glombiewski JA. Efficacy of biofeedback in chronic back pain: a meta-analysis. Int J Behav Med. 2017;24(1):25–41. https://doi.org/10.1007/s12529-016-9572-9.
108. Calderone A, Mazzurco Masi VM, De Luca R, et al. The impact of biofeedback in enhancing chronic pain rehabilitation: a systematic review of mechanisms and outcomes. Heliyon. 2025;11(2):e41917. https://doi.org/10.1016/j.heliyon.2025.e41917.
109. Goessl VC, Curtiss JE, Hofmann SG. The effect of heart rate variability biofeedback training on stress and anxiety: a meta-analysis. Psychol Med. 2017;47(15):2578–86. https://doi.org/10.1017/S0033291717001003.
110. Lehrer PM, Gevirtz R. Heart rate variability biofeedback: how and why does it work? Front Psychol. 2014;5 https://doi.org/10.3389/fpsyg.2014.00756.
111. Lehrer P, Kaur K, Sharma A, et al. Heart rate variability biofeedback improves emotional and physical health and performance: a systematic review and meta analysis. Appl Psychophysiol Biofeedback. 2020;45(3):109–29. https://doi.org/10.1007/s10484-020-09466-z.
112. Jafari H, Courtois I, Van den Bergh O, Vlaeyen JWS, Van Diest I. Pain and respiration: a systematic review. Pain. 2017;158(6):995–1006. https://doi.org/10.1097/j.pain.0000000000000865.
113. Bunzli S, Smith A, Schütze R, O'Sullivan P. Beliefs underlying pain-related fear and how they evolve: a qualitative investigation in people with chronic back pain and high pain-related fear. BMJ Open. 2015;5(10):e008847. https://doi.org/10.1136/bmjopen-2015-008847.
114. Moseley GL. Reconceptualising pain according to modern pain science. Phys Ther Rev. 2007;12(3):169–78. https://doi.org/10.1179/108331907X223010.
115. Nijs J, Wijma AJ, Willaert W, et al. Integrating motivational interviewing in pain neuroscience education for people with chronic pain: a practical guide for clinicians. Phys Ther. 2020;100(5):846–59. https://doi.org/10.1093/ptj/pzaa021.
116. Tatikola SP, Natarajan V, Amaravadi SK, Desai VK, Asirvatham AR, Nagaraja R. Effect of pain neuroscience education+ (PNE+) in people with different mechanisms of chronic pain: a systematic review and meta-analysis. J Body Mov Ther. 2025;41:215–37. https://doi.org/10.1016/j.jbmt.2024.11.016.

117. Lepri B, Romani D, Storari L, Barbari V. Effectiveness of pain neuroscience education in patients with chronic musculoskeletal pain and central sensitization: a systematic review. Int J Environ Res Public Health. 2023;20(5):4098. https://doi.org/10.3390/ijerph20054098.
118. Siddall B, Ram A, Jones MD, Booth J, Perriman D, Summers SJ. Short-term impact of combining pain neuroscience education with exercise for chronic musculoskeletal pain: a systematic review and meta-analysis. Pain. 2022;163(1):e20–30. https://doi.org/10.1097/j.pain.0000000000002308.
119. Zhang Y, Yang C. Influence of pain neuroscience education and exercises for the management of neck pain: a meta-analysis of randomized controlled trials. Medicine. 2024;103(48):e40760. https://doi.org/10.1097/MD.0000000000040760.
120. Cuenca-Martínez F, Suso-Martí L, Calatayud J, et al. Pain neuroscience education in patients with chronic musculoskeletal pain: an umbrella review. Front Neurosci. 2023;17 https://doi.org/10.3389/fnins.2023.1272068.
121. Asmundson GJG, Katz J. Understanding the co-occurrence of anxiety disorders and chronic pain: state-of-the-art. Depress Anxiety. 2009;26(10):888–901. https://doi.org/10.1002/da.20600.
122. Linton SJ. A Transdiagnostic approach to pain and emotion. J Appl Biobehav Res. 2013;18(2):82–103. https://doi.org/10.1111/jabr.12007.
123. Koechlin H, Coakley R, Schechter N, Werner C, Kossowsky J. The role of emotion regulation in chronic pain: a systematic literature review. J Psychosom Res. 2018;107:38–45. https://doi.org/10.1016/j.jpsychores.2018.02.002.
124. Norman-Nott N, Hesam-Shariati N, Wewege MA, et al. Emotion regulation skills-focused interventions for chronic pain: a systematic review and meta-analysis. Eur J Pain. 2024;28(8):1276–93. https://doi.org/10.1002/ejp.2268.
125. Boersma K, Södermark M, Hesser H, Flink IK, Gerdle B, Linton SJ. Efficacy of a transdiagnostic emotion–focused exposure treatment for chronic pain patients with comorbid anxiety and depression: a randomized controlled trial. Pain. 2019;160(8):1708–18. https://doi.org/10.1097/j.pain.0000000000001575.
126. Lumley MA, Schubiner H. Emotional awareness and expression therapy for chronic pain: rationale, principles and techniques, evidence, and critical review. Curr Rheumatol Rep. 2019;21(7):30. https://doi.org/10.1007/s11926-019-0829-6.
127. Dimidjian S, Arch JJ, Schneider RL, Desormeau P, Felder JN, Segal ZV. Considering meta-analysis, meaning, and metaphor: a systematic review and critical examination of "third wave" cognitive and behavioral therapies. Behav Ther. 2016;47(6):886–905. https://doi.org/10.1016/j.beth.2016.07.002.
128. Feliu-Soler A, Cebolla A, McCracken LM, et al. Economic impact of third-wave cognitive behavioral therapies: a systematic review and quality assessment of economic evaluations in randomized controlled trials. Behav Ther. 2018;49(1):124–47. https://doi.org/10.1016/j.beth.2017.07.001.
129. Blasco-Belled A, Tejada-Gallardo C, Alsinet C. Positive psychology interventions can improve mental health for chronic pain patients: a systematic review and meta-analysis. Psychol Health. 2025;40(4):635–51. https://doi.org/10.1080/08870446.2023.2250382.
130. Braunwalder C, Müller R, Glisic M, Fekete C. Are positive psychology interventions efficacious in chronic pain treatment? A systematic review and meta-analysis of randomized controlled trials. Pain Med. 2022;23(1):122–36. https://doi.org/10.1093/pm/pnab247.
131. Iddon JE, Dickson JM, Unwin J. Positive psychological interventions and chronic non-cancer pain: a systematic review of the literature. Int J Appl Posit Psychol. 2016;1(1–3):133–57. https://doi.org/10.1007/s41042-016-0003-6.
132. Scascighini L, Toma V, Dober-Spielmann S, Sprott H. Multidisciplinary treatment for chronic pain: a systematic review of interventions and outcomes. Rheumatology. 2008;47(5):670–8. https://doi.org/10.1093/rheumatology/ken021.
133. Kealy D, Kongerslev MT. Structured group psychotherapies: advantages, challenges, and possibilities. J Clin Psychol. 2022;78(8):1559–66. https://doi.org/10.1002/jclp.23377.
134. Serrat M, Royuela-Colomer E, Auer W, et al. Effectiveness of the FIBROWALK multicomponent therapy in online and outdoor formats for fibromyalgia: a randomized controlled trial (The On&Out study). J Pain. Published online September. 2025;105514 https://doi.org/10.1016/j.jpain.2025.105514.
135. Baños RM, Herrero R, Vara MD. What is the current and future status of digital mental health interventions? Span J Psychol. 2022;25:e5. https://doi.org/10.1017/SJP.2022.2.
136. Beatty L, Lambert S. A systematic review of internet-based self-help therapeutic interventions to improve distress and disease-control among adults with chronic health conditions. Clin Psychol Rev. 2013;33(4):609–22. https://doi.org/10.1016/j.cpr.2013.03.004.
137. Gentili A, Failla G, Melnyk A, et al. The cost-effectiveness of digital health interventions: a systematic review of the literature. Front Public Health. 2022;10 https://doi.org/10.3389/fpubh.2022.787135.
138. Sanabria-Mazo JP, Colomer-Carbonell A, Borràs X, et al. Efficacy of videoconference group acceptance and commitment therapy (ACT) and behavioral activation therapy for depression (BATD) for chronic low back pain (CLBP) plus comorbid depressive symptoms: a randomized controlled trial (IMPACT study). J Pain. 2023;24(8):1522–40. https://doi.org/10.1016/j.jpain.2023.04.008.
139. Gendreau RM, LM MC, Williams DA, et al. Self-guided digital behavioural therapy versus active control for fibromyalgia (PROSPER-FM): a phase 3, multicentre, randomised controlled trial. Lancet. 2024;404(10450):364–74. https://doi.org/10.1016/S0140-6736(24)00909-7.
140. Goudman L, Jansen J, Billot M, et al. Virtual reality applications in chronic pain management: systematic review and meta-analysis. JMIR Serious Games. 2022;10(2):e34402. https://doi.org/10.2196/34402.
141. Matthie NS, Giordano NA, Jenerette CM, et al. Use and efficacy of virtual, augmented, or mixed reality technology for chronic pain: a systematic review. Pain Manag. 2022;12(7):859–78. https://doi.org/10.2217/pmt-2022-0030.
142. VanHouten LE, Greenway TS, Jin J. Stigma of seeking professional psychological help: a person-centered approach to stigma profiles among racially minoritized adults with chronic pain. Stigma Health. Published online January 13. 2025; https://doi.org/10.1037/sah0000615.
143. Kroenke K, Bair MJ, Damush TM, et al. Optimized antidepressant therapy and pain self-management in primary care patients with depression and musculoskeletal pain. JAMA. 2009;301(20):2099. https://doi.org/10.1001/jama.2009.723.
144. Wampold BE. The great psychotherapy debate. 2nd ed. Routledge; 2015. https://doi.org/10.4324/9780203582015.
145. Castaño-Asins JR, Barceló-Soler A, Royuela-Colomer E, et al. Effectiveness of peri-operative psychological interventions for the reduction of postsurgical pain intensity, depression, anxiety and pain catastrophising. Eur J Anaesthesiol. 2025; https://doi.org/10.1097/EJA.0000000000002157.
146. McCracken LM. Personalized pain management: is it time for process-based therapy for particular people with chronic pain? Eur J Pain. 2023;27(9):1044–55. https://doi.org/10.1002/ejp.2091.
147. Scholten S, Glombiewski JA. Enhancing psychological assessment and treatment of chronic pain: a research agenda for personalized and process-based approaches. Curr Opin Psychol. 2025;62:101958. https://doi.org/10.1016/j.copsyc.2024.101958.
148. Burns JW. Mechanisms in psychosocial treatments of chronic pain: what does the evidence tell us? Curr Opin Psychol. 2025;64:102050. https://doi.org/10.1016/j.copsyc.2025.102050.

149. Scholten S, Rubel JA, Glombiewski JA, Milde C. What time-varying network models based on functional analysis tell us about the course of a patient's problem. Psychother Res. 2025;35(4):637–55. https://doi.org/10.1080/10503307.2024.2328304.
150. Linton SJ, Flink IK, Vlaeyen JWS. Understanding the etiology of chronic pain from a psychological perspective. Phys Ther. 2018;98(5):315–24. https://doi.org/10.1093/ptj/pzy027.
151. Day MA, Ehde DM, Sterling M, Jensen MP. How therapist effects shape pain-related outcome improvement in psychological treatments for chronic pain. Curr Opin Psychol. 2025;62:101995. https://doi.org/10.1016/j.copsyc.2025.101995.
152. Theodore BR, Mayer TG, Gatchel RJ. Cost-effectiveness of early versus delayed functional restoration for chronic disabling occupational musculoskeletal disorders. J Occup Rehabil. 2015;25(2):303–15. https://doi.org/10.1007/s10926-014-9539-0.
153. Cleeland CS, Ryan KM. Pain assessment: global use of the brief pain inventory. Ann Acad Med Singap. 1994;23(2):129–38.
154. American Psychiatric Association. Diagnostic and statistical manual of mental disorders. 5th ed. American Psychiatric Association; 2013. https://doi.org/10.1176/appi.books.9780890425596.
155. World Health Organization (WHO). ICD-11: international classification of diseases. 11th ed. WHO; 2022.
156. Miller RP, Kori SH, Todd DD. The Tampa scale: a measure of Kinisophobia. Clin J Pain. 1991;7(1):51.
157. Brown KW, Ryan RM. Mindful attention awareness scale. PsycTESTS Dataset Preprint posted online September 12, 2011. https://doi.org/10.1037/t04259-000.
158. Murphy J, McKellar J, Raffa S, Clark M, Kerns R, Karlin B. Cognitive behavioral therapy for chronic pain among veterans: therapist manual. Department of Veterans Affairs; 2014.
159. Lai L, Liu Y, McCracken LM, Li Y, Ren Z. The efficacy of acceptance and commitment therapy for chronic pain: a three-level meta-analysis and a trial sequential analysis of randomized controlled trials. Behav Res Ther. 2023;165:104308. https://doi.org/10.1016/j.brat.2023.104308.
160. Bontinck J, Chys M, Coppieters I, Meeus M, Cagnie B. Exploration of somatosensory function of patients with acute nonspecific neck pain, through quantitative sensory testing and self-reported symptoms. Clin J Pain. 2023;39(8):377–85. https://doi.org/10.1097/AJP.0000000000001131.
161. Zhu M, Wong SY s, Zhong CC, et al. Which type and dosage of mindfulness-based interventions are most effective for chronic pain? A systematic review and network meta-analysis. J Psychosom Res. 2025;191:112061. https://doi.org/10.1016/j.jpsychores.2025.112061.
162. Gooding H, Stedmon J, Crix D. 'All these things don't take the pain away but they do help you to accept it': making the case for compassion-focused therapy in the management of persistent pain. Br J Pain. 2020;14(1):31–41. https://doi.org/10.1177/2049463719857099.
163. Millard LA, Wan MW, Smith DM, Wittkowski A. The effectiveness of compassion focused therapy with clinical populations: a systematic review and meta-analysis. J Affect Disord. 2023;326:168–92. https://doi.org/10.1016/j.jad.2023.01.010.
164. Barrett D, Brintz CE, Zaski AM, Edlund MJ. Dialectical pain management: feasibility of a hybrid third-wave cognitive behavioral therapy approach for adults receiving opioids for chronic pain. Pain Med. 2021;22(5):1080–94. https://doi.org/10.1093/pm/pnaa361.
165. Norman-Nott N, Briggs NE, Hesam-Shariati N, et al. Online dialectical behavioral therapy for emotion dysregulation in people with chronic pain. JAMA Netw Open. 2025;8(5):e256908. https://doi.org/10.1001/jamanetworkopen.2025.6908.
166. Kohlenberg RJ, Kanter JW, Bolling MY, Parker CR, Tsai M. Enhancing cognitive therapy for depression with functional analytic psychotherapy: treatment guidelines and empirical findings. Cogn Behav Pract. 2002;9(3):213–29. https://doi.org/10.1016/S1077-7229(02)80051-7.
167. Vandenberghe L. A functional analytic approach to group psychotherapy. Behav Anal Today. 2009;10(1):71–82. https://doi.org/10.1037/h0100665.
168. Mostafaie A, Zare H, Alipour A, Farzad VA. Compare the effectiveness of cognitive therapy based on meta-theoretical models and meta-cognitive therapy on pain and thought fusion in patients suffering from chronic pain. Health Psychol. 2018;7(25):35–55.
169. Wells A. Meta-cognition and worry: a cognitive model of generalized anxiety disorder. Behav Cogn Psychother. 1995;23(3):301–20. https://doi.org/10.1017/S1352465800015897.

Part V

Clinical Cases

Therapeutic Approaches with $Alpha_2$ Agonists

33

Elisabeth M. Wang and Matthew A. Wanat

Patient Presentation

Chief Complaint

"I tripped over a cord and fell down the stairs."

History of Present Illness

JS is a 76-year-old Caucasian female who presented to the emergency department 13 hours ago via EMS after reportedly tripping and falling down a flight of stairs in her home. She was found an hour later by her daughter, who called 911 immediately. Upon arrival, she was taken quickly to the operating room for a total right hip arthroplasty (THA). After the procedure, she was transferred to the intensive care unit (ICU) and is intubated and sedated.

Past Medical History

Hypertension and chronic obstructive pulmonary disease

Surgical History

Right THA (12 hours ago)

Family History

Mother: died 14 years ago—type 2 diabetes mellitus, hypertension, heart failure with reduced ejection fraction
Father: died from injuries in a car accident 19 years ago

E. M. Wang · M. A. Wanat (✉)
Department of Pharmacy Practice and Translational Research, The University of Houston College of Pharmacy, Houston, TX, USA
e-mail: MAWanat@uh.edu

Social History

Tobacco—none; alcohol—drinks socially with friends; illicit drug use—intravenous heroin (last known use is unknown)

Immunization History

Unknown

Allergies

No known drug allergies

Home Medications

- Losartan 25 mg PO daily
- Amlodipine 10 mg PO daily
- Hydrochlorothiazide 25 mg PO daily
- Albuterol (90 mcg/actuation) 2 inhalations every 4 hours PRN for shortness of breath
- Fluticasone furoate 100 mcg/umeclidinium 62.5 mcg/vilanterol 25 mcg, one inhalation daily

Current Medications

- Propofol continuous IV infusion 30 mcg/kg/min
- Fentanyl continuous IV infusion 75 mcg/hour
- Heparin 5000 units SQ q8h
- Pantoprazole 40 mg IV daily
- Lorazepam 1 mg IV q2h PRN agitation—1 dose received
- Low-dose insulin sliding scale protocol—no doses received
- Electrolyte replacement protocol—no doses received
- Cefazolin 2 g IV q8h × 3 doses (2 doses received)

J. P. Reinert et al. (eds.), *Adjunctive Analgesic Strategies for the Bedside Clinician and Beyond*,
https://doi.org/10.1007/978-3-032-21675-5_33

Physical Examination

Vital Signs

Tmax since admission: 99.3 °F; BP range: 130–150/80–90 mm Hg; HR range: 80–92 beats/min; Respiratory Rate (RR) 12 breaths/min; Ht 66 inches; 75 kg

General

Intubated and sedated female patient

HEENT

PERRLA; otherwise deferred

Pulmonary

Pressure control mode, pressure control of 10, PEEP of 8, FiO2 60%; CTAB

Cardiovascular

Normal sinus rhythm

Abdomen

Soft, non-tender, symmetrical, and without distention

Genitourinary

Foley catheter noted

Neurologic

Richmond Agitation and Sedation Scale (RASS): –1; CAM-ICU: negative; Care Pain Observation Tool (CPOT): 3

Extremities

Consistent skin color; right hip bandage CDI; RLE swelling; RLE tenderness; pulses 2+ bilaterally

Laboratory Findings

Na = 138 mEq/L	WBC = 8.4 × 10^3/mm^3	Ca = 10.1 mg/dL
K = 3.9 mEq/L	Hgb = 9.2 g/dL	Mg = 1.9 mg/dL
Cl = 98 mEq/L	Hct = 33%	Phos = 3.0 mg/dL
CO_2 = 24 mEq/L	Plt = 150 × 10^3/mm^3	AST = 20 IU/L
SCr = 1.3 mg/dL		ALS = 24 IU/L
BUN = 20 mg/dL		
Glucose = 178 mg/dL		

Learning Assessment Questions

1. Which screening tool indicates JS's pain is not adequately controlled?
   (a) Richmond Agitation and Sedation Scale (RASS)
   (b) Critical Care Pain Observation Tool (CPOT)
   (c) Confusion Assessment Method for the Intensive Care Unit (CAM-ICU)
   (d) Respiratory Rate (RR)

2. JS's family members inform the team that she has a history of opioid use disorder but has never been started on a medication for management. She is switched from propofol to intravenous dexmedetomidine, and the medical team asks if there is any risk with administering a bolus. What side effect would a patient be most likely to experience with a bolus of dexmedetomidine?
   (a) Hypermagnesemia
   (b) Hyponatremia
   (c) Tachycardia
   (d) Hypertension

3. While on therapy with dexmedetomidine, JS experiences bradycardia, which necessitates a dose reduction because of her hemodynamics. In addition to receiving the bolus dose previously, what risk factors were present in JS that may increase her risk of experiencing bradycardia while on dexmedetomidine?
   (a) Baseline chronic bradycardia as an outpatient
   (b) History of coronary artery disease
   (c) Concurrent use of other AV nodal blocking agents
   (d) Advanced age (> 75 years old)

4. Which of the following best explains the mechanism by which $alpha_2$ agonists help decrease opioid use requirements for pain?
   (a) $Alpha_2$ receptor activity at the spinal dorsal horn
   (b) $Alpha_{2B}$ receptor activity in the central nervous system
   (c) $Alpha_{2C}$ receptor activity on vascular smooth muscle to prevent shivering and subsequent pain
   (d) $Alpha_{2A}$ receptor activity causes a startle response, allowing for muscle contraction and breathing variation

5. The team wants to follow up with JS's family members by informing them that JS has a history of opioid misuse, but the patient is still intubated and sedated. What resources, in addition to family information, could be *most* useful to help determine the extent of JS's opioid use?
   (a) Check the state Prescription Drug Monitoring Program portal
   (b) Hold sedation to wake the patient up after a spontaneous breathing trial and determine her use
   (c) Call JS's outpatient pharmacy of record and ask them about her medication fill history
   (d) Check a urine drug screen to assess opioid use

6. After about 36 hours of dexmedetomidine administration, the team extubates JS. Since being taken off the fentanyl continuous infusion, she has been showing signs of opioid withdrawal, including tachycardia, agitation, and tremors. Which of the regimens would be the best option for JS, as buprenorphine is not available at this time?
   (a) Start oxycodone 10 mg PO q6h and oxycodone 5 mg q4h PRN breakthrough pain + continue dexmedetomidine.
   (b) Start oxycodone 10 mg PO q6h + continue dexmedetomidine
   (c) Start clonidine 0.1 mg q6h + wean off dexmedetomidine
   (d) Start ibuprofen 600 mg PO q8h + wean off dexmedetomidine

7. What about—JS is preparing to be discharged from the hospital after a five-day stay post THA. She has restarted her home medications and is receiving acetaminophen 1000 mg q8h for pain but still complains of some right hip pain. Her blood pressure is noted to range from 130–136/78–82 mm Hg after resuming her home medications. Which of the following therapy options would be appropriate to start for adjunct pain control in JS?
   (a) Ibuprofen 800 mg q8h PRN
   (b) Oxycodone 10 mg q8h PRN
   (c) Clonidine 0.1 mg q8h
   (d) Nothing at this time

8. Which of the following is TRUE regarding dosing adjustment considerations for alpha$_2$ agonists?
   (a) Tizanidine requires renal dosing adjustment
   (b) Dexmedetomidine requires hepatic dosing adjustment
   (c) Clonidine does not require renal dosing adjustment
   (d) Tizanidine has a major drug interaction with inhibitors of CYP2A6

Answers

1. B (Critical Care Observation Tool)
   Answer A is incorrect, as the RASS score is validated to assess sedation in critically ill patients. Answer C is incorrect, as the CAM-ICU score is used to assess critically ill patients for delirium. Respiratory rate could be one parameter to help indicate a patient is in pain, but it is not a screening tool, and this patient's RR is within normal limits. Answer B is correct, as the CPOT screening tool is validated to assess pain control in critically ill patients [1–4].

2. D (Hypertension)
   Answer D is correct, as higher dexmedetomidine plasma concentrations with an intravenous bolus can be associated with an increase in blood pressure. The mechanism is postulated to be secondary to peripheral vasoconstriction via alpha-2 receptor agonism in vascular smooth muscle cells. Answers A and B are incorrect, as it is not a commonly reported side effect of dexmedetomidine. Answer C is incorrect, as an IV bolus of dexmedetomidine is more likely to cause bradycardia [5, 6].

3. D (Advanced age)
   Answer D is correct. Advanced age is a risk factor for patients experiencing bradycardia and/or hypotension while on dexmedetomidine. Options A and B are risk factors for experiencing bradycardia but are not relevant or present in JS. Option C would increase the risk of bradycardia, but JS is not on any other agents that block the AV node [7–9].

4. A (Alpha2 receptor activity at the spinal dorsal horn)
   Answer A is correct. It is hypothesized that the analgesic effect of alpha-2 agonists is via activity at the spinal dorsal horn through inhibition of nociceptive neurons, as well as decreasing substance P release. Answers B and C are incorrect as alpha$_{2B}$ receptors are more commonly found in the vascular smooth muscle, while alpha$_{2A}$ and alpha$_{2C}$ receptors are mostly found in the central nervous system. Answer D is incorrect as it is the alpha$_{2C}$ receptor that can produce a startle response [5, 6, 9].

5. A (Check the state Prescription Drug Monitoring Program portal)
   Answer A is likely to be the most useful resource, as the PDMP will provide information on all controlled substance fills in the state database; however, this database would not include information on opioids obtained not from a community pharmacy. B is incorrect because it would be inappropriate to hold sedation to ask this question to the patient. C is incorrect because this option would only provide limited data, if the pharmacy provides the information at all, and would already be obtained by checking the PDMP. Answer D is incorrect because JS has already received opioids as part of her care plan during this hospitalization [10–12].

6. C (Start clonidine 0.1 mg q6h + wean off dexmedetomidine)
   Answers A and B are incorrect, as this patient has a history of opioid use disorder; initiating opioids in this patient could be harmful and would not address the

patient's opioid use disorder. Alternative agents to manage opioid use disorder are recommended. Answer D is incorrect, as ibuprofen should be used in combination with an agent (clonidine, buprenorphine, or methadone) that will manage the patient's opioid withdrawal symptoms. Answer C is correct, as clonidine is recommended in the setting of opioid withdrawal and can help bridge the patient off dexmedetomidine [13, 15].

7 C (Clonidine 0.1 mg q8h)
Ibuprofen would not be the best agent to start in this patient, as she is still hypertensive, and nonsteroidal anti-inflammatory agents can exacerbate hypertension (Answer A is incorrect). Oxycodone would not be the best option to initiate in this patient, as she has a history of opioid use disorder, and this medication could be harmful (Answer B is incorrect). Clonidine would be the best option for this patient, as it can help decrease this patient's pain and address her comorbidities of hypertension and opioid use disorder (Answer C is correct). Answer D is incorrect, as this patient is in pain, and something should be done to help address this [13, 15–17].

8. A (Tizanidine requires a renal dose adjustment)
Tizanidine requires both renal and hepatic dosing adjustments (Answer A is correct). Dexmedetomidine does not require renal dosing adjustments (Answer B is incorrect). Clonidine does require renal dosing adjustment with lower doses recommended in patients with an estimated glomerular filtration rate < 30 mL/min/1.73m^2. Tizanidine has a major drug-drug interaction with concurrent CYP1A2 inhibitors such as ciprofloxacin [5, 6, 9, 14, 15].

References

1. Sessler CN, Gosnell MS, Grap MJ, et al. The Richmod agitation-sedation scale: validity and reliability in adult intensive care unit patients. Am J Respir Crit Care Med. 2002;166(10):1338–44. https://doi.org/10.1164/rccm.2107138.
2. Ely EW, Margolin R, Francis J, et al. Evaluation of delirium in critically ill patients: validation of the Confusion Assessment Method for the Intensive Care Unit (CAM-ICU). Crit Care Med. 2001;29(7):1370–9. https://doi.org/10.1097/00003246-200107000-00012.
3. Tousignant-Laflamme Y, Bourgault P, Gelinas C, Marchand S. Assessing pain behaviors in healthy subjects using the Critical-Care Pain Observation Tool (CPOT): a pilot study. J Pain. 2010;11(10):983–7. https://doi.org/10.1016/j.jpain.2010.01.266.
4. Gelinas C, Johnston C. Pain assessment in the critically ill ventilated adult: validation of the critical-care pain observation tool and physiologic indicators. Clin J Pain. 2007;23(6):497–505. https://doi.org/10.1097/AJP.0b013e31806a23fb.
5. Weerink MAS, Struys MMRF, Hannivoort LN, Barends CRM, Absalom AR, Colin P. Clinical pharmacokinetics and pharmacodynamics of dexmedetomidine. Clin Pharmacokinet. 2017;56(8):893–913.
6. Dexmedetomidine. Lexi-Drugs. UpToDate Lexidrug. UpToDate Inc. https://online.lexi.com. Accessed 28 May 2025.
7. Ice CJ, Personett HA, Frazee EN, Dierkhising RA, Kashyap R, Oeckler RA. Risk factors for dexmedetomidine-associated hemodynamic instability in noncardiac intensive care unit patients. Anesth Analg. 2016;122(2):462–9.
8. Guinter JR, Kristeller JL. Prolonged infusions of dexmedetomidine in critically ill patients. Am J Health Syst Pharm. 2010;67(15):1246–53. https://doi.org/10.2146/ajhp090300.
9. Giovannitti JA Jr, Thoms SM, Crawford JJ. Alpha-2 adrenergic receptor agonists: a review of current clinical applications. Anesth Prog. 2015;62(1):31–9. https://doi.org/10.2344/0003-3006-62.1.31.
10. Dowell D, Ragan KR, Jones CM, Baldwin GT, Chou R. CDC clinical practice guideline for prescribing opioids for pain — United States, 2022. MMWR Recomm Rep. 2022;71(RR-3):1–95.
11. Haegerich TM, Jones CM, Cote PO, Robinson A, Ross L. Evidence for state, community and systems-level prevention strategies to address the opioid crisis. Drug Alcohol Depend. 2019;204:107563.
12. The ASAM national practice guideline for the treatment of opioid use disorder: 2020 focused update. J Addict Med. 2020;14(2S Suppl 1):1–91.
13. Bhatt K, Thompson Quan A, Baumgartner L, Jia S, Croci R, Puntillo K, et al. Effects of a clonidine taper on dexmedetomidine use and withdrawal in adult critically ill patients—a pilot study. Crit Care Explor. 2020;2(11):e0245.
14. Tizanidine. Lexi-Drugs. UpToDate Lexidrug. UpToDate Inc. https://online.lexi.com. Accessed 28 May 2025.
15. Clonidine. Lexi-Drugs. UpToDate Lexidrug. UpToDate Inc. https://online.lexi.com. Accessed 28 May 2025.
16. Ibuprofen. Lexi-Drugs. UpToDate Lexidrug. UpToDate Inc. https://online.lexi.com. Accessed 5 June 2025.
17. Oxycodone. Lexi-Drugs. UpToDate Lexidrug. UpToDate Inc. https://online.lexi.com. Accessed 5 June 2025.

34 Addressing Barriers to Care

Faith S. Wellings

Patient Presentation

Chief Complaint
Severe low back pain and immobility.

History of Present Illness
JP is a 47-year-old Hispanic-American male who presents to the emergency department for the third time this month with severe low back pain and is "barely able to get out of bed." JP relates that he has been dealing with back pain for many years, but it has worsened recently. He experiences occasional pain and/or numbness and tingling radiating down his legs. Other than rest and lying in bed, he has not found anything else that relieves the pain. He does not routinely see his primary care provider and mentions that his provider is "tired of hearing about my back and hasn't given me anything that helps. They suggested physical therapy, but I can't afford the copay, and my insurance only covers so many sessions anyway."

Past Medical History
Back injury after a fall from a ladder 15 years ago, hypertension, and obesity.

Surgical History
L4–L5 Discectomy 3 years ago.

Family History
Noncontributory.

Social History
JP lives approximately 1 h away in a small town with his wife and four children and is self-employed as a building contractor. Occasionally drinks 1–2 beers on weekends; history of opioid use disorder currently in remission. Quit using smokeless tobacco 20 years ago.

Allergies
Ibuprofen ("tears up my stomach").

Home Medications
Amlodipine 10 mg orally daily, buprenorphine 16 mg/naloxone 4 mg once daily.

Physical Examination

Vital Signs
BP 144/80 mmHg, HR 78 bpm, RR 16 breaths/minute, afebrile, SpO2 98% on room air.
Ht: 175 cm Wt: 105 kg.

General
Flat affect and occasional wincing upon movement.

HEENT
Normocephalic and atraumatic, mucous membranes are moist, PERRLA.

Pulmonary
No tachypnea; no wheezing, rales, or rhonchi.

Cardiovascular
Regular rate and rhythm, no murmurs, rubs, or gallops.

Abdomen
Soft, non-tender, no distention, active bowel sounds.

Genitourinary
Deferred, the patient denies any urinary symptoms or incontinence.

F. S. Wellings (✉)
Wilkes University, Wilkes-Barre, PA, USA
e-mail: faith.wellings@wilkes.edu

J. P. Reinert et al. (eds.), *Adjunctive Analgesic Strategies for the Bedside Clinician and Beyond*,
https://doi.org/10.1007/978-3-032-21675-5_34

Neurologic

Alert and oriented. Diminished patellar reflex and diminished sensation on the medial aspect of the right thigh. Positive straight leg raise test.

Extremities

No edema, skin is warm, dry, and intact. Right foot drop is present.

Laboratory Findings

Na = 137 mg/dL	WBC = 9.1 × 10^3/mm^3	Ca = 8.9 mg/dL
K = 3.9 mEq/L	RBC = 4.2 × 10^6/mm^3	Mg = 1.9 mg/dL
Cl = 102 mEq/L	Hgb = 13.1 g/dL	Phos = 2.8 mg/dL
CO_2 = 23 mEq/L	Hct = 39%	AST = 42 IU/L
BUN = 20 mg/dL	Plt = 275 × 10^3/mm^3	ALT = 25 IU/L
SCr = 1.1 mg/dL		Albumin = 3.5 g/dL
Glucose = 97 mg/dL		

Questions

1. Which of the following is true concerning biases and stigmas that may affect JP's care?
   A. Men are more often referred for psychotherapy, while women are more likely to be prescribed analgesics when reporting the same type of pain.
   B. People with racial and ethnic minority backgrounds are often prescribed higher analgesic doses.
   C. People with a history of substance use disorder (SUD) may avoid seeking care because of the stigma associated with the use of SUD medications.
   D. Complementary and integrative medicine approaches are often overutilized, related to provider beliefs about the risks of opioids.
2. Which social determinants of health (SDoH) domain(s) are most relevant for JP?
   A. Economic stability, healthcare access and quality.
   B. Education access and quality, and social and community context.
   C. Neighborhood and built environment.
   D. Health-related quality of life.
3. Which of the following could help improve health outcomes for JP?
   A. Using mobile health (mHealth) applications for education, monitoring, or treatment.
   B. Streamlining all of JP's care so it is provided by his PCP to ensure continuity.
   C. Linking JP's PCP with tele-education led by specialists at academic medical centers.
   D. A and C.
   E. All of the above.
4. What is the most appropriate statement to use when engaging in empathetic communication and building trust with JP?
   A. "You've got this!"
   B. "I understand."
   C. "You're too young to have this much pain!"
   D. "We will work hard to get you the support that you need."
5. Which of the following represents a method to reduce communication barriers related to JP's care?
   A. Actively listening and using appropriate terminology based on health literacy level.
   B. Documenting in the chart that the patient is refusing physical therapy.
   C. Using a phone translation application or Language Line for patient interactions.
   D. All of the above.
6. Which of the following could help improve JP's engagement with managing his pain?
   A. Decision-making guided by hospital policy.
   B. Setting physical goals based on published research.
   C. Gathering patient history using a checkbox form.
   D. Motivational interviewing and action planning.
7. Which of the following elements of the healthcare system could present barriers to optimal pain management in this case?
   A. An open health system formulary.
   B. Insurance coverage caps for non-pharmacologic therapies.
   C. Electronic health record interoperability.
   D. Opioid overdose risk.
8. What strategies could be employed to improve interdisciplinary healthcare team member collaboration when handling complex pain management scenarios?
   A. Tracking adherence to guidelines through medication use evaluations.
   B. Conducting patient satisfaction surveys and sharing results throughout the organization.
   C. Training on situational awareness, emotional regulation, and partnership building.
   D. Encouraging team members to focus on their role and let coworkers focus on their job.

Answers

1. *Correct answer: C*

Rationale: People with a history of substance use disorder (SUD) may avoid seeking care because of the stigma associated with the use of SUD medications [25]. It has been found that men are more likely to be judged to benefit from analgesics, while women are more often recommended for psychotherapy [21, 29]. Research has shown that those from racial and ethnic minority backgrounds are less likely to receive adequate pain treatment and are prescribed pain medications at lower rates and lower doses compared to White patients [13]. Complementary and integrative medicine approaches are often underutilized [16]; this may be related to provider concerns about a lack of high-quality evidence supporting their effectiveness [18].

2. *Correct answer: A*

Rationale: Comprehensive SDoH screening using an appropriate tool is recommended. Given the information provided, the best answer choice is economic stability and healthcare access and quality due to the patient's concerns about affording treatment and the significant distance he may need to travel for services due to living in a distant rural area, both of which represent significant barriers to care [1]. Neighborhood and built environment (answer choice C) could also play a role when considering his work environment in construction, which has significant physical demands and risk of injury and exacerbation of chronic pain [9, 28]; however, this was not the most comprehensive answer. Education access and quality and social and community context should be considered but may not be the highest priority at this time. Health-related quality of life, while significantly influenced by SDoH, is not a social determinant of the health domain itself.

3. *Correct answer: D*

Rationale: Mobile health applications, telehealth visits, provider tele-education, and co-managing patients with experts remotely are beneficial in overcoming barriers to accessing health care and may improve health outcomes. [15, 24, 30]. Consultation with an interdisciplinary pain medicine team and specialists in the management of underlying disease states contributing to pain is recommended whenever possible [25].

4. *Correct answer: D*

Rationale: Physician empathy is correlated with patient trust and has a significant positive impact on outcomes, including pain scores and quality of life [3, 27]. Empathy can be cultivated through healthcare professional training and assessed via several available assessment scales [10, 14, 20, 22, 23]. Affirming statements [17] can help build trust, while invalidating statements may erode patient trust in healthcare providers. Common phrases can unintentionally make others feel unheard, isolated, and/or misunderstood.

5. *Correct answer: A*

Rationale: Actively listening can help build trust and facilitate collaboration between patients and healthcare providers [7, 26]. Using plain language, being specific, and limiting information to key points is recommended based on health literacy and patient education literature [19]. Accurate and unbiased chart documentation is critical in avoiding perpetuation of bias, which could affect future pain management by other providers [6]. Answer choice B exemplifies inaccurate documentation and how future care could be negatively impacted by biased language. Using a phone translation application or Language Line is recommended to help prevent miscommunication and misunderstandings when providing care to individuals with limited English proficiency. The case does not provide enough information to suggest that translation services would be required for this patient, but an assessment should be made to determine if such services may be needed.

6. *Correct answer: D*

Rationale: Motivational interviewing and action planning are ways of encouraging patient autonomy and supporting self-management. Encouraging autonomy has been shown to have a significant effect on pain management behavior [12]. Shared decision-making involves clinicians and patients coming together to discuss the best available practices and consider patient values and preferences when determining a treatment plan [5]. The patient's expectations and goals are key elements of the discussion. Decisions should not be based solely on hospital policy, although policies can help ensure safe and effective treatment. Likewise, published literature should be evaluated, and evidence-based therapies should be utilized whenever appropriate, but patient-centered goals (which may extend beyond physical capabilities) are important. Research has shown that patients often have more to say than what is covered on standardized forms [11].

7. *Correct answer: B*

Rationale: Insurance coverage caps for non-pharmacologic therapies are the most relevant concern for JP, as he expressed frustration regarding the cost and limitation on physical therapy visits. Insurance plans may have coverage restrictions on non-pharmacological treatments (e.g., physical therapy, acupuncture, or cognitive-behavioral therapy), despite evidence supporting their efficacy [2, 8]. An open formulary indicates that the availability of medications is less restricted (vs. a closed formulary, where only specific medications are available/covered, or prior approval may be needed for certain therapies). Electronic health record (EHR) interoperability (i.e., the ability for different EHR systems to exchange data) would theoretically improve communication between healthcare entities/providers, which could have a positive impact on patient management. Opioid overdose risk, although relevant to care decisions, is not an element of the healthcare system.

8. *Correct answer: C*

Rationale: Situational awareness, emotional regulation, and partnership-building trainings are a way to mitigate biases and stigmas, which allows for the development of a team that maintains shared values and respect as core competencies [4, 31]. Tracking adherence to guidelines through medication use evaluations, conducting patient satisfaction surveys, and sharing results throughout the organization, although potentially valuable for assessing healthcare quality and outcomes, are not specifically targeted toward improving healthcare team collaboration (although targeted intervention could arise from the findings). The Interprofessional Education Collaborative (IPEC) Core Competencies for Interprofessional Collaborative Practice include using the "knowledge of one's own role and team members' expertise to address individual and population health outcomes" and applying the "values and principles of the science of teamwork to adapt one's own role in a variety of team settings" rather than remaining siloed in individual roles [31].

A review of content covered in this case may be found in Chap. 26.

References

1. Baker MB, Liu EC, Bully MA, Hsieh A, Nozari A, Tuler M, Binda DD. Overcoming barriers: a comprehensive review of chronic pain management and accessibility challenges in rural America. Healthcare (Basel). 2024;12(17):1765. https://doi.org/10.3390/healthcare12171765.
2. Candon M, Nielsen A, Dusek JA. Trends in insurance coverage for acupuncture, 2010–2019. JAMA Netw Open. 2022;5(1):e2142509. https://doi.org/10.1001/jamanetworkopen.2021.42509.
3. Canovas L, Carrascosa AJ, Garcia M, et al. Impact of empathy in the patient-doctor relationship on chronic pain relief and quality of life: a prospective study in Spanish pain clinics. Pain Med. 2018;19:1304–14.
4. Cascella LM. Improving health equity and addressing bias in pain management. MedPro Group; n.d. Accessed from: https://www.medpro.com/bias-pain-management#:~:text=Some%20strategies%20that%20have%20been%20recommended%20at%20the%20provider%20level,can%20affect%20thinking%20and%20reasoning.
5. Elwyn G, Coulter A, Laitner S, Walker E, Watson P, Thomson R. Implementing shared decision making in the NHS. BMJ. 2010;341:c5146. https://doi.org/10.1136/bmj.c5146.
6. Goddu AP, O'Conor KJ, Lanzkron S, et al. Do words matter? Stigmatizing language and the transmission of bias in the medical record. J Gen Intern Med. 2018;33(5):685–91.
7. Haverfield MC, Giannitrapani K, Timko C, Lorenz K. Patient-centered pain management communication from the patient perspective. J Gen Intern Med. 2018;33(8):1374–80. https://doi.org/10.1007/s11606-018-4490-y.
8. Heyward J, Jones C, Compton W. Coverage of nonpharmacologic treatments for low back pain among US public and private insurers. JAMA Netw Open. 2018;1(6):e183044. https://jamanetwork.com/journals/jamanetworkopen/fullarticle/2705853.
9. Hurwitz EL, Randhawa K, Torres P, et al. The global spine care initiative: a systematic review of individual and community-based burden of spinal disorders in rural populations in low- and middle-income communities. Eur Spine J. 2018;27(Suppl 6):802–15. https://doi.org/10.1007/s00586-017-5393-z.
10. Kelm Z, Womer J, Walter JK, Feudtner C. Interventions to cultivate physician empathy: a systematic review. BMC Med Educ. 2014;14:219–30.
11. Kilborn K, Sommer JL, Reynolds K, Roy R, El-Gabalawy R. The need to say more: a qualitative analysis of added free text to chronic pain patient intake packages. Pain Manag Nurs. 2023;24(2):201–8.
12. Kim R, Kim A. A structural equation model for low Back pain management behavior in patients with spinal disease. Pain Manag Nurs. 2024;26(1):e107–15. https://doi.org/10.1016/j.pmn.2024.10.018.
13. Meghani SH, Byun E, Gallagher RM. Time to take stock: a meta-analysis and systematic review of analgesic treatment disparities for pain in the United States. Pain Med. 2012;13(2):150–74.
14. Miller SR. A curriculum focused on informed empathy improves attitudes toward persons with disabilities. Perspect Med Educ. 2013;2(3):114–25. https://doi.org/10.1007/S40037-013-0046-3.
15. Moreno-Ligero M, Moral-Munoz JA, Salazar A, Failde I. mHealth intervention for improving pain, quality of life, and functional disability in patients with chronic pain: systematic review. JMIR Mhealth Uhealth. 2023;11:e40844. https://doi.org/10.2196/40844.
16. Nahin RL, Rhee A, Stussman B. Use of complementary health approaches overall and for pain management by US adults. JAMA. 2024;331(7):613–5. https://doi.org/10.1001/jama.2023.26775.
17. National Center for Ethics in Health Care Goals of Care Conversations Skills Training for Clinicians. Empathetic responses handout. 2018. Updated June 2018. Retrieved from U.S. Department of Veterans Affairs website: https://www.ethics.va.gov/GoCC.asp. Accessed 20 Jun 2025.
18. Ng JY, Li SY, Cramer H. Perceptions and attitudes regarding complementary, alternative, and integrative medicine among published neurology authors: a large-scale, international cross-sectional survey. BMC Neurol. 2024;24(1):215. https://doi.org/10.1186/s12883-024-03661-9.
19. Oosterhaven J, Pell CD, Schröder CD, et al. Health literacy and pain neuroscience education in an interdisciplinary pain management programme: a qualitative study of patient perspectives. Pain Rep. 2023;8(6):e1093. Published 2023 Oct 18. https://doi.org/10.1097/PR9.0000000000001093.
20. Ratka A. Empathy and the development of affective skills. Am J Pharm Educ. 2018;82(10):1140–3. https://doi.org/10.5688/ajpe7192.
21. Samulowitz A, Gremyr I, Eriksson E, Hensing G. "Brave men" and "emotional women": a theory-guided literature review on gender bias in health care and gendered norms towards patients with chronic pain. Pain Res Manag. 2018;2018:6358624. https://doi.org/10.1155/2018/6358624.
22. Stepien KA, Baernstein A. Educating for empathy: a review. J Gen Intern Med. 2006;21(5):524–30.
23. Sulzer SH, Feinstein NW, Wendland CL. Assessing empathy development in medical education: a systematic review. Med Educ. 2016;50(3):300–10. https://doi.org/10.1111/medu.12806.
24. Thies KM, Anderson D, Beals-Reid C. Project ECHO chronic pain: a qualitative analysis of recommendations by expert faculty and the process of knowledge translation. J Contin Educ Health Prof. 2019;39(3):194–200. https://doi.org/10.1097/CEH.0000000000000264.
25. U.S. Department of Health and Human Services. Pain management best practices Inter-Agency Task Force. 2019. Report: Updates, Gaps, Inconsistencies, and Recommendations. Retrieved from U.S. Department of Health and Human. Services website: https://www.hhs.gov/ash/advisory-committees/pain/reports/index.html.

26. Wiering B, de Boer D, Krol M, Wieberneit-Tolman H, Delnoij D. Entertaining accurate treatment expectations while suffering from chronic pain: an exploration of treatment expectations and the relationship with patient-provider communication. BMC Health Serv Res. 2018;18(1):706. https://doi.org/10.1186/s12913-018-3497-8.
27. Wu Q, Jin Z, Wang P. The relationship between the physician-patient relationship, physician empathy, and patient trust. J Gen Intern Med. 2022;37(6):1388–93. https://doi.org/10.1007/s11606-021-07008-9.
28. Yap ZL, Summers SJ, Grant AR, Moseley GL, Karran EL. The role of the social determinants of health in outcomes of surgery for low back pain: a systematic review and narrative synthesis. Spine J. 2022;22(5):793–809. https://doi.org/10.1016/j.spinee.2021.11.013.
29. Zhang L, Losin EAR, Ashar YK, Koban L, Wager TD. Gender biases in estimation of others' pain. J Pain. 2021;22(9):1048–59. https://doi.org/10.1016/j.jpain.2021.03.001.
30. Zhou C, Crawford A, Serhal E, Kurdyak P, et al. MHPE. The impact of project ECHO on participant and patient outcomes: a systematic review. Acad Med. 2016;91(10):1439–61. https://doi.org/10.1097/ACM.0000000000001328.
31. Zorek JA, Ragucci K, McKearney S, et al. IPEC Core Competencies for Interprofessional Collaborative Practice:Version 3. 2023. Available at: https://www.ipecollaborative.org/. Accessed 20 June 2025.

Case Studies in Art Therapy

35

Giustino Varrassi, Alberto Corriero, Giacomo Farì, Christopher Gharibo, Alena Javurkova, Matteo Luigi Giuseppe Leoni, Filomena Puntillo, and Jaroslava Raudenska

Case Study: Sarah—Chronic Pain and Identity Reconstruction

Patient Profile

- *Name*: Sarah
- *Age*: 42
- *Condition*: Fibromyalgia and chronic fatigue syndrome
- *Setting*: Outpatient rehabilitation clinic

Presenting Issue

Sarah was referred to art therapy after years of struggling with diffuse, persistent pain that had not responded well to pharmacological treatment. Her pain was accompanied by depression and a sense of loss around her career and active lifestyle. She described herself as "a shadow of who I used to be."

Therapeutic Approach

Sarah engaged in a 10-week individual art therapy program. Early sessions focused on body mapping, where she drew outlines of her body and used color and symbols to mark areas of pain, numbness, and emotion. This helped externalize her internal state and facilitated conversations with her physician about her pain distribution. Later sessions introduced narrative collage, where she pieced together images representing her pre-illness self, her current state, and a future she hoped to move toward. Creating these collages helped Sarah articulate her grief and begin to reframe her identity, not just as a person with chronic pain, but as someone still capable of growth and creativity.

Outcome

By the end of the program, Sarah reported a noticeable decrease in her pain-related anxiety and an increased sense of agency. While her physical symptoms remained, she said, "I no longer feel like I'm fighting myself. I'm making room for who I am now."

Case Vignette: Malik—Postoperative Pain in a Pediatric Setting

Patient Profile

- *Name*: Malik
- *Age*: 8
- *Condition*: Recovery from appendectomy
- *Setting*: Pediatric hospital inpatient unit

Presenting Issue

Malik was recovering well medically, but his care team noted high anxiety, uncooperative behavior during wound care, and refusal to speak. He cried whenever staff approached and clutched his abdomen protectively.

G. Varrassi (✉)
Fondazione Paolo Procacci, Rome, Italy

A. Corriero · F. Puntillo
Department of Interdisciplinary Medicine, ICU Section, University of Bari Aldo Moro, Bari, Italy

G. Farì
Department of Experimental Medicine, University of Salento, Lecce, Italy

C. Gharibo
Department of Pain Management, NYU Langone Health, New York, NY, USA

A. Javurkova
Department of Clinical Psychology, University Hospital Kralovske Vinohrady and 3rd Faculty of Medicine, Prague, Czech Republic

M. L. G. Leoni
Department of Medical and Surgical Sciences and Translational Medicine, Sapienza University of Rome, Rome, Italy

J. Raudenska
Department of Nursing, 2nd Faculty of Medicine, Charles University, Prague, Czech Republic

J. P. Reinert et al. (eds.), *Adjunctive Analgesic Strategies for the Bedside Clinician and Beyond*, https://doi.org/10.1007/978-3-032-21675-5_35

Therapeutic Approach
An art therapist visited Malik's room and offered him paper, markers, and stickers. Initially hesitant, Malik began by scribbling angrily. The therapist encouraged him to draw "what the pain looked like," and Malik drew a red monster with sharp teeth. Over time, he added armor to the monster, then a superhero fighting it. This activity evolved into a comic strip in which Malik, as the superhero, defeats the pain monster. In the process, he began speaking about his fear of "the cut" and "people touching me."

Outcome
Following these sessions, Malik became more compliant with dressing changes and verbalized his fears to both the therapist and nurses. His pain ratings decreased, and he became more relaxed during procedures. His mother noted, "It was like he needed a way to say what was happening without using words."

Case Study: Elena—Psychosomatic Pain and Trauma

Patient Profile
- *Name*: Elena
- *Age*: 29
- *Condition*: Unexplained pelvic pain
- *Setting*: Trauma-informed outpatient clinic

Presenting Issue
Elena had visited multiple specialists for chronic pelvic pain that had no clear medical explanation. During her intake, she revealed a history of childhood sexual abuse but had never engaged in therapy.

Therapeutic Approach
Elena's art therapy began with nonthreatening materials like watercolors and soft pastels. Over time, she gravitated toward clay, which allowed her to work with tactile sensations safely. Her therapist used trauma-informed approaches, including grounding exercises and choice-based directives, to ensure emotional safety. Through the creation of abstract sculptures, Elena explored themes of protection, shame, and release. One pivotal session involved sculpting a "shell" with cracks in it that, she said, "held the pain but let it breathe."

Outcome
While Elena's physical pain persisted intermittently, her panic episodes and dissociation decreased significantly. She described feeling "less trapped in my body" and began individual trauma counseling alongside continued art therapy. This case illustrated the complex interface of trauma, somatic pain, and creative healing.

Case Vignette: Thomas—Pain and Loss at End of Life

Patient Profile
- *Name*: Thomas
- *Age*: 71
- *Condition*: Advanced pancreatic cancer
- *Setting*: Hospice

Presenting Issue
Thomas was in palliative care, receiving opioids for intense pain. He expressed regret about his estranged relationship with his son and anxiety about death. He had stopped participating in most activities.

Therapeutic Approach
An art therapist visited with watercolors and asked if Thomas would like to paint anything from memory. He painted a landscape of a lake where he used to fish with his son. This opened a conversation about reconciliation and legacy. Over several sessions, Thomas created a memory box with photos, letters, and small objects for his son. He dictated a letter and asked the therapist to help him transcribe and decorate it. His physical engagement was limited, but his emotional energy increased during sessions.

Outcome
Thomas's pain perception diminished during art-making. He described the sessions as "a peaceful time" and was able to deliver the box to his son before he passed. Hospice staff noted a marked improvement in his mood and spiritual peace.

Composite Case: Group Art Therapy for Women with Migraines

Group Composition
- 6 women aged 25–55
- All were diagnosed with chronic migraines
- Weekly 90-min art therapy sessions for 8 weeks
- Setting: Community health center

Themes and Process

The group used metaphoric imagery to describe their pain, such as "tight coils," "dark spirals," and "exploding suns." Through painting, collage, and mixed media, participants shared their migraine experiences and coping strategies. Sessions incorporated guided imagery, journaling, and group reflection. One particularly impactful activity was the creation of "pain masks" representing how they appear on the outside versus how they feel internally. This fostered empathy and mutual support.

Outcome

At the end of the program, participants reported improved pain tolerance, reduced anxiety, and a stronger sense of community. One participant said, "This group gave my pain a voice and made me feel less alone."

Clinical Reflections

These cases underscore the unique role of art therapy in pain management. The creative process offers a symbolic and safe distance from pain, making it more approachable. Art therapy engages the full spectrum of pain—physical, emotional, and existential—while offering a powerful outlet when words fall short. Crucially, it empowers patients by allowing them to choose materials, symbols, and personal narratives, restoring a sense of agency. Every pain experience is deeply individual, and art therapy honors this uniqueness. Healing emerges not through prescription, but through discovery, one image, symbol, or brushstroke at a time. Group art therapy has been increasingly recognized in peer-reviewed literature for its multifaceted benefits across diverse populations. Recent studies highlight its efficacy in enhancing emotional well-being, fostering social connections, and providing a supportive environment for self-expression [1, 2]. Considering the multiplicity of factors involved in the development of chronic pain [3], the application of art as a support to therapy proves useful in the majority of patients resistant to conventional therapies.

References

1. Aydın M, Kutlu FY. The effect of group art therapy on loneliness and hopelessness levels of older adults living alone: a randomized controlled study. Florence Nightingale J Nurs. 2021;29(3):271–84. https://doi.org/10.5152/FNJN.2021.20224.
2. Yin Y, Ko KS. The effect of group art therapy on acculturative and academic stress of Chinese graduate students in South Korea. Front Psychol. 2023;14:1179778. https://doi.org/10.3389/fpsyg.2023.1179778.
3. Moncada MAA, Tamayo MAN, Encinas MAN, Leoni MLG, Varrassi G. Immuno-Inflammatory Mechanisms in the Chronification of Pain. Pain Ther. 2026 Mar 7. https://doi.org/10.1007/s40122-026-00818-x.

36 Adherence Case Studies

Brian Tasma, Marilee Clemons, Derek Gyori, and Sarah Aldrich Renner

Case 1

Patient Presentation

Chief Complaint
Establishing primary care.

History of Present Illness
A 38-year-old female establishing care in the office with a history of chronic low back pain s/p motor vehicle accident 15 years ago. She reports most recently filling her prescriptions 2 weeks ago for a 4-week supply, but she did not bring her bottles to the office. She reports difficulty affording her medications and traveling to and from appointments, as she shares a car with her roommate. She tried physical therapy about 14 years ago, shortly after a car accident, but did not continue due to challenges with transportation and insurance coverage. She would like to return to physical therapy if she can afford it and obtain transportation. She tries to stay active and walk daily, but this is often limited by her pain. She looked into exercise options near her and did not find anything affordable within walking distance. A previous provider prescribed lidocaine 4% topical patches, but they were too expensive, and she did not try them.

B. Tasma
General Internal Medicine, University of Toledo College of Medicine and Life Sciences, Toledo, OH, USA

M. Clemons
Pharmacy Services, UToledo Health, Toledo, OH, USA

D. Gyori
Pharmacy Services, VA Ann Arbor Healthcare System, Ann Arbor, MI, USA

S. A. Renner (✉)
General Internal Medicine & Pharmacy Practice, University of Toledo College of Pharmacy and Pharmaceutical Sciences, Toledo, OH, USA
e-mail: sarah.aldrich2@utoledo.edu

Past Medical History

- Chronic lumbar radiculopathy
- Rheumatoid arthritis

Surgical History
Cholecystectomy 5 years ago.

Family History
Noncontributory.

Social History
Moved across the state 1 week ago, changed jobs, and has a new insurance policy. Is a never-smoker. Denies any recent alcohol use. Denies any history of illicit drug use.

Immunization History

- Up-to-date.

Allergies

- No known drug allergies.

Home Medications

- Oxycodone/acetaminophen 5 mg/325 mg, 1 tablet by mouth every 8 hours as needed for back pain.
- Methotrexate 7.5 mg, 1 tablet by mouth weekly.
- Abatacept 125 mcg injected subcutaneously once weekly.

J. P. Reinert et al. (eds.), *Adjunctive Analgesic Strategies for the Bedside Clinician and Beyond*,
https://doi.org/10.1007/978-3-032-21675-5_36

Physical Examination

Vital Signs

- BMI: 28 kg/m^2
- Weight: 150 pounds
- Temperature: 98.4 °F
- Blood Pressure: 117/73 mmHg
- HR: 79 BPM

General

Overweight, no apparent distress. Alert and oriented to person, place, time, and situation.

HEENT

Pupils are equally round and reactive to light and accommodation bilaterally.

Pulmonary

Lungs clear to auscultation bilaterally.

Cardiovascular

Regular rate and rhythm. No murmurs.

Abdomen

Soft, nontender, and nondistended. Normal bowel sounds.

Genitourinary

Deferred.

Neurologic

Cranial nerves 2–12 intact. 5/5 strength in the bilateral lower extremities. Antalgic gait favoring the left lower extremity. 2+ Patellar and Achilles reflexes bilaterally. Positive straight right leg raise test.

Musculoskeletal

No spinal deformity. No paraspinal tenderness.

Extremities

No peripheral edema.

Laboratory Findings

Labs not available today (initial visit).

Questions

1. Which of the following is/are the appropriate next step(s) to investigate medication adherence (select all that apply)?
   (a) Send a prescription for the patient's oxycodone/acetaminophen to be filled immediately
   (b) Presumptive testing is followed by confirmatory testing if presumptive testing is negative
   (c) Check the prescription drug monitoring program and claims data
   (d) Refuse to manage the patient's pain medications

Rationale

- Correct answer(s): B, C. Direct and indirect methods of testing for adherence give the provider valuable information on whether the patient is taking their medications and can help confirm the patient is not taking other recreational or illicit substances. Oxycodone may not appear on presumptive testing, so confirmatory testing may be required. The PDMP will give the provider a history of the patient's previous prescription opioid fill history.
- Incorrect answer(s): A, D. Although it is appropriate to manage the patient's pain medications, refilling them immediately would be premature. Utilizing direct and indirect methods of adherence would be appropriate. At that time, sending a prescription refill with instructions to fill closer to the 4-week interval is recommended, as she had her oxycodone/acetaminophen refilled for a 4-week supply 2 weeks ago.

2. Which dimensions of nonadherence is the patient experiencing (select all that apply)?
   (a) Social and Economic
   (b) Patient-Related
   (c) Therapy-Related
   (d) Condition-Related
   (e) Healthcare or System Related

Rationale

- Correct answer(s): A, D, E. The social and economic dimension is correct due to the patient's inadequate insurance coverage, high cost of medications and transportation to appointments, and lack of stable living conditions due to the recent move. Condition-related is correct due to the severity of pain symptoms resulting in a change in her lifestyle. Healthcare or system-related is correct due to the lack of care continuity with changing providers and restricted formularies for some of her medications.
- Incorrect answer(s): B, C. "Patient-related" is incorrect, as she is not actively deciding to be nonadherent and is adherent when her medications and treatments are available. "Therapy-related" is incorrect due to her minimal number of medications and lack of reported side effects or medication concerns.

3. Which of the following issues are related to the patient's nonadherence (select all that apply)?
   (a) Complexity of regimen

(b) High cost of medications
(c) Forgetfulness
(d) Perceived benefit of treatment
(e) Lack of stable living conditions
(f) Access to appointments and follow-up

Rationale

- Correct answer(s): B, E, F. The high cost of medications is correct due to the patient's challenges getting coverage for her therapies and variable insurance coverage. Lack of stable living conditions is correct due to the patient's move. Access to appointments and follow-up is correct due to challenges with transportation to appointments.
- Incorrect answer(s): A, C, D. The complexity of the regimen is incorrect, as the patient only has three medications. Forgetfulness is incorrect, as the patient does not report challenges remembering her medications. Perceived benefit of treatment is incorrect, as the patient reports benefit of pharmacologic and nonpharmacologic therapy when available.

4. Which of the following strategies could be utilized to improve the patient's adherence?
   (a) Medication reminders in a phone application
   (b) Use of manufacturer coupons or assistance programs for high-cost medications
   (c) Review of insurance formulary to find cost-effective alternatives
   (d) Educate the patient on the disease state(s) and expectations for treatment
   (e) Utilize a medication synchronization program

Rationale

- Correct answer(s): B, C, D. Manufacturer coupons or assistance programs would be a correct option to help with the high cost of some of her medications. Reviewing the formulary is correct to determine cost-effective options that may also control her conditions. Educating the patient on her disease states and expectations for treatment is correct, as this could improve her outlook on pharmacological and nonpharmacological therapy and offer additional understanding of navigating her care.
- Incorrect answer(s): A, E. Medication reminders are incorrect, as the patient is not having an issue remembering her medications. Medication synchronization programs, although convenient, are not correct here, as the patient is not having difficulty obtaining/remembering medication prescriptions from the pharmacy.

5. Which nonpharmacological methods would be appropriate to recommend for this patient?
   (a) Confirm insurance coverage and order physical therapy
   (b) Instruct them to attend yoga classes two times daily
   (c) Apply cold/hot packs to the affected area as needed
   (d) Buy a gym membership to walk on a treadmill and lift weights

Rationale

- Correct answer(s): A, C. Confirming insurance coverage and ordering physical therapy is correct since this would be beneficial for the patient's pain, if affordable. Cold/hot packs are correct since these are relatively inexpensive and can be utilized at home to improve pain.
- Incorrect answer(s): B, D. Instructing the patient to attend yoga and buy a gym membership is inappropriate due to the patient's lack of patient transportation and limited funds to afford options not covered by insurance.

6. How would you create a plan to meet goals for nonpharmacological treatments?
   (a) Tell the patient to do all physical therapy exercises daily
   (b) Instruct the patient to lift weights five times per week and assess at follow-up
   (c) Empathize with the struggle of meeting the goal of walking 5/7 days and re-evaluate
   (d) Develop a SMART goal with the patient and assess it at the next visit

Rationale

- Correct answer(s): C, D. Empathizing with the patient about meeting walking goals and developing SMART goals are correct, as these utilize motivational interviewing and goal setting specific to the patient. These options facilitate a patient-centered approach to improving her adherence.
- Incorrect answer(s): A, B. Telling the patient to do physical therapy exercises daily and to lift weights five times weekly is incorrect, as these instructions may not be feasible due to the patient's abilities and do not incorporate the patient's opinions and goals.

Case 2

Patient Presentation

Chief Complaint

Postoperative pain.

History of Present Illness

A 72-year-old male patient with a complex medical history was discharged from the hospital last week, which involved a right knee-replacement surgery. He was provided with a new list of medications but was not scheduled for any follow-up visits. He takes several medications for multiple chronic disease states, including new medications for pain management post-procedure. He is unable to implement the changes at home due to conflicting information and unclear instructions. Consequently, he becomes confused and cannot take his medications as intended. This results in poorly managed postoperative pain and limited ability to participate in physical therapy.

Past Medical History

- Type 2 Diabetes Mellitus
- Hypertension
- Hyperlipidemia
- Chronic Obstructive Pulmonary Disease
- Obesity
- History of NSTEMI (6 years ago)
- Right knee osteoarthritis

Surgical History

Right total knee arthroplasty 1 week ago.

Family History

Father—Coronary artery disease and hypertension.
Mother—Hypertension and type 2 diabetes mellitus.

Social History

Lives alone. The family is located in another state. Is a former smoker who quit 20 years ago. Was smoking 1.5 PPD for 30 years. Denies any recent alcohol use. Denies any history of illicit drug use.

Immunization History

- Due for the zoster vaccine recombinant.

Allergies

- Penicillin (hives).

Home Medications

- Hydrocodone/acetaminophen 5 mg/325 mg, 1 tablet by mouth every 6 hours as needed for pain
- Aspirin 81 mg by mouth daily
- Diclofenac gel 4 grams topically every 6 hours as needed for pain
- Lidocaine 4% topical patch every 12 hours
- Semaglutide 2 mg subcutaneously once weekly
- Metformin 1000 mg by mouth BID
- Atorvastatin 80 mg by mouth daily
- Dapagliflozin 10 mg by mouth daily
- Lisinopril 40 mg by mouth daily
- Metoprolol succinate ER by mouth, 50 mg daily
- Albuterol HFA two puffs every 4 hours as needed for shortness of breath
- Fluticasone furoate, umeclidinium, vilanterol 100/62.5/25 mcg, one puff by mouth once daily

Physical Examination

Vital Signs

- BMI: 30.8 kg/m^2
- Weight: 215 pounds
- Height: 5′10″
- Temperature: 98.6 °F
- Blood Pressure: 152/83 mmHg
- HR: 68 BPM

General

Obese and in pain. Alert and oriented to person, place, time, and situation. Ambulating with a walker.

HEENT

Pupils are equally round and reactive to light and accommodation bilaterally.

Pulmonary

Faint end-expiratory wheezes bilaterally. Decreased breath sounds bilaterally.

Cardiovascular

Regular rate and rhythm. No murmurs.

Abdomen

Soft, nontender, and nondistended. Normal bowel sounds.

Genitourinary

Deferred.

Neurologic

Cranial nerves 2–12 are intact.

Musculoskeletal

The right knee incision site is clean, dry, and intact. No erythema, warmth, or drainage of the right knee. 4/5 strength of the right lower extremity. 5/5 strength of the left lower extremity.

Extremities

No lower extremity edema bilaterally.

Laboratory Findings

Na: 135 mEq/L	AST: 42 IU/L
K: 4.2 mEq/L	ALT: 38 IU/L
Cl: 102 mEq/L	Hgb A1c: 7.4%
CO2: 23 mEq/L	
SCr: 1.02 md/dL	
BUN: 24 mg/dL	
Glucose: 142 mg/dL	

Questions

7. Which dimensions of nonadherence is the patient experiencing (select all that apply)?
   (a) Social and Economic
   (b) Therapy-Related
   (c) Condition-Related
   (d) Healthcare or System Related

Rationale

- Correct answer(s): B, C, D. "Therapy-related" is correct due to the complexity of the patient's medication regimen. "Condition-related" is also correct due to recent surgery and confusion related to his medications as a result of his complex health needs. Finally, "healthcare or system related" is correct due to the challenges with transitions of care after his procedure.
- Incorrect answer(s): A. Social and economic status is not a factor here, as the patient can afford his medications and has access to care.

8. Which of the following issues are related to the patient's nonadherence (select all that apply)?
   (a) Complexity of regimen
   (b) Lack of care continuity
   (c) Lack of understanding
   (d) Medication Cost

Rationale

- Correct answer(s): A, B, C. This patient is not adherent due to the complexity of his medication regimen with multiple medication types, dosing frequencies, and administrative routes. Adherence is also impacted by a lack of care continuity after his recent procedure, and this leads to a lack of understanding of his medications and treatment.
- Incorrect answer(s): D. Cost is not a factor here, as the patient can afford his medications.

9. Which of the following strategies could be utilized to improve the patient's adherence?
   (a) Medication reminders in a phone application
   (b) Review of insurance formulary to find cost-effective alternatives
   (c) Educate the patient on the disease state(s) and expectations for treatment
   (d) Schedule for provider follow-up
   (e) Provide education on the current medication regimen, including adherence strategies

Rationale

- Correct answer(s): C, D, E. Adherence could be improved through disease state education, medication education, and regular follow-up with the provider. Addressing these areas with the patient will reduce confusion and ensure the ability to utilize medications effectively.
- Incorrect answer(s): A, B. The patient is not forgetting to take his medications, so an alarm will not address his misunderstanding. Reviewing the formulary will not help, as the patient currently has access to his medications.

Index

J. P. Reinert et al. (eds.), *Adjunctive Analgesic Strategies for the Bedside Clinician and Beyond*,
https://doi.org/10.1007/978-3-032-21675-5

B

O

T

GPSR Compliance

The European Union's (EU) General Product Safety Regulation (GPSR) is a set of rules that requires consumer products to be safe and our obligations to ensure this.

If you have any concerns about our products, you can contact us on ProductSafety@springernature.com

In case Publisher is established outside the EU, the EU authorized representative is:

Springer Nature Customer Service Center GmbH
Europaplatz 3
69115 Heidelberg, Germany

Batch number: 10731667

Printed by Printforce, the Netherlands